Current Techniques in Vascular Surgery

Edited by

James S. T. Yao, MD, PhD
Magerstadt Professor of Surgery
Northwestern University Medical School
Northwestern Memorial Hospital
Chicago, Illinois

William H. Pearce, MD
Professor of Surgery
Northwestern University Medical School
Chief, Division of Vascular Surgery
Northwestern Memorial Hospital
Chicago, Illinois

McGraw-Hill
Medical Publishing Division

New York St. Louis San Francisco Auckland Bogotá Caracas Lisbon London
Madrid Mexico City Milan Montreal New Delhi San Juan
Singapore Sydney Tokyo Toronto

McGraw-Hill
A Division of The **McGraw-Hill** *Companies*

Current Techniques in Vascular Surgery

1 2 3 4 5 6 7 8 9 0 DOC-DOC 0 9 8 7 6 5 4 3 2 1 0

ISBN:0-07-136501-X

Notice

Medicine is an ever-changing science. As new research and clinical experience broaden our knowledge, changes in treatment and drug therapy are required. The authors and the publisher of this work have checked with sources believed to be reliable in their efforts to provide information that is complete and generally in accord with the standards accepted at the time of publication. However, in view of the possibility of human error or changes in medical sciences, neither the authors nor the publisher nor any other party who has been involved in the preparation or publication of this work warrants that the information contained herein is in every respect accurate or complete, and they disclaim responsibility for any errors or omissions or for the results obtained from use of the information contained in this book. Readers are encouraged to confirm the information contained herein with other sources. For example and in particular, readers are advised to check the product information sheet included in the package of each drug they plan to administer to be certain that the information contained in this work is accurate and that changes have not been made in the recommended dose or in the contraindications for administration. This recommendation is of particular importance in connection with new or infrequently used drugs.

This book was set in Palatino by The PRD Group, Inc.
The editors were Michael P. Medina and Susan Parmentier.
The production supervisor was Phil Galea.
Project management was provided by Spectrum Publishing Services.
The cover designer was Elizabeth Schmitz.
The index was prepared by Joanne Way.

R.R. Donelley & Sons was printer and binder.

This book is printed on acid-free paper.

Cataloging-in-Publication Data for this title is on file at the Library of Congress.

Contents

MANAGEMENT OF CEREBROVASCULAR ISCHEMIA

LOWER EXTREMITY ARTERIAL ISCHEMIA

COMPLEX UPPER EXTREMITY VASCULAR PROBLEMS

MANAGEMENT OF TRAUMA

Contributors

Cameron M. Akbari, MD
Assistant Professor of Surgery
Harvard Medical School
Attending Vascular Surgeon
Beth Israel Deaconess Medical Center
Boston, Massachusetts

Max Amor, MD
Co-Director, Cardiovascular Unit
Interventional Cardiologist
Polyclinique d'Essey
Essey-les-Nancy, France

Richard K. Baer, MD
Medical Director, Medicare Part A
AdminaStar Federal
Chicago, Illinois

William H. Baker, MD, FACS
Professor of Surgery
Stritch School of Medicine
Loyola University Medical Center
Maywood, Illinois

B. Timothy Baxter, MD, FACS
Professor of Surgery, Anatomy and Cell Biology
University of Nebraska Medical Center
Chief of Vascular Surgery
Omaha VA Medical Center
Omaha, Nebraska

Gary J. Becker, MD, FSCVIR, FACC, FACR
Voluntary Professor of Radiology
University of Miami School of Medicine
Assistant Medical Director
Miami Cardiac & Vascular Institute
Miami, Florida

Amardip Bhuller, MD
General Surgery Resident
Indiana University Medical Center
Indianapolis, Indiana

Walter L. Biffl, MD
Assistant Professor of Surgery
University of Colorado Health Sciences Center
Chief of Pediatrics
Denver Health Medical Center
Denver, Colorado

Thomas C. Bower, MD
Associate Professor of Surgery
Director, Vascular Surgery Fellowship Program
Mayo Graduate School of Medicine
Mayo Foundation
Rochester, Minnesota

Kellie R. Brown, MD
Fellow, Division of Vascular Surgery
Medical College of Wisconsin
Milwaukee, Wisconsin

Jon M. Burch, MD
Professor of Surgery
University of Colorado Health Sciences Center
Chief, General and Vascular Surgery
Denver Health Medical Center
Denver, Colorado

Kenneth J. Cherry, Jr., MD
Professor of Surgery
Mayo Medical School
Consultant, Division of Vascular Surgery
Mayo Clinic
Rochester, Minnesota

Andy C. Chiou, MD, MPH
Assistant Professor of Surgery
Uniformed Services University of the Health Sciences, Bethesda, Maryland
Major, USAF Medical Corps
Wilford Hall USAF Medical Center, Lackland Air Force Base
San Antonio, Texas

Lori I. Cindrick, MD
Senior Vascular Fellow
Department of Surgery
Temple University Hospital
Philadelphia, Pennsylvania

Anthony J. Comerota, MD, FACS
Professor of Surgery
Temple University School of Medicine
Chief of Vascular Surgery
Temple University Hospital
Philadelphia, Pennsylvania

Joseph S. Coselli, MD
Professor of Surgery
Baylor College of Medicine
Senior Attending Surgeon
The Methodist Hospital
Houston, Texas

Jack L. Cronenwett, MD
Professor of Surgery
Dartmouth Medical School
Chief, Section of Vascular Surgery
Dartmouth-Hitchcock Medical Center
Lebanon, New Hampshire

Michael C. Dalsing, MD, FACS
Professor of Surgery
Indiana University Medical School
Director of Surgery
Indiana University Medical Center
Indianapolis, Indiana

James L. Ebaugh, MD
Resident, General Surgery
Northwestern University School of Medicine
Resident, General Surgery
Northwestern Memorial Hospital
Chicago, Illinois

James M. Edwards, MD
Associate Professor of Surgery
Division of Vascular Surgery
Oregon Health Sciences University
Staff Surgeon
Portland VA Hospital
Portland, Oregon

Mark A. Farber, MD
Division of Vascular Surgery
Department of Surgery
Assistant Professor
University of North Carolina School of Medicine
Chapel Hill, North Carolina

Samuel R. G. Finlayson, MD, MPH
Assistant Professor
Department of Surgery
Dartmouth Medical School
Attending Surgeon
Dartmouth-Hitchcock Medical Center
Lebanon, New Hampshire

Kathleen D. Gibson, MD
Vascular Surgery Fellow
Division of Vascular Surgery
University of Washington
School of Medicine
University of Washington Medical Center
Seattle, Washington

Peter Gloviczki, MD, FACS
Professor of Surgery
Mayo Medical School
Chair, Division of Vascular Surgery
Mayo Foundation
Rochester, Minnesota

David Green, MD, PhD
Professor of Medicine
Northwestern University Medical School
Director, Hemostasis and
Thrombosis Center
Northwestern Memorial Hospital
Chicago, Illinois

Peter Harris, MD, FRCS
Honorary Lecturer
University of Liverpool
Director of Vascular Services
Regional Vascular Unit
Royal Liverpool University Hospital
Liverpool, United Kingdom

Heitham T. Hassoun, MD
Trauma Research Center Fellow
Resident in General Surgery
Department of Surgery
University of Texas—Houston
Medical School
Houston, Texas

Peter K. Henke, MD
Assistant Professor of Surgery
Section of Vascular Surgery
University of Michigan
Ann Arbor, Michigan

Larry H. Hollier, MD, FACS, FRCS
Professor of Vascular Surgery
Mount Sinai School of Medicine
Surgeon-in-Chief, Chairman
Department of Surgery
Mount Sinai Medical Center
New York City, New York

K. Wayne Johnston, MD, FRCSC, FACS
Professor of Surgery and
R. Fraser Elliott Chair in
Vascular Surgery
University of Toronto
Division Head, Vascular Surgery
Toronto General Hospital
Toronto, Ontario Canada

Corey Jost, MD
Instructor of Surgery
Mayo Medical Center
Clinical Fellow of Vascular Surgery
Saint Mary's Hospital
Rochester, Minnesota

Blair A. Keagy, MD
Professor of Surgery
Chief, Division of Vascular Surgery
University of North Carolina School
of Medicine
Chapel Hill, North Carolina

Todd Kuiken, MD, PhD
Assistant Professor
Northwestern University
Medical School
Director of Amputee Services
Rehabilitation Institute of Chicago
Chicago, Illinois

S. Ram Kumar, MD
Research Fellow
Keck School of Medicine of the University of Southern California
USC University Hospital
Los Angeles, California

Moon Kwoun, MD
Assistant Professor of Surgery
Tufts University School of Medicine
Division of Vascular Surgery
New England Medical Center
Boston, Massachusetts

F. Elizabeth Labombard, RT, RDMS, RVT
Staff Technologist
Dartmouth-Hitchcock Medical Center
Lebanon, New Hampshire

Gregory L. Landry, MD
Assistant Professor of Surgery
Division of Vascular Surgery
Oregon Health Sciences University
Portland, Oregon

Scott A. LeMarie, MD
Assistant Professor of Surgery
Baylor College of Medicine
Attending Surgeon
The Methodist Hospital
Houston, Texas

Michael R. Lepore, Jr., MD
Vascular Surgeon Fellow
Alton Ochsner Clinic
New Orleans, Louisiana

Peter H. Lin, MD
Assistant Professor of Surgery
Emory University School of Medicine
Atlanta, Georgia

Frank W. LoGerfo, MD
William V. McDermott Professor of Surgery
Harvard Medical School
Chairman, Department of Surgery
Chief, Division of Vascular Surgery
Beth Israel Deaconess Medical Center
Boston, Massachusetts

Alan B. Lumsden, MD
Associate Professor of Surgery
Emory University School of Medicine
Head, Division of Vascular Surgery
Emory University Hospital
Atlanta, Georgia

Herbert I. Machleder, MD
Professor Emeritus
Division of Vascular Surgery
Department of Surgery
UCLA School of Medicine
Los Angeles, California

Michael Marin, MD
Division of Vascular Surgery
Department of Surgery
Mount Sinai Medical Center
New York, New York

Jon S. Matsumura, MD, FACS
Assistant Professor of Surgery
Northwestern University Medical School
Chief, Vascular Surgery
Chicago VA Healthcare System, Lakeside Division
Chicago, Illinois

Kenneth L. Mattox, MD
Professor and Vice Chair, Department of Surgery
Baylor College of Medicine
Chief of Staff/Surgery
Ben Taub General Hospital
Houston, Texas

Martin F. McKneally, MD, PhD, FRCSC, FACS
Professor of Surgery
Department of Surgery, Joint Center for Bioethics
University of Toronto
Staff Surgeon
Toronto General Hospital, University Health Network
Toronto, Ontario Canada

Michael A. McKusick, MD
Assistant Professor of Radiology
Mayo Graduate School of Medicine
Department of Vascular & Interventional Radiology
St. Mary's Hospital
Rochester, Minnesota

Gregory L. Moneta, MD
Professor of Surgery, Division of Vascular Surgery
Oregon Health Sciences University
Portland, Oregon

Samuel R. Money, MD, FACS
Clinical Associate Professor of Surgery
Tulane University School of Medicine
Chief, Section of Vascular Surgery
Alton Ochsner Clinic
New Orleans, Louisiana

Frederick A. Moore, MD, FACS
James H. "Red" Duke, Jr. Professor of Surgery and Vice Chairman, Department of Surgery
University of Texas—Houston Medical School
Chief, General Surgery and Trauma & Critical Care
Memorial Hermann Hospital
Houston, Texas

Mark D. Morasch, MD
Assistant Professor
Division of Vascular Surgery
Department of Surgery
Northwestern University Medical School
Active Staff
Northwestern Memorial Hospital
Chicago, Illinois

Junaid Mudaliar, MD
Resident
Department of Vascular Surgery
University of Missouri-Columbia Health Sciences Center
Columbia, Missouri

Ryan D. Nachreiner, MD
General Surgery Resident
Indiana University Medical Center
Indianapolis, Indiana

Thomas F. O'Donnell, Jr., MD
Andrews Professor of Surgery
Tufts University School of Medicine
President and CEO
New England Medical Center
Boston, Massachusetts

Takao Ohki, MD
Assistant Professor of Surgery
The University Hospital for the Albert Einstein College of Medicine
Chief, Endovascular Program
Montefiore Medical Center
Bronx, New York

Kenneth Ouriel, MD
Professor and Chairman, Department of Vascular Surgery
The Cleveland Clinic and Foundation
Cleveland, Ohio

William H. Pearce, MD
Professor of Surgery
Northwestern University Medical School
Chief, Division of Vascular Surgery
Northwestern Memorial Hospital
Chicago, Illinois

John M. Porter, MD
Professor of Surgery, Division of Vascular Surgery
Oregon Health Sciences University
Portland, Oregon

Richard J. Powell, MD
Assistant Professor
Dartmouth-Hitchcock Medical Center
Lebanon, New Hampshire

Joseph Rabin, MD
Albert Einstein College of Medicine
Division of Vascular Surgery, Department of Surgery
Montefiore Medical Center
New York, New York

Chet R. Rees, MD
Attending Vascular and Interventional Radiologist
Department of Surgery
Baylor University Medical Center Hospital
Dallas, Texas

David C. Rice, MB, BCH
Thoracic Surgery Resident
Baylor College of Medicine
Houston, Texas

Thom W. Rooke, MD
Professor of Medicine
Mayo Medical School
Head, Section of Vascular Medicine
Mayo Clinic
Rochester, Minnesota

Vincent L. Rowe, MD
Assistant Professor of Surgery
Keck School of Medicine of the University of Southern California
Chief, Division of Vascular Surgery
USC University Hospital
Los Angeles, California

Robert B. Rutherford, MD, FASC
Emeritus Professor of Surgery
University of Colorado
Silverthorne, Colorado

Martin A. Schreiber, MD
Assistant Professor of Surgery
Baylor College of Medicine
Trauma Director
Ben Taub General Hospital
Houston, Texas

Anton N. Sidawy, MD, MPH
Professor of Surgery
George Washington and Georgetown Universities
Chief, Surgical Service
VA Medical Center
Washington, District of Columbia

David Silver, MD
Professor Emeritus
University of Missouri-Columbia
Staff Surgeon
University of Missouri-Columbia Health Sciences Center
Columbia, Missouri

Michael Sobel, MD, FACS
Professor and Chief, Vascular Surgery Section
Upstate Medical University of New York, Syracuse
Chief of Surgery
Syracuse VA Medical Center
Syracuse, New York

James C. Stanley, MD
Professor of Surgery
University of Michigan
Head, Section of Vascular Surgery
University of Michigan, University Hospital
Ann Arbor, Michigan

David L. Steed, MD
Professor of Surgery
University of Pittsburgh
Director, Wound Healing/Limb Preservation Clinic
University of Pittsburgh
Pittsburgh, Pennsylvania

D. Eugene Strandness, Jr., MD
Professor of Surgery
Vascular Surgery
University of Washington School of Medicine
Seattle, Washington

Apostolos K. Tassiopoulos, MD
Vascular Fellow
Department of Surgery
Loyola University Medical Center
Maywood, Illinois

Lloyd M. Taylor, Jr. , MD
Professor of Surgery, Division of Vascular Surgery
Oregon Health Sciences University
Portland, Oregon

Robert W. Thompson, MD
Associate Professor of Surgery, Cell Biology & Physiology, and Radiology
Department of Surgery
Washington University School of Medicine
Attending Surgeon
Barnes–Jewish Hospital
St. Louis, Missouri

Jonathan B. Towne, MD
Professor, Surgery
Medical College of Wisconsin
Chairman, Vascular Surgery
Froedtert Memorial Lutheran Hospital
Milwaukee, Wisconsin

Srinivas Tummala, MD
Fellow
Vascular Interventional Radiology
Miami Cardiac and Vascular Institute
Miami, Florida

William D. Turnipseed, MD
Professor
University of Wisconsin Medical Center
Chief, Vascular Surgery
University Health Sciences Center
Madison, Wisconsin

Gilbert R. Upchurch, Jr., MD
Assistant Professor of Surgery
Section of Vascular Surgery
University of Michigan
Ann Arbor, Michigan

S. Rao Vallabhaneni, FRCS(Ed), FRCS
Regional Vascular Unit
Royal Liverpool University Hospital
Liverpool, United Kingdom

Frank J. Veith, MD
Professor of Surgery
Albert Einstein College of Medicine
Chief, Vascular Surgical Services
Montefiore Medical Center
Bronx, New York

Daniel B. Walsh, MD
Professor of Surgery
Dartmouth Medical School
Vice Chair, Department of Surgery
Dartmouth Hitchcock Medical Center
Lebanon, New Hampshire

Fred A. Weaver, MD
Professor of Surgery
Keck School of Medicine of the University of Southern California
Chief, Division of Vascular Surgery
University of Southern California University Hospital
Los Angeles, California

Marshall W. Webster, MD
Mark M. Ravitch Professor of Surgery
University of Pittsburgh
Executive Vice Chair, Department of Surgery
University of Pittsburgh School of Medicine
Pittsburgh, Pennsylvania

Wayne F. Yakes, MD
Director, Vascular Malformation Center
Radiology Imaging Associates Swedish Medical Center
Englewood, Colorado

Osvaldo Junti Yano, MD
Vascular Surgery Fellow
Mount Sinai Medical Center
New York, New York

James S. T. Yao, MD, PhD
Magerstadt Professor of Surgery
Northwestern University Medical School
Acting Chair, Department of Surgery
Northwestern Memorial Hospital
Chicago, Illinois

Foreword

A QUARTER CENTURY OF NORTHWESTERN VASCULAR SYMPOSIA—A REFLECTION

As we enter the new millennium, this annual symposium on vascular surgery is a quarter-century old. This is indeed a landmark achievement for continuing education in vascular surgery. Having been involved from the very beginning in the planning of each meeting and the publication of the compendium books, I would like to reflect on the progress and changes in the practice of vascular surgery in the past 25 years.

John J. Bergan, former Chief of the Division of Vascular Surgery, Northwestern University Medical School, first conceived the idea of this continuing education initiative. The main objective is to address a specific topic of vascular disease and to bring together national and international surgeons to present their experience in their chosen field. With support from a generous education grant from Scholl, Inc., the first symposium was held on December 2, 1976, at the Drake Hotel, and the topic was *Venous Problems.* We dedicated the symposium to honor Dr. Geza de Takats, a pioneer vascular surgeon from Chicago (Figure 1). The symposium represented the first meeting attended by international experts to address a specific and much neglected subject in vascular disease. The meeting was a great success with Mayor Richard J. Daley in attendance for the opening ceremony (Figure 2). He proclaimed the first day of the meeting as Dr. Geza de Takats Day in Chicago. Nineteen years later, his son, Richard M. Daley, visited us during the 1995 symposium on *Arterial Surgery: Management of Challenging Problems* to honor another great surgeon, Dr. Michael DeBakey. He presented to Michael DeBakey a certificate of honorary citizenship of Chicago (Figure 3).

One of the unique features of the Northwestern Symposium is the publication of a book at the time of the meeting. We did not publish the book, *Venous Problems,* at the first meeting because of the printing process. It was published by YearBook Publishers 2 years later. No publication was made in connection with the 1977 symposium, *Correctable Cerebral Ischemia*; instead, the entire meeting was recorded onto a videotape. In

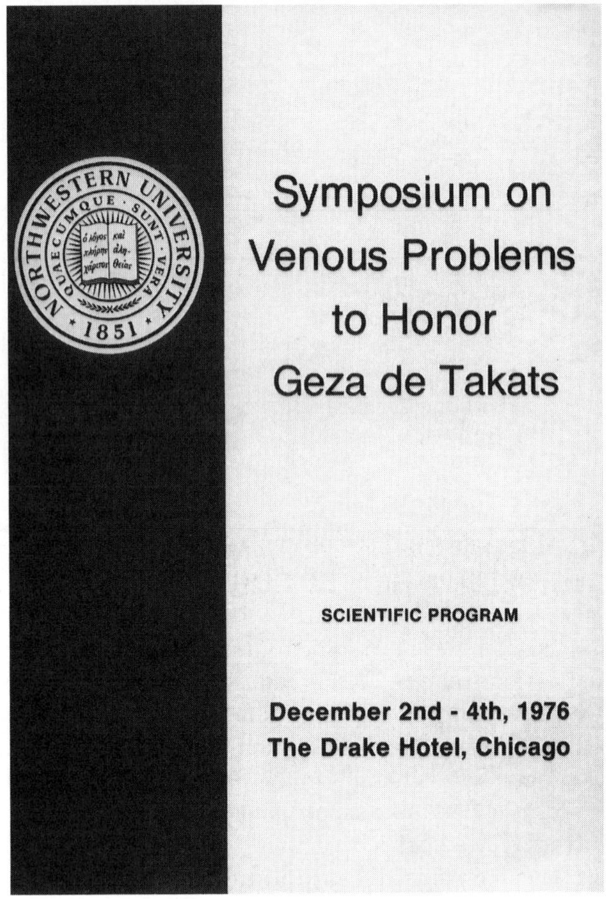

Figure 1. Cover of the first program book.

1978, Grune & Stratton, Inc., introduced the rapid printing process and thus began the publication of a book at the meeting. *Gangrene and Severe Ischemia of the Lower Extremities* made its first appearance on time at the meeting December 7–9, 1978. For the next 23 years, we have successfully published a book containing all presentations at the time of the meeting.

Table 1 shows the titles of the symposia presented over the last 25 years. We are grateful to the invited faculty members of the symposia for making them possible. We are also grateful to W. L. Gore Co. for the generous education grant to make the books available for registrants at the meetings. We have worked with publishers such as W. B. Saunders, Appleton & Lange, and currently with McGraw-Hill.

Over the last 25 years, there have been significant changes in the practice of vascular surgery. In reviewing the contents of the 24 books we have published, I am amazed at these changes. We started the symposia on the subject of venous disease with *Venous Problems* in 1976, and subsequently repeated the subject in 1984, with *Surgery of the*

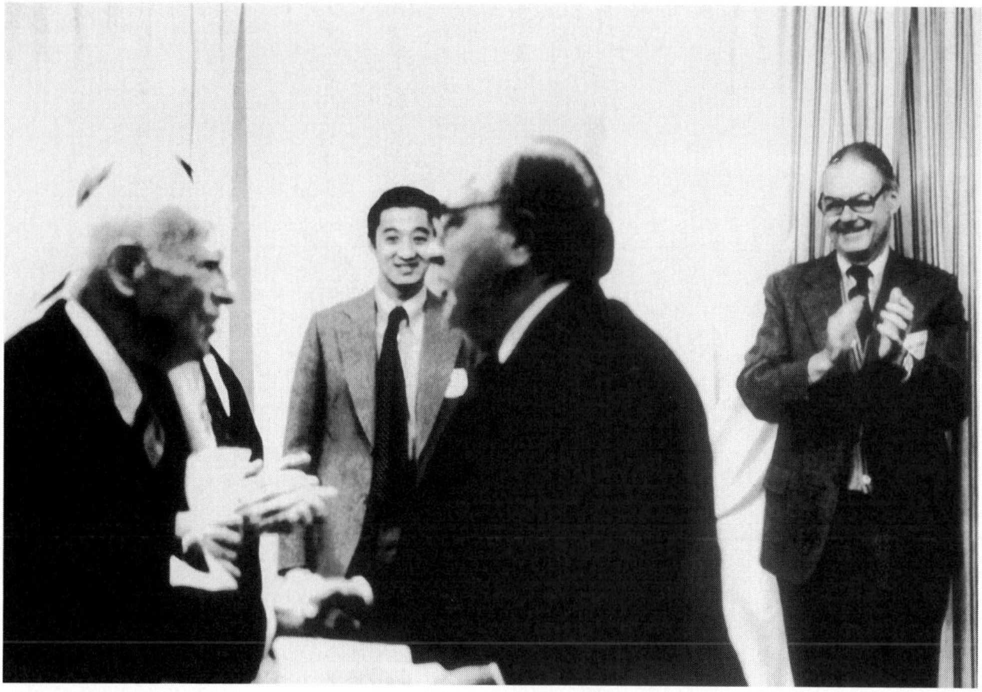

Figure 2. Mayor Richard J. Daley and Dr. Geza de Takats at the first symposium (1976). Left to right: Geza de Takats, James S. T. Yao, Richard J. Daley, and James E. Eckenhoff (Dean of Northwestern University Medical School).

Veins, and in 1990, with *Venous Disorders.* In 1976, presentations on diagnosis of deep vein thrombosis were dominated by indirect noninvasive testing using various types of plethysmographs or transcutaneous Doppler examination. Also popular was the I-125 fibrinogen uptake technique. At present, all of these techniques are obsolete and have been replaced by direct examination with the duplex scan. The I-125 fibrinogen technique provided valuable information on the natural history of deep vein thrombosis but, because of possible virus infection, the technique has now completely disappeared from clinical use. Not only is duplex scan currently the test of choice in the diagnosis of acute deep vein thrombosis, it also offers new information on venous valvular function. The use of low-dose heparin was just beginning to be used as a preventive measure for acute deep vein thrombosis in 1976. In the 1990 symposium on *Venous Disorders,* we discussed clinical trials of low molecular weight heparin for prevention of deep vein thrombosis. Currently, treatment of acute deep vein thrombosis has evolved to the introduction of outpatient treatment by fractionated heparin as an acceptable practice. Vena cava interruption has also taken a great leap, from umbrella to percutaneous placement of filter and, recently, bedside placement of filter with guidance by intravascular ultrasound.

Have we made significant advances in operative approaches in the surgical treatment of venous problems? Perhaps not much. One of the newest techniques is venous

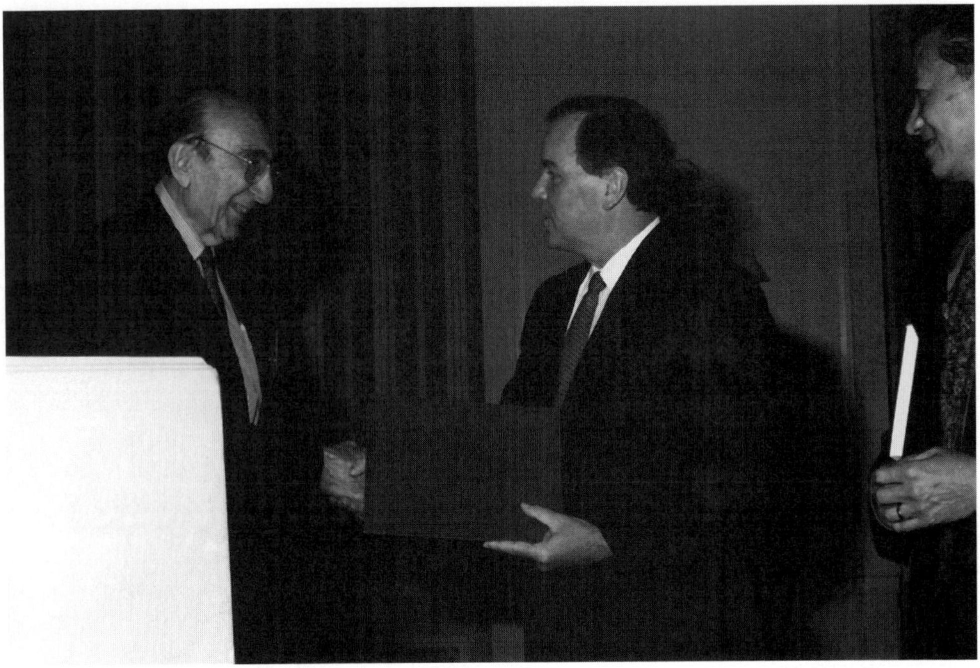

Figure 3. Mayor Richard M. Daley and Dr. Michael DeBakey at the 1995 symposium. Left to right: Michael DeBakey, Richard M. Daley, and James S. T. Yao.

valve repair, which was discussed in the first symposium in 1976. In the symposia on *Surgery of the Veins* and on *Venous Disorders,* we called attention to valve transplantation and transposition and the expanded experience with valve repair. In recent years, stent placement and balloon angioplasty have become favored ways to treat venous compression in thoracic outlet or iliac vein compression syndrome. Venous bypass with or without A-V fistula remains an enigma, and the procedure is not a routine practice of most vascular surgeons. The laparoscopic technique for perforator interruption is now under trial to determine the efficacy of the minimally invasive procedure. In any event, treatment of chronic venous insufficiency continues to be a challenge to vascular surgeons. The treatment of lymphedema is also static and the newer approach is intense physiocompression treatment. To a certain extent, one may conclude the treatment of chronic leg swelling is by proper elastic support.

No publication was made on the second symposium entitled *Correctable Cerebral Ischemia.* We repeated this topic in 1982 symposium on *Cerebrovascular Insufficiency.* It is interesting to note that oculoplethysmography, digital subtraction arteriography, and extracranial–intracranial (EC-IC) bypass, a popular practice in 1982, have now all but disappeared in the diagnosis and treatment of cerebral ischemia. Plaque hemorrhage and cerebral protection during carotid endarterectomy were popular topics for debate. The NASCET study had not yet begun, and the role of carotid endarterectomy has always been questioned by neurologists. Although we have not dedicated a symposium

TABLE 1. NORTHWESTERN VASCULAR SURGERY SYMPOSIA

Year	Symposium Title
1976	*Venous Problems*
1977	*Correctable Cerebral Ischemia*
1978	*Gangrene and Severe Ischemia of the Lower Extremities*
1979	*Surgery of the Aorta and Its Body Branches*
1980	*Operative Techniques in Vascular Surgery*
1981	*Arterial Aneurysms*
1982	*Cerebrovascular Insufficiency*
1983	*Evaluation and Treatment of Upper and Lower Extremity Circulatory Disorders*
1984	*Surgery of the Veins*
1985	*Reoperative Arterial Surgery*
1986	*Vascular Surgical Emergencies*
1987	*New Developments in Arterial Surgery*
1988	*Surgery of the Aorta*
1989	*Techniques in Arterial Surgery*
1990	*Venous Disorders*
1991	*Technologies in Vascular Surgery*
1992	*Long-Term Results in Vascular Surgery*
1993	*Aneurysms: New Findings and Treatment*
1994	*Advances in Treatment of Ischemic Extremities*
1995	*Arterial Surgery: Management of Challenging Problems*
1996	*Vascular Surgery: Twenty Years of Progress*
1997	*Techniques in Vascular and Endovascular Surgery*
1998	*Practical Vascular Surgery*
1999	*Modern Vascular Surgery*
2000	*Vascular Surgery 2000*

to cerebral ischemia in recent years, the subject was incorporated in subsequent symposia. With the passage of time and several multicenter trials (NASCET, ECST, VA study, ACAS, CASANOVA), carotid endarterectomy has emerged as the treatment of choice for prevention of stroke. In diagnostic testing, the duplex is now the standard test of choice for patients suspected to have carotid stenosis. For arteriography, the improved imaging capability of the MRA has nearly replaced the standard contrast arteriography. Surgery may be done with duplex alone, provided the noninvasive laboratory has good quality control of diagnostic accuracy, or when in question, one may supplement with MRA. At present, lurking behind the scene of treatment of carotid stenosis is the angioplasty and stent placement, a technique unheard of in the 1980s. The initiation of a much-needed multicenter trial is now in progress to establish the safety and efficacy of this new technique.

Extremity ischemia is common. We have examined this specific topic beginning in 1978 with *Gangrene and Severe Ischemia of the Lower Extremities,* in 1983 with *Evaluation and Treatment of Upper and Lower Extremity Circulatory Disorders,* and in 1994 with *Ad-*

vances in Treatment of Ischemic Extremities. In 1978, femorotibial vein graft was just beginning and *in-situ* vein graft was not even mentioned. There were a few who advocated the use of umbilical vein prosthesis as alternate conduit. The late result of formation of aneurysm has eliminated this type of graft from clinical use. Hemodynamic studies using Doppler ultrasound or electromagnetic flowmeter were common practice. The latter is no longer in use in the operating room. In 1983, infrainguinal bypass continued to develop with the introduction of a variety of techniques such as bypass to distal arteries or to isolated popliteal arteries and the composite-sequential bypass grafts. Several investigators introduced the concept of endothelial cell seeding of prosthetic grafts, but the technique has never been proved for clinical application. The by-product of endothelial cell research, however, is good—it led many vascular surgeons into the study of molecular biology, and thus began the stage of research in biotechnology. In the 1994 symposium on *Advances in Treatment of Ischemic Extremities,* we saw significant progress made since 1978. Critical ischemia by clinical and noninvasive tests had been defined. Infrainguinal revascularization had included aggressive surgical approaches with pedal artery bypass, free-tissue transfer, *in-situ* vein graft with various techniques for valve cutting, and vein cuff for prosthetic graft. We also had learned that bypass to distal arteries offers limb salvage for the diabetic population. We were also more knowledgeable about hematologic problems and their influence on graft patency. Graft surveillance by duplex scan to detect significant graft stenosis prior to graft thrombosis had become standard practice to extend graft patency. Refinement of MRA or on-table arteriography had gradually replaced the need for contrast catheter arteriography in most patients.

No procedures offer more technical challenge than aortic surgery and its major branches. In 1979, we began with a symposium on *Surgery of Aorta and Its Body Branches,* and then revisited the topic in 1988, with *Surgery of the Aorta.* Vascular surgeons have always maintained a special interest in aneurysm formation and its treatment. We have devoted two symposia to this subject: *Arterial Aneurysms* in 1981, and in 1993, *Aneurysms: New Findings and Treatment.* In the late 1970s, computed tomography (CT) scan was just starting to become the diagnostic test of choice. We have now entered into ultrafast CT with 3D arteriography, eliminating the use of catheter arteriography. Significant progress has been made in the treatment of thoracoabdominal aortic aneurysm. Balloon angioplasty, with or without stent placement, gradually replaced surgery as the treatment of choice for segmental stenosis of iliac arteries. Interest in the retroperitoneal approach to aortic aneurysm grafting has been reactivated and is of use in patients with a hostile abdomen. Two significant advances have been made in aortic aneurysm: (1) the understanding of pathogenesis of aneurysm formation, and (2) the endovascular graft. In 1981, there was only a single presentation about elastase as a factor of aneurysm formation. In the 1990s, the use of molecular biology has provided great insight into aneurysm formation. We are now armed with information on genetic basis of aneurysm formation, collagen and elastin metabolism, and the interaction with enzymes such as metalloproteinase (MMP-9) in the pathogenesis of aneurysm. We also have a much better understanding of the role of inflammatory cells in arterial wall pathology. The second advance is the introduction of endovascular graft. The FDA has now approved two endovascular grafts for clinical use, and only long-term follow-up will determine the efficacy of this new and innovative treatment.

Recurrent stenosis or reocclusion of bypass constitute a great part of re-do procedures in vascular surgery. Surgical emergencies can also be challenging. We dedicated two symposia, *Reoperative Arterial Surgery* in 1985 and *Vascular Surgical Emergencies* in 1986, to these two topics.

Surgical technique is always a popular topic for practicing vascular surgeons, and participants always welcome the opportunity to learn from master technical surgeons. In 1980, we initiated a symposium on *Operative Techniques in Vascular Surgery* and again in 1989 on *Techniques in Arterial Surgery.* As technology became an integral part of the surgical armamentarium, we examined new technology in 1991 in *Technologies in Vascular Surgery.* With emerging technology such as endoluminal graft and minimally invasive or scope-assisted procedures taking a foothold in the practice, we updated surgical technique in 1997 and expanded the title to *Techniques in Vascular and Endovascular Surgery.* We reviewed the use of angioscopy, intravascular ultrasound, genetic engineering, thrombolytic therapy, laser, and atherectomy. Laser ablation of atherosclerotic plaque, a technique greeted with great enthusiasm in the 1980s, has faded completely, as has atherectomy. Unless the long-term results are positive, new techniques will not stand the test of time, and it is expected that the current interest in endovascular graft will meet with similar scrutiny.

In recent years, we have changed the focus of the symposium to the overall practice of vascular surgery rather than on a specific disease. These include symposia on *Long-Term Results in Vascular Surgery* (1992), *Arterial Surgery: Management of Challenging Problems* (1995), *Vascular Surgery: Twenty Years of Progress* (1996), *Practical Vascular Surgery* (1998), and *Modern Vascular Surgery* (1999). This is done to keep pace with rapid development in the treatment and diagnosis of carotid, aorta, and upper and lower extremity ischemia; aneurysm; and venous problems. We hope this annual review provides updated and balanced information for our participants.

We are thankful for the many leaders in vascular surgery who give up their time to join the faculty of this symposium and to prepare a manuscript for publication. We are also honored to have had the opportunity to dedicate several symposia to outstanding vascular surgeons: Edwin J. Wylie (*Cerebrovascular Insufficiency*, 1982), Stanley Crawford (*Aneurysms: New Findings and Treatments*, 1993), D. Emerick Szilagyi (*Advances in Treatment of Ischemic Extremities*, 1994), Michael DeBakey (*Arterial Surgery: Management of Challenging Problems*, 1995), and most recently, Jesse Thompson (*Techniques in Vascular and Endovascular Surgery*, 1997).

After 25 years of involvement in the symposium, I continue to view vascular surgery as a very challenging surgical specialty. Over this period, we have seen the birth of the board certification of vascular surgery, the development of regional vascular societies, and practice and clinical pathways to shorten hospital stays. In research, large animal experimentation has been replaced by molecular biology and transgenic animal studies. Bench-to-bedside treatment using growth factor or gene transfer is now a reality. Advances in surgery rely on the development of technology, and it is expected that more innovative techniques will be introduced to treat vascular disease. It is indeed a privilege to have participated in the growth of this specialty over the past 25 years.

James S. T. Yao

Acknowledgments

After 19 years as Director of the Office of Continuing Medical Education, Paula Puntenney has announced her departure from the Medical School effective in July 2000. Not only will the Medical School miss her dearly, but the Division of Vascular Surgery has also lost a great organizer for the annual Vascular Symposium. Her charms and great leadership will be sorely missed. I am sure many participants who have known her for years share our sadness in the loss of a great person and tireless worker. We thank Paula for her unrelenting support, and wish her every success in her new adventures.

We also would like to thank Lynnette Dangerfield, Jan Goldstein, and Sara Minton for secretarial assistance, and Susan Parmentier for her superb editorial skill and effort.

1

Carotid Endarterectomy without Arteriography

Kathleen D. Gibson, MD, and
D. Eugene Strandness, Jr., MD

INTRODUCTION

After the development and refinement of carotid endarterectomy (CEA) in the 1950s and 1960s, the number of these procedures performed in the United States progressively increased. By 1985, it was estimated that 107,000 extracranial vessel endarterectomies were performed at nonfederal hospitals in the United States, making it the most common peripheral vascular procedure performed.[1] Despite its popularity, the efficacy and safety of CEA for the prevention of stroke compared to medical management was questioned, and calls were made for prospective randomized trials. The North American Symptomatic Carotid Endarterectomy Trial (NASCET)[2] and the European Carotid Surgery Trial (ECST)[3] confirmed the benefit of endarterectomy in the prevention of stroke in symptomatic patients with a high-grade carotid stenosis. The benefit of endarterectomy in asymptomatic patients is more controversial. The largest trial conducted in asymptomatic patients, the Asymptomatic Carotid Atherosclerosis Study (ACAS), reported a benefit of surgical therapy over medical management in patients with carotid stenosis >60%.[4] Because these trials have shown a benefit of CEA, precise estimation of the degree of stenosis of the carotid bulb is of critical importance.

Edgar Moniz and colleagues[5] pioneered the use of arteriography in the visualization of the cerebral circulation in 1937. Arteriography of the carotid arteries was found to reliably indicate the extent of carotid stenosis and was used as the sole preoperative diagnostic modality until the development of duplex ultrasonography (DUS) in the 1970s and 1980s.[6,7] DUS is now the most extensively used screening tool for carotid disease.

More recently, computerized tomographic angiography (CTA) and magnetic resonance angiography (MRA) have also been used as noninvasive imaging tools for the preoperative planning of CEA. All three of these modalities have been used as either an adjunct to or a replacement for the traditional preoperative carotid arteriogram.

Although many surgeons now routinely perform CEAs without preoperative angiography, controversy continues regarding the prudence of this approach. Questions also remain regarding which noninvasive imaging technique is best suited as a replacement for angiography before CEA.

PREOPERATIVE CAROTID ASSESSMENT: ARTERIOGRAPHY

Cerebral arteriography was long considered the gold standard for imaging the carotid arteries. The morbidity and mortality associated with angiography must be included in the overall risk estimate for CEA when it is used preoperatively. In the ACAS trial, nearly one-half of the neurologic morbidity was secondary to complications of arteriography.[4] In a review of eight prospective and seven retrospective studies of cerebral arteriography in patients with "mild" cerebrovascular disease, Hankey and colleagues[8] found the overall risk of transient ischemic attack (TIA) or stroke to be 4% and permanent neurologic deficit to be approximately 1%. It also appears that cerebral arteriography may be more hazardous in patients with a history of TIA or evolving stroke.[9,10] A study by Teodotou and colleagues[9] estimated the risk of neurologic complication to be 4.5% in patients with TIAs and 7.7% in patients with stroke in evolution.[9] Other investigations are in agreement with these findings—that the overall risk of neurologic complication attributed to arteriography ranges from 1% to 10%.[9–14] These risks may equal or exceed the risk of neurologic complication secondary to operative CEA.

Less morbid complications of arteriography include contrast-associated nephropathy, which has an incidence of between 0% and 20%,[15] and contrast media allergy, which occurs in up to 7.4% of patients.[16] Local complications such as hematomas are reported in between 2% and 7% of patients.[8,11,14] Pseudoaneurysms, nerve, and vessel injuries secondary to cerebral angiography are rare but potentially serious complications.

Efforts at cost containment have become increasingly important in our current health-care environment. Cerebral arteriography is the most expensive of the preoperative carotid imaging modalities. A study by Garrard and colleagues[17] in 1997 found that routine arteriography prior to endarterectomy increased total patient charges by 43%. These investigators estimated that if the numbers of carotid arteriograms were decreased by 50%, it could save the health-care system $276 million per annum. Ammar[18] conducted a cost-containment study at the University of Kansas–Wichita in which the use of preoperative arteriography was reduced from 100% to 22%. The estimated savings at that institution with the decreased use of arteriography, subtracting charges for repeated duplex scanning, was $1.6 million over a 1-year period of time.[18]

It is also important to remember there is inter- and intraobserver variability in the interpretation of cerebral arteriograms. A study of 99 patients with a history of TIAs found the mean absolute difference in estimate of carotid stenosis was 8% to 9.5%. Clinically important differences that could potentially change patient management occurred between 3% and 6% of the time.[19]

Whereas carotid arteriography is often considered the gold standard against which other methods of estimating carotid stenosis are compared, the true gold standard is the

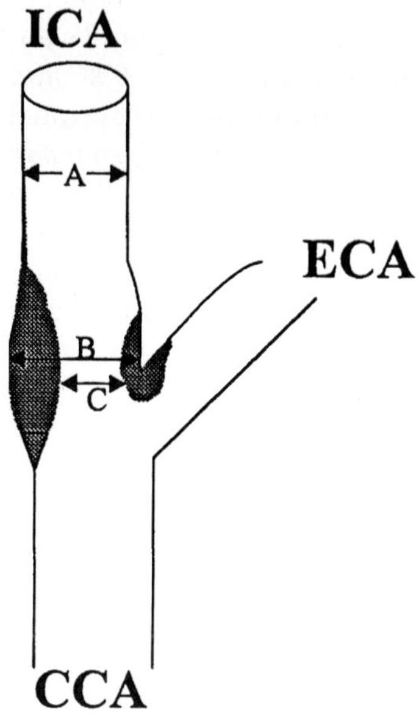

Figure 1–1. Methods for assessing carotid stenosis in the NASCET and ECST. NASCET % diameter stenosis = (1 − C/A) × 100; ECST % diameter stenosis = (1 − C/B) × 100 (Refs. 2, 3).

pathologic lesion itself. Several studies that defined the degree of carotid stenosis using *ex-vivo* measurements of carotid plaques have found that conventional arteriography underestimates the degree of stenosis present, and in fact correlates less well with pathologic plaque burden than either DUS or MRA.[20–22] An additional pitfall in the determination of degree of carotid stenosis by arteriography is that the criteria for measurement of stenosis have not been standardized. NASCET used the ratio of the artery diameter at the stenosis to the distal normal ICA, whereas ECST used the ratio of the diameter at the stenosis to the estimated true bulb width (Figure 1–1).[2,3] The disparity in estimation of stenosis using the two methods is most pronounced when grading lesser degrees of stenosis. Nicolaides and colleagues[23] estimated that 70%, 77%, and 83% ECST stenoses correspond to 47%, 60%, and 70% NASCET stenoses, respectively.

Even though arteriography remains the most expensive, invasive, and morbid modality for imaging the carotid artery, it is the most widely applied. Given the dependence of patient benefit on the accurate estimation of stenosis, many surgeons have been reluctant to proceed with endarterectomy without preoperative arteriography. If any imaging technique is to replace arteriography, it must, in addition to being less expensive and less morbid, have proven accuracy in the estimation of the degree of carotid stenosis.

DUPLEX ULTRASONOGRAPHY

Duplex ultrasonography has become the most widely applied diagnostic screening tool used for evaluation of the carotid artery. It is noninvasive, inexpensive, widely available, and provides both anatomic and hemodynamic information. The accuracy of DUS in detecting carotid stenosis has been evaluated in numerous studies in comparison to angiograms or to pathologic specimens. When compared to angiography as a gold standard, the sensitivity of DUS in detecting carotid stenosis ranges from 93% to 99% and the specificity from 71% to 98%.[24–27] Moneta and colleagues[28] found that the maximal overall accuracy of DUS for detection of a 60% or greater stenosis was 90% when using peak systolic and end diastolic velocity criteria. Some authors have suggested that the addition of color-flow imaging may further improve the accuracy of DUS in determining degree of carotid stenosis.[29–31] The comparison of DUS to arteriography in quantification of carotid stenosis may not be entirely valid, as several recent studies have shown that DUS correlates more closely with *ex-vivo* plaque specimens than arteriography, which tends to underestimate the degree of stenosis.[20,21,32]

Errors in duplex interpretation can occur in the presence of unusual anatomy, such as vessel kinks or densely calcified plaques. Typically, a vascular technologist should be able to recognize the technical limitations of the exam in these situations, and recommend confirmatory testing with other imaging modalities. It has long been known that DUS has limitations in accurately assessing the origin of the arch vessels, the carotid siphon, and the intracerebral circulation. In the past, some have argued that these limitations mandate arteriography prior to endarterectomy in order to avoid missing possible lesions in these areas. The frequency of lesions in these areas, however, is not common, and the clinical importance of these lesions even when present is questionable. A 1987 study by Akers et al.[33] reviewed 1000 arteriograms performed for the evaluation of extracranial vascular disease and found significant lesions in only 1.8% of the studies. More recently, Kadwa and colleagues[34] found aortic branch disease in 14.7% of patients undergoing evaluation for endarterectomy, but also found that all of the lesions had been suspected prior to the angiogram because of arm pressure differences or abnormalities seen with duplex scanning. The presence of intracranial disease likewise rarely alters clinical management or short- or long-term outcomes of patients with significant extracranial carotid stenosis.[35,36] Akers et al.[37] found carotid siphon lesions in 6% and intracranial aneurysms in 2% of patients undergoing intracranial arteriography for carotid disease. None of the patients had symptoms attributable to these lesions, and the intracranial findings did not alter clinical management.

Like other diagnostic imaging modalities, DUS is subject to both operator and interpretive errors. One of the greatest problems with DUS has been the lack of standardized protocols between different diagnostic vascular laboratories. Although many laboratories have used criteria developed at the University of Washington (Table 1–1),[38] the stenosis categories defined by these duplex velocity criteria did not include the cutoff points found in the NASCET, ECST, or ACAS. For this reason, a number of investigators have developed new duplex velocity criteria to correlate with the thresholds used in randomized clinical trials.[28,39–44] Our institution uses the parameters developed by Moneta and colleagues[28] to correlate duplex velocity defined stenoses with the levels found in randomized trials. The ratio of the peak systolic velocity (PSV) in the internal carotid artery to the PSV in the common carotid artery (ICA/CCA ratio) is calculated. Values >4.0 are predictive of carotid stenosis of >70% (overall accuracy, 88%) as used in the NASCET,[41] and values >3.2 are predictive of >60% carotid stenosis (overall accuracy, 89%) as used in the ACAS.[28]

TABLE 1–1. DUPLEX ULTRASOUND CLASSIFICATION OF CAROTID STENOSIS[a]

Lumen Diameter Reduction[b]	Peak Systolic Frequency (Velocity)[c]	End Diastolic Frequency (Velocity)	Spectral Waveform
None	<4 kHz (<125 cm/sec)		Minimal to no spectral broadening, normal boundary layer separation
<50%	<4 kHz (<125 cm/sec)		Loss of boundary layer separation
50–79%	>4 kHz (>125 cm/sec)		Marked spectral broadening
80–99%	>4 kHz (>125 cm/sec)	>4.5 kHz (>140 cm/sec)	Marked spectral broadening
Occlusion			No flow in ICA, flow in CCA to zero at end diastole ipsilaterally, occlusive "thump"

[a] From Strandness.[38]
[b] Based on arteriographic measurement of stenosis, comparing residual ICA lumen diameter to the estimated diameter of the carotid bulb.
[c] Based on 5-MHz pulsed Doppler with 60° angle of insonation.

The accuracy of DUS as a preoperative imaging modality in the treatment of carotid disease is highly dependent on the consistency and quality of the vascular laboratory. As such, proper training and accreditation is essential. The Intersocietal Commission for the Accreditation of Vascular Laboratories (ICAVL) mandates vascular laboratories fulfill specific criteria prior to accreditation. Laboratories that meet these requirements are accredited for a period of 3 years.[45]

MAGNETIC RESONANCE ANGIOGRAPHY

Magnetic resonance angiography (MRA) is a diagnostic imaging modality that has been available only since the early 1990s. MRA is noninvasive and does not subject the patient to ionizing radiation, and can also provide information regarding the carotid siphon and the intracranial circulation. A number of studies have compared MRA to conventional angiography in assessing the degree of carotid stenosis. Studies to date have found sensitivities of MRA versus conventional cerebral angiography in the range of 84% to 100% and specificities ranging from 64% to 98%.[27,46–49] Some authors have noted that MRA overestimates the degree of carotid stenosis compared to conventional angiography.[50,51] Pan and colleagues[20] found that stenosis measurements obtained with MRA actually correlated with histologic stenosis better than conventional angiography.

Given that MRA is noninvasive and provides reasonable accuracy in estimating degree of carotid stenosis, one might postulate that it could be substituted for DUS or conventional angiography in the preoperative workup of patients with carotid disease. There are distinct disadvantages to MRA, however. It is not widely available, and is contraindicated for patients with certain types of metallic implants (i.e., pacemakers), patients with intraocular metal fragments, patients whose weight exceeds the capacity of the MR table, and patients with claustrophobia.

Although there is considerable overlap in the ranges of sensitivity and specificity in estimating degree of stenosis with MRA versus DUS, a prospective study by Jackson and colleagues[46] concluded that the specificity of DUS is significantly better than MRA in determining a 60% or greater carotid artery stenosis. A study by Modaresi and colleagues[52] found that MRA was less sensitive than DUS in distinguishing between severe stenosis and complete occlusion of the carotid artery. Some authors have advocated the performance of CEA without conventional arteriography with use of preoperative DUS and MRA. The authors assert that the imaging modalities are complementary, and that MRA confirms DUS findings and adds additional information regarding the intracranial circulation.[47,48,53,54] Others, however, argue that MRA rarely changes clinical decision making over DUS alone in patients with carotid disease and is therefore rarely indicated.[55,56] MRA is considerably more expensive than DUS,[57,58] and therefore must add relevant information to clinical decision making in order to warrant its use in conjunction with DUS.

COMPUTED TOMOGRAPHIC ANGIOGRAPHY

Computed tomographic angiography (CTA) is the most recently developed technique for imaging the carotid artery. Although noninvasive, CTA does subject the patient to both IV contrast and radiation, is more costly than DUS, and is not yet widely available. It is able to accurately assess the degree of stenosis in areas of arterial wall calcification, and images are obtained more quickly than MRA.[59,60] In estimating a carotid stenosis >70%, CTA has a sensitivity in the range of 88% to 100% and specificity in the range of 92% to 100% compared to conventional arteriography.[61–63] CTA shows poorer correlation with conventional angiography in arteries with mild to moderate stenosis.[64] The role of CTA as a sole preoperative imaging technique prior to CEA has not been defined, but some have suggested that it has a role as a confirmatory test rather than conventional arteriography when the findings of DUS or MRA are ambiguous.[65]

CAROTID ENDARTERECTOMY WITHOUT ARTERIOGRAPHY

The performance of CEA without preoperative arteriography remains controversial. Several authors, including the principal investigator of NASCET, have asserted that conventional arteriography is mandatory prior to endarterectomy.[66–69] Reasons given for this assertion include concerns that DUS cannot reliably distinguish occlusions from high-grade stenoses[67] and that DUS lacks precision to accurately assess a patient's risk of stroke.[66,68] Some of these concerns arose from DUS studies performed in the NASCET. There was no standardization of equipment or criteria, however, among participating NASCET centers performing DUS.[70]

Multiple investigations have been performed addressing the question of whether CEA can be safely performed without preoperative arteriography.[25,71–79] The results of 10 studies supporting this approach are displayed in Table 1–2. Studies in which patients underwent both conventional arteriography and DUS found that arteriography

TABLE 1–2. CAROTID ENDARTERECTOMY WITHOUT ARTERIOGRAPHY

Authors	Year	N^a	Design	Imaging Studies[b]	Results
Goodson et al.[71]	1987	78	Retrospective	DUS + CA	Comparison of preop imaging to OR findings: DUS 99% sensitive, CA 91% sensitive
Wagner et al.[72]	1991	753	Retrospective	DUS + selective CA	No significant difference in morbidity and mortality in patients undergoing preop DUS alone (n = 255) v. those undergoing preop CA (n = 484)
McKittrick et al.[73]	1993	114	Retrospective	DUS + selective CA	CA changed operative plan in 2/58 patients who had CA + DUS. Intraop findings did not correlate with DUS in one patient and with CA in one patient.
Dawson et al.[25]	1993	94	Prospective	DUS + CA	Clinical exam + DUS sufficient for preop planning in 93% patients.
Cartier et al.[74]	1993	130	Retrospective	DUS	Operative findings agreed with preop DUS 96% cases. One chronic and 5 fresh ICA thromboses in OR. Fresh thromboses successfully revascularized.
Chervu and Moore[75]	1994	110	Retrospective	DUS + selective CA	Operative findings and DUS concurred in all cases. CA found 2 intracranial or siphon lesions with no change in operative plan.
Mattos et al.[76]	1994	167	Retrospective	DUS + CA	CA altered clinical management in 4% patients.
Shifrin et al.[77]	1996	109	Retrospective	DUS	Intraop findings differed from DUS in 2 patients: one total occlusion 26 days post DUS, one missed kink requiring reimplantation.
Loftus et al.[78]	1998	494	Prospective	DUS + selective CA	CA performed in 35 patients. Periop CVA rate 4.2%, 1.3% in last year of study. No procedures abandoned secondary to unexpected findings.
Ballotta et al.[79]	1999	99	Prospective	DUS + CA	CA altered clinical management in 2% patients: DUS overestimated stenosis in one patient, and diagnosed ICA occlusion in one artery with "string sign".

[a] Number of carotid arteries
[b] DUS = duplex ultrasound; CA = conventional arteriography.

altered operative plans in only 2% to 7% of cases.[25,76,78] Dawson et al.[25] concluded that patients should undergo arteriography on the basis of atypical duplex findings or in cases in which the clinical symptoms and DUS findings did not concur. Series in which DUS was used as a sole preoperative imaging modality or in which arteriography was used selectively reported neurologic complications in 1.8% to 4.2% of patients,[72–75,77] rates that are similar to published data in patients undergoing routine preoperative arteriography prior to endarterectomy.

As patients are at risk for neurologic events not only during endarterectomy but during cerebral angiography as well, the use of noninvasive preoperative imaging with selective use of angiography may decrease the overall stroke rate in patients being managed for cerebrovascular disease. In 1995, Kuntz and colleagues[80] performed a morbidity analysis to determine if the 5-year stroke risk could be reduced in asymptomatic patients with suspected carotid disease with the use of preoperative DUS or MRA rather than conventional angiography. Using a methods-of-decision analysis, the investigators accounted for the risk of neurologic events in patients misdiagnosed by MRA or DUS (using accuracies for MRA and DUS compared to arteriography) and concluded that the preoperative use of MRA or DUS rather than arteriography as a preoperative imaging modality would decrease the 5-year risk of stroke by 8 to 10 per 1000 patients.

INDICATIONS FOR PREOPERATIVE ARTERIOGRAPHY

In the majority of patients with carotid disease, preoperative imaging with DUS alone is both safe and cost-effective. However, there are specific circumstances in which arteriography is warranted. DUS exams obtained in a vascular lab that is not accredited or has not validated the criteria they use to grade stenosis should be viewed with caution. In such cases, patients should have a repeat DUS in a credible lab if possible, or have preoperative arteriography if evaluation in a reliable lab is not available. If the DUS is technically limited by calcifications, kinks, or coils, or if the patient's symptoms are not consistent with the DUS findings, confirmatory testing with alternative imaging modalities should be obtained.

A frequently quoted limitation of DUS is the differentiation of total carotid occlusion from high-grade stenosis. The ability to distinguish a "string sign" from a total occlusion can be critical in the management of a symptomatic patient. Three studies have investigated the accuracy of DUS to detect carotid occlusions. In comparison to conventional angiography, the accuracy of DUS to detect total occlusion is 97% to 98%, with positive predictive value of 92.5% to 96%, and negative predictive value of 98% to 99%.[81–83] Although uncommon, a false-positive diagnosis of carotid occlusion in a symptomatic patient has potentially devastating consequences, as such an individual remains at high risk for stroke. A confirmatory arteriogram, therefore, is prudent in a symptomatic individual, but probably not necessary in an asymptomatic patient if the DUS was of high quality with no technical limitations. In patients with a contralateral occlusion, DUS tends to overestimate the degree of stenosis on the ipsilateral side.[84,85] Although preoperative arteriography is not necessary in these patients, awareness of this overestimation and use of alternative duplex parameters to grade the degree of stenosis on the ipsilateral side, as outlined by Fujitani et al.[86] and AbuRahma et al.,[87] are important. Patients with bilateral disease should have a repeat DUS scan prior to operation on the second side, as the velocity in the unoperated side may change.[88]

There are several other circumstances in which preoperative arteriography is warranted. Most surgeons would agree that angiography is indicated in nonatherosclerotic diseases of the carotid arteries, such as a dissection or fibromuscular dysplasia; in radiation-induced carotid disease; or for preoperative planning in patients with recurrent disease after endarterectomy. Patients with evidence of significant intrathoracic or vertebrobasilar arterial disease on physical exam or DUS with symptoms attributable to such lesions should also undergo arteriography.

CONCLUSIONS

Carotid endarterectomy without preoperative arteriography is safe, cost-effective, and may decrease patient morbidity and mortality. Although preoperative arteriography is necessary in some patients, the decision regarding which patients require arteriography should be straightforward on the basis of physical exam, patient symptoms, and noninvasive studies. The use of noninvasive imaging as a sole preoperative planning modality mandates high-quality examinations performed by experienced and well-trained personnel.

REFERENCES

1. Pokras R, Dyken ML. Dramatic changes in the performance of endarterectomy for diseases of the extracranial arteries of the head. *Stroke.* 1988;19:1289–1290.
2. Beneficial effect of carotid endarterectomy in symptomatic patients with high-grade carotid stenosis. North American Symptomatic Carotid Endarterectomy Trial Collaborators. *N Engl J Med.* 1991;325:505–507.
3. Randomised trial of endarterectomy for recently symptomatic carotid stenosis: final results of the MRC European Carotid Surgery Trial (ECST). *Lancet.* 1998;351:1379–1387.
4. Endarterectomy for asymptomatic carotid artery stenosis. Executive Committee for the Asymptomatic Carotid Atherosclerosis Study. *JAMA.* 1995;273:1421–1428.
5. Moniz E, Lima A, deLacerda R. Hemiplegies par thrombose de la carotide interne. *PresseMed.* 1937;45:977.
6. Barber FE, Baker DW, Nation AW, Strandness DE Jr, Reid JM. Ultrasonic duplex echo-Doppler scanner. *IEEE Trans Biomed Eng.* 1974;21:109–113.
7. Blackshear WM Jr, Phillips DJ, Thiele BL, et al. Detection of carotid occlusive disease by ultrasonic imaging and pulsed Doppler spectrum analysis. *Surgery.* 1979;86:698–706.
8. Hankey GJ, Warlow CP, Sellar RJ. Cerebral angiographic risk in mild cerebrovascular disease. *Stroke.* 1990;21:209–222.
9. Theodotou BC, Whaley R, Mahaley MS. Complications following transfemoral cerebral angiography for cerebral ischemia. *Surg Neurol.* 1987;28:90–92.
10. Heiserman JE, Dean BL, Hodak JA, et al. Neurologic complications of cerebral angiography. *AJNR.* 1994;15:1401–1407.
11. Davies KN, Humphrey PR. Complications of cerebral angiography in patients with symptomatic carotid territory ischaemia screened by carotid ultrasound. *J Neurol Neurosurg Psychiatry.* 1993;56:967–972.

12. Leow K, Murie JA. Cerebral angiography for cerebrovascular disease: the risks. *Br J Surg.* 1988;75:428–430.
13. Earnest F 4th, Forbes G, Sandok BA, et al. Complications of cerebral angiography: prospective assessment of risk. *AJR.* 1984;142:247–253.
14. Dion JE, Gates PC, Fox AJ, Barnett HJM, Blom RJ. Clinical events following neuroangiography: a prospective study. *Stroke.* 1987;18:997–1004.
15. Porter GA. Contrast-associated nephropathy. *Am J Cardiol.* 1989;64:22E–26E.
16. Mikkonen R, Kontkanen T, Kivisaari L. Acute and late adverse reactions to low-osmol contrast media. *Acta Radiol.* 1995;35;72–76.
17. Garrard CL , Manord JD, Ballinger BA, et al. Cost savings associated with nonroutine use of carotid angiography. *Am J Surg.* 1997;174:650–654.
18. Ammar AD. Cost-efficient carotid surgery: a comprehensive evaluation. *J Vasc Surg.* 1996; 24:1050–1056.
19. Young GR, Sandercock PAG, Slattery J, Humphrey PRD, Smith ETS, Brock L. Observer variation in the interpretation of intra-arterial angiograms and the risk of inappropriate decisions about carotid endarterectomy. *J Neurol Neurosurg Psychiatry.* 1996;60:152–157.
20. Pan XM, Saloner D, Reilly LM, et al. Assessment of carotid artery stenosis by ultrasonography, conventional angiography, and magnetic resonance angiography: correlation with *ex vivo* measurement of plaque stenosis. *J Vasc Surg.* 1995;21:82–89.
21. Alexandrov AV, Bladin CF, Maggisano R, Norris JW. Measuring carotid stenosis: time for a reappraisal. *Stroke.* 1993,24:1292–1296.
22. Eckstein HH, Post K, Hoffmann E, Hupp T, Allenberg JR. Determination of the degree of stenosis of the internal carotid artery in the surgical specimen after eversion TEA: comparison with angiography and c-w-Doppler ultrasound. *Vasa.* 1995;24:176–183.
23. Nicolaides AN, Shifrin EG, Bradbury A, et al. Angiographic and duplex grading of internal carotid stenosis: can we overcome the confusion? *J Endovasc Surg.* 1996;3:158–165.
24. Hames TK, Humphries, Ratliff DA, Birch SJ, Gazzard VM, Chant AD. The validation of duplex scanning and continuous wave Doppler imaging: a comparison with conventional angiography. *Ultrasound Med Biol.* 1985;11:827–834.
25. Dawson DL, Zierler RE, Strandness DE Jr, Clowes AW, Kohler TR. The role of duplex scanning and arteriography before carotid endarterectomy: a prospective study. *J Vasc Surg.* 1993;18:673–683.
26. Taylor DC, Strandness DE, Jr. Carotid artery duplex scanning. *J Clin Ultrasound.* 1987;15:635–644.
27. Polak JF, Bajakian RL, O'Leary DH, Anderson MR, Donaldson MC, Jolesz FA. Detection of internal carotid artery stenosis: comparison of MR angiography, color Doppler sonography, and arteriography. *Radiology.* 1992;182:35–40.
28. Moneta SL, Edwards JM, Papanicolaou G, et al. Screening for asymptomatic internal carotid artery stenosis: duplex criteria for discriminating 60% to 99% stenosis. *J Vasc Surg.* 1995; 21:989–994.
29. Londrey GL, Spadone DP, Hodgson KJ, Ramsey DE, Barkmeier LD, Sumner DS. Does colorflow imaging improve the accuracy of duplex carotid evaluation? *J Vasc Surg.* 1991;13:659–663.
30. Bray JM, Galland F, Lhoste P, et al. Colour Doppler and duplex sonography and angiography of the carotid artery bifurcations. Prospective, double blind study. *Neuroradiology.* 1995; 37:219–224.
31. Branas CC, Weingarten MS, Czeredarczuk M, Schafer PF. Examination of carotid arteries with quantitative color Doppler flow imaging. *J Ultrasound Med.* 1994;13:121–127.
32. Goodson SF, Flanigan DP, Bishara RA, Schuler JJ, Kikta MJ, Meyer JP. Can carotid duplex scanning supplant arteriography in patients with focal carotid territory symptoms? *J Vasc Surg.* 1987;5:551–557.

33. Akers DL, Markowitz IA, Kerstein MD. The value of aortic arch study in the evaluation of cerebrovascular insufficiency. *Am J Surg*. 1987;154:230–232.
34. Kadwa AM, Robbs JV, Abdool-Carrim ATO. Aortic arch angiography prior to carotid endarterectomy. Is its continued use justified? *Eur J Vasc Endovasc Surg*. 1997;13:527–530.
35. Mackey WC, O'Donnell TF, Jr, Callow AD. Carotid endarterectomy in patients with intracranial vascular disease: short-term risk and long-term outcome. *J Vasc Surg*. 1989;10:432–438.
36. Mattos MA, van Bemmelen PS, Hodgson KJ, Barkmeier LD, Ramsey DE, Sumner DS. The influence of carotid siphon stenosis on short- and long-term outcome after carotid endarterectomy. *J Vasc Surg*. 1993;17:902–911.
37. Akers DL, Bell WH 3rd, Kerstem MD. Does intracranial dye study contribute to evaluation of carotid artery disease? *Am J Surg*. 1988;156:87–90.
38. Strandness DE, Jr. *Duplex Scanning in Vascular Disorders, 2nd Ed.* New York: Raven Press Ltd.; 1993;113–157.
39. Faught WE, Mattos MA, van Bemmelen PS, et al. Color-flow duplex scanning of carotid arteries: new velocity criteria based on receiver operator characteristic analysis for threshold stenoses used in symptomatic and asymptomatic carotid trials. *J Vasc Surg*. 1994;19:818–828.
40. Winkelaar GB, Chen JC, Salvian AJ, Taylor DC, Teal PA, Hsiang YN. New duplex ultrasound criteria for managing symptomatic 50% or greater carotid stenosis. *J Vasc Surg*. 1999;29:986–994.
41. Moneta GL, Edwards JM, Chitwood RW, et al. Correlation of North American Symptomatic Carotid Endarterectomy Trial (NASCET) angiographic definition of 70% to 99% stenosis with duplex scanning. *J Vasc Surg*. 1993;17:152–159.
42. Beebe HG, Salles-Cunha SX, Scissons RP, et al. Carotid arterial ultrasound scan imaging: a direct approach to stenosis measurement. *J Vasc Surg*. 1999;29:838–844.
43. AbuRahma AF, Robinson PA, Strickler DL, Alberts S, Young L. Proposed new duplex classification for threshold stenoses used in various symptomatic and asymptomatic carotid endarterectomy trials. *Ann Vasc Surg*. 1998;12:349–358.
44. Carpenter JP, Lexa FJ, Davis JT. Determination of sixty percent or greater carotid artery stenosis by duplex Doppler ultrasonography. *J Vasc Surg*. 1995;22:697–705.
45. Zierler RE. Vascular surgery without arteriography: use of Duplex ultrasound. *Cardiovasc Surg*. 1999;7:74–82.
46. Jackson MR, Chang AS, Robles HA, et al. Determination of 60% or greater carotid stenosis: a prospective comparison of magnetic resonance angiography and duplex ultrasound with conventional angiography. *Ann Vasc Surg*. 1998;12:236–243.
47. Turnipseed WD, Kennell TW, Turski PA, Acher CW, Hoch JR. Combined use of duplex imaging and magnetic resonance angiography for evaluation of patients with symptomatic ipsilateral high-grade carotid stenosis. *J Vasc Surg*. 1993;17:832–840.
48. Scarbino T, Carriero A, Magarelli N, et al. MR angiography in carotid stenosis: a comparison of three techniques. *Eur J Radiol*. 1998;28:117–125.
49. Young GR, Humphrey PR, Shaw MD, Nixon TE, Smith ET. Comparison of magnetic resonance angiography, duplex ultrasound, and digital subtraction angiography in assessment of extracranial internal carotid artery stenosis. *J Neurol Neurosurg Psychiatry*. 1994;57:1466–1478.
50. Riles TS, Eidelman EM, Litt AW, Pinto RS, Oldford F, Schwartzenberg GW. Comparison of magnetic resonance angiography, conventional angiography, and duplex scanning. *Stroke*. 1992;23:341–346.
51. Buijs PC, Klop RB, Eikelboom BC, et al. Carotid bifurcation imaging: magnetic resonance angiography compared to conventional angiography and doppler ultrasound. *Eur J Vasc Surg*. 1993;7:245–251.

52. Modaresi KB, Cox TC, Summers PE, et al. Comparison of intra-arterial digital subtraction angiography, magnetic resonance angiography, and duplex ultrasonography for measuring carotid artery stenosis. *Br J Surg*. 1999;86:1422–1426.
53. Huston J, Nichols DA, Luetmer PH, et al. MR angiographic and sonographic indications for endarterectomy. *Am J Neuroradiol*. 1998;19:309–315.
54. Saouaf R, Grassi CJ, Hartnell GG, Wheeler H, Suojanen JN. Complete MR angiography and Doppler ultrasound as the sole imaging modalities prior to carotid endarterectomy. *Clin Radiol*. 1998;53:579–586.
55. Erdoes LS, Marek JM, Mills JL, Berman SS, Whitehill T, Hunter GC. The relative contributions of carotid duplex scanning, magnetic resonance angiography, and cerebral arteriography to clinical decision making: a prospective study in patients with carotid occlusive disease. *J Vasc Surg*. 1996;23:950–956.
56. Ozaki CK, Irwin PB, Flynn TC, Huber TS, Seeger JM. Surgical decision making for carotid endarterectomy and contemporary magnetic resonance angiography. *Am J Surg*. 1999; 178: 182–184.
57. Melissano G, Castellano R, Mazitelli S, Zoppei G, Chiesa R. Safe and cost-effective approach to carotid surgery. *Eur J Vasc Endovasc Surg*. 1997;14:164–169.
58. Vanninen R, Manninnen H, Soimakallio S. Imaging of carotid artery stenosis: clinical efficacy and cost-effectiveness. *Am J Neuroradiol*. 1995;16:1875–1883.
59. Sameshima T, Futami S, Morita Y, et al. Clinical usefulness of and problems with three-dimensional CT angiography for the evaluation of arteriosclerotic stenosis of the carotid artery: comparison with conventional angiography, MRA and ultrasound sonography. *Surg Neurol*. 1999;51:301–309.
60. Marks MP, Napel S, Jordan JE, Enzmann DR. Diagnosis of carotid artery disease: preliminary experience with maximum-intensity–projection spiral CT angiography. *Am J Roentgenol*. 1993; 160:1267–1271.
61. Simeone A, Carriero A, Armillotta M, et al. Spiral CT angiography in the study of the carotid stenosis. *J Neuroradiol*. 1997;24:18–22.
62. Leclerc X, Godefroy O, Lucas C, et al. Internal carotid arterial stenosis: CT angiography with volume rendering. *Radiology*. 1999;210:673–682.
63. Marcus CD, Ladam-Marcus VJ, Bigot JL, Clement C, Baehrel B, Menanteau BP. Carotid arterial stenosis: evaluation at CT angiography with the volume-rendering technique. *Radiology*. 1999;211:775–780.
64. Link J, Brossmann J, Grabener M, et al. Spiral CT angiography and selective digital subtraction angiography of internal carotid artery stenosis. *Am J Neuroradiol*. 1996;17:89–94.
65. Cinat ME, Pham H, Vo D, Gordon I, Wilson SE. Improved imaging of carotid artery bifurcation using helical computed tomographic angiography. *Ann Vasc Surg*. 1999;13:178–183.
66. Barnett HJM, Eliasziw M, Meldrum HE. The identification by imaging methods of patients who might benefit from carotid endarterectomy. *Arch Neurol*. 1995;52:827–833.
67. Bomstein NM, Beloev ZG, Norris JW. The limitations of diagnosis of carotid occlusion by Doppler ultrasound. *Ann Surg*. 1988;207:315–317.
68. Eliasziw M, Rankin RN, Fox AJ, Haynes RB, Barnett HJM. Accuracy and prognostic consequences of ultrasonography in identifying severe carotid artery stenosis. North American Symptomatic Carotid Endarterectomy Trial (NASCET) Group. *Stroke*. 1995;26:1747–1752.
69. Gender JW, Lamparello PJ, Riles TS, Giangola G, Imparato AM. Is duplex scanning sufficient evaluation before carotid endarterectomy? *J Vasc Surg*. 1989;9:193–201.
70. Strandness DE, Jr. Angiography before carotid endarterectomy. *Arch Neurol. Neurol*. 1995; 52:832–833.
71. Goodson SF, Flanigan DP, Bishara RA, Schuller JJ, Kitkta MJ, Meyer JP. Can carotid duplex

scanning supplant arteriography in patients with focal carotid territory symptoms? *J Vasc Surg.* 1987;5:551–557.

72. Wagner WH, Treiman RL, Cossman DV, Foran RF, Levin PM, Cohen JL. The diminishing role of diagnostic arteriography in carotid disease: duplex scanning as definitive preoperative study. *Ann Vasc Surg.* 1991;5:105–110.
73. McKittrick JE, Cisek PL, Pojunas KW, Blum GM, Ortgiesen P, Lim RA. Are both color-flow duplex scanning and cerebral arteriography required prior to carotid endarterectomy? *Ann Vasc Surg.* 1993;7:311–316.
74. Carrier R, Cartier P, Fontaine A. Carotid endarterectomy without angiography. The reliability of Doppler ultrasonography and duplex scanning in preoperative assessment. *Can J Surg.* 1993;36:411–416.
75. Chervu A, Moore WS. Carotid endarterectomy without arteriography. *Ann Vasc Surg.* 1994;8:296–302.
76. Mattos MA, Hodgson KJ, Faught WE, et al. Carotid endarterectomy without angiography: is color-flow duplex scanning sufficient? *Surgery.* 1994;116:776–783.
77. Shifrin EG, Bomstein NM, Kantarovsky A, et al. Carotid endarterectomy without angiography. *Br J Surg.* 1996;83:1107–1109.
78. Loftus IM, McCarthy MJ, Pan H, et al. Carotid endarterectomy without angiography does not compromise operative outcome. *Eur J Vasc Endovasc Surg.* 1998;16:489–493.
79. Ballotta E, Da Giau G, Abbruzzese E, et al. Carotid endarterectomy without angiography: can clinical evaluation and duplex ultrasonographic scanning alone replace traditional arteriography for carotid surgery workup? A prospective study. *Surgery.* 1999;126:20–27.
80. Kuntz KM, Skillman JJ, Whittemore AD, Kent KC. Carotid endarterectomy in asymptomatic patients—is contrast angiography necessary? A morbidity analysis. *J Vasc Surg.* 1995;22:706–716.
81. Kirsch JD, Wagner LR, James EM, et al. Carotid artery occlusion: positive predictive value of duplex ultrasonography compared with arteriography. *J Vasc Surg* 1994;19:624–629.
82. Mansour MA, Mattos MA, Hood DB, et al. Detection of total occlusion, string sign, and preocclusive stenosis of the internal carotid artery by color flow duplex scanning. *Am J Surg.* 1995;170:154–158.
83. AbuRahma AF, Pollack JA, Robinson PS, Mullins D. The reliability of color duplex ultrasound in diagnosing total carotid artery occlusion. *Am J Surg.* 1997;174:185–187.
84. Busuttil SJ, Franklin DP, Youkey JR, Elmore JR. Carotid duplex overestimation of stenosis due to severe contralateral disease. *Am J Surg.* 1996;172:144–148.
85. Van Everdingen KJ, van der Grond J, Kappelle LJ. Overestimation of a stenosis in the internal carotid artery by duplex sonography caused by an increase in volume flow. *J Vasc Surg.* 1998;27:479–485.
86. Fujitani RM, Mills JL, Wang LM, Taylor SM. The effect of unilateral internal carotid arterial occlusion upon contralateral duplex study: criteria for accurate interpretation. *J Vasc Surg* 1992;16:459–468.
87. AbuRahma AF, Richmond BK, Robinson PA, Khan S, Pollack JA, Alberts S. Effect of contralateral severe stenosis or carotid occlusion on duplex criteria of ipsilateral stenoses: comparative study of various duplex parameters. *J Vasc Surg.* 1995;22:751–762.
88. Abou-Zamzam AM, Jr., Moneta GL, Edwards JM, Yeager RA, Taylor LM, Porter JM. Is a single preoperative duplex scan sufficient for planning bilateral carotid endarterectomy? *J Vasc Surg.* 2000;31:282–288.

2

Magnetic Resonance Angiography Alone for Carotid Artery Surgery

William D. Turnipseed, MD

The traditional role of contrast arteriography in preoperative evaluation of patients with physical findings or symptoms suggestive of cerebral vascular insufficiency has changed considerably as less invasive methods of vascular imaging have become available. Although contrast arteriography remains the most accurate method of obtaining high-quality imaging of the cerebral vascular system, its interventional nature and cost render it inappropriate for routine screening and surveillance purposes. Despite better fluoroscopy, use of smaller catheters, and digital computer enhancement, contrast arteriography adversely affects cost–benefit formulas that assess outcome in treatment of patients with cerebral vascular disease.[1] Although postangiographic risk for death or a stroke remain quite low (0.1–1%), transient morbidity [associated with catheter induced hemorrhage (2%), embolization (2%), or allergic reactions to injected the contrast media (3%)] is not uncommon.[2] Clinical studies, such as the Asymptomatic Carotid Atherosclerosis Study (ACAS) trial, suggest that arteriography can be almost as dangerous as carotid surgery, accounting for nearly half the strokes that were reported in the entire study (1.2% out of 2.3%)[3]. Furthermore, x-ray arteriography is expensive ($5,000 = technical + professional charges + ambulatory surgery) and costs almost as much as carotid endarterectomy (CEA) itself. The major argument against continued use of traditional contrast arteriography in the assessment of cerebral vascular disease continues to be risk exposure cost and poor patient acceptance. Recent experience with magnetic resonance imaging (MRI) suggests that physiological characterization and anatomic display of cerebral vascular circulation can be obtained without the necessity of vascular catheters or injection of contrast agents. Magnetic resonance arteriography (MRA) uses an electronic field to create differential atomic signals in soft tissues. A variety of MRI techniques have been devised to provide arterial imaging based on functional blood-flow patterns and velocities. Arterial image acquisition is most commonly achieved using time-of-flight (TOF) or phase-contrast (PC) pulse sequences. Two-dimensional (2D) TOF, the most commonly used technique, is a gradient recall procedure that uses radio frequency pulses to suppress signals from surrounding soft tissue, and is based on the concept of blood flowing into a given field of view appears bright in relationship to adjacent saturated soft tissues. The other image acquisition technique used in MRA is PC sequencing. Image signal intensity in PC arteriography (PCA) is ultimately proportional to blood-flow velocity. PC sequences are programmed to assign a specific MR signal phase to each velocity of blood flow. Faster moving protons in blood accumulate greater phase shift relative to slowly flowing blood. PCA relies on the physical principal that spins moving in the direction of a bipolar magnetic field gradient acquire a phase shift proportional to their velocity and gradient amplitude and duration. TOF imaging is most commonly used to evaluate the brachiocephalic and cervical carotid arteries, whereas PC imaging is used to evaluate the complex flow patterns of the intracranial circulation and to acquire flow velocity data. Advantages of 2D TOF include minimum saturation effects at normal flow velocities, short acquisition time, and an increased sensitivity to low-flow states in the circulation. The major disadvantage of TOF is susceptibility to inplane flow artifacts and intervoxel dephasing (Flow void), which tends to overestimate the severity of stenoses. The use of three-dimensional image acquisition (3D TOF), which uses much thicker volume slabs than 2D TOF (3–8 cm in thickness vs. 1.5 mm for 2D TOF) can be used to increase spacial resolution and eliminate image artifacts. The combination of 2D and 3D TOF imaging allows for detection of low flow and also improves spatial resolution.

PCA is often performed, in addition to TOF imaging, in order to confirm the presence of stenotic lesions in areas of complex geometric flow and determine flow velocity data. Two-dimensional PCA is sensitive to fast or slow flow, has shorter scan times, and better documentation of vessel morphology with less sensitivity to complex flow pattern artifacts. PCA using 3D volume acquisitions can decrease the amount of intervoxel dephasing in turbulent flow areas of the intracranial circulation. Image data can be retrospectively processed and projected into any desired plane so that oblique views of intracranial aneurysms and arteriovenous malformations can be obtained. Three-dimensional PC images also can be used to create directional flow images, making it possible to obtain physiologic as well as anatomic information about blood flow through the intracranial circulation.[4]

The recent use of 3D TOF image acquisition in conjunction with intravenous injection of paramagnetic contrast agents has improved the accuracy and utility of MRA significantly. Digital subtraction of source images enables processing very similar to digital arteriography. Paramagnetic contrast agents, such as gadolinium, are heavy metal analogs that are chelated with dialthalene triamene pentacedic acid (DTPA). Combined use of 3D TOF and gadolinium or similar contrast agents has resulted in significant reduction in flow-void artifacts, elimination of inplane flow defects, and reduced imaging time as well as improved spatial resolution. When these arterial imaging techniques are used in combination, overall accuracy of MRA compared with traditional contrast arteriography ranges from 92% to 98%, depending on the field of view interrogated. Sensitivity ranges from 83% to 97% and specificity ranges from 92% to 98%.[3,5,6]

One of the major issues regarding contemporary use of MRA has to do with whether it can be used as a sole diagnostic test and effectively eliminate the use of contrast arteriography and possibly noninvasive testing. Few would argue that MRA can provide more information about patients with cerebrovascular disease than duplex imaging. Unlike duplex testing, which is limited to assessment of extracranial vessels and perhaps the carotid siphon, the combination of MRI and MRA can be used to image the brain and screen for intracranial pathology, such as silent cortical ischemia, hemorrhage, tumor, and aneurysms. MRA can be used to determine intracranial directional flow patterns to quantitate regional hemispheric blood flow characteristics and provide high-quality imaging of the extracranial circulation.[7–9] Clinicians who champion the solitary use of duplex imaging would suggest that in most clinical settings, the additional information derived from MRA adds little to treatment plans or outcome, and therefore is unnecessary. This is overstated simplification of clinical fact.

It seems more appropriate to suggest that there is a need to determine the minimum amount of information required for safely treating patients with signs and symptoms of cerebrovascular disease. The most appropriate use of pretreatment diagnostic testing depends in a large part on whether the patient is symptomatic. For any test to be used effectively in management decision making, its shortcomings and limitations must be clearly understood, and the consequences of such deficiencies considered in the evaluation of both symptomatic and asymptomatic patients.

Clearly, appropriate treatment of patients with acute symptoms of cerebral insufficiency depends on clinical assessment and confirmation of cause. The use of MRI/MRA in the setting of acute neurologic injury is attractive because extent of brain injury as well as abnormalities in the brachiocephalic circulation can be determined quickly without interventional risk exposure or delay in diagnosis. Cerebral diffusion MRI studies can identify early ischemic injury and/or parenchymal bleeds, while more conventional T2 weighted tests can identify abnormalities, such as old stroke, tumor, arteriovenous malformation or intracranial aneurysm. MRA is very accurate for detection of carotid occlusion, acute dissection, complex plaque, and high-grade stenoses. This information can be critical to clinicians planning acute-care strategies. Unfortunately, inappropriate patient selection may result in poor-quality imaging studies and the need for additional diagnostic testing, which can cause treatment delays, increased cost, and increased risk exposure. Therefore, MRI/MRA testing should be performed in only those individuals with acute neurologic symptoms of possible vascular origin who are conscious, able to follow verbal instructions, and able to hold still on command. These MRA tests should not be performed in agitated, claustrophobic, or unstable and acutely ill patients.

Pretreatment evaluation of patients with remote symptoms of cerebral ischemia or asymptomatic cervical bruits invariably differs from assessment of the acutely symptomatic patient. The most appropriate evaluation of patients with symptomatic or high-risk carotid occlusive disease varies somewhat based on available diagnostic resources. In centers in which ultrasonography and high-quality MRI/MRA are available, it is possible to avoid the use of contrast arteriography and CT scans in up to 95% of all cases. However, the reality of current practice would strongly suggest that MRA will never replace duplex ultrasonography (DUS) as a screening and surveillance tool. Ultrasound-based testing is extremely accurate for detection of hemodynamically significant cervical carotid disease. It is safe, cost-efficient, and well suited for repetitious use. Duplex testing is effective in discriminating between normal and diseased carotid and vertebral arteries, it can distinguish hemodynamically insignificant disease from high grades of stenosis, and it allows for morphologic assessment of carotid plaque.[10]

Ultrasonography should be the first test performed in patients with cervical bruits or remote hemispheric symptoms suggestive of cerebral ischemia. Because DUS is safe and extremely accurate as a diagnostic screening procedure (93%), it is unreasonable to subject patients to unnecessary risks associated with contrast arteriography or to the greater expense of MRA when DUS can provide equivalent triage information.[11] Whether duplex testing alone is appropriate for the planning of interventional management in such patients is controversial. A common scenario involves the patient with recent symptoms of cerebral ischemia, asymptomatic cervical bruits, or high comorbid risk factors for stroke who is referred to a surgeon with duplex testing in hand. The problem for the treating physician is whether to depend on the information from such a test. Unfortunately, duplex imaging is very operator dependent, and accuracy rates vary tremendously from laboratory to laboratory. In our experience, when follow-up tests in our own laboratories were performed, we found that nearly one-half of all referral studies sent with patients to our clinic vary at least one disease category from what was originally stated. The practice of basing surgical decisions on DUS alone demands high diagnostic test accuracy, clearly documented disease category classifications, and continued quality assurance. When good-quality images are obtained by skilled technicians in accredited diagnostic facilities, treatment of patients with stable or transient nondisabling hemispheric symptoms and ipsilateral carotid disease does not require additional vascular imaging.[10]

MRI/MRA can be very helpful as a confirmatory test when asymptomatic patients with suspected high-grade carotid artery disease are referred from uncredentialed diagnostic laboratories. In our practice, MRA is most commonly used in conjunction with Duplex imaging. The most commonly performed MRA technique is 2D and 3D TOF with contrast enhancement. MRA can be particularly helpful in the assessment of patients with focal hemispheric symptoms and Duplex evidence of hemodynamically insignificant disease. MRA is routinely performed when Duplex testing suggests bilateral high-grade occlusive disease, ipsilateral or contralateral occlusions, or when high cervical bifurcations, torturous carotid vessels, or densely calcified arteries are encountered, making interpretation difficult.[12]

In conclusion, the use of MRA as a sole diagnostic test is not indicated in most clinical settings. As a solitary test it has the greatest clinical potential for use in the setting of acute cerebral vascular ischemia. The ability to detect brachiocephalic arterial disease and simultaneously identify pathologic changes in the brain are of great importance in this situation. More commonly, MRA will be used in concert with Duplex testing.[7,13,14] When asymptomatic patients are referred with carotid ultrasounds suggesting significant occlusive disease, MRA provides a safe and accurate confirmation that surgery is indicated. MRA should always be performed when Duplex testing is technically inadequate or when complex patterns of extracranial occlusive disease may alter interpretational accuracy. Duplex testing as a sole preoperative test is most appropriate in patients who have documented ipsilateral high-grade occlusive disease and focal nondisabling symptoms of cerebral insufficiency.[1,9,12,15,16]

REFERENCES

1. Cronenwett JL, Birkmeyer JD, Nackman GB, et al. Cost-effectiveness of carotid endarterectomy in asymptomatic patients. *J Vasc Surg.* 1997;25(2):298–309.
2. Turnipseed WD. Diagnosis of carotid stenosis. In: Yao J, Pearce W, eds. *Progress in Vascular Surgery.* Stamford CT: Appleton & Lange; 1997:63–73.
3. Anonymous. Endarterectomy for asymptomatic carotid artery stenosis. Executive Committee for the Asymptomatic Carotid Atherosclerosis Study [see comments]. *JAMA* 1995;273(18):1421–1428.
4. Anderson CM, Edelman RR, Turski PA. *Clinical Magnetic Resonance.* New York: Raven Press; 1993.
5. Turnipseed WD, Grist TM. *Role of Magnetic Resonance Angiography in Peripheral Vascular Disease. Advances in Vascular Surgery.* St. Louis, MO: Mosby, 1998:155–170.
6. Prince MR. Gadolinium-enhanced MR aortography. *Radiology* 1994;191(1):155–164.
7. Turnipseed WD, Kennell TW, Turski PA, Acher CW, Hoch JR. Magnetic resonance angiography and duplex imaging: noninvasive tests for selecting symptomatic carotid endarterectomy candidates. *Surgery* 1993;114(4):643–648.
8. Turski PA, Levine R, Turnipseed W, Kennell T. MR angiography flow analysis. Neurovascular applications. [Review] [38 refs]. *Magn Res Imag Clin Nor Am.* 1995;3(3):541–555.
9. Nehler MR, Moneta GL, Lee RW, Edwards JM, Taylor LM, Jr., Porter JM. Improving selection of patients with less than 60% asymptomatic internal carotid artery stenosis for follow-up carotid artery duplex scanning. *J Vasc Surg.* 1996;24(4):580–585.
10. Strandness DE, Jr. Carotid endarterectomy without angiography. In: Yao J, Pearce W, eds. *Progress in Vascular Surgery.* Stamford, CT: Appleton & Lange; 1997:99–108.
11. Strandness DE, Jr. Angiography before carotid endarterectomy—no. *Arch Neurol.* 1995;52(8): 832–833.
12. Abou-Zamzam AM, Jr., Moneta GL, Edwards JM, Yeager RA, Taylor LM, Jr., Porter JM. Is a single preoperative duplex scan sufficient for planning bilateral carotid endarterectomy? *J Vasc Surg.* 2000;31(2):282–288.
13. Patel MR, Kuntz KM, Klufas RA, et al. Preoperative assessment of the carotid bifurcation. Can magnetic resonance angiography and duplex ultrasonography replace contrast arteriography? *Stroke* 1995;26(10):1753–1758.
14. Polak JF, Kalina P, Donaldson MC, O'Leary DH, Whittemore AD, Mannick JA. Carotid endarterectomy: preoperative evaluation of candidates with combined Doppler sonography and MR angiography. Work in progress [see comments]. *Radiology* 1993;186(2):333–338.
15. Moneta GL, Edwards JM, Chitwood RW, et al. Correlation of North American Symptomatic Carotid Endarterectomy Trial (NASCET) angiographic definition of 70% to 99% internal carotid artery stenosis with duplex scanning. *J Vasc Surg.* 1993;17(1):152–157.
16. van Everdingen KJ, van der GJ, Kappelle LJ. Overestimation of a stenosis in the internal carotid artery by duplex sonography caused by an increase in volume flow [see comments]. *J Vasc Surg.* 1998;27(3):479–485.

3

Preoperative Arterial Duplex Mapping With Limited Intraoperative Arteriography for Planing Lower Extremity Bypass

Richard J. Powell, MD, Daniel B. Walsh, MD, and F. Elizabeth Labombard, RT, RDMS, RVT

Contrast arteriography, which was first described by dos Santos in 1929, is considered a prerequisite prior to proceeding with lower extremity arterial bypass grafting. Arteriography has long been considered the gold standard for defining the arterial anatomy in selecting both a source of arterial inflow and a distal outflow artery for bypass grafting. However, as advances in both arterial duplex mapping and intraoperative fluoroscopic imaging have been made, it is now possible to proceed safely with lower extremity arterial bypass grafting without preoperative arteriography.

The purpose of this report is to describe our technique of preoperative arterial duplex mapping used in conjunction with limited intraoperative arteriography to obtain the information necessary to proceed with lower extremity revascularization without the use of preoperative arteriography.

PREOPERATIVE ARTERIOGRAPHY

Preoperative arteriography has been the most commonly used procedure to define the arterial anatomy prior to proceeding with lower extremity bypass. This procedure has been widely used with relatively good accuracy and safety over many years. However, as vascular surgery has developed, it is now commonplace to perform complex revascularization procedures to pedal and tarsal arteries. Procedures such as these require an accurate assessment of the distal target arteries with regards to quality of the artery and run-off. In the performance of preoperative arteriography, one of the biggest obstacles faced by the interventionist is how to obtain adequate visualization of the distal arterial anatomy in the lower extremity in the presence of multilevel occlusive disease. The use of digital subtraction arteriography (DSA) along with selective catheterization and intra-arterial vasodialators has improved the ability to visualize these distal vessels. Nonetheless, arteriography is a two-dimensional (2D) image attempting to examine a three-dimensional (3D) process. As most vascular surgeons are well aware, arteriography frequently underestimates the degree of occlusive disease in the arterial circulation due to posterior plaques, which might not be visualized on anterior and oblique views. This impression is supported by the available literature. A study by Kohler et al.[1] shows that aortoiliac arteriography had an accuracy of 70% for the detection of significant arterial stenosis when compared with intra-arterial pressure measurements.[1] In addition, the visualization of lower extremity arteries in patients with multilevel arterial occlusive disease has been shown to be inadequate in up to 70% of cases.[2]

Other limitations of arteriography include its invasive nature. The overall major complication rate has been reported to be 3%.[3] These complications include vascular injury, such as pseudoaneurysm formation, dissection, and distal embolization. In addition, patients who require femoral distal bypass grafting are frequently diabetics with impaired renal function. Diabetics are particularly prone to contrast-induced renal failure, which can occur in up to 15% of these patients, although only a small number will go on to require dialysis.[4]

PREOPERATIVE DUPLEX ARTERIAL MAPPING

Kohler and coworkers[1] first described the use of duplex arterial mapping in 1987 and compared this to arteriography for the localization and classification of arterial stenoses. For detecting stenoses that were >50% reduction in diameter, duplex scanning had a positive predictive value of 80% and a negative predictive value of 93%. These results were similar to reported comparisons between two different radiologists reading the same arteriogram. Moneta and coworkers[5] compared lower extremity arterial duplex mapping to arteriography in a blinded fashion. These investigators found that arterial duplex mapping had a sensitivity ranging from 89% in the iliac vessels to 67% in the popliteal artery for detecting a stenosis of >50%. In the tibial vessels, the overall sensitivity for predicting tibial artery occlusion was 90% in the anterior and posterior tibial arteries and 82% in the peroneal artery. A meta-analysis of 71 studies evaluating arterial duplex scanning in comparison to arteriography has similarly shown that duplex ultrasonography accurately defines the lower extremity arterial anatomy.[6] In this study, the specificity for the detection of a stenosis >50% in the aortoiliac segment was 86% and the detection of an occlusion was 97%. In the femoropopliteal tract, there was an 80% sensitivity for the detection of a stenosis, with a specificity of 96%. Similarly, in the infrageniculate arteries the sensitivity and specificity was 83% and 84%, respectively.

Since this time, numerous reports have documented the use of colorflow duplex arterial mapping to plan lower extremity revascularization procedures. Ligush and coworkers[7] prospectively compared operations predicted by duplex ultrasound scanning and operations predicted by conventional arteriography. Of the actual operations performed, 83% were correctly predicted by duplex ultrasound scanning, whereas 90% were correctly predicted by arteriography. Their conclusion was that duplex ultrasound scanning can reliably predict infrainguinal reconstruction strategies. Similarly, Ascher and coworkers[8] have shown that duplex ultrasound scanning may be a safe alternative to arteriography for 89% of patients presenting with critical ischemia in need of an infrageniculate bypass.

At the noninvasive vascular laboratory at the Dartmouth–Hitchcock Medical Center, patients are examined in the supine position with the head of the examination table raised comfortably. When the examination is to include iliac arteries, patients are instructed to have clear liquids the evening prior to the examination and to take nothing by mouth after midnight. Both the Siemens Q2000 and the ATL 3000 HDI color duplex ultrasound machines are used for duplex arteriography. Depending on the instrument available and the patient's body habitus, a 3.5 or 5 MHz curved linear array transducer is used for the evaluation of the common iliac arteries, identification of the internal iliac arteries, and interrogation of proximal segments of the external iliac arteries. In larger or more obese patients, these low-frequency probes are occasionally required for visualization of the distal superficial femoral artery and above-the-knee popliteal segments. A 5-MHz linear array transducer is used for the distal external iliac artery; the common femoral artery; its bifurcation; and the superficial femoral, popliteal, and tibial arteries to the ankle. A 7.5-MHz linear array transducer is usually preferable for interrogation of the pedal arterial circulation.

Although examinations are frequently individualized based on previously determined conditions, our general approach focuses on answering several questions related to the lower extremity arterial circulation:

1. Are there significant stenoses present within the lower extremity arterial circulation?
2. Where are these stenoses located? What is their length and degree of severity?
3. Are there total occlusions within the circulation? Where are they?
4. Is the inflow to the lower extremity adequate for supporting a bypass?
5. Is there vein of adequate quality and length to achieve successful bypass of the lesions found with duplex arteriography?

The most often used criterion for the identification of a significant stenosis except at bifurcations is a focal increase in peak systolic velocity of the least 100%. At bifurcations, due to the absence of published criteria, we define a significant stenosis as a strikingly high peak systolic velocity followed by a marked decrease in peak systolic velocity. Significant turbulence or a significantly different or flattened waveform immediately distal to the bifurcation should make one suspicious for the presence of significant disease.

When sonographic visualization of the arterial circulation is optimal, absence of flow is diagnostic of occlusion. Frequently, dense fibrosis and calcified plaque may obscure segments of the vessel lumen. In these circumstances, a diseased but patent vessel cannot be excluded entirely. A Doppler waveform configuration that does not change significantly from above to below the nonvisualized segment makes occlusion unlikely. The findings of all abruptly flattened, slowly rising, low-velocity waveforms is equally nonspecific, but also likely to be indicative of total or near-total occlusion. The generalized assessment of the arterial walls and plaque morphology is performed using B-mode ultrasound. Qualitative descriptors such as "mild," "moderate," "severe," "dense," "calcified," "irregular," "diffuse," and "echolucent" are used to alert the physician to the general condition of the artery as seen during the ultrasound examination.

Assessment of possible target arteries for bypass involves the determination of the quality of the outflow bed. Continuity of vessels, the presence of significant disease, and evidence of good collateral circulation are determined using Doppler, B-mode, and colorflow examinations. Peak and end diastolic velocities are measured in possible target arteries. Because the inflow is usually severely compromised in these patients, peak systolic velocities offer little in selecting the optimal target artery. In the lab at the Dartmouth–Hitchcock Medical Center, close attention is given to the resistive index. We believe that robust diastolic flow suggests evidence of good distal perfusion, but we have not yet established precise criteria for this evaluation. The diameter of the target vessel and presence or absence of atherosclerotic plaque is also noted.

INTRAOPERATIVE ARTERIOGRAPHY

Because of the difficulties involved in the selection of a distal arterial target for lower extremity bypass grafting in patients with multilevel arterial occlusive disease, some authors[2,9,10] suggest the use of intraoperative arteriography as a means to better define the lower extremity arterial anatomy. In a review of 22 patients who underwent a lower extremity bypass procedure, Zatina and coworkers[9] found that the appropriate bypass procedure could be performed with a combination of intraoperative arteriography and preoperative duplex mapping. A more recent study that addresses this issue was published by Huber and coworkers,[10] who compared intraoperative arteriography to traditional preoperative arteriography in 114 extremities in 104 consecutive patients who required infrageniculate bypass grafting. They found that intraoperative arteriography altered the operative plan in 24% of patients. Changes in the planned bypass procedure included selection of a more distal anastomosis site in 13% and selection of a more proximal anastomosis site in 4% of patients. Selection of a different artery for the distal anastomosis occurred in 3% of patients and amputation rather than bypass occurred in 2% of patients. More importantly, intraoperative arteriography resulted in bypass rather than planned amputation in 42% of patients who were deemed unreconstructible based on their preoperative arteriogram. Intraoperative arteriography was performed using an x-ray plate wrapped in sterile plastic that was positioned beneath the extremity. Inflow occlusion was used while a 23-gauge butterfly needle was placed into the predicted target vessel or most proximal patent segment of the arterial tree. From 12 to 20 mL of Ionic contrast was used while images were obtained using a Philips BV 29 portable x-ray unit. These investigators found that this procedure on average added an additional 13 min to the operative procedure.

The technique of intraoperative arteriography depends largely on what sort of equipment is available to the surgeon. At the present time, many units are equipped with highly sophisticated C-arm fluoroscopy units, which are capable of performing digital subtraction arteriography, road mapping, and have relatively high resolution. C-arm units can now come equipped with a 12-in. image intensifier, which decreases the need for multiple stepwise arteriograms when performing full-length lower extremity arteriography. In addition, newer models are now capable of more than 1 MB of resolution and have pulse-chase capability, which allows for the documentation of the arteriographic anatomy of the entire lower extremity following a single bolus of contrast.

At Dartmouth, we have largely replaced preoperative arteriography with a combination of preoperative duplex arterial mapping and intraoperative arteriography, which is performed using a mobile C-arm fluoroscopy unit with DSA capability and a 12-in. image intensifier. The portions of the arterial tree that are imaged are based on information obtained from the preoperative arterial duplex map. When planning a vascular procedure on the lower extremity—particularly a lower extremity bypass graft—the critical information that must be acquired prior to proceeding with the bypass includes adequacy of inflow and a suitable outflow artery. Adequacy of inflow can typically be evaluated by physical examination and determining the quality of the femoral pulse. In addition, we routinely perform intraoperative pressure measurements in the common femoral artery both before and after performance of the bypass and compare this with aortic pressure. Finally, we use duplex arteriography of the iliac artery in order to uncover possible flow-limiting lesions prior to surgery. If the duplex arterial map of the iliac artery appears unremarkable and there is no significant pressure gradient in the common femoral artery, then there is usually no need to image the iliac arteries intraoperatively. An important technical note is to be sure that if a sheath or angiocath is used to measure the pressure, the surgeon must make sure the tip of the catheter is in the common femoral artery and not the external iliac artery or a lesion could be missed. Next, a suitable recipient distal vessel for the bypass must be identified. We use arterial duplex mapping to do this. If the arterial duplex mapping is a good-quality study and identifies an adequate outflow vessel, then we proceed with surgery without additional intraoperative arteriography other than limited arteriography of the outflow vessel at the time that the artery is dissected out. If the duplex arterial map is a limited study or poor-quality study, typically due to heavy arterial calcification, then we proceed with full lower extremity arteriography. To perform this, we do a selective catheterization of the most distal visualized vessel on duplex arterial map. Most often, this means placement of a catheter in the common femoral artery, either through an ipsilateral retrograde cannulation of the common femoral artery or through a contralateral femoral artery puncture. Arteriography is performed using digital subtraction arteriography and non-ionic contrast material, typically with boluses of 20 cc of contrast per injection. Most often, we are able to image the entire lower extremity using <80 cc of contrast. Again, duplex arterial mapping can be used to direct the arteriographic examination of the lower extremity to only those portions of the lower extremity arterial anatomy that require visualization. For instance, if the superficial femoral artery is known to be occluded on duplex arterial mapping, then there is no need to image this area using conventional intraoperative arteriography. In situations of superior femoral artery (SFA) occlusion, we routinely begin our examination from the knee down. Occasionally, it is impossible to obtain good-quality arteriography of the infrageniculate vessels from the common femoral artery due to poor collateralization from the profunda femoris artery. In these situations, we usually dissect out the most proximal vessel that appears to have flow based on duplex ultrasound, such as the below-the-knee popliteal artery or tibial–peroneal trunk, and perform arteriography through the vessel using inflow occlusion. These images are then collected and stored as a part of the patient's permanent record in the same folder that the patient's duplex studies are stored. This allows us to review both the patient's previous arteriograms as well as their duplex studies at the same time that patients are seen in the clinic.

Using the above-mentioned approach, we have performed infrageniculate lower extremity bypass in 23 patients using duplex arterial mapping alone. There was no difference in graft patency at 1 year when compared to patients who underwent bypass graft placement following preoperative arteriography. During the time from 1998–2000, we performed approximately 160 lower extremity revascularization procedures with duplex arterial map and limited intraoperative arteriography.

In conclusion, we have found preoperative arterial duplex mapping combined with limited intraoperative arteriography to be an effective technique in evaluating the lower extremity arterial anatomy prior to proceeding with lower extremity bypass. In addition, familiarity with this equipment prepares the surgeon to handle situations such as combined inflow insufficiency, which can frequently be treated with an endovascular procedure, and outflow disease, which frequently warrants bypass surgery. The flexibility that intraoperative arteriography offers allows the surgeon to tailor the angiographic evaluation based on the patient's physical examination, symptoms, and duplex arterial mapping so that the surgeon can obtain adequate information to proceed with the procedure, yet limit the incidence of complications and cost typically seen with routine preoperative arteriography.

REFERENCES

1. Kohler TR, Nance DR, Cramer MM, et al. Duplex scanning for diagnosis of aortoiliac and femoropopliteal disease: a prospective study. *Circulation.* 1987;76:1074–1080.
2. Patel KR, Semel L, Clauss RH. Extended rate for limb salvage with intraoperative prereconstruction angiography. *J Vasc Surg.* 1988;7:531–537.
3. Hessel SJ, Adams DF, Abrams HL. Complications of angiography. *Radiology.* 1981;138:273.
4. Gomes AS, Baker JD, Martin-Paredero V, et al. Acute renal dysfunction after major arteriography. *AJR.* 1985;145:1249.
5. Moneta GL, Yeager RA, Antonovic R, et al. Accuracy of lower extremity arterial duplex mapping. *J Vasc Surg.* 1992;15:275–284.
6. Koelemay MJW, Hartog D, Prins MH, et al. Diagnosis of arterial disease of the lower extremities with duplex ultrasonography. *Br J Surg.* 1998;83:404–409.

7. Ligush J, Reavis SW, Preisser JS, et al. Duplex ultrasound scanning defines operative strategies for patients with limb-threatening ischemia. *J Vasc Surg.* 1998;28:482–491.
8. Ascher E, Mazzariol F, Hingorani A, et al. The use of duplex ultrasound arterial mapping as an alternative to conventional arteriography for primary and secondary infrapopliteal bypasses. *Am J Surg.* 1999;178:162–165.
9. Zatina MA, Schroder WB, Wilkerson DK, et al. Can intra-operative prebypass arteriography substitute for the preoperative arteriogram? *J Vasc Surg.* 1991;5:143–149.
10. Huber TS, Back MR, Flynn TC, et al. Intraoperative prebypass arteriography for infragenicu-late revascularization. *Am J Surg.* 1997;174:205–209.

4

Magnetic Resonance Imaging to Replace Arteriography for Lower Extremity Ischemia

William H. Pearce, MD, and Andy C. Chiou, MD, MPH

INTRODUCTION

The basic requirement for patients undergoing lower extremity revascularization is the identification of an adequate inflow vessel and a recipient target vessel with optimal outflow. A variety of techniques have been used over the past several decades to access the aortoiliac segment and the distal runoff vessels (Table 4–1). The minimal requirement for an inflow vessel is one, without an identifiable hemodynamically significant stenosis. A significant proximal stenosis produces a hemodynamic failure despite a patent vascular graft.[1] The selection of a distal runoff vessel varies depending on an adequate length of venous conduit and the indication for the procedure. In patients undergoing femoropopliteal reconstructions for disabling claudication, the surgical procedure of choice is an above-the-knee popliteal artery bypass. In patients with critical limb ischemia, the bypass is carried to the vessel with the greatest outflow to the foot. In patients with rest pain, it is acceptable to perform a bypass to an isolated segment with only collateral blood flow to the foot. However, in patients with gangrene or ulcers, a bypass beyond all obstructions is mandatory. Restoration of pulsatile flow to the foot is the goal. In addition, when performing femoropopliteal or femorodistal bypasses, reconstruction of the profunda artery is usually performed in conjunction. Therefore, techniques that evaluate both the profunda and the femoropopliteal segment are needed.

TABLE 4-1 PLANNING LOWER EXTREMITY REVASCULARIZATION

Physical Exam
Segmental Limb Pressures
Angiography
Duplex Scan
CT Angiography
MRA—Gadolinium Enhanced
—Time-of-Flight

ANGIOGRAPHY

Contrast arteriography was the first technique available for evaluating the arterial system. Initially, arteriography was performed via a translumbar approach. In addition, the image was in only a single plane (anterioposterior). These single-plane images were found to greatly underestimate arterial stenosis, particularly of the iliac and profundafemoris vessels. Later, biplanar arteriography would solve this problem. Originally, angiography was performed using rapid changing of cassettes or long films to image tibial and pedal vessels. Unfortunately, this technique required accurate timing of the contrast bolus to visualize tibial and pedal vessels. Timing errors were common and patients were deemed nonreconstructable based on these inadequate images. With the development of the Seldinger technique, distal vessels could be cannulated selectively. Reactive hyperemia and intra-arterial vasodilators improve tibial and pedal visualization.

With the advent of digital subtraction angiography (DSA), the need for accurate timing of the contrast bolus was decreased, as the fluoroscope was continuously imaging the lower extremity. DSA also significantly decreased the amount of contrast needed. Current arterial DSAs provide excellent views of outflow vessels. However, in patients with unilateral disease, identification of patent pedal vessels is sometimes difficult, again because of timing errors. Despite the advent of DSA and the lessening of requirements for contrast material, nephrotoxicity continues to be a concern. Finally, whether conventional arteriography or DSA is performed, arterial injury may occur.

ULTRASOUND

Ultrasound evaluation of the lower extremity is the most common noninvasive technique for evaluating lower extremity blood flow. Segmental limb pressures and duplex ultrasounds are often combined to identify hemodynamically significant lesions in the aortoiliac and femoropopliteal segments.[2,3] Recently, interest has increased in the use of ultrasound duplex imaging as the sole imaging modality prior to lower extremity revasculariization.[4,5] The aortoiliac segment and the peripheral vessels can be seen with the duplex ultrasound scan in the majority of patients. In a prospective study of patients undergoing lower extremity revascularization, Ramaswami et al.[4] found that ultrasound was able to diagnose aortoiliac and femoropopliteal disease in 80% of patients. The duplex criteria was of peak systolic velocity ratio (PSVR) of >2 in lesions of <5 cm used to identify hemodynamically significant disease. The most common reasons that the iliac arteries were not visualized were the presence of bowel gas, patient size, and tortuosity of the vessel. Visualization of the femoropopliteal was possible in 100% of patients, and in 97% of patients, the popliteal bifurcation was identified. In a similar study, Kohler et al.[5] found duplex scanning compared favorably with angiography. Unfortunately, problems can occur at the trifurcation and in areas of heavy calcification. When evaluating the foot, pedal vessels are poorly seen because of the close proximity of the vessel to the surface. It is also difficult to select the single vessel that has the best outflow, particularly when evaluating the perineal artery. In a comparative study between arteriography and duplex arterial mapping, Wain et al.[6] found that duplex scanning was accurate and predictive in 90% of patients undergoing infrainguinal bypasses. The duplex was accurate in identifying the above-the-knee popliteal segment as the site of the anastomosis femoropopliteal bypass. However, for tibial vessels the duplex was accurate in only 24% of patients. Arteriography was still required for tibial reconstruction. For example, the perineal artery splits just above the ankle to provide collateral blood flow to the pedal vessels. Therefore, a proximal posterior tibial artery may appear to be the best patent tibial vessel, however, it has no direct connection with the foot, whereas the perineal artery may directly communicate through its major collateral branches. Wain and coworkers[6] concluded that the use of duplex ultrasound scanning was excellent for patients with above-the-knee bypasses but was poor for distal bypasses. More extensive studies are needed to determine feasibility and long-term patency of grafts placed based solely on the information provided by duplex scanning.

Finally, it does not appear that duplex scan alone is sufficient for revision of lower extremity bypass grafts. Arteriography was much more accurate in this setting.[7]

COMPUTERIZED TOMOGRAPHY ANGIOGRAPHY

Recently, computerized tomographic angiography (CTA) has been advocated for proximal aortoiliac imaging. Unfortunately, this technique uses a large contrast bolus and, similar to lower extremity arteriography, imaging must be timed with the bolus. For this reason, resolution of arteries beyond the iliac is poor. For proximal lesions it may be of some benefit.

MAGNETIC RESONANCE ANGIOGRAPHY

Recently, magnetic resonance angiography (MRA) has become available as a noninvasive technique to image peripheral vessels. With standard two-dimensional time-of-flight (2D TOF), peripheral vessels appear as black holes. Using a variety of techniques, one is able to presaturate the blood entering the field of interest to produce an arterial image. In a prospective comparative study of DSA and TOF-MRA, Hoch et al.[8] found that the two techniques were comparable. The MRA accurately predicted 90% of suprainguinal and 95% of infrainguinal bypass procedures. These values compared favorably to DSA, which predicted 100% of suprainguinal disease and 85% of infrain-

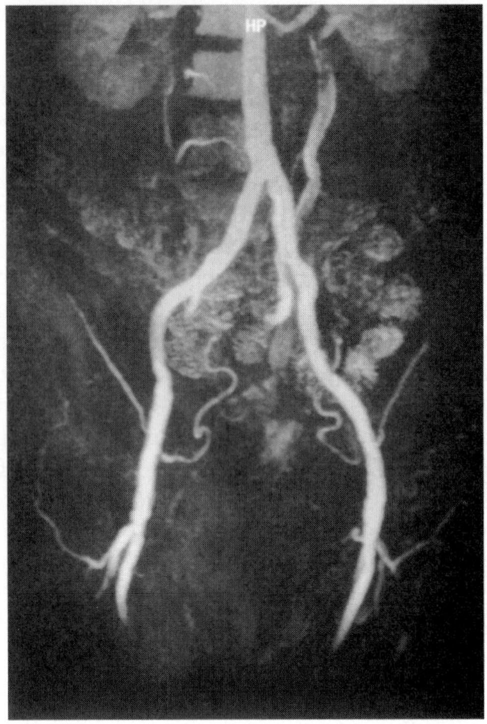

Figure 4–1. Three-dimensional (3D) gadolinium (Gd)-enhanced MRA of the aortoiliac segment in a patient with distal ischemia. Note the high-resolution pictures of the aorta and its major branches.

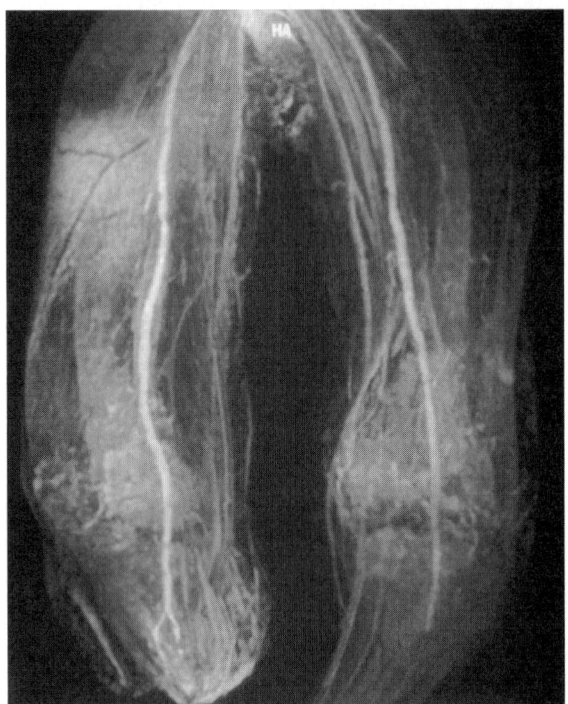

Figure 4–2. Gd contrast-enhanced femoropopliteal segment demonstrating an intact femoropopliteal artery.

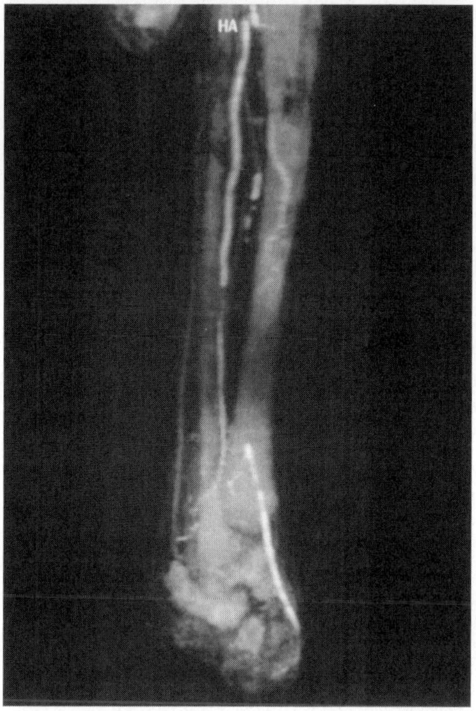

Figure 4–3. Distal MRA in the patient's right lower extremity that demonstrates tibial artery occlusion and a patent peroneal and dorsalis pedus artery.

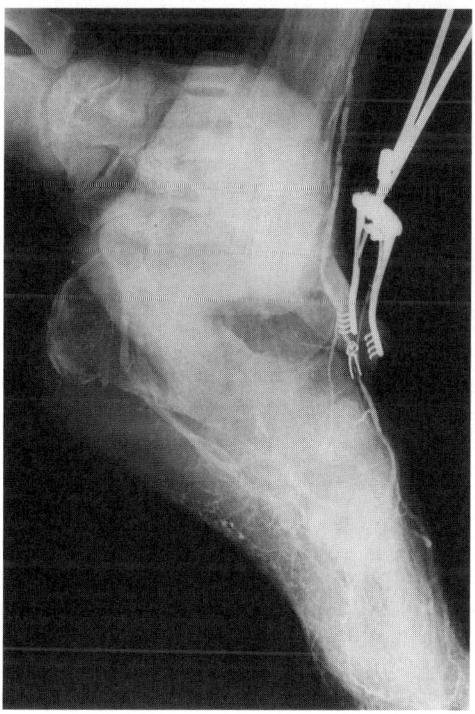

Figure 4–4. Intraoperative arteriogram of the pedal vessels demonstrating the same vessel as was seen with MRA (Fig. 4–3).

guinal disease. These results were confirmed by Carpenter et al.[9] who also used 2D TOF–MRA-based studies. The difference between the studies is that Hoch et al.[9] used EKG-triggered 2D TOF to eliminate pulsation artifacts; however, they did not find that this new technique improved accuracy. Intraoperative prebypass angiography (IPA) is a technique that is frequently used when no tibial or pedal vessel is identified. Combining IPA with MRA (2D TOF) is only logical. Huber and colleagues[10] compared this combination with conventional arteriography and found that MRA + IPA was accurate and cost-effective.

Gadolinium (Gd)-enhanced three-dimensional (3D) MRA is a recent development that provides higher resolution with multi-planer reconstruction (Figures 4–1 through 4–4). Comparative studies using Gd-enhanced high resolution 3D techniques have shown that MRA-Gd compares also favorably with DSA. No false negative findings were seen in the iliac femoropopliteal arteries in a report by Winterer et al.[11] Between 10% and 16% of mild stenosis and 14% and 16% of high-grade stenosis were overread by MRA when compared to DSA. Undergrading of stenosis did not occur in the iliac or femoropopliteal system, but did in the crural system, with an occurrence rate of 14%. Gd-enhanced 3D MRA can be reconstructed and viewed in three dimensions. This feature avoids the single-plane view provided by standard angiography. The primary limitation of this technique is the restricted body area covered by the coil. The development of a moving table that would allow tracking of a single contrast bolus will obviate some of the problems associated with the limited anatomic region viewed.[12] In addition, this would diminish the background signal by contrast medium already within the tissue. Other artifacts that limit the usefulness of this technique include respiratory variation, metallic artifacts, and venous superimposition.

Contrast-enhanced MRA is also effective in detecting arterial graft complications. MRA-Gd when compared to angiography was 91% sensitive and 97% specific for detecting graft stenosis.[13] Errors occurred with timing and metal artifacts. Metallic stents may be problematic in the arterial system. Ferromagnetic stents such as Palmaz produce significant artifact. However, ZA-stents (Cook and other nonferromagnetic stents) produced an artifact.[14]

COMMENT

With the rapid change in imaging technology, patients are no longer required to undergo contrast arteriography. Our current algorithm for the evaluation of patients with lower extremity ischemia includes a physical examination (Figure 4–5) followed by MRA. Based on this study, the patients are separated into those with proximal disease and those with distal disease. Patients with proximal disease undergo operative, medical, or endovascular procedures. Interestingly, since 1995, the number of patients undergoing aortoiliac angioplasty has decreased dramatically. The tendency to perform aortoiliac angioplasty is greater when a catheter is already within the iliac system. Long-segment angioplasties of the external iliac have poor outcome and have been abandoned. In addition, there has been a high rate of failure of patients undergoing kissing aortic stent. Therefore, based on these studies, we are more likely to perform a

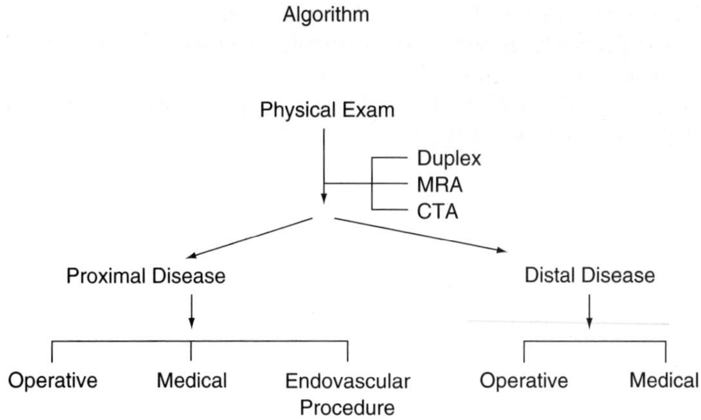

Figure 4–5. Algorithm demonstrating an MRA-based approach to patients with lower extremity ischemia. A physical exam is performed that initially localizes the primary lesion. MRA is then performed to determine whether the patient is a candidate for an endovascular or operative procedure.

unilateral stent with a crossover femorofemoral graft, aortic replacement, or axial bifemoral grafts depending on the patient's comorbidities. Patients with proximal or distal disease are also treated medically based on the symptoms. Patients who are found to have predominately distal disease undergo either operative or medical management. For patients in whom a lower extremity vascularization is planned, contrast-enhanced MRA has replaced conventional angiography except for pedal vessels. With the development of moving gantries within the MR machine, more accurate imaging may be performed in these vessels. To date, Gd has not been associated with known complications. Unfortunately, MRA-Gd is limited to those patients without pacemakers and other metallic implants.

REFERENCES

1. Buchbinder D, Pasch AR, Schuler JJ, et al. Efficacy of femorofemoral bypass for intermittent claudication. Clinical and hemodynamic assessment. *Am J Surg.* 1986;152(2):215–219.
2. Rutherford RB, Lowenstein DH, Klein MF. Combining segmental systolic pressures and plethysmography to diagnose arterial occlusive disease of the legs. *Am J Surg.* 1979;138:211.
3. Johnston KW. Role of Doppler ultrasonography in determining the hemo-dynamic significance of aortoiliac disease. *Can J Surg.* 1978;21:319.
4. Ramaswami G, Al-Kutoubi A, Nicolaides A, et al. The role of duplex scanning in the diagnosis of lower limb arterial disease. *Ann Vasc Surg.* 1999;13(5):494–500.
5. Kohler T, Nance D, Cramer MM, et al. Duplex scanning for diagnosis of aortoiliac and femoropopliteal disease: a prospective study. *Circulation.* 1987;(76):1074–1080.
6. Wain RA, Berdejo GL, Delvalle WN, et al. Can duplex scan arterial mapping replace contrast arteriography as the test of choice before infrainguinal revascularization? *J Vasc Surg.* 1999;29(1):100–107.

7. Landry GJ, Moneta GL, Taylor LM, Jr., et al. Duplex scanning alone is not sufficient imaging before secondary procedures after lower extremity reversed vein bypass graft. *J Vasc Surg.* 1999;29(2):270–280.
8. Hoch J, Kennell T, Hollister M, et al. Comparison of treatment plans for lower extremity arterial occlusive disease made with electrocardiography-triggered two-dimensional time-of-flight magnetic resonance angiography and digital subtraction angiography. *Am J Surg.* 1999;178:166–173.
9. Carpenter J, Golden M, Barker C, Holland G, Baum R. The fate of bypass grafts to angiographically occult runoff vessels detected by magnetic resonance angiography. *J Vasc Surg.* 1996;23(3):483–489.
10. Huber T, Back M, Ballinger R, et al. Utility of magnetic resonance arteriography for distal lower extremity revascularization. *J Vasc Surg.* 1997;26(3):415–423.
11. Winterer JT, Laubenberger J, Scheffler K, et al. Contrast-enhanced subtration MR angiography in occlusive disease of the pelvic and lower limb arteries: results of a prospective intraindividual comparative study with digital subtraction angiography in 76 patients. *J Comp Assist Tom.* 1999;23:583–589.
12. Ho VB, Prince MR, Dong Q. Magnetic resonance imaging of the aorta and branch vessels. *Cor Art Dis.* 1999;10(3):141–149.
13. Bendib K, Berthezene Y, Croisille P, Villard J, Douek PC. Assessment of complicated arterial bypass grafts: value of contrast-enhanced subtraction magnetic resonance angiography. *J Vasc Surg.* 1997;26(6):1036–1042.
14. Schurman K, Vorwerk D, Bucker A, et al. Magnetic resonance angiography of nonferromagnetic iliac artery stents and stent-grafts: a comparative study in sheep. *Cardio Interv Rad.* 1999;22(5):394–402.

5

Issues Related to Conflict of Interest in Vascular Surgery

K. Wayne Johnston, MD, FRCSC, FACS, and Martin F. McKneally, MD, PhD, FRCSC, FACS

INTRODUCTION

Why has conflict of interest become an issue? Trust in the medical profession and scientific research is based on two assumptions: First, the assumption that physicians will put the interest of patients above their own; and second, that science is conducted in an honest and unbiased way. The expansion of the role of industrial funding of research and the increased opportunity for physicians to become entrepreneurial players in the pharmaceutical and medical device market threatens the validity of these assumptions. Furthermore, there is an unresolved incongruity between business ethics and the ethics of medicine. The ethics of medicine gives high value to patient care, teaching, and research. Early and wide disclosure of the results of scientific research is valued in the professional community as an important component of a cooperative universal quest for understanding of biology and the conquest of disease. Communication of new findings at meetings and in journals is admired and socially rewarded by promotion and professional respect. Linkage to monetary reward is very loose. In contrast, the ethics of business gives high value to returning a profit to investors. The results of scientific research are valued in the business community as proprietary trade secrets that must be protected in order to gain an advantage over competitors in the marketplace.

The incongruity of business and medical ethical values leads to misunderstanding and occasionally to conflict. Physicians who are perceived as entrepreneurial capitalists may be subjected to public humiliation. Companies that withhold or repress the dissemination of scientific information that might help in the conquest of disease may be subjected to public criticism. The importance of developing a common set of standards and values is illustrated dramatically by the debate about ownership of the human genome.[1–3] Dialog leading to agreement on intellectual property rules is needed; this will require compromise and a new social construct.

Because financial interests may bias an individual's actions and decisions, thereby undermining trust, it is important to consider how to minimize the influence of real or perceived self-interest and thereby protect the integrity of the profession. The perception of interference with primary duties damages the reputation of the profession, even when no such interference occurs. Identifying and managing conflicts of interest is a complex task. The purpose of this chapter is to define conflict of interest and suggest approaches that are helpful in recognizing, avoiding, and dealing with situations that may represent a conflict of interest. In suggesting a framework for approaching this issue, we recognize that we do not have a complete solution. In writing this chapter, we relied on a number of important sources that can serve as a source for additional reading.[4–6]

DEFINITION

Conflicts commonly arise in day-to-day relationships. Brody states

> The existence of conflicting loyalties has always been a part of the patient–physician relation. Physicians have, in addition to their obligation to any individual patient, obligations to their other patients, to their families, to themselves, to society, their religion, etc. Like everyone else, physicians live in a tangled web of conflicting obligations.[7]

Conflict of interest is defined as a circumstance or situation in which professional judgment, decisions, or actions concerning a primary interest (e.g., appropriate patient care) tends to be unduly influenced by a secondary interest (e.g., financial gain). The primary interests or concerns of physicians in their most general form are the health of patients, the integrity of research, and the education of students and colleagues. Secondary interests are not illegitimate; they include financial gain, professional advancement, prestige, power, and the interests of family and friends and others. Trust in the medical profession is based on a covenant that requires professionals to put their primary interests above secondary gains when conflicts arise.

There is nothing unethical, deceitful, or fraudulent about having a conflict of interest; however, it is expected that the professional will take appropriate steps to manage the conflict to prevent it from unduly influencing the way in which patient care, research, and teaching are conducted. Individuals who are involved with exciting new areas of research are often those who have broad interests or relationships. However, problems arise if the secondary interests influence or appear to influence their primary responsibility in ways that undermine the integrity of the professional role.

The secondary interest that is most easily discussed and analyzed is financial interest. It serves as a surrogate for other secondary interests. We follow this convention in this chapter, alluding from time to time to other secondary interests when applicable.

Bioethics

The ethic of medicine is characterized by a covenant of trust; patients trust that their interests will be ranked above the personal and financial interests of their physicians.

Thompson's landmark essay, "Understanding financial conflicts of interest," clarifies the primary obligations of the medical profession as (1) providing care, (2) performing valid research, and (3) teaching.[5] The profession enjoys the privileges of self-regulation and social status as part of a covenant with society. The public has come to rely on physicians to live up to these professional obligations. In general, these expectations are met and the profession enjoys a high level of respect and trust compared to other groups.

Professional judgment is trusted by patients and society because of the fiduciary duty physicians accept to rank their primary interests above such secondary interests as personal gain, promotion, fame, or other benefits. This fiduciary duty derives from the covenant of trust and the principle of justice that reasonable expectations should be met, particularly by those who have professed their intention to serve patients and society in this way.

Law

There is a large body of legal opinion that governs the conduct of lawyers, security traders, and financial agents who serve as trustees. The law generally requires trustees to act to protect the best interests or well-being of the less-powerful or less-informed party in the relationship. This so-called fiduciary duty has been extended from financial trusteeship to the trust relationship in other unbalanced power relationships, including those between physicians and patients, teachers and students, and clergy and laity. In some jurisdictions, conflicts of interest have been prohibited by law; for example, the 1991 Regulated Health Professions Act of Ontario prohibits members of the health-care profession from practicing "while the member is in a conflict of interest." In general, the courts have held to the "reasonable person rule": If the conflict of interest were publicly known, would any reasonable person conclude that professional judgment would not be influenced by the secondary interest? The logical extension of this rule is that disclosure of a conflicting secondary interest is a defensible approach to managing a conflict. The standards to which lawyers and judges hold themselves are considerably more stringent than those that apply in medicine. Recusal (i.e., the removal of oneself from the responsibility of judging a case) is required if there is the slightest possibility of secondary gain for the judge based on the outcome of a trial. The acceptance of even the most trivial of gifts by a judge would lead to severe penalties, including disbarment.

Policy

Medical societies, pharmaceutical manufacturers' associations, and scientific journals often have clearly defined policies regarding conflicts of interest. These generally recommend disclosure or prohibition as an approach to managing conflict. The Council on Ethical and Judicial Affairs of the American Medical Association (AMA) specifies the level of subsidies and gifts that are acceptable for members and the arm's length relationship between manufacturers and physicians that is required for subsidization of educational events. Although the AMA allows gifts of minimal value to physicians, the Canadian Medical Association (CMA)[8] stipulates a strict prohibition of personal gifts to physicians from the pharmaceutical industry. The policy also discourages investment in pharmaceutical companies "if knowledge about the success of the company . . . might inappropriately affect the manner of their practice or their prescribing behaviour".[8] The policy further states that the results of surveillance studies "will be made available for publication in a peer reviewed journal within a reasonable period".[8]

MAKING A JUDGMENT ON THE POTENTIAL SERIOUSNESS OF CONFLICT

The potential severity of a conflict depends on multiple factors. First, the value of the secondary gain. If a very large profit or benefit will accrue to the professional, the risk of unintentional or intentional bias is proportionally increased. For this reason, threshold values have been set by various organizations at arbitrary but generally low levels. Secondary gain is more likely to be influential if the benefit to the individual is large and if it occurs immediately. Sometimes doctors do not recognize the seductive interference or secondary gain when the value of the gift is small (it's only a trip, meal, etc.). Second, the extent of discretion and accountability in professional choice. If the author of an authoritative review article is choosing among a large number of scientific papers to highlight the most important ones, some journals require disclosure of the financial links of the author to the companies in question. Similarly, if large-scale discretionary professional judgments are made, such as which institutions are chosen for a clinical trial, there is greater risk that secondary interests will influence the decisions if they are unreviewed. Transparency can be achieved by external review or by blinding. Third, the seriousness of the harm that may result if the conflict of interest is not properly managed. If a professional judgment will have a profound public impact, there is a need for more rigorous standards for management of the conflict. For example, the editor of a major authoritative journal has a powerfully influential voice that can influence practice, public policy, and market performance of products and procedures. Some journals—notably, the *New England Journal of Medicine*—require complete divestiture of financial interests in the biomedical industry as a condition of holding the position of Editor-in-chief.

APPROACHES TO DEALING WITH CONFLICT OF INTEREST

Voluntary Measures

Ideally, physicians should have the good judgment to be aware that their decisions may be biased because of secondary interests. Based on their strength of character, they should eliminate bias or remove themselves from the conflicted situation. In small communities, virtue and local reputation may protect professional judgment from conflicts of interest. Thompson[5] emphasizes how difficult it is to "determine what motives have influenced a professional decision . . . even in one's own case, and all the more so in the case of people one does not know personally".[8] For this reason, external regulation has been developed by many organizations.

Regulations Regarding Disclosure

Regulations by the profession provide more assurance than individual discretion. The most common regulation used by medical organizations and medical journals is the requirement that all financial linkages that might be affected by the outcome of a report must be disclosed. Disclosure of financial linkages places the responsibility for discounting or assessing the probable influence of secondary gain to the reader or listener. Although this is more helpful than keeping the financial relationship secret, it is an incomplete remedy. If authors specify what steps were taken to minimize the potentially confounding effects of bias, their claims may be strengthened. Common techniques include blinding as to treatment assignment or outcome, independent statistical review, and independent assessment using generally accepted techniques of measurement and analysis. Transparency (i.e., the likelihood that deviation from proper procedure will be detectable) is increased if the data are stored and analyzed in an objective third-party facility. This is particularly pertinent for trials of pharmaceuticals. Company control of data, analysis, and release of results to the public reduces the transparency of pharmaceutical trials. Other methods of increasing credibility include explicit discussion of how conflicts were managed.

Regulations Regarding Abstention

Program committees, executive committees, and editorial boards may require that members abstain from voting on, or even abstain from discussion of papers, projects, or contracts when there is a clear-cut conflict of interest. More influential positions may require divestiture or prohibition from participation. This is particularly common in appointments or elections to government office to protect the public and the office holder from the appearance or the practice of biased awards of government contracts.[5]

FINANCIAL CONFLICTS THAT SHOULD BE DISCLOSED

In disclosing if an individual or a family member has a financial conflict of interest, the following activities or relationships with biomedical companies, device manufacturers, or pharmaceutical companies are considered to be relevant:

- officer, board member, trustee, owner, or employee of a company
- stock, stock options, or bond holder (including immediate family)
- paid consultancy, scientific advisory committee membership, or lecturer for a company
- patent is held
- research grants from a company. (Note that grant support may be a source of conflict of interest irrespective of whether it is from industry or the public sector. Conflict arises because grants provide overhead to support the institution, and in addition may provide a "profit" to support other unrelated research projects for the investigator, thereby potentially contributing to academic advancement.)

A modified version of the form used by the American Urological Association to disclose an individual's relationships with each company follows.

In relation to company	Self	Family member	Business partner
Owner or employee			
Board member, officer, trustee			
Investment in company			
Paid consultant or advisor			
Investigator for company			
Research grant to support scientific study			
Paid by company as meeting participant, lecturer			
Patent held			

SOME EXAMPLES OF CONFLICT

Authorship

Although many regard modern-day science as an exact discipline, unfortunately, studies are carried out by humans who may make errors or may be biased. In an ideal study, bias may be reduced by blinding the investigators and randomizing the patients; however, this is possible in only a small number of studies. Recently, major journals have recognized the importance of conflict of interest in publication.[9,10] Sponsorship of a drug study by industry is associated with a more favorable report of the drug's efficacy. For example, when the drug clozapine was compared to typical antipsychotic drugs for the treatment of schizophrenia, the study is that reported some kind of connection with the manufacturer of the drug reported significantly better results and fewer side effects. In contrast, nonsponsored studies reported equivocal findings.[11] In analyzing the results of studies on the efficacy of calcium channel blockers, Stelfox et al.[12] reported that the studies were more likely to be supportive if the authors had a financial relationship with manufacturers of the drugs. In order to determine if a financial relationship was present, the authors contacted the researchers and inquired if they had received consultation fees, funds to support research, support to attend a symposium, a speaking fee, or an employment relationship. Of the authors who were supportive of the use of calcium channel blockers, 96% had financial relationships with manufacturers, whereas those who did not have a financial relationship were either neutral (60%) or critical (37%) of the use of calcium channel blockers. Of concern, only 2 of the 70 articles reviewed disclosed the authors' potential conflict of interest. A study aimed at determining the factors that influenced the conclusions in published review articles on the impact of passive smoking concluded that funding by the tobacco industry was an important determinant of the conclusions. Of the variables examined, only the presence of an affiliation with the tobacco industry was related to the conclusion that passive smoking was not harmful.[13,14] *The New York Times* reported a $5 million plan to identify and recruit "neutral" scientists to create doubt about global warming.[15] Although this type of financial support is common in politics and business, to financially support scientists who have a particular opinion is alarming because it may bias a scientists opinions and hence damage the trust that the results of scientific work is reliable.

Journal of Vascular Surgery

This issue of conflict of interest affects authors, reviewers, and editors. Recent changes in policy concerning disclosure of conflict of interest by authors publishing articles in the *Journal of Vascular Surgery* is discussed first, and the equally important problem of managing competitive interests by reviewers and editors follows.

Authors. The editors noted that the *Journal of Vascular Surgery* had a very low level of disclosure of financial interests (i.e., equity holdings, honoraria, patents, consultancies, or scientific advisory board memberships) and aimed to improve the rate of disclosure by implementing the new policy that specifically questioned the financial relationships with products mentioned in the paper. In the July 1999 issue of the *Journal of Vascular Surgery,* the editors[16] announced that

> As of this issue, the *Journal of Vascular Surgery* will join many other major medical journals in requiring authors to disclose financial and other potential competitive interests. . . . Because some degree of competition of interest is inescapable in most papers, the most practical approach to reducing the risk that the overall quality of a paper is reduced by unconscious biased decisions in the design, implementation, analysis, or discussion of the research is to ask the authors to disclose potential competitive interests to the readers. Through disclosure, competitive interests are made transparent. Consequently the readers can assess the magnitude of the competition and add this to their overall interpretation of the published work. (p. 200)

Leaving it up to the reader to read the author's statement of disclosure and determine the extent of a potential conflict of interest is only a partial solution to the problem, but is better than none.

In implementing this policy, the editorial office routinely requests clarification of possible conflict of interest for all papers that have been accepted for publication, and does not just request information if the editors suspect a conflict of interest. It is important to note that letters to the editor and other correspondence may be biased, and these authors also must be asked to declare potential conflicts of interest. Through disclosure, conflicts of interest are made visible and more transparent. Consequently, the readers can determine if a conflict is present and assess the magnitude of the conflict; hence, readers can choose whether to use this information in their overall interpretation of the published work.

Because progress in the vascular surgery is in part related to advances in the application of new technology and drugs, it is important to publish articles describing the results. At the *Journal of Vascular Surgery,* potential conflicts of interest are not considered in the review process.

What action should be taken if an author does not disclose a potential conflict of interest? If the oversight is because the individual was not aware of the policies of the *Journal* or the *Journal* office failed to request full disclosure of all conflicts of interest, then a simple publication of a correction is appropriate. However, if conflicts have been deliberately concealed or the author intentionally chose not to declare the conflict because he/she had not been influenced by financial interests, then the editors will publish a statement indicating that the paper may be unreliable because the authors failed to meet the standards of disclosure required by the *Journal.*

Reviewers. The editors aim to select reviewers that do not have competing interests. If the paper is accepted for publication, the authors are asked to fully disclose any potential financial conflict of interest. This information is made available to the readers.

Editors. The editors of the *Journal of Vascular Surgery* are expected to divest themselves of competitive financial interests and provide a detailed declaration of their potential conflicts of interest to the Joint Council on an annual basis. It is difficult to minimize conflict of interest by reviewers; however, they are asked to exempt themselves from a review if they have a competing financial or professional relationship that might bias their review. Members of the editorial board annually declare their conflicts of interest to the editors, and this information is considered in aiming to select unbiased reviewers.

Involvement in Administration of the Vascular Societies

The Joint Council of the Society for Vascular Surgery and the North American chapter of the International Society for Cardiovascular Surgery have adopted a policy on conflict of interest. Specifically, it is deemed to be inappropriate for a member of council to influence the society's decisions on an issue related to a product or company if the member has a financial interest in the company. Thus, at an executive or committee meeting of the society, the member should abstain from discussing issues that might have an impact (positive or negative) on a company or one of its competitors.

Educational Programs

In order to reduce the conflict of interest in the organization of educational programs, the following approaches should be considered.[17–19] Control over the scientific content of any program and the selection of presenters must be in the hands of an organizing committee that is not influenced by industry. A specific company should not pay the expenses and honoraria for individual invited speakers, but may contribute to support the overall expenses of the meeting. If an author has a conflict of interest that might bias his/her decisions in the design, analysis, presentation, or discussion of the research study, then the audience should be informed of this by the authors.

A Company Offers to Sponsor a Speaker for Rounds

It may appear to be a great opportunity to accept a company's offer to provide a well-known speaker for rounds; however, problems arise if the company chooses the individual. In order to maintain their independent professional judgment so that they can best meet their patients' needs, physicians should be free from unbiased information. Thus, in developing an educational program, the physicians responsible for its organization must have complete control over the content of the meeting and selection of the speakers so that the information is provided in a format that is free from bias.

Relationships with Industry

Pharmaceuticals

Pharmaceutical companies spend large sums of money each year in the marketing to individual physicians, including gifts, entertainment, travel subsidies, sponsoring teaching activities, and others. Pharmaceutical representatives recognize that they are among the last of the door-to-door salesmen and take pride in their effectiveness. Although medical associations have published guidelines on relationships between physicians and the pharmaceutical industry, a recent study raises concern. The authors observed that meetings with drug company representatives, company sponsorship of Continuing Medical Education (CME) events, funding for travel or lodging, and attending presentations by speakers who were sponsored by the drug company were associated with a change in prescribing patterns.[20] Thus, in developing more rigorous guidelines to manage the interaction between physicians and the pharmaceutical industry, it seems appropriate for professional associations to develop definitions, standards of behavior, and a consensus process to address the issues—we are just at the beginning of this process, which must be worked out collaboratively.

Medical Devices

The major advances in research have provided great opportunities for translating basic research into commercial products. Increasingly, clinicians have developed relationships with industry to investigate the exciting potential applications of new drugs and devices. Indeed, universities have encouraged the relationships because of the "profits" that may ensue. Collaborations between industry and clinicians are generally beneficial; however, there are major potentials for conflict of interest.

Details of the potential conflicts are described elsewhere in this book and in recent publications.[20,21] In brief, the clinician has a primary responsibility to the patients under their care in the study, but conflicts arise because of their relationships with and responsibilities to others: the sponsoring company, hospital, and University; other coinvestigators; and the scientific community at large. When an investigator has a close relationship with an industry that may result in financial or academic gain (publication, promotion, tenure, grant renewal), it may be difficult to exhibit unbiased objectivity in carrying out and reporting on the results of the investigations. Indeed, it is not possible to completely eradicate the potential rewards from a relationship with industry. The sponsoring institution (including the clinical edge of the department, administration, Institutional Review Board (IRB)) may be in a similar conflict, but they must also develop policies to ensure that their employees are not in conflict between their professional responsibilities and personal gains.

The integrity and credibility of physicians is eroded when they endorse products or present data favoring a particular manufacturer if they receive secondary benefits from the manufacturer. When a professional is perceived as promoting rather than evaluating a pharmaceutical or medical device, the respect of their peers and their reputation in the medical community may be damaged.

Clinical Studies

Entering One's Own Patients in a Clinical Study

In any clinical study, there is a potential conflict of interest between serving the best interest of the patient and solving the scientific question. When a physician asks his/her own patients to enter a clinical study, this conflict of interest may be compounded by the imbalance of power inherent in the doctor–patient relationship. Entry into a study requires that the following criteria be met[22]: The study must be scientifically valid and approved by an ethics review committee. When entering a patient into a randomized treatment study, the physician must be reassured that the alternative treatments fall within the options accepted and recommended by the profession as a whole. It is ethical to offer patients entry into a study if the profession remains divided over the best choice of treatment options (i.e., if a state of professional uncertainty exists in the informed medical community as to which treatment is unequivocally best). Freedman[23] describes this as "clinical equipoise." His formulation provides a sound moral basis for physicians to enter patients into a trial even if they are personally biased toward one treatment (e.g., "If she were my wife, she'd have a radical mastectomy"). Stringent disclosure of the alternative treatments is mandatory in order to avoid coercion. Consent to participate must be voluntary and without coercion that the patient's decision might adversely affect their subsequent care. The patient must be free to withdraw from the study at any time. It is expected that patients be informed of the results if the data might affect their subsequent management and that the results of a study will be made available for publication within a reasonable period of time.

It may be tempting to enter a patient in a study who otherwise might not be "perfectly" eligible. Disregarding one of the eligibility criteria in order to enter a patient into a trial may invalidate the results of the study. Entering a patient who would otherwise be ineligible for the study risks jeopardizing a study that was developed with broad agreement between the funding group, the patients, and the investigators in order to provide scientifically valid and generalizable knowledge. Violating a research protocol brings lasting discredit when it is made public. This was dramatically illustrated by the professional and public response to the actions of Dr. Roger Poisson (who enrolled ineligible subjects in the NSABP trials of breast cancer treatment).[24] Violations of trust and loss of integrity usually induce irremediable distrust. In some circumstances, patients who do not qualify for a research protocol can be offered the new treatment outside the study on compassionate grounds.

Being Paid for Recruitment of Patients into a Research Study

It is inappropriate for a physician to accept payment for recruiting a patient for enrollment in a research study. After a patient has been recruited into a study, it is quite appropriate for a physician to be remunerated at a fair hourly rate for time spent to explain the study, obtain consent, complete the data forms, and so on. However, to accept financial incentives in order to recruit a patient risks jeopardizing the patient's trust that their doctor will provide unbiased advice and put the patient's interest first. Physicians' advanced knowledge of the medical options contributes to their fiduciary responsibility to put the patients' interests ahead of their opportunity for personal gain.

Self-Referral and Prescribing Treatment

The public does not expect physicians to prescribe medications or treatments primarily to increase sales or reap personal profits. It is widely recognized that the opportunity to profit has a subtle, insidious, and often unrecognized effect on prescribing patterns and treatment decisions.[25] Furthermore, physician-owned diagnostic and treatment facilities have been documented to be overutilized by their physician owners.

To remove or minimize these effects, professional organizations generally recommend against the ownership of stock in pharmaceutical companies or medical device companies and self-referral. The best test of what to do is transparently public defensibility (i.e., "Would I be comfortable with public disclosure of my ownership or profit?").

Managed Care

In a fee-for-service practice, conflict may arise because performing additional procedures maximizes the physician's income. This model may encourage overutilization. In contrast, in the managed-care environment, the patient may not recognize that the gatekeeper physician can increase his/her income or the group income by withholding medical care. In managed care, the insurers' financial risks and benefits are shared with the physicians and are controlled by the gatekeepers, who limit access to expensive specialist, diagnostic, and therapeutic interventions. In both circumstances, the physician–patient relationship may be compromised by the conflict between the physician's financial interests and the best interests of his/her patients. Many recent articles address the ethic issues raised by managed care.[26–28]

CONCLUSIONS

This chapter discusses some of the issues related to conflict of interest in vascular surgery. Conflict of interest in dealing with primary responsibilities that include patient care, research, and education is a situation that occurs when a secondary interest, such as a financial interest, influences or appears to influence the primary interest. Disclosure of financial conflicts is important in dealing with this situation, but other approaches are also discussed. Examples are discussed in which the physician–patient relationship may be compromised by the conflict between the physician's financial interests and the best interests of his/her patients.

Informal Glossary

Bias. A tendency or prejudice that prevents impartial consideration of a question.

Clinical equipoise. A state of professional uncertainty within the informed medical community about the best treatment for a condition.

Competition. A contest for some prize or advantage. Competitions imply the possibility of varying degrees of success (from L.: *com petere*—to seek together).

Conflict. A battle or fight between incompatible forces. Conflicts imply contradiction or the opposition of incompatible forces or claims (from L.: *conflictus*—collision).

Interest. Concern, stake, relationship, or involvement that may bring advantage or detriment. Vested interests are firmly established and noncontingent claims. *Best interest* implies greatest benefit or advantage (from *inter esse*—to be between or among).

Fiduciary. Fiduciary agents, such as physicians, teachers, and lawyers, are entrusted to care for the interests of those who are vulnerable, less informed, or less powerful. Fiduciaries are expected by society to give priority to the interests entrusted to them (from L.: *fiducia*—trust).

Transparent. Easily discerned and understood; open, obvious, evident. (In physics, *transparency* means transmitting without distortion.)

REFERENCES

1. Thomas SM. Genomics: the implications for ethics and education. *Br Med Bull.* 1999; 55(2):429–445.
2. Marshall E. Genome sequencing. Talks of public–private deal end in acrimony [news]. *Science.* 2000;287(5459):1723–1725.
3. "The human genome itself must be freely available to all humankind" [news]. *Nature.* 2000;404(6776):325.
4. Spece RG, Shimm DS, Buchanan AE. *Conflicts of Interest in Clinical Practice.* New York: Oxford University Press, 1996.
5. Thompson DF. Understanding financial conflicts of interest [see comments]. *N Engl J Med.* 1993;329(8):573–576.
6. Lemmens T, Singer PA. Bioethics for clinicians: 17. Conflict of interest in research, education and patient care [see comments]. *CMAJ.* 1998;159(8):960–965.
7. Brody B. Special ethical issues in the management of PVS patients. *Law Med Health Care.* 1992;20(1–2):104–115.
8. Physicians and the pharmaceutical industry (update 1994). Canadian Medical Association [see comments]. *CMAJ.* 1994;150(2):256A–256F.
9. Smith R. Conflict of interest and the *BMJ* [editorial] [see comments]. *BMJ.* 1994;308(6920):4–5.
10. Smith R. Beyond conflict of interest. Transparency is the key [editorial] [see comments]. *BMJ.* 1998;317(7154):291–292.
11. Wahlbeck K, Cheine M, Essali MA. Clozapine vs "typical" neuroleptic medication for schizophrenia. In: *Cochrane Collaboration. Cochrane Library Issue 4.* Oxford: Update Software, 1998.
12. Stelfox HT, Chua G, O'Rourke K, Detsky AS. Conflict of interest in the debate over calcium-channel antagonists [see comments]. *N Engl J Med.* 1998;338(2):101–106.
13. Barnes DE, Bero LA. Industry-funded research and conflict of interest: an analysis of research sponsored by the tobacco industry through the Center for Indoor Air Research [see comments]. *J Health Polit Policy Law.* 1996;21(3):515–542.
14. Barnes DE, Bero LA. Why review articles on the health effects of passive smoking reach different conclusions [see comments]. *JAMA.* 1998;279(19):1566–1570.
15. Cushman JH Jr. Industrial group plans to fight climate treaty. *The New York Times* 1998; April 26:A1.
16. Johnston KW, Rutherford RB. Disclosure of competition of interest [editorial]. *J Vasc Surg.* 1999;30(1):200–202.
17. Physicians and the pharmaceutical industry. American College of Physicians. *Ann Intern Med.* 1990;112(8):624–626.

18. Gifts to physicians from industry [editorial] [see comments]. *JAMA.* 1991;265(4):501.
19. Wazana A. Physicians and the pharmaceutical industry: is a gift ever just a gift? [see comments]. *JAMA.* 2000;283(3):373–380.
20. Rutherford RB. Problems with the dissemination of up-to-date information on the results of endograft repair for abdominal aortic aneurysm [comment] [see comments]. *J Vasc Surg.* 1999;29(6):1167–1169.
21. Rutherford RB, Johnston KW. Potential problems with industry-supported clinical research. *J Vasc Surg.* 2000;31(5):1066–1076.
22. Weijer C, Dickens B, Meslin EM. Bioethics for clinicians: 10. Research ethics [see comments]. *CMAJ.* 1997;156(8):1153–1157.
23. Freedman B. Equipoise and the ethics of clinical research. *N Engl J Med.* 1987;317(3):141–145.
24. Weijer C. The breast cancer research scandal: addressing the issues [editorial]. *CMAJ.* 1995;152(8):1195–1197.
25. Cohen L. Issue of fraud raised as MD self-referral comes under spotlight in Ontario. *CMAJ.* 1996;154(11):1744–1746.
26. Freeman VG, Rathore SS, Weinfurt KP, Schulman KA, Sulmasy DP. Lying for patients: physician deception of third-party payers. *Arch Intern Med.* 1999;159(19):2263–2270.
27. Axelrod DA, Goold SD. Maintaining trust in the surgeon–patient relationship: challenges for the new millennium. *Arch Surg.* 2000;135(1):55–61.
28. Meyers C. Managed care and ethical conflicts: anything new? *J Med Ethics.* 1999; 25(5):382–387.

6

Clinical Trials and the Approved Use of New Medical Devices

Jon S. Matsumura, MD, and Richard K. Baer, MD

INTRODUCTION

In 1965, the Social Security Act (SSA) was signed by President Lyndon B. Johnson, establishing the Medicare program that provides for health insurance for Americans 65 years and older and certain other patient groups. In developing the SSA, Congress provided Medicare payment for services based on principles of reasonableness and medical necessity as well as safety and effectiveness.[1] Congress also provided for a number of Medicare program exclusions, such as routine physical examinations, eyeglasses, hearing aids, and, except under certain specific programs, services that are experimental or investigational.[2] In the 35 years since the establishment of the Medicare program, several major forces have reshaped health care. These include (1) the evolution of the Health Care Financing Administration (HCFA) into a dominant role in setting national payment policies for new treatments, which are then emulated by other insurers; (2) the regulatory power of the Food and Drug Administration (FDA) to determine premarket approval for the sale of new devices guided by standards of evidence-based medicine; (3) a plethora of scientific breakthroughs that allow rapid development of new medical devices; and (4) the emergence of a competitive, profit-driven private sector seeking to develop and market these medical devices for use in new treatments. This chapter discusses the regulatory pathways for coverage of new medical devices, with particular attention to reimbursement issues pertinent to clinical trials, subsequent approved uses, and off-label use of medical devices.

MEDICARE POLICY: NATIONAL AND LOCAL

HCFA administers the Medicare program for 39 million beneficiaries through a number of contractors. Medicare Part A, which pays for hospital, skilled nursing, home health, end stage renal disease, and other institutional services, is administered by fiscal intermediaries. Medicare Part B, which pays for physician services and the services of other nonphysician practitioners, is administered by carriers.

Most claims submitted to Medicare are for standard treatments and FDA-approved uses of medical devices, and are paid without further consideration. However, new medical devices are constantly being introduced into the market, and many are quite expensive. Only a limited number of national coverage policies governing Medicare coverage for new devices have been set by HCFA. In situations in which a national coverage policy exists, contractor medical directors have no discretion to deviate from the national policy. In general, however, the national coverage process moves too slowly to address adequately the needs of physicians wishing to use new and emerging technologies. Therefore, most decisions regarding coverage for new treatments are decided by the local Medicare contractors. When an HCFA national coverage policy does exist, it has the advantage of reducing the geographic differences and possible disparities in coverage that may arise by local coverage decisions.

An example of this is the HCFA directive to contractor medical directors to deny payment for carotid stenting, which is currently considered investigational.[3,4] Unfortunately, there is often no national policy for investigational devices and off-label use of approved devices. In order to make informed coverage decisions on a local basis, carriers and fiscal intermediaries have formed advisory committees [i.e., Carrier Advisory Committee (CAC) and Intermediary Advisory Committee (IAC)] composed of members of the physician and provider communities. Although the CAC and IAC may provide information to the Medicare contractor about the prevailing local practice patterns and preferences for utilization of a particular new technology, the result is that there are often regional differences in the determination of Medicare coverage for new procedures, especially in the early phase, when physician consensus is lacking and published data is scarce.

The CAC's consideration of a draft Medicare policy to cover noncoronary vascular stents used for FDA off-label indications illustrates the important advisory role played by the Committee. There are few labeled uses for stents in the vascular system, and these are for selective stenting of the iliac artery following failed angioplasty. No stents are currently approved for use in the renal arteries, brachiocephalic arteries, femoral arteries, or any veins. The Governmental Affairs Committee from the Society of Cardiovascular and Interventional Radiology, the Society for Vascular Surgery, and the International Society for Cardiovascular Surgery provided an advisory role through the local CAC on suggested indications and limitations of coverage for off-label use of noncoronary vascular stents. In making these types of coverage determinations, Medicare contractors find it beneficial to use the expertise of national provider associations and "policy/position papers or recommendations made by pertinent national and/or local specialty societies."[5]

Evidence-Based Medicine

Ideally, all decisions in medical practice would be based on well-conducted, adequately powered clinical trials that clearly demonstrate safety and efficacy and result in FDA approval of the device. Levels of quality of medical evidence have been classified by

Sackett.[6] It is not practical or possible for physicians always to meet the highest standards of evidence-based medicine for all the circumstances they meet in clinical practice. Physicians are confronted with uncommon problems that have not yet been subjected to rigorous evaluation, or they may encounter old problems that have never undergone rigorous testing in which new, alternative therapies may be considered. Clearly, the best option is to enroll patients into well-structured clinical trials to obtain necessary data to use as the basis for sound decisions in the future. Unfortunately, due to the rapid advance of technology and past difficulty in financing large clinical trials, there is a paucity of high-quality evidence in many areas of medical decision making.

At times, medical practice and physician consensus oppose what the best-quality published data suggest. For example, the use of primary iliac stenting was compared to selective stent placement by the Dutch Iliac Stent Trial Group.[7] This randomized trial showed that there were no substantial differences in clinical results between a strategy of selective iliac stenting and primary stenting, although the latter procedure was more expensive. Despite this evidence, many physicians continue to practice primary stenting based on unpublished data and cohort studies that demonstrate positive results with primary stenting that seem to surpass historical controls with selective stenting. Certainly there are individual patient situations in which primary stenting would be considered good medical judgment by a majority of physicians, but the best published evidence suggests that this approach is not the best for all patients.

More difficulty occurs when physician practice progresses so far that clinical equipoise is questioned. Using the previous example, there is inadequate clinical data to support FDA approval of a labeled use for primary stenting and, at the same, clinicians remain so convinced of its benefit that they are unwilling to enroll patients in clinical trials to evaluate the efficacy of selective stenting. This is rather reminiscent of the situation in the early 1980s regarding carotid endarterectomy for symptomatic and asymptomatic carotid stenosis. Although there are several potential solutions to the problem of using devices for unlabeled indications, including denial of payment and criminal investigations for physicians who bill fraudulently for these procedures, a more ideal solution is to proceed with clinical trials that assess the effectiveness of these new therapies. The North American Symptomatic Carotid Endarterectomy Trial and the Asymptomatic Carotid Artery Surgery study demonstrate the type of data that can be gained from rigorous trials that evaluate the efficacy of a controversial treatment.[8,9] In some cases, scientific testing shows that therapies are ineffective and patients are spared from treatments that are not only costly, but may also be dangerous. An example of one such high-profile and expensive treatment is ablative chemotherapy and bone marrow transplantation for advanced metastatic breast cancer, which was not shown to be superior to standard treatment in several randomized trials. Clearly, all physicians have an essential responsibility to engage in the testing of new therapies in adequately powered and well-conducted clinical trials prior to widespread application. It is important to note that for most new devices, registry studies and cohort studies are unlikely to provide the level of medical evidence necessary to gain FDA approval, and to ensure medical populations of the safety and efficacy of new technologies.

Clinical Trials and Medicare Coverage: Interagency Agreement

Adequately powered clinical trials, however, are expensive and difficult to organize and carry out. On November 1, 1995, the FDA and HCFA developed an interagency letter of agreement that responded to patients' and physicians' needs for rapid development of new devices and industry's needs to have assistance in conducting clinical trials on improvements to existing devices. In the past, any device undergoing an FDA clinical trial was essentially considered to be experimental in nature and not eligible for Medicare coverage. This agreement resulted in a policy in which the FDA designates certain new devices with an Investigational Device Exemption (IDE). Category A devices are technologies for which there is little previous technology (i.e., it was an experimental device in a completely new class and not eligible for Medicare coverage). Category B devices are devices that are refinements or improvements of existing technologies and, although considered investigational, according to the interagency agreement would be considered eligible for Medicare coverage. The agreement stipulated that coverage is conditional on continuing FDA approval of the clinical trial, local supervision by the Institutional Review Boards, use of the device in accordance with the clinical trial protocol, and absence of established Medicare national policy to the contrary. Some carrier medical directors request specific preapproval for each investigational device exemption (IDE) prior to submitting claims.

In addition, the interagency policy stipulated specific billing practices to be followed, including use of the "-QA"modifier for Current Procedural Terminology (CPT) codes and filing of physician claims to the carrier with the IDE number in item 23 of the HCFA 1500 form. Hospitals follow a similar procedure for the UB-92 claim form. From personal experience, we have found that cooperation between investigators and local Medicare contractor medical directors is a productive, mutually educational experience. Many clinicians may be unaware of the specific requirements for billing these clinical trials, but information from a Medicare Part B bulletin in Illinois specifically outlines provider responsibilities (Figure 6–1).[5] Specifically, providers are responsible for knowing the rules and regulations governing the services they bill to the Medicare program.

With the development of this interagency agreement, there is now a reasonable mechanism through which high-quality data can be obtained to evaluate the safety and

PROVIDERS RESPONSIBLE for KNOWING GUIDELINES

A provider is responsible to know the rules and regulations that apply to all services he/she bills to the Medicare Program. According to the Medicare Carriers Manual, Section 7103.1E.1, "In general, the physician should have known a policy or rule if the policy or rule is in the Federal regulations . . ." The provider is also responsible to know the rules and regulations that are made available through publications from the carrier which include, but are not limited to, the *Medicare Part B Provider Handbook*, the *Medicare B Bulletin*, and mailings sent periodically to all or individual providers.

Figure 6–1. Provider responsibilities for billing clinical trials *(excerpted from Medicare B Bulletin for Illinois, September 1996, p. 3).*

effectiveness of new medical devices used in the vascular territories. Physician investigators now have a better opportunity to work with the industry to initiate and complete these much-needed clinical trials. A recent executive order by President Clinton may further expand Medicare coverage of clinical investigations.

APPROVED USE OF NEW DEVICES

The IDE process is a primary avenue through which industry sponsors gain a premarket approval to sell new medical devices. This usually involves one to three phases of clinical trials to evaluate the safety and effectiveness of the new device. When a premarket approval (PMA) is granted, specific FDA labeling accompanies the device outlining the indications for use as well as cautionary statements and warnings. The labeling may appear as the *instructions for use* (IFU). Often, the clinical trial is designed with multiple inclusion and exclusion criteria that form the initial basis for indications for approved uses of the devices. If these clinical trials are sufficiently successful, the FDA approves the medical devices for use in vascular beds, where the clinical trial has demonstrated their safety and effectiveness. The medical device amendments of the Federal Food, Drug, and Cosmetic Act, as amended by the Safe Medical Devices Act of 1990, specifically defines *safety* as reasonable assurance, based on valid scientific evidence, that the probable benefits to health, under the conditions of intended use, outweigh any probable risk. *Effectiveness* is defined as reasonable assurance that, in a significant proportion of the population, the use of the device for its intended uses and conditions of use, when labeled, will provide clinically significant results.[10] Often, additional restrictions on the indications are placed in the labeling based on findings from the clinical trials. For example, clinical trials that led to the recent PMA of an endovascular graft excluded patients with aneurysm rupture. Because there was no adequate data currently available to substantiate its safety and efficacy for patients with this critical problem, the labeling does not include ruptured aneurysms. For nonruptured aneurysms, the clinical trial did detect advantages as well as potential complications of the new procedure compared to the standard operative repair. These new findings resulted in the FDA panel recommending approval conditional on several other requirements, including initiation of a training program for physicians who would use the device, provision of a patient-friendly educational brochure, and continued surveillance of the existing patients for up to 5 years to obtain further data long-term safety and effectiveness.

Investigational device exemptions are not limited to large corporate sponsors, but may actually be physician initiated as well. These investigator-initiated IDEs are less likely to lead to a PMA. A third regulatory process is the less-known humanitarian device exemption pathway (HDE). The HDE provides regulatory relief for medical devices where the anticipated use of the device will occur in <4,000 patients worldwide on an annual basis. The FDA has recognized that adequately powered clinical trials could not feasibly be performed in many of these cases. Furthermore, the cost of performing those clinical trials could never be recouped by industry sponsors because of the limited number of sales of the device if an approval was obtained. These devices may be desperately needed by patients, but because the number of affected patients is so few, the devices had not been developed, much like orphan drugs that are not developed for rare medical conditions.

OFF-LABEL USE

Physicians using FDA-approved medical devices for an off-label indication may practice medicine as their training and judgment dictate, but should submit to Medicare claims only for procedures that are safe and effective, and not investigational or experimental. Technically, Medicare does not cover off-label uses of medical devices unless the contractor grants a specific exception. The difficulty arises when medical practice outpaces the availability of adequate data to judge safety and efficacy of new technologies. An illustrative example is the use of stents for the treatment of malignant superior vena cava obstruction. Physicians should consult with their Medicare contractor medical directors on an individual basis when a potentially controversial off-label use of a device is being considered.

In the course of treating an individual patient, physicians often come to a medical decision that the patient's best course of treatment involves the use of a medical device for an indication other than that for which it was labeled. In current clinical practice, off-label use of medical devices, particularly in noncoronary stents, has become widespread and, many would argue, has become the standard of care. Purists, wishing to base clinical decision making on evidence-based medicine, argue that inadequate data exist to support the evolution of a standard of care in this manner, still a large number of physicians believe that off-label use of a device in a particular instance without adequate clinical trials is entirely appropriate.

In fact, many specialty societies have formulated policy statements to support off-label use of medical devices for specific indications. Private industry is pleased to be able to make sales of their products for both labeled and off-labeled indications, although they are not permitted by the FDA to market devices for off-label indications. A potential conflict arises when off-label use becomes so predominant that it becomes accepted as the preferred treatment without adequate data to support its use. When clinical practice reaches this point, there is the danger that companies may even become unwilling to support clinical trials evaluating a device's effectiveness because the study might result in data showing that the device is ineffective or unsafe. Renal artery stenting using biliary and coronary stents in an off-label application is a prime example of how years of widespread off-label use have evolved into a commonplace treatment. Although renal artery stenting was rarely used, a Dutch randomized trial was published showing relatively little benefit of renal artery angioplasty compared to modern medical management of mild to moderate hypertension. Clearly, this is one of many areas that is ripe for responsible and thorough investigation using clinical trials.

SUMMARY

New medical devices will no doubt play a major role in the future improvement in medical care in the United States. Although many medical devices will obtain FDA approval for a variety of indications, there may be situations in which off-label uses of FDA-approved devices are also likely to be dangerous, ineffective, or inappropriate. Although individual physicians should be allowed to continue to make the best medical decisions in a given situation, it is only through properly designed and conducted clinical trials that adequate evidence will be gained and disseminated for determining the safe and appropriate indications for new medical devices. For Category B devices, HCFA and the FDA have provided a payment mechanism for which interested investigators and corporate sponsors can conduct much-needed clinical trials. Investigators and industry partners must rise to fulfill this responsibility in this new era of evidence-based medicine.

REFERENCES

1. SSA Sec. 1862(a)(1)(A).
2. SSA Sec. 1862(a)(1)(D).
3. HCFA Pub 6 Coverage Issues Manual 50-32.3.
4. Bettmann MA, Katzen BT, Whisnant J, et al. Carotid stenting and angioplasty: a statement for healthcare professionals from the Councils on Cardiovascular Radiology, Stroke, Cardio-Thoracic and Vascular Surgery, Epidemiology, and Prevention, and Clinical Cardiology, American Heart Association. *Circulation.* 1998;97(1):121–123.
5. Medicare B Bulletin for Illinois, p. 3, September 1996.
6. Sackett DL. Evidence-based medicine. *Semin Perinat.* 1997;21(1):3–5.
7. Tetteroo E, van der Graaf Y, Bosch JL, et al. Randomised comparison of primary stent placement versus primary angioplasty followed by selective stent placement in patients with iliac-artery occlusive disease. *Lancet.* 1998;351:1153–1159.
8. North American Symptomatic Carotid Endarterectomy Trial Collaboration. Beneficial effect of carotid endarterectomy in symptomatic patients with high grade carotid stenosis. *N Engl J Med.* 1991;325:445–453.
9. Executive Committee for the Asymptomatic Carotid Atherosclerosis Study. Endarterectomy for asymptomatic carotid artery stenosis. *JAMA.* 1995;275:1421–1428.
10. Food and Drug Administration National Institutes of Health, Meeting of: *Circulatory System Devices Panel.* June 23, 1999.

7

Issues Related to Industry Supported Clinical Research

Robert B. Rutherford, MD, FACS

INTRODUCTION

Device manufacturers and pharmaceutical companies are now a very significant source of clinical research funding. It is important to appreciate that although industry–clinician relationships may foster important research, they can potentially compromise an investigator's scientific integrity and even affect patient safety. The professional and financial rewards that may result from a successful clinical trial can be significant, and this may compromise in an insidious way the clinician's primary responsibilities to the patient, to his or her institution, and to the vascular community as a whole. This article addresses issues that may arise when the company sponsoring a study is primarily in charge of the design, conduct, and analysis of the study or is in control of the study data. These circumstances raise potential conflicts for the clinical investigator and may create problems for others (e.g., the patient, institutional research boards (IRBs), regulatory bodies, the scientific community, and the clinicians whose practice is a focus of the trial). These problems include financial conflict of interest; contractual limitations on the investigator's right to publish trial data and improper practices in the presentation and publication of the trial data in the form of delay in reporting adverse events; avoiding publication of negative trials, in which the device or drug proves to be no better or worse than the nontreatment control or a current standard treatment; or multiple publications.

Many of the views expressed in this chapter have been developed and reported in greater detail by the author in an editorial,[1] and some of the more critical statements are quoted directly.

ADVANTAGES OF INDUSTRY-SUPPORTED CLINICAL RESEARCH AND ITS POTENTIAL PITFALLS

Increasingly, scientific investigators in all specialties have come to rely on support from industry to carry out their research. University support for clinical research is diminishing, and support from national funding agencies and charitable foundations is difficult to obtain. Currently, much of the total National Institutes of Health (NIH) budget is going to targeted areas, often promoted by requests for proposal (RFPs). The development of new devices and their clinical testing is almost impossible to do independently in a university setting, and few patents are coming from universities. Most innovators or inventors soon seek venture capital or the support of a large established company. In addition, most surgical investigators feel fortunate to be able to obtain funding from industry to carry out research. Such research supports their academic development and promotion. In reading the *curriculum vitae* of young faculty, it is impressive how much of their research funding support is now coming from industry. Investigators also recognize that such corporate-funded clinical research is generally less demanding than peer-reviewed funding in terms of the application and approval process. The company usually supplies the research protocols, including the necessary background information, along with prototype IRB applications and patient consent forms. Funding allows research associates to be hired to help with the recruiting of patients and the collecting and reporting of patient data. In many multicenter trials, the company processes and analyzes the data centrally, and in the larger trials this would be difficult for a principle investigator to do. In spite of these and other advantages from industry-supported research, there are also some risks, and not all are obvious to the potential investigator—particularly the problems that might be encountered with the control of scientific data by the industry sponsor.

The Basis for Potential Conflicts between the Investigator and the Industry Sponsor

In carrying out a clinical research study, both the investigator and the company share the desire that the new technology (typically a device or drug) will significantly improve the diagnosis or treatment of patients. Both sides hope and expect that the joint venture will reflect well on themselves and their institutions. However, both the company and the investigator have other, differing objectives in carrying out the same research project, and these may come into conflict. In funding research, the company also has the underlying objective to increase or maintain profit for the shareholders, and the importance of this goal is understood by their coordinators of clinical research. Furthermore, in return for investment in a research project, the company must protect its proprietary interests. These objectives are promoted or protected in contractual agreements between the investigator and the company.

In accepting a research contract, the individual investigator may become involved in developing and testing a potential significant diagnostic or therapeutic advance, but may have other goals that could potentially result in conflict. As physicians, investigators have a primary responsibility to proper patient care and safety. As a researcher, the primary goal is acquisition of knowledge, to be published and applied where possible for the good of patients. In pursuing these goals, the clinical investigator must have ready access to the data, be able to verify the results and their analysis, and be able to report those results in a timely and accurate fashion. The company also has responsibilities in regard to patient safety, but in the analysis and reporting of results, a conflict with their financial and proprietary interests may arise that, depending on how it is solved, may ultimately put the company and the investigator at odds.

Financial Conflict of Interest

Contractual agreements for participation in company-sponsored clinical research typically do not provide a means to give investigators appropriate credit or reward for their innovative ideas or constructive advice, which may significantly improve the ultimate design of a device or determine the success of a trial. However, those involved in early device development or those who move from the principle investigator (PI) of the trial to running the post-trial clinical programs may be rewarded with stock options. Alternatively, an investigator's trial experience may engender such faith in the drug's or device's ultimate success that they may purchase stock. The American Medical Association (AMA) has recommended that "in order to avoid criticism that the decisions an investigator makes during the study might have been biased by financial conflict of interest and the concern that the validity of the scientific data may have been jeopardized, the investigator should not hold stock or stock options in the sponsoring company or be an officer of the company."[2] The *Journal of Vascular Surgery* published a conflict of interest document for members of the joint vascular societies[3] that applies to publications, presentations, and committee membership. Investments in mutual funds that are managed by others may be overlooked, but all known holdings in the company, including those by close family members or practice partners, should be declared, so as to alert the audience or readers of potential competition of interest. Although the above AMA recommendation cautions against doing research for a company in which one has stock, stock may be offered after completion of the research in recognition of contributions to the development or testing of a device or drug. This is not wrong, but failure to disclose this when presenting or publishing about the device or drug is inappropriate, and has led to increasing public criticism, as exemplified by the recent media coverage of the Heart Port device[4] and coronary stents.[5]

Restrictive Research Contracts

Nondisclosure agreements protect the company against the investigator divulging proprietary information, which is appropriate. They also may contain clauses that impose inappropriate restrictions on when and how the investigator may publish data from the trial. This has created problems for a number of investigators, only a few of which have become well known.[6,7] The company's lawyers, to protect their client's proprietary interests, usually draw up such agreements, and only occasionally are the investigator's rights addressed as well. Knowing that it may be a one-sided agreement, investigators should read over all contracts and pay particular attention to certain details [e.g., be sure one's access to the data and right to publish important aspects (with coinvestigators) is not restricted by the agreement]. Clauses in the contract dealing with publication rights, confidentiality, intellectual property, access to data, and conflict resolution in particular should be carefully reviewed by the institution as well as the investigator to ensure patient safety through prompt access to data and to guard the scientific freedom of the investigator. Not only should this be done by an individual researcher, but also by a responsible administrator in the researcher's hospital, research institute or university. It is important that there be institutional policies and procedures that define the responsibilities for scrutinizing a contract. Ideally, the terms of the contract with (the company) should be determined at the outset when the study design and methods, including measurement, modeling, and analytical strategies are being developed. The investigators or their duly-formed steering committee should retain the rights to modify the conduct of the trial as appropriate, determine the scientific conclusions, and publish or otherwise disseminate the results of the study and their conclusions, regardless of outcome. Such study contracts exist,[8] but many are restrictive. Finally, it would be of great help if medical and surgical societies collaborated and obtained legal advice in drawing up generic confidentiality documents and clinical research contracts, and in so doing identified items that should be included in research contracts—items that would be viewed as fair and standard practice and would protect the rights of scientific investigators, patients, and institutions as well as the sponsoring company. At the very least, it is important to define the right to have access to data and to present and publish the data in a timely fashion, irrespective of the results of the study.

Developing Clinical Research Protocols

Having a research protocol already drawn up by the sponsoring company along with supporting information and suggested patient consent forms is very convenient. The research protocol can and should serve as a useful starting place for discussions between the sponsor of the research and the principle investigator or potential collaborating investigators from other institutions. Investigators should not simply accept the drafted protocol, but rather should take an active role in improving it. It may lack endpoints that are objective enough, have too favorable exclusion and inclusion criteria, lack appropriate controls or suggest using comparisons with historical controls, not be analyzed on an intent-to-treat basis, have too short a follow-up or fail to include a cost-analysis or quality-of-life assessment, or other features that might prevent conclusive and meaningful results or produce data that cannot be generalized or will not be accepted by one's peers. Even though some companies hire experienced trialists as consultants, investigators involved in the study are more likely to have detailed knowledge of the key clinical issues involved. They should work together to ensure proper stratification, comparable study groups, accurate power estimates, definitions of what constitutes a reportable complication, and gathering and analyzing the data in a format that is compatible with standardized reporting practices.

Payments to Investigators and Institutions

Industry-sponsored research tends to pay well, generally better than most research funding agencies and foundations. It often amounts to more than an even compensation for one's "percent of effort" vis à vis other university income and an even reimbursement for actual research costs. Therefore, some profit may accrue from industry-supported research. Also, industry is less likely to impose controls on how the money may be spent. Furthermore, in being reimbursed for running a clinical trial, the investigator faces a potential conflict of interest—specifically, the conflict of ensuring that the individual patient's rights to receive the most appropriate medial care are guaranteed and the investigator's self-interest in obtaining a "maximum" profit.[9]

Clinicians should expect to be reimbursed fairly for their time spent managing the patients and the project, the salaries of study coordinators and fellows, overhead, and miscellaneous expenses. The AMA recommends that remuneration of the investigator should be commensurate with the efforts, and that the institution that pays the direct and indirect costs should administer funds. However, it seems reasonable that the "profit" could be used for salary support of research assistants or to assist funding other research or educational programs or trainees. Most institutions have mechanisms to prevent faculty from personally receiving and spending the excess monies generated from a research study. The investigator must be aware of the institutions policies on the use of the profit for academic purposes; unfortunately, these are often vague. The IRB should be informed of funding agreements and the investigator should disclose to it if he/she has any other relationship with the sponsoring company such as stockholder, corporate officer, or paid consultant.

The Role of the Institutional Review Board

The IRB has an important role in moderating the company–investigator agreements as well as its major role in protecting the patient. The IRB must ensure that the study design is scientifically valid and approve the ethics of the study to ensure that patients are properly enlisted, receive appropriate informed consent, have a low risk–benefit ratio if enrolled in the study, are not subjected to unnecessary procedures, and that the financial arrangements are appropriate. In addition, however, the IRB should be in a position to monitor the study as it progresses. In order to safeguard patient care, the investigator must have data from the sponsoring company to be able to communicate the results of the safety of continuing the study to the IRB on a regular basis. In order to fulfill its obligation, the IRB must be independent of the sponsor, investigator, and institution.

Data Collection and the Analysis and Control of Data

Even if an individual is the principle instigator (PI) of a trial, he or she may not have the ability, time, or resources to coordinate a major trial and collect and analyze all the data. Oftentimes the company initiates the trial and arrangements are usually made for them to produce the data collection forms, only one copy of which is retained by each institution's PI. The company's need for the data required to file for FDA approval is clear. The major issue is the investigator's access to the overall data. Individual investigators normally have access to their own data, but in addition, the investigators as a group or through a data monitoring committee must be able to monitor the actual data and particularly be aware of adverse events.

If the company controls the data and does not provide full analysis to the investigators at frequent intervals, including the details of complications or adverse reactions, the investigators may not be able to fulfill their ethical and moral responsibility to the patients and their responsibilities to the IRB and institutions. An appropriately constituted *data monitoring committee* that includes representation from both the company and the investigators is the optimum approach so that fully analyzed data, be it positive or negative, is made readily available to the investigators.

Data Analysis

Unfortunately, it has become increasingly apparent to journal editors that some speakers and primary authors of manuscripts presented at national and regional meetings have reviewed only the summarized analysis of the data that was supplied by the company. They have not reviewed the raw data or performed or checked the statistical analyses and cannot supply the additional information requested by discussants or reviewers.

For proprietary reasons, device manufacturers and pharmaceutical companies rarely release the full details of their sponsored research, but beyond this there is a perception that they may be selective about the data from clinical studies that they choose to make public. The company and its consultants are unlikely to hide unfavorable data for any significant period of time, but even if that were not the case, they may not be knowledgeable enough to determine unilaterally which relationships to explore to uncover other potentially significant observations. Thus, using data summarized by company officials or anyone with a vested interest in the outcome, can lead to many problems.

Examples of the control of industry of trial data appear to be becoming more common: The long-completed and oft-presented European randomized trial claiming advantages for primary iliac stenting with the Palmaz device over percutaneous transluminal angioplasty (PTA) alone that was never published;[10] a paper being withdrawn from the 1998 American Venous Forum meeting because the company that sponsored the study did not reply to repeated requests to supply the necessary background information (the denominators, if you will) to put the study findings in proper perspective in sufficient time to allow presentation;[11] using summarized data obtained from a company consultant as the basis for an analysis of the cost effectiveness of an aortic endograft device when access to the complete data was denied after the results of the preliminary analysis were unfavorable.[12] These experiences emphasize the importance of the author/investigator's access to the raw data. Furthermore, providing the investigators with a breakdown of data by participating institution is mandatory so that it can be checked against the raw data kept by individual investigators.

Ideally, data that allows subjective interpretation should not be interpreted primarily by any one person or by person(s) with a vested interest in the outcome of the study. When the results of a trial depend significantly on the interpretation of diagnostic studies, arrangements should be made for these studies to be independently interpreted by blinded individuals (i.e., in a core laboratory) who have no vested interest in the outcome and are independent of company or investigator interference. Even core laboratories are usually supported by the study sponsor, so the blinding process must be carefully enforced.

Interim Data Release

There may be a long delay between completion of a trial and its required follow-up, analysis of the data, submission of a manuscript, and publication of the final results. With nonrandomized studies of new devices, preliminary interval reports of the progress of the trial are possible and may even be desirable. Unfortunately, many of the early reports contain soft data and are presented with enthusiastic bias, often appearing to promote further recruitment of patients. Such updates of data are rarely critical and usually present summarized data supplied by the company. This deprives the vascular surgical community, who can attend a limited number of meetings, of objective updates of trials that could help in patient management decisions [e.g., open abdominal aortic aneurysm (AAA) repair vs. referral to an endograft trial, and if the latter, which one.] This dilemma could be avoided because, in a properly constructed prospective device evaluation, the data are collected in a way that is suitable for submission to the FDA and for publication; consequently, there is no reason why interim data releases, such as presentations at symposia, should not contain objective data and be reported using standard reporting practices. Although it has been accepted—in drug trials, at least—that no data should be released until the end of the study, when the precalculated power of the study is appropriate, regular, objective, and complete disclosure of the outcomes of new devices is needed to assess the failure rate and complications, particularly significant adverse events. Even periodic investigators meetings may not fulfill this need when the data is prepared and presented by company officials, or the investigators are instructed not to disseminate the data, a not uncommon practice. An appropriately constituted publications committee should also oversee interim data releases and presentations, and these should be based on the above considerations.

Delay in Reporting Adverse Events

Significant delays may occur between the initial discovery of device-specific problems and their eventual dissemination at meetings or in published reports. Reports of serious complications should be circulated immediately by the company to all investigators, who then have a responsibility to notify their patients, institution, and IRB. In a recent editorial,[13] the author emphasized the importance of promptly disseminating information if a problem is noted that potentially reflects on the design or deployment of the device, in this case aortic endografts. There have been some prompt disclosures: the hook fractures in the Endovascular Technologies endograft trial[14] and the problem of late rupture of aortic aneurysms "repaired" with the AneuRx device.[15,16] However, this was not the case when fabrication flaws were detected in the Min Tec Stentor graft[17]; and when it was mentioned in an analysis of the Eurostar data,[18] the device was not identified by name. Then there is the problem of Vanguard grafts developing fabric erosions and endoleaks, leading in some cases to aortic rupture. A case report of this was first published in June 1999.[19] By the time this case report was finalized, the company had reported in a letter to their endograft implanters that 5 other cases existed, but there are now 12 and an analysis of these adverse events has still not been published.

This experience brings up the issues of whether it is the company's or the investigator's responsibility to disseminate information about adverse events, who should be the recipients of such information (only potential device implanters vs. the vascular community), what is the appropriate middle ground between premature allegations of device failures and significantly delayed disclosure, and whether it is appropriate to accede to company requests not to identify complications by device in registry presentations and publications. These have been the subjects of a recent exchange in letters to the editors of the *Journal of Vascular Surgery*.[20,21] It is the author's view that although the company has a responsibility to report adverse events promptly to the appropriate agencies as well as their investigators and customers, the investigators have a responsibility to report them promptly to their IRBs, and when it appears to be more than a spurious event, to present and publish them, with journal editors expediting publication in the interest of patient safety and broadly informing the vascular community.

Not Reporting Negative Trials

There is a tendency not to submit negative results for publication, and it is also often difficult to get negative trials published. Just like surgeons with poor results, companies are not likely to want to report negative trials. However, in some instances the research contract appears to give the company the right to block publication. An investigator was obliged to step to the podium at the American Heart Association (AHA) meeting and announce that he was being prevented from presenting the results of the study by the pharmaceutical company sponsor.[22] Permission was withdrawn the evening before presentation. Because of contractual agreements with the investigators, the industry sponsor maintained a right to block public disclosure. In an editorial discussing this incident,[23] it was pointed out that the signed AHA abstract submission document was also binding regarding presentation, and that informed consent documents generally include such statements as "the patients and their families have agreed to participate in an activity with risk and have the right to be assured that the results of the study will be transmitted to the scientific community in a timely fashion." The authors of the editorial maintained "that these other documents (and the informed consent in particular) may also have legal standing as contracts, and that inappropriate delays or limitations in the scope of presentations may represent breaches of these contracts." Although it is reassuring to be told that reporting adverse events or negative trials and their patient safety implications will take legal precedence over contractual agreements restricting publication without company permission, most investigators are leery of legal entanglements and fear they do not have the resources for long litigations. However, the investigator's institution, having endorsed the contract and having it signed by a responsible administrator, would undoubtedly share in legal expenses. In addition, a formally stated position by a number of scientific societies in support of this principle is necessary, and would help relieve the investigator's dilemma and mitigate such contractual restrictions in the future.

A company may not have included a clause to prevent disclosure, but if it controls the pooled data, it can effectively prevent publication, unless all the investigators pool each of their institutions' data, for each investigator has the right to publish their own data. This right was observed a few years ago, when a group of investigators who had recruited by far the most cases in a negative trial finally decided to exercise their right to present and publish the results from their own center[24] when it became apparent that the company was not going to have the overall trial data published. Following the presentation, company officials tried unsuccessfully to undermine that publication through telephone contact with the editors of the journal in which it was to be published. When told that it was undergoing peer review and if accepted would be published, they then asked to publish an article as rebuttal, but declined when they found it would have to be peer reviewed. They settled for a letter to the editor when the article was published[25] and two seemingly spontaneous letters were submitted by others,[26,27] one of whom had a contract with the study sponsor, Curative Technologies, Inc. The primary author's reply[28] effectively dismissed their objections, but this example serves to demonstrate the extent a study sponsor might go to prevent or oppose publication of a negative trial.

To not allow publication of results interferes with the investigator's right to report scientific data from a trial in a timely fashion regardless of outcome, and also with the patient's right to know the outcome because this information may modify their management. Although an investigator has the right to publish the data, there are responsibilities that include ensuring that sufficient time has been allowed to complete the analysis of the data, particularly from more complex trials, confirming that the company is unwilling to publish or assist in publishing this data, and if partial data is being reported, that it is likely to be representative of the whole.

Multiple Publications

One of the problems with multiple publications of the same longitudinal data is that subsequent accounts may have different starting points, ostensibly because the device itself has undergone redesign, but this practice hides "the learning curve." Although it is reasonable to show the impact that improvements in the device or the skills of those implanting it have on the results, it is more appropriate to present the entire experience and carry out subgroup analysis in order to provide the reader with the full picture. Detailed publications covering results, complications, and special aspects of a device are clearly justified, but others in which essentially the same data is revisited with a somewhat different discussion are clearly examples of *salami slicing,* a term used to describe multiple publications of the same data. In this regard, the editors of surgical journals soon plan to publish a joint position paper on "Duplicate and Fraudulent Publications."[29] It maintains that to avoid being considered a duplicate publication, a manuscript must extend an original, published database by substantially more than 50% *and* offer information that is new and different from the original publication. Simply extending the numbers of cases is not acceptable. A manuscript that analyzes the original data in a completely different way, to prove or disprove a different hypothesis, is also an exception to this label. To avoid these problems with clinical trials, a publications committee should decide ahead of time how to present the data fairly to avoid multiple publications and should resist company pressures to broadly publish similar data.

Publication Committees

Many trials form publication committees from among the principle investigators with the intent of fairly dividing up the publication of data emanating from a trial and organizing the publication. This is an appropriate mechanism if it is properly set up and run by the principle investigators. It should be constituted at the outset of the study and be made up of a few respected investigators, or members of a Scientific Advisory Board (if there is one) and a representative or two of the company. There are a number of examples of industry-supported trials ignoring this need, or company officials bypassing the committee,[1] but the point is that investigators should insist that an appropriate publication committee be formed *at the outset* and see that it is proactive, not perfunctory.

CONCLUSIONS

The aim of clinical research trials is to develop safe and effective methods for managing patients' diseases. It is important not to lose sight of this goal in attempting to solve some of the problems identified above. The solutions are not easy because of the complex relationships involved, but, as more and more technical advances are coming to trial, the balance seems to have shifted to a point where industry is exerting more control and the busy clinical investigator is less able to defend his or her rights as a research scientist. It is important that investigators be aware of these potential pitfalls and their need to avoid them, and it is time for clinical research investigators to band together and take a stand against inappropriate control of clinical trials and their data by industry. The pendulum must swing back to a more balanced position, and it is in need of a concerted push.

REFERENCES

1. Rutherford RB, Johnston KW. Potential problems with industry-supported research. *J Vasc Surg*. 2000;31:1066–1076.
2. Council on Scientific Affairs and Council on Ethical and Judicial Affairs, American Medical Association. Conflicts of interest in medical center/industry research relationships, *JAMA*. 1990;263:2790–2793.
3. Johnston KW, Hertzer NR, Rutherford RB, Smith III, RB, Yao JST. Joint Council guidelines for disclosure of conflict of interest. *J Vasc Surg*. 2000;32:213–215.
4. King, RT Jr. The doctor as a stockholder. *The Wall Street Journal,* May 5, 1999; A1.
5. Eichenwald K, Kolata G. Hidden interest—a special report. When physicians double as entrepreneurs. *New York Times,* Financial/Business section. November 30, 1999.
6. Phillips RA, Hoey J. Constraints of interest: lessons at the Hospital for Sick Children. *CMAJ*. 1998;159:955–957.
7. Olivieri NF, Brittenham GM, McLaren CE, et al. Long-term safety and effectiveness of iron-chelation therapy with deferiprone for thalassemia major. *NEJM*. 1998;339:417–423.
8. Etchells E, McLeod RS, Greets W, et al. Economic analysis of low-dose heparin vs. the low-molecular-weight heparin Enoxaparin for prevention of venous thromboembolism after colorectal surgery. *Arch Int Med*. 1999;159:1221–1228.
9. Shimm D, Spece R. Industry reimbursement for entering patients into clinical trials: legal and ethical issues. *Ann Intern Med*. 1991;115:148–151.
10. Richter, GM. Results of a randomized trial of iliac PTA vs. primary stenting. *J Vasc Intervent Radiol*. 1993;4:30. (abstract only)
11. Jones DN Jr, Nehler MR, Merli G, et al. The incidence of adequate surveillance exams in a

multi-center trial of deep venous thrombosis prophylaxis. Abstract submitted and accepted for the 1998 American Venous Forum meeting. Presentation withdrawn.

12. Sternburgh WC III, Money SR. Hospital costs of endovascular vs. open repair of abdominal aortic aneurysms: a multicenter study. *J Vasc Surg.* 2000;31:237–244.
13. Rutherford RB. Problems with the dissemination of up-to-date-information on the results of endograft repair for abdominal aortic aneurysm. *J Vasc Surg.* 1999;29:1167–1169.
14. Bernhard VM. Development of the endovascular prosthesis. *Bull Am Coll Surg.* 1996;81:20–21.
15. Politz JK, Newman VS, Stewart MT. Late abdominal aortic aneurysm rupture after AneuRx repair: a report of three cases. *J Vasc Surg.* 2000;31:599–606.
16. Zarins CK, White RA, Fogarty TJ. Aneurysm rupture following endovascular repair using the AneuRx stent graft. *J Vasc Surg.* 2000;31:960–970.
17. Riepe G, Heilberger P, Umscheid T, et al. Frame dislocation of body middle rings in endovascular stent tube grafts. *Eur J Vasc Endovasc Surg.* 1999;17:28–34.
18. Buth J, Harris PL, Miahle C. Eurostar endovascular registry: success rates, complications, significance of endoleaks, and is suture breakage in stent grafts important? Montefiore Symposium on Current Critical Problems, New Horizons and Techniques in Vascular and Endovascular Surgery, Nov. 19, 1998.
19. Krohg-Sørensen K, Brekke M, Drolsum A, Kvernebo K. Periprosthetic leak and rupture after endovascular repair of abdominal aortic aneurysm. The significance of device design for long term results. *J Vasc Surg.* 1999;29:1152–1158.
20. Harris PR, Buth J. Regarding "Problems with the dissemination of up-to-date-information on the results of endograft repair for abdominal aortic aneurysm." Letter to the editors. *J Vasc Surg.* 1999;30:767–768.
21. Rutherford RB. Reply to letter regarding "Problems with the dissemination of up-to-date information on the results of endograft repair for abdominal aortic aneurysm." *J Vasc Surg.* 1999;30:768–769.
22. Clarke WM, Raps EC, Tong DC, Kelley RE. Cervene in acute ischemic stroke: Results of a phase III randomized efficacy study. *Stroke.* 1999;30:234. (abstract)
23. Goldstein LB, Brott TG, Kothari RU, Smith WS. Clinical stroke trials: guarding against bias. *Stroke.* 1999;30:1165–1166.
24. Krupski WC, Reilly LM, Perez S, Moss KM, Crombleholme PA, Rapp JH. A prospective randomized trial of autologous platelet derived wound healing factors for the treatment of chronic non-healing wounds: A preliminary report. *J Vasc Surg.* 1991;14:526–532.
25. Loss LF, Deitrick GA III, Duff RG. Letter to the editor re: a prospective randomized trial of autologous platelet derived wound healing factors for the treatment of chronic non-healing wounds: a preliminary report. *J Vasc Surg.* 1992;16:125–126.
26. Glover JL. Letter to the editor re: a prospective randomized trial of autologous platelet derived wound healing factors for the treatment of chronic non-healing wounds: a preliminary report. *J Vasc Surg.* 1992;16:124–125.
27. Dosick SM. Letter to the editor re: a prospective randomized trial of autologous platelet derived wound healing factors for the treatment of chronic non-healing wounds: a preliminary report. *J Vasc Surg.* 1992;16:125.
28. Krupski WC. Reply to letters to the editor re: a prospective randomized trial of autologous platelet derived wound healing factors for the treatment of chronic non-healing wounds: a preliminary report. *J Vasc Surg.* 1992;16:126–128.
29. Statement on Duplicate and Fraudulent Submission and Publication. To be published simultaneously in 19 surgical journals by their editors.

8

The CPT Process and New Vascular Surgery CPT Codes

Anton N. Sidawy, MD, MPH

The Current Procedural Terminology (CPT) is a listing of descriptive terms and codes for reporting medical services and procedures. In 1961, the responsibility of putting together nomenclature for disease was passed to the American Medical Association (AMA), which published the first edition of CPT in 1966. The second edition was published in 1970, and contained expanded codes describing procedures in surgery, medicine, and the specialties. In addition, the five-digit code was introduced in the second edition. The third edition was developed by an editorial board and published in 1973. The currently used fourth edition was first published in 1977, and represented significant updates in medical technology. In 1983, AMA and the Health Care Financing Association (HCFA) agreed to use CPT as part of HCFA Common Procedures Coding System (HCPCS) to report services for Part B of the Medicare program. In 1984, annual publication of CPT started. HCFA mandated the use of CPT codes to report outpatient procedures in 1987, when a procedure aiming to update CPT was also introduced to keep pace with the rapidly changing medical environment. In 1992, evaluation and management (E&M) codes were added to CPT.[1]

CPT EDITORIAL PANEL

The CPT Editorial Panel, which is made up of 16 physicians, is authorized to update CPT. Eleven of the 16 physicians are nominated by the AMA and one physician from each of BC/BS, Health Insurance Association of America, HCFA, and American Hospital Association. Of the 11 AMA seats, 8 are regular seats with a tenure of two 4-year terms; the 5 remaining seats are rotating seats and have 2-year terms each. The rotating seats allow for multidisciplinary input. The Executive Committee of the Panel includes the chairman, the vice chairman, and three other members elected by the entire panel. The AMA provides administrative staff support to the Panel. The staff is highly knowledgeable and very helpful. Staff members are readily available to help while an application is put together by providing suggestions on the appropriate language used in the nomenclature of a code or the most appropriate location in the CPT book for the new code to be housed. The Editorial Panel meets quarterly to address about 350 topics a year relating mainly to emerging technology.[2]

CPT ADVISORY COMMITTEE

The Advisory Committee is made up primarily of physicians nominated by national medical specialty societies represented in the AMA house of delegates. The Advisory Committee's primary role is to serve as a resource to the Editorial Panel by reviewing coding issues and by giving advice on appropriate nomenclature relevant to the Advisory member's specialty. In addition, the Advisory Committee provides opinions on the appropriateness of procedures under consideration for new codes. It also provides assistance in the preparation of technical education material and literature pertaining to coding. Members of the Advisory Committee help educate providers in their specialty on the use and benefits of CPT coding.[2] In addition, the Advisory Committee member, working in concert with various members of his or her specialty, puts together the application designed to introduce revisions of codes or new codes. Sometimes, the Advisory member works with members of other specialties to coproduce applications for codes used usually by various specialties (i.e., codes describing endovascular repair of AAA). Our National Vascular Societies are represented on the Advisory Committee.

THE APPLICATION PROCESS

An application for a new CPT code or a change or revision of an existing code can be submitted by physicians, medical specialty societies, state medical societies, or third-party payors. The process is initiated by submitting a rather lengthy application in which the coding change is proposed with full description of the code and, if new, where it should be housed. It is beneficial to have more than one society supporting the application, which contains many questions that should be answered accurately. Some examples are: Is the procedure FDA approved? What CPT codes are currently used to report the procedure, and why they are not adequate to report it? What is the incidence of the disease that the procedure is designed to diagnose/treat? How long has the procedure been provided for patients? How often does a physician in the specialty perform the procedure or service? In addition, a detailed vignette that describes the preoperative, intraoperative, and postoperative work should be included, describing in detail the skill and time involved in performing the procedure. Supporting documents such as operative reports, published articles in medical journals, and additional published literature that would further explain the request should be appended to the application.[1,2]

Once the application is submitted, the AMA staff reviews the application in detail. If the staff determines that the issue has been addressed by the panel, the staff corresponds with and informs the requestor of the panel's decision. However, if the staff feels that the request is new or new information was provided on a request that has been addressed by the Panel, the request is referred to appropriate members of the Advisory Committee. If those members agree that no new code is needed, the staff advises the requestor on how to use existing codes. If all advisors agree that a new code should be considered or a change should be made, or if two or more advisors disagree, the issue is referred to the Editorial Panel.[1]

The CPT Panel meets quarterly to address about 350 issues a year. The panel actions can result in one of three outcomes: (1) Add a new code or revise an existing one; (2) table an item to obtain further information; or (3) reject an item. Once a revision of a code or a new code is approved by the Editorial Panel, it is introduced in the CPT book. Usually, new CPT codes are implemented on January 1 of each year for federal programs. However, other third-party payors may not implement the new codes on the same date.[1]

NEW VASCULAR CPT CODES

In the following paragraphs recently approved CPT codes relating to vascular surgery are delineated. Although this chapter provides a source in which recently approved vascular codes are grouped together, it is very important to note that the reader, before using these codes, should consult the most recent CPT book published by the AMA for accurate description of the code.

Please note that the "+" sign is used to indicate "add-on" code, "●" is used to indicate a new code in the version of CPT being discussed, and "▲" is used to indicate a revised code.

NEW CODES IN THE 1999 CPT BOOK[3]

Upper Extremity Vein for Bypasses

+●35500 Harvest of upper extremity vein, one segment, for lower extremity bypass (for harvest of more than one vein segment, see 35682 and 35683)

Note: In CPT 2000, the add-on code sign (+) was inadvertently deleted, and the code was revised by cardiac surgery to include the use of upper extremity vein for coronary artery bypass

Composite Bypasses

+▲35681 Bypass graft, composite, prosthetic and vein (do not report with 35682 and 35683)

Note from author: In CPT 1999, this code was revised to add "prosthetic and vein"

+●35682 Autogenous composite, two segments of veins from two locations (do not report with 35681 and 35683)

+●35683 Autogenous composite, three segments of vein from two or more locations (do not report with 35681 and 35682)

Thrombectomy of Bypass Graft

▲35875 Thrombectomy of arterial or venous graft (other than hemodialysis graft or fistula) (for thrombectomy of hemodialysis graft or fistula, see 36831, 36833)

35876 with revision arterial or venous graft

Note from author: In CPT 1999, the code 35875 was revised to add "(other than hemodialysis graft or fistula)"

Thrombectomy and Revision of AV Access

●36831 Thrombectomy, arteriovenous fistula without revision, autogenous or nonautogenous dialysis graft (separate procedure)

▲36832 Revision, arteriovenous fistula, without thrombectomy, autogenous or nonautogenous dialysis graft (separate procedure)

Note from author: In CPT 1999, this code was revised to add "without thrombectomy."

●36833 With thrombectomy, autogenous or nonautogenous dialysis graft (separate procedure)

NEW CODES IN THE 2000 CPT BOOK[4]

Revision of Lower Extremity Bypasses

●35879 Revision, lower extremity arterial bypass, without thrombectomy, open; with vein patch angioplasty

●35881 with segmental vein interposition

Autogenous AV Access

●36819 Arteriovenous anastomosis, open; by basilic vein transposition

▲36821 Direct, any site (e.g., Cimino type) (separate procedure)

APPROVED CODES FOR THE 2001 CPT BOOK

Endovascular AAA repair has been performed under investigational protocols. Because there are no codes to describe such repairs, there has been no uniformity in coding these procedures. Recently, however, two endovascular devices were approved by the FDA for general use. Therefore, an application was submitted to create codes that describe various components of endovascular repair of AAA. The CPT Editorial Panel recently approved a new family of 14 codes. These codes follow the rules of *component coding*, meaning that more than one code is needed to describe a complete endovascular AAA repair. It is crucially important for vascular surgeons and their coders to familiarize themselves with the new family of codes and their accurate application. Because endovascular placement of prosthesis for AAA repair requires many different steps, component coding provides the flexibility needed for more accurate coding. Although these codes **cannot** be used until *CPT 2001* is published, the purpose of describing these codes in this chapter is to make the reader aware of what to expect, and to start planning for using these codes.

Endovascular AAA Prosthesis Implantation Codes

●34800 Endovascular repair of infrarenal abdominal aortic aneurysm or dissection; using aortoaortic tube prosthesis

●34802 using modular bifurcated prosthesis (one docking limb)

●34804 using unibody bifurcated prosthesis

+●34808 Endovascular placement of iliac artery occlusion device (list separately in addition to code for primary procedure)
(for radiological supervision and interpretation, use 75952 in conjunction with 34800, 34802, 34804, 34808)

Femoral and Iliac Artery Surgical Exposure

●34812 Open femoral artery exposure for delivery of aortic endovascular prosthesis, by groin incision; unilateral
(for bilateral procedure, use modifier "-50")

+●34813 Placement of femorofemoral prosthetic graft during endovascular aortic aneurysm repair (list separately in addition to code for primary procedure)
(use in conjunction with code 34812)

●34820 Open iliac artery exposure for delivery of endovascular prosthesis or iliac occlusion during endovascular therapy, by abdominal or retroperitoneal incision, unilateral
(for bilateral procedure, use modifier "-50")

Placement of Extension Prosthesis

●34825 Placement of proximal or distal extension prosthesis for endovascular repair of infrarenal abdominal aortic aneurysm; initial vessel

+●34826 each additional vessel (list separately in addition to code for primary procedure)
(Use 34826 in conjunction with code 34825)
(Use codes 34825 and 34826 in addition to codes 34800–34808 as appropriate)
(For staged procedure, use modifier "-58")
(For radiological supervision and interpretation, use 75953)

Open Repair of AAA Following Unsuccessful Endovascular Repair

●34830 Open repair of infrarenal aortic aneurysm or dissection, plus repair of associated arterial trauma, following unsuccessful endovascular repair; tube prosthesis

●34831 aortobi-iliac prosthesis

●34832 aortobifemoral prosthesis

Radiological Supervision and Interpretation (S&I) Codes

●75952 Endovascular repair of infrarenal abdominal aortic aneurysm or dissection, radiological supervision and interpretation
(For implantation of endovascular grafts, to be used with 34800–34808)

●75953 Placement of proximal or distal extension prosthesis for endovascular repair of infrarenal abdominal aortic aneurysm, radiological supervision and interpretation
(For implantation of endovascular extension prosthesis, to be used with 34825, 34826)

Other Codes that Can be Used During Endovascular AAA Repair

Other codes can also be used to describe important steps of this procedure. For example, placement of catheters in the aorta is important in placing the endovascular device; therefore, the already established code 36200 is used to describe this part of the procedure. Obviously, because catheters can be placed from both femoral arteries, the modifier "-50" for bilateral procedures can be added. Other procedures performed during endovascular AAA repair should be reported using already established codes. Examples of such procedures are angioplasty of native arteries with or without stent placement, arterial embolization, intravascular ultrasound, or renal arteriography and angioplasty.

Endovascular AAA Coding Example

Placement of endovascular prosthesis with one docking limb using surgical exposure of bilateral femoral arteries would be described using the following codes:

1. Modular bifurcated with one docking limb: 34802
2. Bilateral femoral exposure: 34812 and 34812-50
3. Placement of aortic catheters: 36200 and 36200-50
4. Radiological S&I: 75952

If a proximal extension is used, then the codes 34825 and 75953 are also added to the above. The flexibility of component coding becomes apparent if and when low-profile carriers are manufactured to allow percutaneous deployment of endovascular prosthesis. Then, femoral artery exposure codes are not used.

REFERENCES

1. CPT Process. Division of Payment Programs, Department of Coding and Nomenclature, American Medical Association, Chicago, IL, 1997.
2. Current Procedural Terminology. American Medical Association web site, http:/www.-assn.org/med-sci/cpt/process.htm.
3. CPT 1999. AMA CPT Editorial Staff. American Medical Association, Chicago, IL, 1998.
4. CPT 2000. AMA CPT Editorial Staff. American Medical Association, Chicago, IL, 1999.

9

Impact of Endovascular Technology on Decision Making for Abdominal Aortic Aneurysms

Jack L. Cronenwett, MD, and
Samuel R. G. Finlayson, MD, MPH

INTRODUCTION

Elective repair of abdominal aortic aneurysms (AAAs) is performed to prolong life in patients at risk for rupture. As with any prophylactic intervention, this requires a careful comparison of the risk and benefit—in this case, the risk of aneurysm rupture versus the risk of surgical repair. Furthermore, life expectancy must be considered because the benefit of aneurysm repair occurs incrementally over subsequent years whereas the risk of surgery occurs immediately. Finally, individual patient preferences vary considerably, from great fear of aneurysm rupture to great fear of surgical complications. For these reasons, decision making for elective AAA repair is complex. It has been further complicated by the introduction of endovascular technology, which has been shown to substantially reduce operative morbidity and, in some cases, operative mortality, because of its less invasive nature.[1,2] This has led to speculation about whether the threshold diameter for elective AAA repair should be reduced for endovascular repair. Theoretically, this would seem to be a logical conclusion. For any given-sized aneurysm, patients with lower operative risk stand to benefit more from elective repair. However, it is difficult to estimate the magnitude of this effect. How important is the reduced risk of endovascular repair compared with open repair? Should patients who would normally undergo elective, open AAA repair at a diameter of 5 cm undergo endovascular repair at a diameter of 4 cm? We have used decision analysis modeling to address these questions.

Decision Analysis Model

To understand the potential impact of endovascular surgery, one must first determine how the introduction of endovascular technology might change the balance of risks and benefits of early AAA repair. Endovascular technology does not change aneurysm rupture risk or patient life expectancy. Instead, it reduces surgical risk and may substantially change patient preference for a less-invasive operation. To investigate this effect, we have used decision analysis, a powerful technique that allows multiple variables to be studied individually, to determine their influence on the optimal decision. We used a Markov decision model of AAA disease for hypothetical patients for whom we could vary age, health status, aneurysm size, and operative risk.[3] In our model, each hypothetical patient cohort progresses in 1-month cycles, during which they are exposed to age- and disease-specific risks of death, aneurysm size–specific risks of rupture, and risks of surgery if this occurs. Based on this simulation, life expectancy for a given management strategy can be calculated as the average number of years of life accumulated by hypothetical patients in that cohort. In order to account for differences in quality of life that might result from operative morbidity, benefit is reported in quality-adjusted life years (QALYs), in which absolute survival is reduced based on patients' assessment of the impact of permanent complications, such as stroke or renal failure.

Probabilities for events experienced by patients in our decision analysis model were derived from the recent literature. One of the most important variables in the model is AAA rupture risk, which is difficult to estimate accurately, particularly in individual patients. Most surgeons estimate rupture risk based on AAA diameter. Among contemporary studies, the annual rupture rate ranged from 0% to 1% for aneurysms <4 cm diameter, from 0% to 12% for aneurysms 4 to 4.9 cm, and up to 25% for aneurysms >5 cm[3]. For our estimate, we used population-based data from Olmstead County, Minnesota, where the annual rupture risk was 1% per year for AAAs 4.0 to 4.9 cm in size, 11% per year for AAAs 5.0 to 5.9 cm in size, and 26% for AAAs 6 to 6.9 cm in size.[4] It is important to emphasize, however, that factors besides AAA diameter influence rupture risk in any given patient.[5] Other important risk factors for aneurysm rupture include smoking, chronic pulmonary disease (CPD), hypertension, rapid expansion, and a strong family history. Recently, female gender[6] and eccentric aneurysm shape[7] have also been found to be important predictors of rupture. Unfortunately, it is not possible to quantitate the influence of each of these factors on aneurysm rupture. For this reason, we have simplified our model to include only aneurysm diameter as the indicator of rupture risk. When considering individual patients, however, it is important to recognize that the presence of other risk factors for rupture increases the risk of any given size AAA. For our model, we assumed an average aneurysm expansion rate of 10% of the diameter per year.[8,9]

To estimate the mortality of elective open AAA repair, we used the age-stratified mortality risk from the Medicare claims data from 1995 in our model, where the overall 30-day mortality risk was 5.2%, but ranged from 3.0% for patients age 65 to 69 to 10.2% for patients over age 80.[3] This contrasts dramatically with the mortality from ruptured AAA repair in the same Medicare population, which averaged 46%, ranging from 35% for patients age 65 to 69, to 58% for patients over age 80.[3] Many other detailed risk estimates, such as morbidity of renal failure or stroke after open surgery and risk of death before surgery for AAA rupture, were derived from the literature and included in our model.

To estimate the morbidity and mortality of endovascular AAA repair, we used recent results from large series, including the US multicenter phase-II trials of the EVT and AneuRx endografts. Thus, for our base-case estimate, we used an elective operative mortality of 1% for endovascular repair, associated with a 5% need for early conversion to open repair, and a late conversion rate of 1%/year, based on a compilation of other recent publications.[1,2,10] Operative mortality was estimated at 11% for early conversion and at 7% for late conversion based on a large series.[11] Other factors, such as time to recovery after endovascular vs. open repair were also modeled. Because patients with AAAs have other comorbid diseases that shorten life expectancy compared with a normal population, we reduced expected survival using population-based studies of survival after successful AAA repair. We further reduced estimated life expectancy based on any permanent morbidities that resulted from surgery, to calculate quality-adjusted life expectancy. To simulate a subgroup of patients in poor health, we doubled the odds of expected operative mortality and reduced life expectancy to that of patients 8 years older.[3]

In order to determine the impact of all of these variables on decision making for AAAs, we used the decision model to calculate the optimal threshold diameter at which open vs. endovascular AAA repair would optimize quality-adjusted life expectancy. We then examined the impact of each variable over a range of plausible estimates (sensitivity analysis) to determine whether changes in this variable would have an important impact on the optimal threshold diameter at which to recommend elective AAA repair by either the open or endovascular technique.

RESULTS OF DECISION ANALYSIS

As expected, our model demonstrated that the optimal threshold diameter for endovascular AAA repair was always smaller than that for open repair because of the reduced surgical risk for endovascular repair.[3] However, for most patients, we found that the difference in optimal threshold diameter for open vs. endovascular repair was small, and did not exceed the 3 mm for men in average health up to age 80 (Table 9–1).

TABLE 9–1. OPTIMAL THRESHOLD DIAMETER FOR ELECTIVE AAA REPAIR

	Men in Average Health		Men in Poor Health	
Age (years)	*Endovascular (cm)*	*Open (cm)*	*Endovascular (cm)*	*Open (cm)*
60	4.6	4.6	4.7	4.7
70	4.7	4.8	4.9	5.0
80	4.9	5.1	5.7	8.1

In men of average health starting with 4 cm AAAs, compared with open surgery, endovascular surgery reduced the optimal threshold diameter from 4.6 to 4.6 cm (no change) at age 60; from 4.8 to 4.7 cm at age 70; and from 5.1 to 4.9 cm at age 80. For open surgery, this agrees with our previous analysis[12] and decision models by others[13] that indicated that life expectancy is optimized in most patients when AAAs are electively repaired at a diameter of 4.5 to 5 cm. The explanation for this finding is that AAA rupture risk appears to increase dramatically at a diameter of approximately 5 cm.[14] Again, it is important to emphasize that other risk factors for AAA rupture besides diameter can influence this threshold in individual patients. For example, in women, for whom risk of rupture appears to be higher, we would apply a slightly lower optimal threshold diameter, but cannot accurately quantitate this difference. Finally, it must be acknowledged that our estimates of outcome after endovascular repair are limited by the available literature. Some have suggested that these results will improve with more experience. However, even if we optimized our estimates for the outcome of endovascular repair (operative mortality 0.5%, permanent morbidity 0.5%, early conversion 1%, late conversion 0%), the optimal threshold for endovascular repair in 70-year-old men is only reduced to 4.6 cm compared with 4.7 cm in our base-case scenario. Thus, it is unlikely that future improvements in endovascular AAA repair will substantially change the threshold for recommending elective repair.

The finding that endovascular repair does not reduce optimal threshold diameter by more than several millimeters may initially be surprising. Many surgeons have estimated that the benefit of endovascular repair would lower the optimal threshold diameter considerably. The explanation for our finding is that the risk of aneurysm rupture has a much greater influence on optimal threshold diameter than does the small difference in elective operative mortality between open and endovascular repair.

The overall benefit of endovascular repair compared to open repair was consistent in our model, but was also relatively small. With an operative mortality of 1% in our model, endovascular repair always improved life expectancy compared with open repair, which had an average operative mortality of 5%. However, this benefit of endovascular repair was in the range of 0.1 to 0.4 QALYs, an improvement in life expectancy of only several months.[3] In comparison, a very effective procedure, such as coronary bypass surgery in 55-year-old men with three-vessel disease and severe angina provides a survival benefit of 1.4 QALYs compared with medical therapy.[15] Carotid endarterectomy in symptomatic patients of age 65 provides a survival benefit of 0.35 QALYs,[16] whereas endarterectomy in asymptomatic patients of average age 67 provides a survival benefit of 0.25 QALYs.[17] Thus, endovascular AAA repair provides a survival benefit over open AAA repair that is comparable to other commonly performed vascular operations. This survival benefit of endovascular vs. open AAA repair varies as a function of age, which in our model is directly related to life expectancy. Thus, for 60-year-old men at low operative risk for open AAA repair, endovascular repair provided a survival benefit of only 0.1 QALYs, whereas for 80-year-old men at higher operative risk for open repair the survival benefit for endovascular repair increased to 0.3 QALYs compared with open repair (Fig. 9–1).

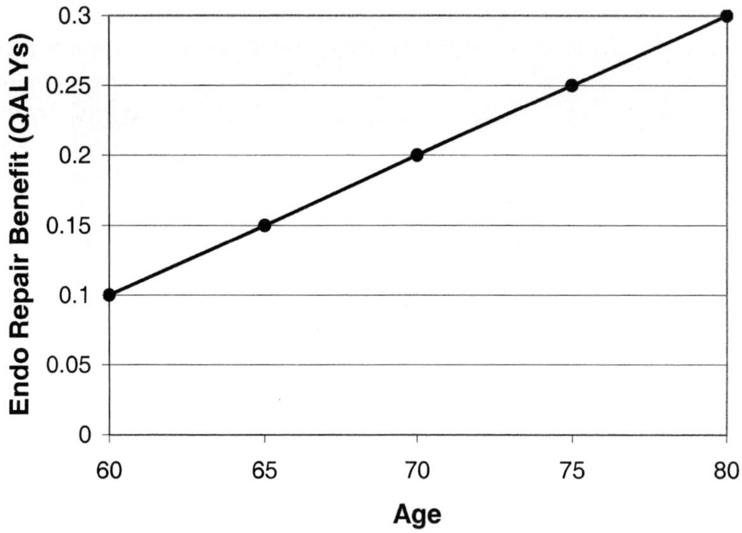

Figure 9–1. The quality-adjusted survival benefit of endovascular vs. open AAA repair increases with age as a result of increased operative mortality of open AAA repair in older men.

INFLUENCE OF SPECIFIC VARIABLES ON DECISION MAKING

Sensitivity analysis allowed us to measure the effect of individual variables in our model. For example, if we assumed a very low AAA rupture risk (odds reduced by twofold), the optimal threshold diameter for elective repair was increased, but only by 2 mm for both endovascular and open repair.[3] Varying the probability of early conversion after endovascular repair from 1% to 15% did not substantially change the benefit of endovascular surgery compared to open repair. The advantage of endovascular repair depends largely on the lower initial operative mortality. If this exceeds 3.5% or if the annual failure rate of endovascular repair (such as from endoleaks) exceeds 6% per year, the advantage of endovascular repair compared with open repair disappears. However, these estimates are well above the current range reported in the literature, suggesting that endovascular repair affords an improved survival benefit even after the long-term results of this procedure are better defined. In most cases, the benefit of endovascular repair compared with open repair depends on the difference in operative mortality of the two procedures (Fig. 9–2).

What about patients in poor health, patients with limited life expectancy and who have higher operative risk? Such patients are assumed to be ideal candidates for endovascular repair. In fact, our model demonstrated that the optimal threshold diameter for elective repair in such patients could be substantially lower for endovascular than open AAA repair. For example, in 80-year-old men in poor health, the optimal threshold diameter for elective open repair is 8.1 cm, whereas for endovascular repair it was substantially lower, at 5.7 cm.[3] However, because of the poor overall life expectancy in

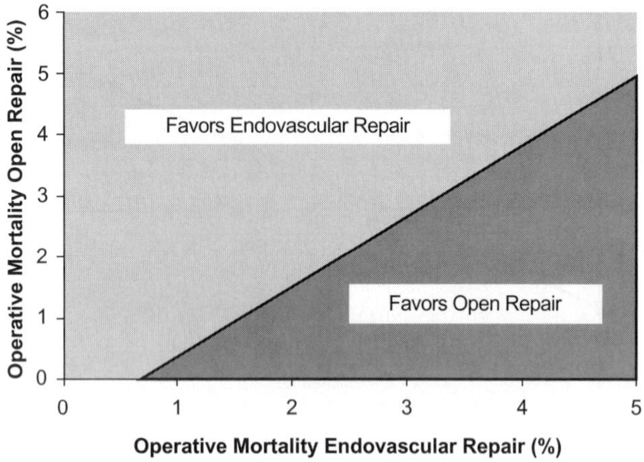

Figure 9–2. Two-way sensitivity analysis showing the effect of operative mortality on the optimal choice between endovascular and open AAA repair. Survival benefit favors endovascular and open repair in the shaded areas as shown, depending on the estimated operative mortality of each procedure.

such patients, the benefit of endovascular repair at this lower, optimal threshold diameter was only 0.2 QALYs, compared with open repair at the higher threshold diameter. This points out the irony that older, high-risk patients who benefit most from endovascular repair actually achieve only a small improvement in life expectancy after AAA repair because of death from other causes.

COST CONSIDERATIONS

How does the cost of new endovascular technology influence decision making for endovascular vs. open AAA repair? Because of development and production expenses, it is clear that endovascular grafts cost substantially more than conventional grafts used for open repair. Recent estimates of hospital costs for open AAA repair are approximately $12,500, compared with $20,000 for endovascular repair.[18] This is a substantial disincentive for hospitals to use the endovascular technique because this cost approaches or may exceed reimbursement.[18] However, cost analyses require a broader perspective than hospital costs alone and must account for differences in the benefit achieved by endovascular repair. Such a cost-effectiveness analysis has been reported by Patel et al.,[19] who demonstrated the cost-effectiveness ratio for endovascular compared to open repair to be $23,000 per QALY of additional survival. This is well within the range of cost-effectiveness, when compared with other generally accepted medical treatments. As expected, effectiveness of endovascular repair was specifically dependent on a substantial reduction in the combined mortality and long-term morbidity of endovascular compared with open repair, as described above. Thus, despite the higher device costs for endovascular AAA repair, this procedure appears cost-effective when compared to open repair. However, as also noted above, the benefit of endovascular repair compared to open repair is smaller than generally appreciated, which makes patient preferences an important consideration when making this decision.

SUMMARY

Endovascular AAA repair appears to reduce operative morbidity and mortality, shorten hospital stay, and allow more rapid recovery. For these reasons, patient preferences will promote the use of endovascular repair. Our finding of a net survival benefit of endovascular compared to open AAA repair suggests that the endovascular technique is optimal for patients in whom both approaches are feasible. However, our model is still limited by the lack of knowledge concerning long-term outcome of endovascular surgery, including the implications of both primary and secondary endoleak, and their potential impact on the risks and costs of subsequent intervention requirements. Despite this limitation, however, modeling over the plausible range of possible events suggests that endovascular repair retains a small benefit over open repair for most patients, and especially for those at higher operative risk. Overall, however, the impact of endovascular repair on the optimal threshold diameter for elective AAA repair is small, usually only several millimeters, or within the range of error of most imaging techniques. For high-risk patients, the impact on optimal threshold diameter is greater, but the benefit remains small. Thus, our results suggest that the optimal threshold for elective AAA repair remains in the range of 4.5 to 5.0 cm diameter for most patients, and that the introduction of endovascular technology should not significantly alter the indications for elective AAA repair.

REFERENCES

1. Zarins CK, White RA, Schwarten D, et al. AneuRx stent graft versus open surgical repair of abdominal aortic aneurysms: multicenter prospective clinical trial [see comments]. *J Vasc Surg*. 1999; 29(2):292–305; discussion 306–308.
2. Goldstone J, Brewster D, Chaikof E. Endoluminal repair versus standard open repair of abdominal aortic aneurysm: early results of a prospective clinical comparison trial. In 46th Scientific Meeting of the International Society for Cardiovascular Surgery. 1998.
3. Finlayson SR, et al. Should endovascular surgery lower the threshold for repair of abdominal aortic aneurysms? *J Vasc Surg*. 1999;29(6):973–985.
4. Reed WW, Hallett JW, Jr., Damiano MA, et al. Learning from the last ultrasound. A population-based study of patients with abdominal aortic aneurysm. *Arch Intern Med*. 1997; 157(18):2064–2068.
5. Cronenwett J, Krupski W, Rutherford R. Abdominal aortic and iliac aneurysms. In Rutherford R, ed. *Vascular Surgery*, Philadelphia, WB Saunders Co. 2000.
6. Brown LC, Powell JT. Risk factors for aneurysm rupture in patients kept under ultrasound surveillance. UK Small Aneurysm Trial Participants. *Ann Surg*. 1999;230(3):289–296; discussion 296–297.
7. Vorp DA, Raghavan ML, Webster MW. Mechanical wall stress in abdominal aortic aneurysm: influence of diameter and asymmetry [published erratum appears in *J Vasc Surg*. 1998;Aug. 28(2):272]. *J Vasc Surg*. 1998;27(4):632–639.

8. Cronenwett JL, Sargent SK, Wall MH, et al. Variables that affect the expansion rate and outcome of small abdominal aortic aneurysms. *J Vasc Surg.* 1990;11(2):260–268; discussion 268–269.
9. Limet R, Sakalihassan N, Albert A. Determination of the expansion rate and incidence of rupture of abdominal aortic aneurysms. *J Vasc Surg.* 1991;14(4):540–548.
10. Blum U, Voshage G, Lammer J, et al. Endoluminal stent-grafts for infrarenal abdominal aortic aneurysms [see comments]. *N Engl J Med.* 1997;336(1):13–20.
11. Jacobowitz GR, Lee AM, Riles TS. Immediate and late explantation of endovascular aortic grafts: the endovascular technologies experience. *J Vasc Surg.* 1999;29(2):309–316.
12. Katz DA, Littenberg B, Cronenwett JL. Management of small abdominal aortic aneurysms. Early surgery vs watchful waiting. *JAMA.* 1992;268(19):2678–2686.
13. Michaels JA. The management of small abdominal aortic aneurysms: a computer simulation using Monte Carlo methods. *Eur J Vasc Surg.* 1992;6(5):551–557.
14. Brown PM, Pattenden R, Vernooy C, et al. Selective management of abdominal aortic aneurysms in a prospective measurement program. *J Vasc Surg.* 1996;23(2):213–220; discussion 221–222.
15. Wong JB, Sonnenberg FA, Salem DN, et al. Myocardial revascularization for chronic stable angina. Analysis of the role of percutaneous transluminal coronary angioplasty based on data available in 1989 [see comments]. *Ann Intern Med.* 1990;113(11):852–871.
16. Kuntz KM, Kent KC. Is carotid endarterectomy cost-effective? An analysis of symptomatic and asymptomatic patients. *Circulation.* 1996;94(9 Suppl):II194–II198.
17. Cronenwett JL, Birkmeyer JD, Nackman GB, et al. Cost-effectiveness of carotid endarterectomy in asymptomatic patients. *J Vasc Surg.* 1997;25(2):298–309; discussion 310–311.
18. Sternbergh WC 3rd, Money SR. Hospital cost of endovascular versus open repair of abdominal aortic aneurysms: a multicenter study. *J Vasc Surg.* 2000;31(2):237–244.
19. Patel ST, Haser PB, Bush HL, Jr., et al. The cost-effectiveness of endovascular repair versus open surgical repair of abdominal aortic aneurysms: a decision analysis model. *J Vasc Surg.* 1999;29(6):958–972.

10

Lessons Learned from European Endovascular Graft Registry

S. Rao Vallabhaneni, FRCS, and
Peter L. Harris, MD, FRCS

INTRODUCTION

Endovascular repair of abdominal aortic aneurysms is applicable in a rising proportion of aneurysm patients as the experience of physicians increases and the range of devices expands. Successful deployment of the endograft can be achieved in more than 97% of the patients with a 30-day mortality rate ≦3%.[1] Operative mortality has been low despite a tendency to select patients with a relatively high incidence of major comorbidities for this treatment. Therefore, the short-term benefits of this approach are not really points of issue.

The primary objective of treatment in the long-term is to prevent the death of the patient as a result of rupture of the aneurysm. Therefore, rupture and death from rupture are noncontentious primary or "hard" end-points for the evaluation of long-term results. A requirement to undertake open surgery in order to replace the endoluminal device with a conventionally sutured graft, for whatever reason, is also unequivocal evidence of failure of the endovascular procedure, and therefore a valid primary end-point. Worldwide experience of endovascular aneurysm repair (EVAR) spans less than one decade, and the vast majority of patients with endografts have been treated within the last year or two. Published reports on the longer-term results of treatment of infrarenal aortic aneurysms using intraluminal endografts have been based on relatively small numbers of patients with a short duration of follow-up.[2–5] The crucial issue continues to be the long-term efficacy of EVAR, and in this chapter we address this with reference to data available from the Eurostar database.

THE EUROSTAR PROJECT

In most European countries, access to endovascular devices has been less restricted than in other parts of the world, most notably the United States. For this reason, Europe represented a very suitable setting for a study that aims to recruit as many patients as possible as quickly as possible in order to develop a database large enough to assess the efficacy of intra-aortic stent grafting within the shortest time possible. The EUROSTAR[6] (EUROpean collaborators on Stent-graft Techniques for Abdominal Aortic Aneurysm Repair) Project was launched in 1996 as a large-scale multicentered international study with the objective of collating information on the results of endovascular treatment of abdominal aortic aneurysms (AAAs). By January 2000, physicians from 88 centers in 16 European countries had registered a total of 2194 patients, making it one of the most successful registries of this type. In order to eliminate bias due to selective reporting, the study protocol requires that all eligible patients be notified to the Data Registry Centre at least 24 hr prior to their operation. Data is collected prospectively, using a standardized protocol for follow-up and reporting of events. The Eurostar database has now reached a size that for the first time allows quantification of the risk and the significance of risk factors in terms of the hard endpoints[7] for evaluation of EVAR.

Patients, Aneurysms, Endografts, and Follow-up[8]

The mean age of the patients was 70.4 yr (range 37–92 yr) with a male : female ratio of 11 : 1. The operative risk profile of the patients according to the ASA classification included ASA 1, 188 (8.9%); ASA 2, 808 (38.1%); ASA 3, 972 (46%); and ASA 4, 153 (7.2%). Smoking, hypertension, and cardiac disease were the most prevalent risk factors. Five hundred sixty-seven patients had had previous laparotomy, 282 patients were considered to be unfit for conventional open surgery, and 89 patients were considered to be unfit for general anaesthesia.

Contrast-enhanced computed tomography (CT) scanning combined with calibrated angiography was the method of choice for preoperative assessment with the majority of the physicians. The mean maximal transverse diameter of the aneurysms was 56.29 mm (range 18–150 mm). The mean of the neck diameters of the aneurysms was 22.61 mm (range 10–40 mm), and the mean neck length was 27.9 mm (range 5–110 mm). There were associated aneurysms of the common iliac arteries in 35% of the patients.

Only devices with European regulatory approval (CE mark) were eligible for inclusion in the study. Bifurcated endovascular stent/grafts were used in 92% of the patients (2017). The make and manufacturer of the devices are shown in Table 10–1.

Patients were assessed clinically and by contrast-enhanced CT scans at 1, 3, 6, 12, and 18 months after operation and at yearly intervals thereafter. Color Duplex ultrasound examination with or without contrast enhancement was also undertaken in a number of centers. Aortography, although mandatory according to the original study protocol at 12 months, was subsequently undertaken only when indicated by the results of CT imaging and at the discretion of the responsible physician. Plain x-rays were included in the follow-up since 1998 to detect impending problems from stent/graft

TABLE 10–1. MAKE AND MANUFACTURER OF STENT–GRAFTS USED IN PATIENTS FROM THE EUROSTAR DATABASE

Device	Number of Patients (%)
Stentor (Mintec, La Ciotat, France)	336 (15.4)
Vanguard (Boston Scientific/Meadox Medical, Oakland, NJ)	869 (39.9)
AneuRx (Medtronic, Sunnyvale, CA)	389 (17.8)
Talent (World Medical, Sunrise, FL)	290 (13.3)
Zenith (Cook, Indianapolis, IN)	123 (5.6)
Ancure (Endovascular Technologies, Menlo Park, CA)	58 (2.7)
Excluder (WL Gore, Flagstaff, AZ)	77 (3.5)
Other	38 (1.7)

distortion and suture breakage leading to strut dislocations. Data reported to the Data Registry Centre included all adverse events.

EARLY RESULTS

The early results were encouraging, with a high rate (97.8%) of successful deployment of the endoluminal device. Conversion to open repair was undertaken at the time of the initial procedure in 28 patients (1.3%). There were 113 deaths in the first postoperative month, giving a 30-day mortality rate of 2.1%. The operative mortality rates were favorable compared to open repair, with 1.0% for ASA 2 patients and 1.6% for ASA 1 patients. The mortality was higher for patients in ASA classes 4 and 3 patients at 9.2% and 2.2%, respectively, indicating that death was related primarily to comorbidity. The overall technical success rate as defined by the Ad Hoc Committee of the SVS/ISCVS[9] was 72%. However, the crucial issue for the evaluation of the technique has been the long-term efficacy.

INTERMEDIATE TO LONG-TERM FOLLOW-UP

Considerable attention has been focused on secondary or "soft" end-points, including endoleak,[10] persistent endoleak,[1] and secondary intervention.[11] However, evidence to confirm that any of these represents a reliable indicator of the eventual outcome of treatment is lacking. A secondary intervention to correct or prevent an impending complication in itself does not represent a failure of EVAR, but the study of secondary interventions is relevant for several reasons: They are important to prevent failure in terms of the hard end-points. They are not always minor and may be associated with a mortality risk. They appear to be required in a much higher proportion of patients compared to the conventional repair, and therefore may influence the outcome of clinical trials. Finally, there are financial implications that must be taken into account in calculations of the overall cost of the treatment.

The size of the Eurostar cohort made it possible for the first time to quantify not only the incidence of late rupture, death, and conversion, but also to elucidate the risk factors for these events.[7]

LATE RUPTURE AND DEATH FROM LATE RUPTURE

Lumsden et al.[12] confirmed there is some risk that the aneurysm may still rupture following endovascular repair. A total of 15 patients registered with EUROSTAR developed unequivocal evidence of rupture of their aneurysm at intervals from 1 to 24 mo after operation (mean 14 mo) based on findings at reoperation, CT images, or the results of postmortem examination. The peak incidence of rupture occurred at 18 mo after operation (range 3–24 mo). Emergency open surgery was undertaken in 8 patients, 5 of whom survived. There were no survivors among the patients who were not subjected to emergency operation. Another 10 patients died suddenly from unknown causes, at least 3 of whom had aneurysms with a maximal diameter in excess of 6 cm shortly before their death. Although cardiac and other causes are possible, rupture of the aneurysm is likely to account for some of these 10 deaths. If account is taken only of those patients in whom the diagnosis was confirmed, the cumulative rupture rate, calculated by life table analysis, approximates to 1.0% per annum.

It has been reported previously that rupture following endovascular aneurysm repair is associated with a lower mortality risk than might be expected otherwise.[13] The present small series of 8 patients who underwent emergency open repair following rupture, 5 (63%) of whom survived, might be considered to support this contention. However, another 7 patients who were not operated on died also, giving an overall mortality rate of 67%, which is in line with expectations following rupture of an AAA.[14]

LATE CONVERSION

Conversion to open repair of an aneurysm previously treated by endovascular repair is a serious undertaking. In the EUROSTAR series, this procedure was undertaken in 31 patients. The average cumulative rate of conversion was 2.1% per year, with a peak incidence at 18 mo. The mortality rate associated with all operations for conversion to open repair was 19%. This is approximately six times higher than that associated with primary open repair of an AAA. Therefore, it is not a procedure to be undertaken lightly. The responsible physician must be convinced that the risk of rupture of the aneurysm or other life- or limb-threatening disaster is substantially greater than the risk of conversion before recommending this course of action to the patient.

THE RISK FACTORS FOR LATE RUPTURE AND LATE CONVERSION

The risk factors for late rupture and late conversion are shown in Table 10–2. The Eurostar experience has drawn attention to some expected but some surprising risk fac-

TABLE 10–2. RISK FACTORS FOR LATE RUPTURE AND LATE CONVERSION

Proximal endoleak
Mid-graft endoleak
Type II endoleak
Distal endoleak
Kinked endograft
Stent migration
Stent thrombosis

tors for late rupture and late conversion. The importance of proximal fixation site endoleak and therefore the urgent need to correct this problem are confirmed. By contrast, distal fixation site endoleak did not have a significant impact on the risk of rupture. It is possible that distal endoleaks do not increase the pressure within the sac of the aneurysm (endotension) to a dangerously high level; but it is also the case that endoleaks at this site can usually be resolved by relatively minor secondary endovascular procedures. This does not usually apply to proximal fixation site endoleaks.

Oversewing of the infrarenal side branches is an integral part of conventional open surgery. Occluding them is not a routine part of endovascular treatment, and type II endoleaks due to perfusion of the sac from these vessels are seen in 10% to 20% of patients. Some resolve spontaneously, and their clinical implications are uncertain. The Eurostar finding that type-II endoleak is a significant risk factor for rupture of the aneurysm has renewed interest in prophylactic management of aortic side branches. Preoperative embolization of selected patent side branches at one center failed to show any significant impact during the follow-up.[15] To reduce the incidence of type-II endoleaks, a policy of preoperative side branch embolization would appear to require targeting of all infrarenal side branches. This is technically very difficult to achieve. There are reports from one center, independent of Eurostar, claiming encouraging results in terms of preventing type-II endoleaks by inserting an absorbable into a gelatin or polyvinyl alcohol sponge in the perigraft space.[16]

Contraction of the sac in its longitudinal dimension following its effective exclusion from arterial pressure[17] and radial forces generated by blood flowing through curved or angulated grafts results in kinking of intra-aneurysmal stent/grafts. Kinking causes stent/graft thrombosis after a critical angle, leading to limb ischaemia. More importantly, it can result in disassociation of the components of modular devices, causing a midgraft endoleak or precipitate a distal fixation site endoleak. A direct relationship between kinking of the device and the risk of eventual rupture of the aneurysm has been shown by the Eurostar data.[7] Kink resistance should be an important feature of future generations of endovascular stent/grafts.

Stent migration is also a device-related issue that Eurostar found to be significantly associated with rupture of the aneurysm and that similarly must be addressed by appropriate improvements in the design of endoluminal stent/grafts.

It is important to take account of the fact that, inevitably, reports from Eurostar reflect mainly the earliest generations of endovascular devices and especially those associated with Vanguard I and II (Boston Scientific Corporation/Meadox Medical, Oakland, NJ). It is possible that the newer generations of endografts will perform differently, but this remains to be proved.

ENDOTENSION, THE MAIN ENEMY

Most of the early reports of EVAR concentrated on the presence or absence of an endoleak. The rationale for using endoleak as an indicator of failure of treatment is based on an assumption that in its presence, aneurysms will continue to expand and eventually rupture. However, it is well established now that the correlation between the presence or absence of endoleak and postoperative change in the morphology of the aneurysm sac is poor.[18] Furthermore, rupture and expansion of aneurysms after endovascular repair without detectable endoleak have been well documented. The Laplace Principle tells us that it is pressure, or *endotension*,[19,20] rather than flow within the aneurysm sac that causes it to expand and rupture. Endotension may be present in the absence of detectable flow.[18] As a concept, endotension purely denotes the distending forces still acting on the walls of a treated aneurysm. Its importance is that, if untreated, it may lead to eventual rupture. It is a pathophysiological phenomenon for which there is no clinically safe method of direct measurement over long term into the follow-up. Therefore, the presence or absence of endotension must be inferred from the morphologic changes in the treated aneurysm. Continued expansion or reexpansion of the sac postoperatively is a sure indication of endotension, and therefore a strong indication for secondary intervention.

SECONDARY INTERVENTIONS AND IMPLICATIONS FOR FOLLOW-UP

Nearly one-third of the cohort underwent a cumulative total of 266 secondary interventions, not counting the late conversions, by 48 mo of follow-up. There were 60 secondary interventions within 30 days of the primary EVAR. The remainder were undertaken after this time, and there is no sign of a decline in the incidence with time up to 48 mo. Transfemoral interventions formed the bulk (82% of the total), whereas transabdominal interventions (4.1%) and extra-anatomical secondary interventions (13.9%) contributed to the rest.

The rates of secondary intervention surprisingly remained constant, at approximately 10% per annum throughout the follow-up without any signs of abatement. This suggests that a structured and methodical follow-up is mandatory for the life of an EVAR recipient.

MORTALITY FOLLOWING EVAR

Aneurysm-related mortality accounts for around 1.5% of all deaths following open aneurysm repair, according to published reports.[21] In the Eurostar cohort of 2194, there were 161 deaths between 1 and 48 mo after EVAR. The causes of death were as follows: cardiac, 28.6%; malignancy, 18.6%; cerebrovascular, 6.8%; respiratory, 3.1%; renal, 1.8%; other, 22.3%; and aneurysm-related mortality, 11.8%. *Aneurysm-related mortality* was defined as death resulting directly from rupture of the repaired aneurysm or another complication of the aneurysm >30 days after repair or death within 30 days of a secondary intervention undertaken solely to rectify a complication of repair. There were a total of 19 deaths from aneurysm-related causes: 9 patients died following proved rupture of their treated aneurysm, 3 died from presumed rupture of their aneurysm, and a further 7 patients died following late conversion (3), graft sepsis (2), and secondary intervention (2). Sudden death of uncertain cause occurred in 10 patients as mentioned earlier, in whom rupture of AAA is a possibility but not proved. Non-aneurysm-related causes of death were comparable to published reports of survival after open repair. However, the proportion of aneurysm-related mortality (11.8%) was appreciably higher than that reported after open repair. These results may reflect the learning curve experience of the teams involved, but continued caution is advisable regarding expectations of outcome from EVAR.

CONCLUSION

The European experience has no doubt contributed significantly to the current understanding of EVAR. It also demonstrates that large databases can be managed successfully across nations for expeditious clinical evaluation of medical techniques. The initial enthusiasm spurred on by low operative mortality rates and faster recovery has been dampened by the emergence of intermediate-term results showing a high risk of both serious and minor late adverse events. Elucidation of the risk factors to guide clinical practice and the further evolution of stent/graft design points the way to improved results in the future. In this way, the Eurostar experience has been and continues to be an important source of information for the medical fraternity and the endovascular grafting industry.

REFERENCES

1. Cuypers P, Buth J, Gevers E, et al. Realistic expectations for patients with stent–graft treatment of abdominal aortic aneurysms. Results of a European multicentre registry. *Eur J Vasc Endovasc Surg*. 1999;17(6):507–516.
2. Matsumara JS, Pearce WH. Early clinical results and studies of aortic aneurysm morphology after endovascular repair. *Surg Clin N Am*. 1999;79(3):529–540.
3. Chuter TA, Gordon RL, Reilly LM, et al. Abdominal aortic aneurysm in high-risk patients: short- to intermediate-term results of endovascular repair. *Radiology*. 1999;210(2):361–365.
4. Zarins CK, White RA, Schwarten D, et al., for the investigators of the Medtronic AneuRx Multicenter Clinical trial. *J Vasc Surg*. 1999;29:292–308.
5. Becquemin J-P, Lapie V, Favre J-P, Rousseau H, for the French Vanguard study group. Midterm results of a second generation bifurcated endovascular graft for abdominal aortic aneurysm repair: the French Vanguard trial. *J Vasc Surg*. 1999;30:209–218.

6. Harris PL, Buth J, Mialhe C, Myhre HO, Norgren L. The need for clinical trials of endovascular abdominal aortic aneurysm stent graft repair: the EUROSTAR project. EUROpean collaborators on Stent-graft Techniques for abdominal aortic Aneurysm Repair. *J Endovasc Surg.* 1997;4(1):72–79.
7. Harris PL, Vallabhaneni SR, Desgranges P, Becquemin J-P, Laheij RJF, on behalf of the Eurostar Collaborators. Late rupture, conversion and death following endovascular repair of infra-renal aortic aneurysm: incidence and risk factors. *J Vasc Surg.* (in press).
8. Progress report including the data of the overall patients cohort Eurostar Data Registry Centre January 2000. *www.esvs.org/esvs/eurostarwebsite.html*
9. Ahn SS, Rutherford RB, Johnston KW, et al. Reporting standards for infrarenal endovascular aneurysm repair. *J Vasc Surg.* 1997;25:405–410.
10. Cuypers P, Buth J, Tielbeek A, Gardien M, Idu M. Endovascular abdominal aortic aneurysm repair. First experiences regarding 20 patients in Eindhoven. *Ned Tijdschr Geneeskd.* 1997;141(28):1385–1390.
11. May J, White GH, Waugh R, et al. Adverse events after endoluminal repair of abdominal aortic aneurysms: a comparison during two successive periods of time. *J Vasc Surg.* 1999;29:32–39.
12. Lumsden AB, Allen RC, Chaikof EL, et al. Delayed rupture of aortic aneurysms following endovascular stent grafting. *Am J Surg.* 1995;170:174–178.
13. May J, White GH, Waugh R, et al. Rupture of abdominal aortic aneurysms: a concurrent comparison of outcome of those occuring after endoluminal repair versus those occuring *de novo. Eur J Vasc Endovasc Surg.* 1999;18:344–348.
14. Kantonen I, Lepäntalo M, Brommels M, et al., and the Finnvasc Study group. Mortality in ruptured abdominal aortic aneurysms. *Eur J Vasc Endovasc Surg.* 1999;17:208–212.
15. Anbarasu A, Gould DA, McWilliams RG, et al. Experience and follow-up of aortic side-branch embolisation in AAA endovascular repair. Presented at IOS2000–Imaging, Oncology, Science. 22–24 May 2000, Birmingham, UK.
16. Maclerewicz J, Hopkinson BR. Vascular Surgical Society of Great Britain and Ireland: prevention of limbar artery endoleaks following endovascular abdominal aortic aneurysm repair with the selective use of absorbable gelatin sponge. *Br J Surg.* 1999;86(5):697.
17. Harris P, Brennan J, Martin J, et al. Longitudinal aneurysm shrinkage following endovascular aortic aneurysm repair: a source of intermediate and late complications. *J Endovasc Surg.* 1999;6(1):11–16.
18. Gilling-Smith GL, Martin J, Sudhindran S, et al. Freedom from endoleak after endovascular aneurysm repair does not equal treatment success. *Eur J Vasc Endovasc Surg.* 2000;19(4):421–425.
19. Gilling-Smith G, Brennan J, Harris P, et al. Endotension after endovascular aneurysm repair: definition, classification and strategies for surveillance and intervention. *J Endovasc Surg.* 1999;6:305–307.
20. White GH, May J, Petrasek P, Waugh R, Stephen M, Harris J. Endotension: an explanation for continued AAA growth after successful endoluminal repair. *J Endovasc Surg.* 1999;6:308–315.
21. Johnston KW. Nonruptured abdominal aortic aneurysm: six-year follow-up results from the multicentre prospective Canadian aneurysm study. *J Vasc Surg.* 1994;20(2):163–170.

11

Treatment of Abdominal Aortic Aneurysms in Patients with Significant Comorbidities

Marshall W. Webster, MD

INTRODUCTION

In the nearly 50 years since the initial open resection of an abdominal aortic aneurysm (AAA) by Dubost, great strides have been made in the operative techniques and graft materials available to vascular surgeons, including the ability to manage intraoperatively many complex aneurysms, such as inflammatory AAA, or aneurysms with associated anatomic abnormalities, such as a horseshoe kidney. The mortality from elective AAA resection in most hospitals is <5%, and is frequently reported as 2% to 3%.[1]

Corresponding dramatic advances in the medical management of chronic diseases, such as coronary artery atherosclerosis and chronic obstructive pulmonary disease, have now made it possible to undertake resection of AAA in patients who might previously have been considered high, or even prohibitive, operative risks. Although the endovascular repair of AAA holds great promise of reducing operative risk, many patients are as yet not manageable by this emerging technology. Ultimately, however, these endovascular techniques may extend even further the number of patients with associated medical diseases who may be repaired with reasonable safety. In fact, there may ultimately be no absolute contraindication to repair of AAA when the indications are appropriate.

The majority of patients with AAA, simply by virtue of the age of onset of this disease alone, have some degree of concomitant diseases. Nearly all patients with AAA have a history of past or current cigarette smoking. Significant coronary artery disease is present in approximately one-half of all patients with AAA. Obesity is common, although in the elderly, malnutrition may be evident, and anemia is not unusual.

Hypertension is frequent. Clinical dehydration may be present in patients who have undergone angiography in the previous 24 to 48 hr. Electrolyte abnormalities, such as hypokalemia, may be found secondary to the medical treatment of other underlying disorders. There is also the potential of impaired wound healing from chronic steroid use.

GENERAL EVALUATION AND CONSIDERATIONS

The need for a careful history and physical examination is never more important than in this setting. A full recognition of underlying medical conditions, as well as their past and present therapy, is vital for determining if further preoperative evaluation is required and for careful preoperative preparation. Routine preoperative laboratory tests should include electrolytes, BUN, creatinine, CBC with differential, and platelet count. A baseline electrocardiogram and chest x-ray should be routine. Most patients have computerized axial tomography or magnetic resonance imaging of their AAA preoperatively, and these studies may detect associated abnormalities such as intrabdominal malignancies. Appropriate medical consultation and specialty support pre- and postoperatively should be obtained. Steyerberg et al.[2] attempted to develop a numeric clinical prediction rule for operative risk based primarily on a meta-analysis of published series of AAA resections, but this does not really replace the approach to any specific patient. Regrettably, this preoperative assessment is not possible in patients requiring emergency surgery for a ruptured or leaking AAA.

Age alone should not be considered a major contraindication to elective aortic resection. A number of reported series[3–5] have found only modest increase in morbidity and mortality from elective resection in octogenarians if they are otherwise in good health. Life expectancy, however, may be a consideration. Patients older than 80 years on average have a higher severity of illness score, and coexisting illnesses may be the explanation for the minimal increased risk rather than age per se. Individuals 80 years old have an expected life expectancy of 6 to 8 years. Even a moderately increased surgical risk, regardless of age, may not be acceptable in a patient with a limited life expectancy and possibly marginal indications for AAA repair. Large AAAs (>6 cm diameter) are always a more compelling indication for surgery than smaller ones, and symptomatic or rapidly expanding AAA are always a serious concern.

Regardless of the associated medical problems, a carefully planned and performed technical operation, minimizing blood loss and tissue trauma, reduces the likelihood of postoperative complications. Monitoring pulmonary wedge pressure with a Swan–Ganz catheter and cardiac function with transesophageal echocardiography assists in optimizing intraoperative management. Similarly, attentive monitoring and care postoperatively, especially regarding fluid replacement, with early ambulation, minimizing nasogastric tubes, and good prophylaxis for venous thromboembolism are all important for reducing postoperative complications, which may cascade in the patient with serious underlying medical conditions or loss of reserves.

CARDIAC DISEASE

In general, the most common and serious medical disorder increasing the risk of resection of AAA is coronary artery disease. The landmark study by Hertzer et al.[6] from the Cleveland Clinic established the high prevalence of coronary atherosclerosis in this population through a large series of patients who underwent routine coronary angiography preoperatively. Although routine cardiac catheterization is not recommended today, the appropriate strategy for detecting potentially critical myocardial ischemia and predicting postoperative cardiac events still remains somewhat controversial.

Rational strategies for cardiac assessment have recently been outlined by Wakefield and Stanley[7] and by Won et al.[8] In general, asymptomatic patients without a history of angina, myocardial infarction, congestive heart failure, significant dysrhythmias, or diabetes, and who have a normal electrocardiogram do not require a formal cardiac evaluation. Patients with a history suggesting myocardium at risk for possible perioperative infarction or who have had a prior myocardial infarction should undergo, at a minimum, physiological testing for reversible perfusion abnormalities. Most commonly, this is by thallium scanning. Although some nuclear cardiology laboratories are unwilling to perform exercise thallium testing on patients with AAA, preferring pharmacologic stress testing (adenosine), this does not appear to be a justified concern,[9] at least for aneurysms <6 cm in diameter. Our bias is to proceed with exercise thallium scanning unless claudication or some other limiting condition exists. When thallium scanning or stress (dobutamine) echocardiography suggests myocardium at risk, cardiac catheterization and coronary angiography are necessary preoperatively, with intervention by angioplasty or coronary bypass if indicated. Despite some concern over an increased risk of AAA rupture in patients undergoing other operative procedures, especially coronary bypass, that risk does not seem excessive and is outweighed by the risk of myocardial infarction perioperatively in patients with untreated myocardial ischemia undergoing AAA resection.[6,10] Concurrent coronary bypass and AAA resection is not recommended by most surgeons, but AAA resection should not be delayed unduly following coronary revascularization.

Overall, the patients at highest risk are those with a recent myocardial infarction (<3 months) and patients with a history of congestive heart failure or a low ejection fraction (<35%). These patients represent the most formidable challenges, and elective aneurysm repair should be undertaken only with careful consideration and good cardiology support, as well as specialized intraoperative management and postoperative care.

In all patients undergoing peripheral vascular operations, including AAA resection, several large controlled trials have unequivocally demonstrated that beta blockade substantially reduces the risk of perioperative coronary events and should be used in all patients unless there is a specific contraindication.[11,12] Patients with cardiac valvular disease, especially aortic stenosis, or who have had prosthetic valve replacements frequently require special management and manipulation of anticoagulation during the perioperative period.

Patients with hypertension for whom there is the suspicion that the etiology may be renal vascular disease should undergo appropriate testing and ultimately angiography if indicated, so that renal revascularization may be considered at the time of resection of the aneurysm. This is rarely required, and adding a renal artery bypass increases the overall operative risk of aneurysm resection.

PULMONARY DISEASE

Traditionally, patients with chronic obstructive pulmonary disease, especially patients who are oxygen dependent, have been considered at very high or even prohibitive risk from operation. The paradox is that this patient group may also be the one at highest risk of spontaneous AAA rupture if treated expectantly. Fortunately, with careful management, resection can be undertaken with only minimally increased risk. In the preoperative evaluation, a good pulmonary history is important. Patients should attempt to discontinue tobacco use weeks or months prior to surgery, although most patients with end stage pulmonary disease and oxygen dependency have already stopped smoking. If no pulmonary symptoms are present, and the patient is able to walk up several flights of stairs without dyspnea, no further pulmonary evaluation is required. Patients who are symptomatic require more formal pulmonary function tests and baseline blood gas measurements while breathing room air. Patients at high risk from operation because of pulmonary insufficiency are those who are oxygen dependent, have a PaO_2 $\leq$60 mmHg, $PaCO_2$ $\geq$45 mmHg, forced expiratory volume in 1 sec (FEV_1) $\leq$50% of predicted, and forced vital capacity (FVC) $\leq$75% of predicted.

Meticulous preoperative preparation with breathing exercises, elimination of underlying pulmonary infectious processes, and use of bronchodilator therapy and steroid therapy in selected patients reduces the likelihood of postoperative complications. A clinical pathway that emphasizes limited perioperative fluid administration, early extubation, pulmonary toilet, and early ambulation is important. Epidural anesthesia for relief of postoperative pain and improved ventilation is helpful. In these pulmonary cripples, as well as many other medically precarious patients, a retroperitoneal incision for AAA resection may reduce the risk of complications.[13] Using these adjuncts, we recently reported a series of 14 consecutive oxygen-dependent patients who underwent AAA resection with no mortality and minimal morbidity.[14] All patients were extubated within 24 hr and no patient developed pneumonia. Only one patient was in the intensive care unit for more than 24 hr. During this period, four additional patients were denied operation as prohibitive risks. Given this experience and that of others,[2] chronic pulmonary insufficiency should not be considered a contraindication to surgery if the AAA resection is warranted, based on objective parameters. The further refinement of endovascular techniques may nearly eliminate the special risks of this group of patients.

GASTROINTESTINAL DISEASE

Patients who have underlying chronic gastrointestinal disorders such as peptic ulcer disease, inflammatory bowel disease, or chronic hepatic failure must be assessed appropriately. Postoperative control of gastric acid production and compensation for longstanding steroid administration and preoperative correction of malnutrition and coagulopathies are essential. Patients with cirrhosis and even moderate hepatic failure, especially patients with ascites and coagulopathy, represent very high operative risks, and should be accepted for operation with great caution. If required, simultaneous liver transplantation and resection of AAA may be undertaken with some success, and has been performed in at least three patients in our institution.

HEMATOLOGIC DISORDERS

In the past, severe congenital and acquired coagulopathies, particularly hypocoagulable states such as hemophilia, have been considered nearly absolute contraindications to operations of the magnitude of AAA resection. Modern diagnostic capabilities identifying specific bleeding abnormalities and specific factor replacement therapy have made resection feasible for nearly all patients with disorders of the intrinsic and extrinsic coagulation pathways and the thrombocytopenias, regardless of etiology.[15,16] It should be noted that the AAA alone, when associated with intraluminal thrombus, may induce a fibinolytic state.[17] Close collaboration with a hematologist and a specialized blood bank are critical to successful management of the severe coagulopathies.

UROLOGIC AND RENAL DISORDERS

Chronic renal failure, although always a concern, should not represent an undue risk with careful intraoperative management.[2] The greatest risk is worsening renal function due to a transient reduction of renal blood flow during cross-clamping of the aorta, or from atheroembolism at surgery. Patients with low-grade renal failure should be informed about the possibility of requiring permanent renal dialysis postoperatively. Patients who are already on chronic renal hemodialysis must have the operation coordinated with timely preoperative and postoperative dialysis, as well as planning for the chronic anemia typically encountered in this patient group. Patients on chronic ambulatory peritoneal dialsysis (CAPD) require temporary or permanent vascular access for postoperative care, although if a retroperitoneal resection can be accomplished, continued CAPD may be a possibility.

Patients with active urinary tract infections should have culture-specific antibiotic treatment prior to elective resection and placement of a prosthetic aortic graft. If, during routine preoperative evaluation of an asymptomatic patient, a urine specimen shows bacteruria, appropriate preoperative antibiotic coverage may be adequate without delaying operation. If there is concern, however, delay may be suggested while further evaluation and treatment are considered.

PRIOR ORGAN TRANSPLANTATION

Today, with the rapidly growing transplant recipient population, many patients are being encountered with AAA who have had prior heart, liver, or kidney transplantation.

Heart transplant patients, especially patients who have been transplanted for ischemic cardiomyopathy, seem particularly prone to develop aortic aneurysms. The technical details of operative management of transplant recipients are beyond this review,[18] but the medical management of immunosuppression is critical to success and requires the expertise of a transplant surgeon or internist of the appropriate specialty. With appropriate medical management, these patients can be operated on without excessive risk. We reported eight heart transplant patients with an infrarenal AAA who underwent successful resection without mortality and only one episode of transient cardiac rejection.[19] The special technical requirements and options in management of renal transplant patients who must have AAA resection have been well described.[20]

DERMATOLOGIC

A variety of skin disorders may raise concern about wound healing or graft infection, and consultation with a dermatologist is helpful. The most frequently encountered problem is psoriasis, but this does not seem to pose any special risk with standard skin preparation, and wound healing is usually favorable.

CONCOMMITANT MALIGNANCIES

During the preoperative evaluation of patients with AAA, concurrent malignancies of the gastrointestinal, respiratory, or genitourinary tract may be discovered, or conversely, the incidental presence of an AAA may be found during the work-up of a patient with a solid tumor. The management of these complex situations requires a highly individualized approach and takes into account the relative risk to the patient of the AAA and the tumor. Patients with evidence of metastatic disease who have received optimal treatment can be considered for resection of the AAA if their life expectancy from the tumor exceeds the risk of rupture of the AAA, often a difficult judgment. Older patients with prostatic cancer most commonly fit into this group. Similarly, patients who have had primary treatment of their malignancy and who appear to be disease free may undergo resection of the AAA if any side effects of tumor treatment, such as leucopoenia from chemotherapy, have resolved.

The simultaneous operative resection of intra-abdominal malignancies and AAA is also a difficult decision, but can be justified in some circumstances. Simultaneous resection of malignancies of the gastrointestinal tract is especially controversial because of the risk of peritoneal contamination. Patients with concomitant colorectal cancer and AAA should always undergo staged procedures, the order depending on the circumstances, but in general, the cancer takes precedence.[21] With concomitant gastric cancer, one stage treatment has been described in several patients interestingly using two incisions—a retroperitoneal incision for the AAA and a standard transperitoneal incision for the gastric tumor resection.[22]

The concurrent presence of a renal malignancy and an AAA is a surprisingly common circumstance. Simultaneous resection may be justified in these patients. We reported 10 patients who have had simultaneous resection of an AAA and a renal cell carcinoma, with 1 death.[23] This single-stage approach should be reserved for carefully selected patients.

SUMMARY

Advances in the management of patients with AAA and coexisting chronic medical diseases now make it possible to resect aneurysm in all but the most severely ill. With the maturation of endovascular techniques, this may be even more achievable. Nonetheless, aneurysm repair is a major surgical procedure, never to be undertaken lightly. At present, more than 60% of all deaths following elective AAA resection are cardiac in origin. The decision to operate should be based on clear indications for resection, and not just the ability to complete a tour de force.

REFERENCES

1. Lloyd WE, Paty PSK, Darling RC III, et al. Results of 1000 consecutive elective abdominal aortic aneurysm repairs. *Cardiovasc Surg.* 1996;4:724–726.
2. Steyerberg EW, Kievet J, Van Otterloo JCA, van Bockel JH, Eijkemans MJC, Habbema JDF. Perioperative mortality of elective abdominal aortic aneurysm surgery. A clinical prediction rule based on literature and individual patient data. *Arch Intern Med.* 1995;155:1998–2004.
3. Falk V, Vettelschoz M, Walther T, Autschbach R, Dalichau H, Mohr FW. Surgical treatment of abdominal aortic aneurysms in octogenarians. *Cardiovasc Surg.* 1996;4:727–731.
4. Kazmers A, Perkins AJ, Jacobs LA. Outcomes after abdominal aortic aneurysm repair in those ≥80 years of age. Recent veterans affairs experience. *Ann Vasc Surg.* 1998;12:106–112.
5. Glock Y, Smile E, Dalous P, et al. Abdominal aortic aneurysmectomy in octogenarian patients. *J Cardiovasc Surg.* 1990;31:71–76.
6. Herzter NR, Beven EG, Young JR, et al. Coronary artery disease in peripheral vascular patients. A classification of 1000 coronary angiograms and results of surgical management. *Ann Surg.* 1984;199:223–233.
7. Wakefield TW, Stanley JC. Cardiopulmonary assessment for major vascular reconstructive procedures. In: Haimovici H, ed. *Vascular Surgery,* 4th ed. Cambridge, MA: Blackwell Science; 1996:209–223.
8. Won A, Acosta JA, Browner D, Hye RJ. Validation of selective cardiac evaluation prior to aortic aneurysm repair. *Arch Surg.* 1998;133:833–838.
9. Best PJ, Tajik AJ, Gibbons RJ, Pellikka PA. The safety of treadmill exercise stress testing in patients with abdominal aortic aneurysms. *Ann Intern Med.* 1998;129:628–631.
10. Durham SJ, Steed DL, Moosa HH, Makaroun MS, Webster MW. Probability of rupture of an abdominal aortic aneurysm after an unrelated operative procedure. A prospective study. *J Vasc Surg.* 1991;13:248–252.
11. Poldermans D, Boersma E, Bax JJ, et al. The effect of bisoprolol on perioperative mortality and myocardial infarction in high-risk patients undergoing vascular surgery. *N Engl J Med.* 1999;341:1789–1794.
12. Mangano DT, Layug EL, Wallace A, Tateo I. Effect of atenolol on mortality and cardiovascular morbidity after noncardiac surgery. *N Engl J Med.* 1996;335:1713–1720.

13. Kirby LB, Rosenthal D, Atkins CP, et al. Comparison between the transabdominal and retroperitoneal approaches for aortic reconstruction in patients at high risk. *J Vasc Surg.* 1999;30:400–406.
14. Eskandari MK, Rhee RY, Steed DL, et al. Oxygen-dependent chronic obstructive pulmonary disease does not prohibit aortic aneurysm repair. *Am J Surg.* 1999;178:125–128.
15. Arroyo A, Porto J, Gesto R. Congenital factor VII deficiency in a patient with an abdominal aortic aneurysm. *J Vasc Surg.* 1996;24:288–290.
16. Kobayashi M, Matsushita M, Nishikimi N, Sakurai T, Takamatsu J, Nimura Y. Treatment for abdominal aortic aneurysm in a patient with hemophilia A. A case report and review of the literature. *J Vasc Surg.* 1997;25:945–948.
17. Yamazumi K, Ojiro M, Okumura H, Aikou T. An activated state of blood coagulation and fibrinolysis in patients with abdominal aortic aneurysm. *Am J Surg.* 1998;175:297–301.
18. Ammori BJ, Madan M, Bodenham AR, Gough MJ. A review of the management of abdominal aortic aneurysms in patients following cardiac transplantation. *Eur J Endovasc Surg.* 1997;14:185–190.
19. Muluk SC, Steed DL, Makaroun MS, et al. Aortic aneurysm in heart transplant patients. *J Vasc Surg.* 1996;22:689–696.
20. Jebara VA, Fabiani J-N, Moulonguet-Deloris L, et al. Abdominal aortic aneurysmectomy in renal transplant patients. *Tex Heart Inst J.* 1990;17:240–244.
21. Nora JD, Pairolero PC, Nivatvongs S, Cherry KJ, Hallet JW, Gloviczki P. Concomitant abdominal aortic aneurysm and colorectal carcinoma: priority of resection. *J Vasc Surg.* 1989;9:630–636.
22. Komori K, Okadome K, Funahashi S, Itoh H, Sugimachi K. Surgical strategy of concomitant abdominal aortic aneurysm and gastric cancer. *J Vasc Surg.* 1994;19:573–576.
23. Konety BR, Shuman B, Webster MW, Steed DL, Bahnson RR. Simultaneous radical nephrectomy and repair of abdominal aortic aneurysm. *Urology.* 1996;47:813–818.

12

Endovascular Grafts for Ruptured Aneurysms

Takao Ohki, MD, Joseph Rabin, MD, and Frank J. Veith, MD

STANDARD OPEN REPAIR FOR RUPTURED ANEURYSMS AND ITS LIMITATIONS

The first successful repair of a ruptured infrarenal abdominal aortic aneurysm (AAA) was reported in 1954.[1] Since then, several important advances have been made in the nonsurgical care of patients with ruptured aneurysms, including the transportation of these patients, their critical care, the management of their cardiac dysfunction, and their pharmacologic support. Despite these advances, the operative mortality rates have not significantly improved, and they still range from 24% to 70%.[2–17] This is due, in part, to the fact that the basic surgical techniques for repairing ruptured AAAs have changed very little, even though some minor improvements have been introduced. These improvements include supraceliac clamping, suturing the graft within the aneurysm without excising the aneurysm, more frequent use of tube grafts, and the use of lower porosity prostheses.[3,4,6–11,13] The requirements of general anesthesia, a large surgical incision, the amount of dissection, and the accompanying invasiveness and blood loss required for open repair may be responsible for the poor outcome, because they have, for the most part, remained unchanged.

LIMITATIONS AND BENEFITS OF ENDOVASCULAR GRAFT REPAIR FOR RUPTURED ANEURYSMS

The use of endovascular grafts (EVGs) to treat a variety of arterial pathology, including elective AAAs, iliac artery aneurysms, occlusive disease, and traumatic lesions, has had promising short and midterm results.[18–27] Although theoretically EVGs are appealing because they are minimally invasive, their use in the treatment of ruptured AAAs or iliac artery aneurysms had been limited to a single case report.[28] One of the major reasons for the limited use of EVGs in this acute setting is due to the need for preoperative measurements of the aneurysmal and adjacent arterial anatomy so that an appropriate size and configuration of the graft can be selected, and this resulting delay has been deemed inappropriate in the urgent setting of ruptured AAAs.

EXPERIENCE AT THE MONTEFIORE MEDICAL CENTER IN NEW YORK WITH ENDOVASCULAR REPAIR OF RUPTURED AAAS

Vascular Innovation "One Size Fits Most" Graft

In order to eliminate the need for preoperative measurements and fabrication of grafts, we developed the Vascular Innovation (VI) graft (Vascular Innovation Inc., Toledo, OH), which facilitates intraoperative customization.[29,30] This graft is constructed by suturing a Palmaz stent (P5O14, Cordis, Warren, NJ) to a standard wall ePTFE graft (6 mm × 40 cm, IMPRA, Tempe, AZ) (Figs. 12–1, 12–2).[29] This stent–graft combination

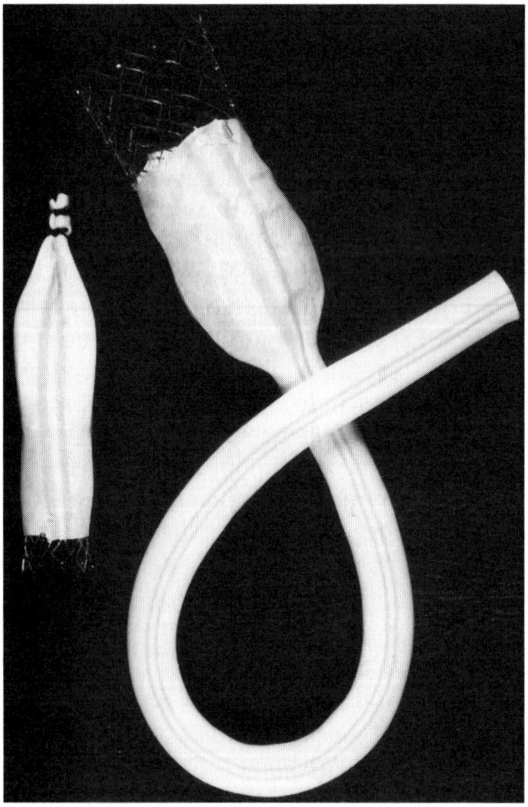

Figure 12–1. The Vascular Innovation graft. An extra-large Palmaz stent is attached to the PTFE graft.

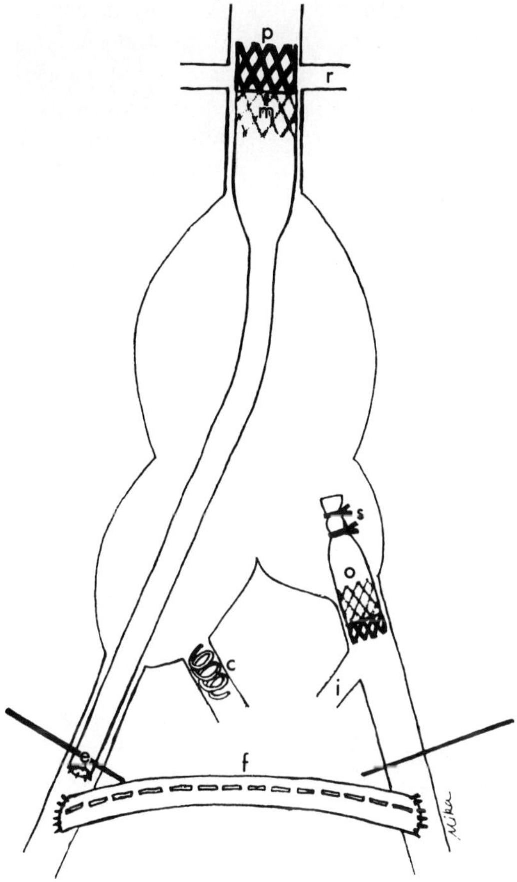

Figure 12–2. Schematic drawing illustrating deployment of the VI graft. The VI graft is fixed within the proximal neck with a large Palmaz stent (p). The cranial end of the graft is denoted by a metallic marker (m) attached to the graft. In this example, the bare portion of the stent is deployed across the orifice of the renal arteries so that the graft is implanted immediately below the renal arteries (r). An endoluminal anastomosis (e) is performed at the distal end of the EVG. The occluder device (o) is always deployed in the contralateral common iliac artery to preserve at least one internal iliac artery (i). c, embolization coil; f, femoro-femoral bypass; s, suture to occlude the end of the occluder.

is then mounted onto a large percutaneous transluminal angioplasty (PTA) balloon (Maxi LD 25 mm × 4 cm, Cordis) and inserted into a 16-Fr sheath (Cook Inc., Bloomington, IN). An occluder device (for occlusion of the opposite common iliac artery) is constructed by attaching a Palmaz stent (P4014 or P308) to an ePTFE graft that is closed at one end by ligatures. This occluder device is also mounted onto a PTA balloon and inserted into either a 12- or a 16-Fr sheath. These grafts are prefabricated and are kept sterile for emergent use.

Obtaining Proximal Control

In hemodynamically unstable patients, an occlusion balloon (Occlusion Catheter, Meditech, Oakland, NJ) is inserted through the brachial artery and inflated in the suprarenal aorta (Fig. 12–3). In order to maintain vasoconstriction, which is often released with the induction of general anesthesia, this procedure is performed under local anesthesia. In many cases, this vasoconstriction is the key function in maintaining the blood pressure above a lethal level.

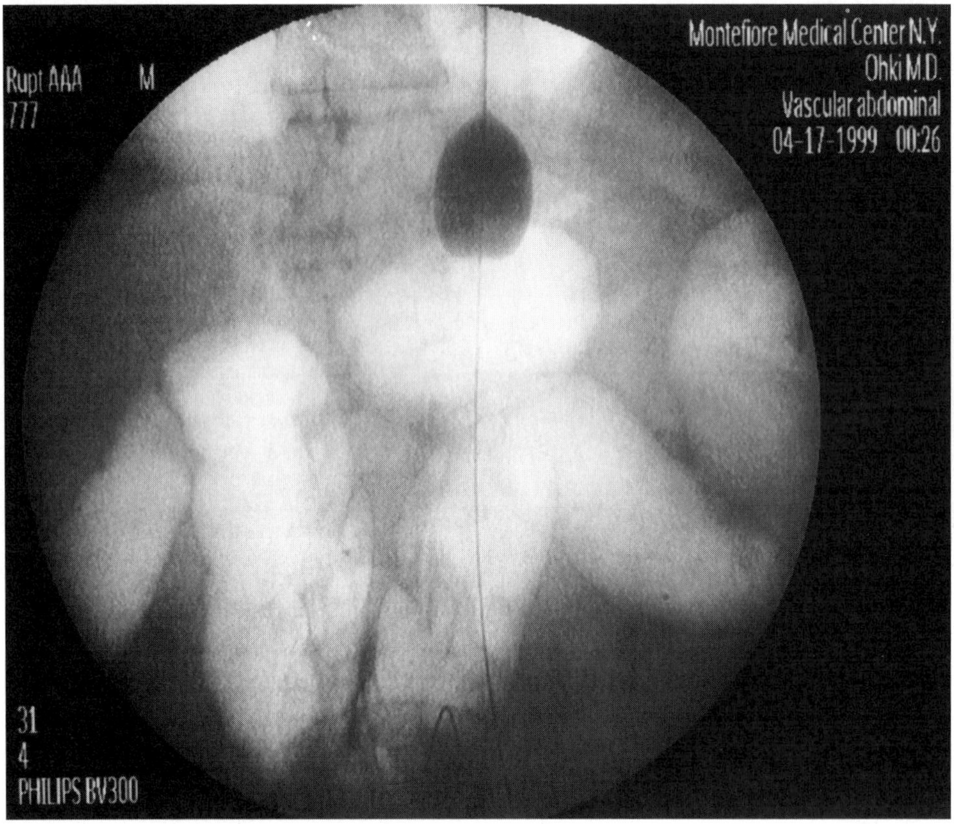

Figure 12–3. Fluoroscopic view of a proximal occlusion balloon introduced through the brachial artery.

Intraoperative Angiogram

Under general anesthesia, both common femoral arteries are exposed and introducer sheaths are inserted. In those cases in which a preoperative computed tomography (CT) scan or angiogram was not performed, an aortogram is obtained first, using a portable fluoroscope (OEC Model 9800, OEC Medical, Salt Lake City, UT, or BV 300, Philips, The Netherlands) and the Acist contrast power injector system (Acist Medical Systems, Eden Prairie, MN). A decision that is based on several criteria is then made regarding the feasibility of an endovascular repair (Table 12–1).

TABLE 12–1. EXCLUSION CRITERIA FOR ENDOVASCULAR REPAIR

Proximal neck diameter larger than 28 mm
Pararenal AAAs (neck length shorter than 10 mm)
Bilateral, long iliac artery occlusions
Mycotic aneurysm

Technique for Deploying the VI Graft[30]

Either before or after deployment of the VI graft, coil embolization of the hypogastric artery ipsilateral to the side of graft insertion is performed. The VI graft delivery system is inserted into the aorta over a superstiff wire that is placed in the ascending thoracic aorta. Once the graft is inserted into the proximal aneurysm neck, the delivery sheath is retracted. In order to confirm appropriate positioning in regard to the renal arteries, a repeat angiogram is performed using a pigtail catheter introduced via the contralateral femoral artery. Inflation of the deployment balloon expands the stent and fixes the VI graft within the proximal neck. By varying the inflation pressure, the VI graft is able to accommodate a wide range of proximal neck diameters ranging from 15 to 28 mm (Fig. 12–4). In each case, the length of the graft is 40 cm so that the distal end of the graft always emerges from the introduction arteriotomy site. The graft is then cut to the appropriate length and hand-sewn endoluminally within the common femoral or distal external iliac artery (Fig 12–5). For AAAs, the VI graft is placed within the proxi-

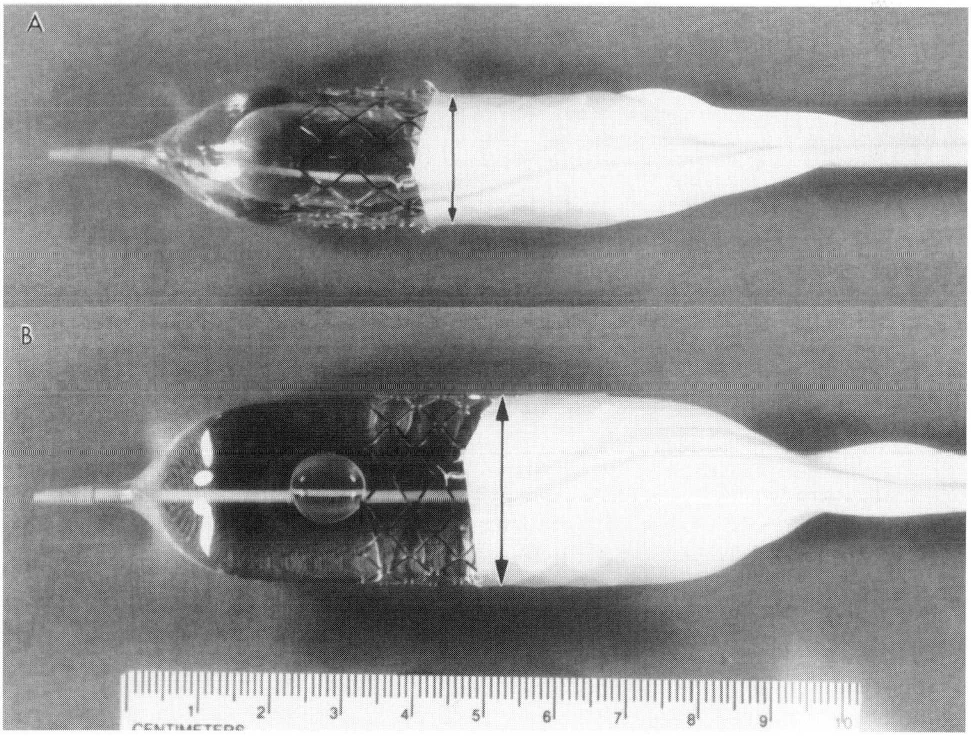

Figure 12–4. Method for customizing the proximal stent diameter of the Vascular Innovation graft intraoperatively. (**A**) When the deployment balloon is inflated to 2 ATM, the stent is expanded to 20 mm in diameter (*small arrow*). (**B**) Due to the compliant nature of the balloon, at 6 ATM of inflation pressure the stent is expanded to 28 mm (*large arrow*). (*From Ohki T, Veith FJ, Sanchez LA, et al., Endovascular graft repair of ruptured aortoiliac aneurysms. J Am Coll Surg 1999;189:102–113, with permission.*)

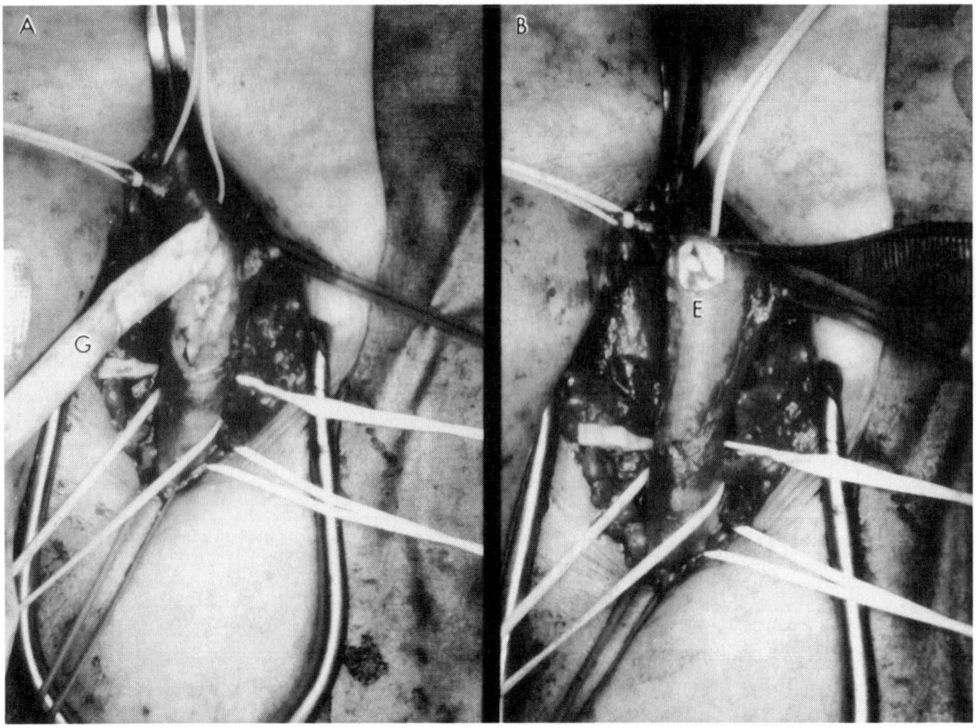

Figure 12–5. Method for customizing the length of the VI graft intraoperatively. (**A**) In each case, the EVG is made long enough so that the distal end of the graft (G) emerges from the arteriotomy site. (**B**) The graft is cut to the appropriate length as it emerges from the femoral artery and an endoluminal anastomosis (E) is carried out. (*From Ohki T, Veith FJ, Sanchez LA, et al. Endovascular graft repair of ruptured aortoiliac aneurysms. J Am Coll Surg 1999;189:102–113, with permission.*)

mal neck and the occluder device is placed in the opposite common iliac artery, thereby preserving at least one hypogastric artery. In addition, a femorofemoral bypass is performed (Figs. 12–6, 12–7). For iliac aneurysms with a proximal common iliac neck, the main EVG is placed from that neck to the common femoral or external iliac artery.

PATIENTS

Ten patients (9 male, 1 female) with ruptured AAAs were treated using the VI graft. There were 6 AAAs (5 true, 1 false) and 4 iliac artery aneurysms (2 true, 2 false). The mean age of the patients was 68 yr. All 10 patients were deemed to be at high-risk for open surgical treatment because of comorbid disease [8 patients with COPD requiring home oxygen (EF <20%) and 2 patients with hostile abdomens (multiple abdominal operations with pelvic irradiation)]. Seven patients were transferred to our institution from other hospitals after developing symptoms, including acute onset of abdominal or back pain, syncope, or external bleeding. In each case, another surgeon

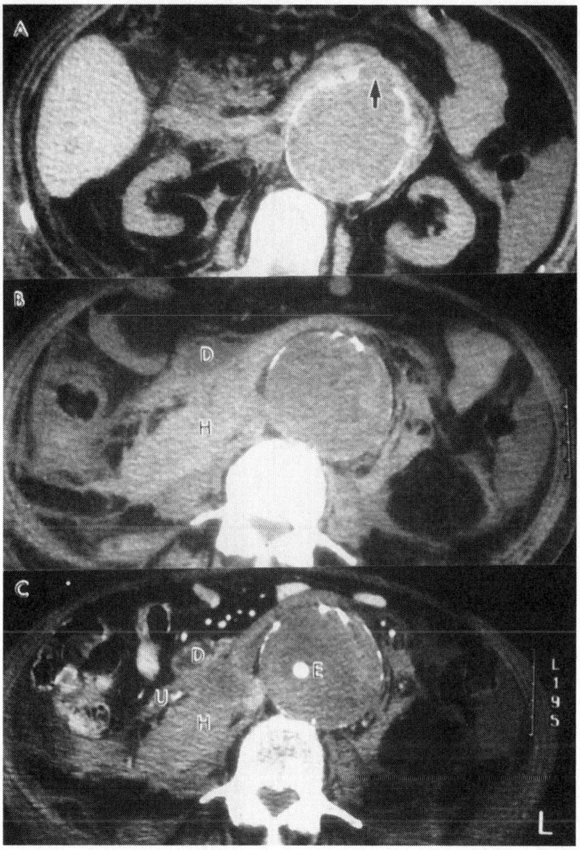

Figure 12–6. CT scan images of a ruptured AAA. This 71-year-old male was admitted to another hospital for medical treatment of his pneumonia secondary to chemotherapy for leukemia. His other comorbid diseases included severe COPD requiring home oxygen and congestive heart failure with an ejection fraction of 25%. The patient experienced a sudden onset of severe abdominal pain which a CT scan confirmed to be a ruptured AAA. Due to his coexisting diseases, standard repair was deemed prohibitive and he was transferred to our institution. On arrival, his systolic blood pressure was 75 mm Hg and his hematocrit was 18%. (**A**) Preoperative CT scan reveals a possible rupture site (*arrow*) in the AAA. (**B**) Preoperative CT scan showing the more distal portion of the AAA. The AAA measures 7.5 cm in diameter. In addition, a large hematoma (H) can be seen in the right retroperitoneal space, which is displacing the duodenum (D). (**C**) Postoperative enhanced CT scan. Contrast is confined within the EVG (E) with evidence of complete aneurysmal exclusion. The ureter, which is displaced by the large hematoma, is visualized. Despite his comorbid condition, he was extubated 6 hr following the procedure and was able to eat on the second postoperative day. (*From Ohki T, Veith FJ, Sanchez LA, et al. Endovascular graft repair of ruptured aortoiliac aneurysms. J Am Coll Surg 1999;189:102–113, with permission.*)

considered the patient to be unsuitable for standard surgery and best treated by an EVG. No patient in this series had cardiac arrest or required cardiopulmonary resuscitation preoperatively, although 2 required endo-tracheal intubation and ventilator support.

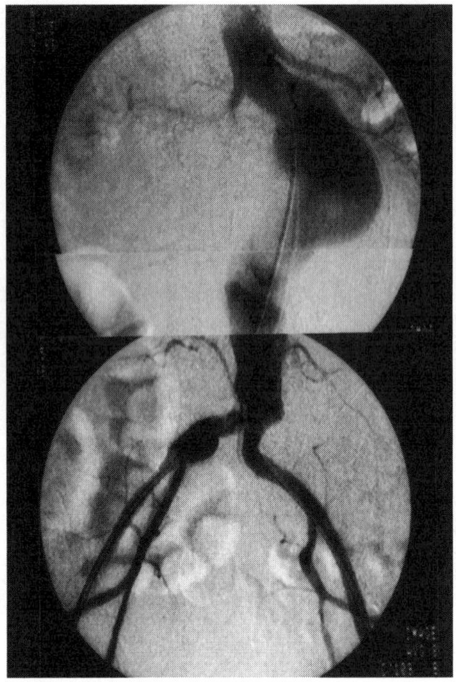

A

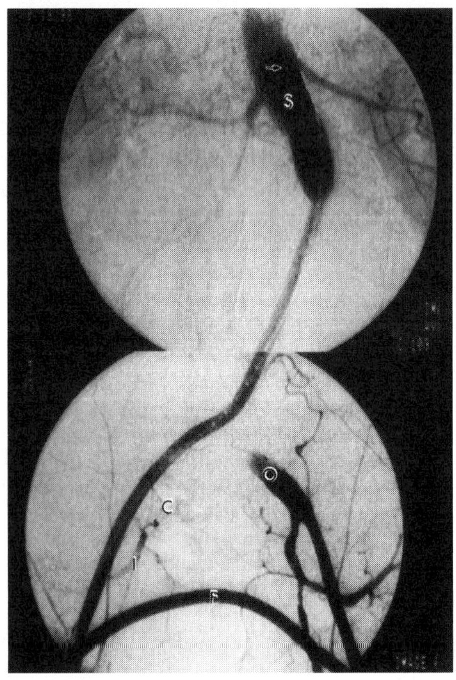

B

Figure 12–7. Intraoperative angiogram of the patient described in Figure 12–6. (**A**) Preoperative angiogram reveals a large AAA and a small common iliac aneurysm. (**B**) Completion angiogram. The AAA is completely excluded with no evidence of an endoleak. The bare portion of the proximal stent (S) is placed above the renal arteries, and the cranial end of the graft, which is denoted by the gold marker (*arrow*), is placed immediately below the renal arteries. The right internal iliac artery is opacified by retrograde flow. C, embolization coils; O, occluder device; F, femorofemoral bypass. (*From Ohki T, Veith FJ, Sanchez LA, et al. Endovascular graft repair of ruptured aortoiliac aneurysms. J Am Coll Surg 1999;189: 102–110, with permission.*)

OUTCOME

Because of sustained hemodynamic instability, four cases required rapid proximal arterial control that was obtained either by the use of a proximal occlusion balloon or by the rapid deployment of the EVG. In all cases, the EVG was deployed successfully at the target site with complete exclusion of the ruptured aneurysm and no evidence of an endoleak. All patients experienced resolution of their preoperative symptoms. The mean operative time was 5 hr and the mean blood loss was 800 mL. One patient died in the operating room from cardiac arrest due to a preexisting acute myocardial infarction. Another patient died 3 weeks postoperatively from multiple organ failure. One patient required evacuation of a hematoma through a limited retroperitoneal incision 7 days postoperatively. There were three surgical complications, including one postoperative MI and two groin wound infections that required drainage but healed without graft involvement. The mean length of hospital stay was 7 days. One graft occluded 2 mo postoperatively and an axillofemoral bypass was required. However, this patient's aneurysm continued to be excluded successfully from the circulation until she died from her preexisting cervical cancer. During a mean follow-up of 15 mo, 2 patients died from preexisting comorbid disease that was unrelated to their EVG repair. There are no signs of an endoleak in the remaining 5 survivors, and each graft continues to be functional at a mean follow-up of 22 mo.

COMMENTS

We developed the VI graft to eliminate the need for precise preoperative measurements. This was possible due to the use of a compliant stent deployment balloon and also because the graft length is always made longer than required and then cut to the proper length *in situ,* as described above.

One potential disadvantage of EVG repair for ruptured AAAs is that it may take longer to achieve proximal arterial control compared with standard repair. However, in the past we used an occlusion balloon, which can be inserted from the brachial artery when such immediate control was required. More liberal use of this technique may further expand the indications for EVG repair in the treatment of ruptured aneurysms.

Potential Advantages of EVG Repair in the Treatment of Ruptured AAAs

Several potential advantages to EVG repair of ruptured aneurysms include the ability to obtain proximal control prior to the introduction of general anesthesia, the ability to deploy the graft from a remote access site, reduced blood loss, and minimizing hypothermia by eliminating laparotomy.

Ability to Obtain Proximal Control Prior to the Induction of General Anesthesia

Patients with ruptured AAAs may initially be severely hypotensive. However, many patients, especially those who are able to get to a hospital, may have their blood pressure stabilized at a nonlethal level. This is mainly due to vasoconstriction, which is the human body's response to hypotension. It is not uncommon for this vasoconstriction to be released during the induction of general anesthesia, which results in a sudden drop in blood pressure. Therefore, a relatively stable patient may become severely hypotensive, mandating urgent application of proximal cross-clamping. This, as well as the presence of a hematoma that may distort the intra-abdominal anatomy (see next section), further pose technical difficulties in the repair of ruptured AAAs. However, a guidewire can be inserted in the abdominal aorta through a percutaneous puncture under local anesthesia, thereby maintaining the vasoconstriction. Once the guidewire is inserted in the aorta, the patient can then safely undergo induction of general anesthesia because proximal control can be rapidly and safely obtained by introducing a brachial occlusion balloon over the previously placed guidewire.

Ability to Deploy the Graft from a Remote Access Site

EVGs can be inserted and deployed through a remote access site, thereby obviating the need for laparotomy and, more importantly, eliminating the technical difficulties that are encountered when performing a standard repair in this setting. The anatomy of the retroperitoneal structures is often distorted and obscured because of a large hematoma, which may lead to technical difficulties as well as inadvertent injury of the inferior vena cava, the left renal vein or its genital branches, the duodenum, or other surrounding structures. These iatrogenic injuries have been the cause of significant operative morbidity and mortality following standard surgery for ruptured aneurysms.[5,7–10,12] In contrast, EVG repair is performed within the arterial tree, which is unaffected by extravasated blood or previous operative scarring. Thus, the degree of technical difficulty encountered when treating a ruptured aneurysm with an EVG is similar to that for elective cases. Moreover, this approach completely eliminates the risk of inadvertent injury to surrounding structures.

Reduced Blood Loss

In our experience, EVG repair for ruptured AAA was accomplished with a relatively small amount of blood loss (800 mL) compared with that reported for open, ruptured AAA repair. The blood loss during elective EVG repair has also been reported to be less than that for open repair.[31] This advantage is more important in patients with ruptured aneurysms because these patients have already lost a significant amount of blood following rupture, and disseminated intravascular coagulation (DIC) secondary to blood loss is a devastating complication. There are several reasons why this limited blood loss was possible, including the fact that EVG repair does not release the tamponade effect within the retroperitoneum and other surrounding structures. In addition, back-bleeding from the iliac and lumbar arteries and bleeding from the anastomotic suture lines and from the iatrogenic venous injury, which are the main sources of blood loss during standard repair, can be completely eliminated during EVG repair.

Minimizing Hypothermia by Eliminating Laparotomy

Hypothermia secondary to poor perfusion and laparotomy can exacerbate coagulopathy, which is one of the causes of mortality following open surgical repair. EVG repair can minimize the extent of hypothermia by avoiding laparotomy.

CONCLUSIONS AND FUTURE TRIALS

The relatively low mortality rate (20%) and the short length of hospital stay (7 days) in this group of patients are encouraging because this study was carried out only in high-risk patients who were nonsurgical candidates. These results show that EVG repair of ruptured AAAs and iliac artery aneurysms is feasible and effective in selected cases. However, before the widespread use of this technique is adopted, further device refinements and longer follow-up are needed. In addition, whether the more liberal use of proximal occlusion balloons will permit the treatment of larger cohorts of patients, including those who are more hemodynamically unstable, remains to be demonstrated.

We are currently conducting a prospective, nonrandomized study to evaluate the feasibility, safety, and effectiveness of a new approach in the treatment of ruptured AAAs.[32] This approach is characterized by the following: (1) limited fluid resuscitation to prevent rebleed from the aneurysm; (2) routine brachial wire placement under local anesthesia prior to the induction of general anesthesia; (3) deployment of a proximal occlusion balloon over this wire in patients with low blood pressure or in patients who deteriorate after induction of general anesthesia; (4) depending on the anatomic characteristics of the aneurysm, the performance of either EVG repair with the VI graft or a standard open repair. We have already enrolled 12 patients in this study. The preliminary results appear promising, and to date we have not lost any patients.

ACKNOWLEDGMENTS

Supported by grants from the U.S. Public Health Service (HL 02990-04), the James Hilton Manning and Emma Austin Manning Foundation, and the Anna S. Brown Trust.

REFERENCES

1. Gerbode F. Ruptured abdominal aortic aneurysm: a surgical emergency. *Surg Gynecol Obstet.* 1954;98:759–764.
2. Ernst CB. Abdominal aortic aneurysms. *N Engl J Med.* 1993;328:1167–1172.
3. Wakefield TW, Whitehouse WM, Wu SC. Abdominal aortic aneurysm rupture: statistical analysis of factors affecting outcome of surgical treatment. *Surgery.* 1982;91:586–595.
4. Donaldson MC, Rosenberg JM, Bucknam CA. Factors affecting survival after ruptured abdominal aortic aneurysm. *J Vasc Surg.* 1985;2:564–570.
5. Shackleton CR, Schechter MT, Bianco R, Hildebrand KD. Preoperative predictors of mortality risk in ruptured abdominal aortic aneurysm. *J Vasc Surg.* 1987;6:583–589.
6. Ouriel K, Geary K, Green RM, Fiore W, Geary JE, DeWeese JA. Factors determining survival after ruptured aortic aneurysm: the hospital, the surgeon, and the patient. *J Vasc Surg.* 1990;11:493–496.
7. Crawford ES. Ruptured abdominal aortic aneurysm: an editorial. *J Vasc Surg.* 1991;13:348–350.
8. Johansen K, Kohler TR, Nicholls SC, Zierler RE, Clowes AW, Kazmers A. Ruptured abdominal aortic aneurysm: the Harborview experience. *J Vasc Surg.* 1991;13:240–247.

9. Harris LM, Faggioli GL, Fiedler R, Curl GR, Ricotta JJ. Ruptured abdominal aortic aneurysms: factors affecting mortality rates. *J Vasc Surg.* 1991;14:812–820.
10. Gloviczki P, Pairolero PC, Mucha P. Ruptured abdominal aortic aneurysms: repair should not be denied. *J Vasc Surg.* 1992;15:851–859.
11. Marty-Ane CH, Alric P, Picot MC, Picard E, Colson P, Mary H. Ruptured abdominal aortic aneurysm: influence of intraoperative management on surgical outcome. *J Vasc Surg.* 1995;22:780–786.
12. Panneton JM, Lassonde J, Laurendeau F. Ruptured abdominal aortic aneurysm: impact of comorbidity and postoperative complications on outcome. *Ann Vasc Surg.* 1995;9:535–541.
13. Darling RC, Cordero JA, Chang BB. Advances in the surgical repair of ruptured abdominal aortic aneurysms. *Cardiovasc Surg.* 1996;4:720–723.
14. Farooq MM, Freischlag JA, Seabrook GR, Moon MR, Aprahamian C, Towne JB. Effect of the duration of symptoms, transport time, and length of emergency room stay on morbidity and mortality in patients with ruptured abdominal aortic aneurysms. *Surgery.* 1996;119:9–14.
15. Lazarides MK, Arvanitis DP, Drista H, et al. POSSUM and APACHE II scores do not predict the outcome of ruptured infrarenal aortic aneurysms. *Ann Vasc Surg.* 1997;11:155–158.
16. Halpern VJ, Kline RG, DiAngelo AJ, Cohen JR. Factors that affect the survival rate of patients with ruptured abdominal aortic aneurysms. *J Vasc Surg.* 1997;26:939–948.
17. Dardik A, Burleyson GP, Bowman H, et al. Surgical repair of ruptured abdominal aortic aneurysms in the state of Maryland: factors influencing outcome among 527 recent cases. *J Vasc.* 1998;28:413–421.
18. Parodi JC, Palmaz JC, Barone HD. Transfemoral intraluminal graft implantation for abdominal aortic aneurysms. *Ann Vasc Surg.* 1991;5:491–499.
19. Blum U, Voshage G, Lammer J, et al. Endoluminal stent-grafts for infrarenal abdominal aortic aneurysms. *N Engl J Med.* 1997;336:13–20.
20. Marin ML, Veith FJ, Cynamon J, et al. Initial experience with transluminally placed endovascular grafts for the treatment of complex vascular lesions. *Ann Surg.* 1995;222:1–17.
21. Ohki T, Marin ML, Veith FJ, et al. Endovascular aorto-uni-iliac grafts and femoro-femoral bypass for bilateral limb threatening ischemia. *J Vasc Surg.* 1996;24:984–997.
22. Marin ML, Veith FJ, Panetta TF, et al. Transluminally placed endovascular stented graft repair for arterial trauma. *J Vasc Surg.* 1994;20:466–473.
23. Ohki T, Marin ML, Veith FJ. Use of endovascular grafts to treat non-aneurysmal arterial disease. *Ann Vasc Surg.* 1997;11:200–205.
24. May J, White GH, Yu W, et al. Concurrent comparison of endoluminal versus open repair in the treatment of abdominal aortic aneurysms: analysis of 303 patients by life table method. *J Vasc Surg.* 1998;27:213–220.
25. Yusuf SW, Whitaker SC, Chuter TAM, et al. Early results of endovascular aortic aneurysm surgery with aortouniiliac graft, contralateral iliac occlusion, and femorofemoral bypass. *J Vasc Surg.* 1997;25:165–172.
26. Ohki T, Veith FJ, Sanchez LA, Marin ML, Cynamon J, Parodi JC. Varying strategies and devices for endovascular repair of abdominal aortic aneurysms. *Semin Vasc Surg.* 1997;10:242–256.
27. Yuan JG, Marin ML, Veith FJ, et al. Endovascular grafts for the treatment of para-anastomotic aneurysm. *J Vasc Surg.* 1997;26:210–221.
28. Yusuf SW, Whitaker SC, Chuter TA, Wenham PW, Hopkinson BR. Emergency endovascular repair of leaking aortic aneurysm. *Lancet.* 1994;344:1645.
29. Ohki T, Veith FJ. Minimally invasive vascular surgery. In: Brooks DC, ed. *Current Review of Minimally Invasive Surgery,* 3rd edition. Current Medicine, Inc., Philadelphia, 1998;125–136.
30. Ohki T, Veith FJ, Sanchez LA, et al. Endovascular graft repair of ruptured aorto-iliac aneurysms. *J Am Coll Surg.* 1999;189:102–123.

31. Zarins CK, White RA, Schwarten D, et al. AneuRx stent graft versus open surgical repair of abdominal aortic aneurysms: multicenter prospective clinical trial. *J Vasc Surg.* 1999;29: 292–305.
32. Ohki T, Veith FJ. Endovascular grafts and other image guided catheter based adjuncts to improve the treatment of ruptured aortoiliac aneurysms. *Ann Surg*, 2000 (in press).

13

Factors Influencing the Growth of Aortic Aneurysm:

Potential for Pharmacologic Treatment

B. Timothy Baxter, MD and Robert W. Thompson, MD

INTRODUCTION

Abdominal aorta aneurysm (AAA) is a common entity effecting 2% of the general population and resulting in at least 15,000 deaths per year from rupture and exsanguination.[1] What is most alarming is an increase in the incidence of AAA at a time when mortality related to atherosclerotic cardiovascular disease is decreasing.[2] Aneurysmorrhaphy is effective in preventing aneurysm rupture, but population-based studies indicate that elective operative mortality actually exceeds 5%.[3] Detection of small aneurysms (3.5–5.5 cm) by ultrasound is accurate and inexpensive. Unfortunately, screening it is not currently considered cost-effective for two reasons: (1) the majority of aneurysms detected by screening are small and do not warrant immediate surgical intervention, and (2) there is no effective medical treatment to inhibit the growth of these small aneurysms. An effective treatment that prevented or slowed the growth of small aneurysms could make screening cost-effective and reduce AAA-associated mortality.

The natural history of AAA is progressive expansion. The growth rate is exponential, increasing as aneurysm diameter increases. Diameter is the single best predictor of rupture risk. A small 3.5 cm AAA growing at an average rate (0.4 cm/yr) will reach 5.5 cm in 5 yr. Pharmacologic therapy that inhibited growth by only 50% would extend the time from detection of a small AAA to consideration for aneurysm repair beyond 10 years. The impact of inhibiting aneurysm expansion by varying degrees is shown in Figure 13–1. Aortic aneurysms typically occur in the sixth through the eighth decades

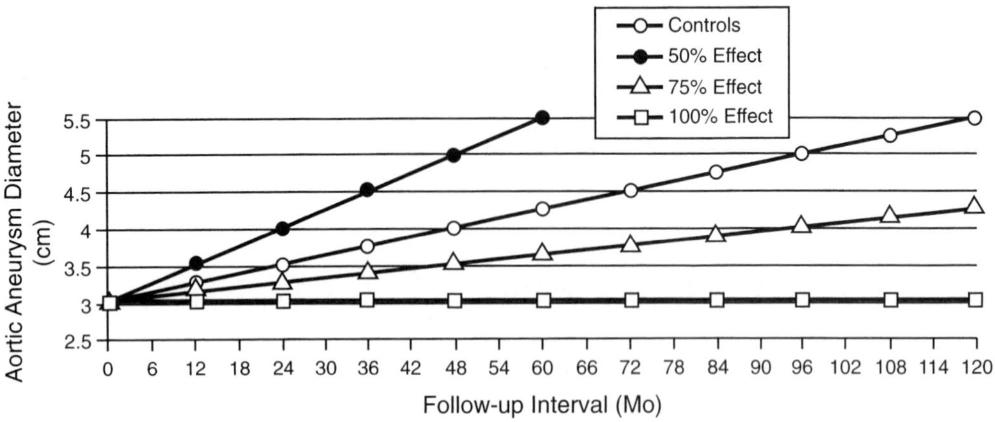

Figure 13–1. The effects of varying degrees of inhibition of aortic aneurysm expansion. A 3.0-cm abdominal aortic aneurysm (AAA) would be expected to reach 5.5 cm in 5 yr based on average growth. This would be extended to 10 yr if this growth rate were decreased by 50%. Inhibition of 50% or more would extend the time it took for a 3.0-cm aneurysm to reach 5.5 cm, well beyond the life expectancy of most AAA patients. *(Modified from Thompson RW and Baxter BT. MMP inhibition in abdominal aortic aneurysms. Rationale for a prospective randomized clinical trial. Ann N Y Acad Sci. 1999;878:159–178.)*

of life in a patient population with significant coexistent cardiovascular and cerebral vascular disease. The mortality from all causes in this group is 6–7% year. Effective pharmacotherapy would have two important benefits: (1) It would increase detection of AAA by making screening cost-effective; and (2) it would reduce the need for repair of many aneurysms by preventing them from reaching a critical size. These measures could prevent most AAA-associated mortality.

Breakthroughs in basic pathophysiology and pharmacology have led to effective medical therapy for diseases that could only be controlled by surgery in the past. Peptic ulcer disease is perhaps the best paradigm for this progression from surgical to medical therapy. Remarkable advances in our understanding of AAA pathophysiology have occurred in the past several years. The critical role of inflammatory cells and a family of matrix-degrading enzymes (matrix metalloproteinases, or MMPs) have been elucidated through animal models that closely recapitulate human disease. General inhibition of MMPs inhibits the growth of experimental AAA.[4] Propranolol has hemodynamic and biochemical effects that suggest it may also inhibit AAA growth.[5] Targeting the immune response reduces aortic dilatation in acute animal models.[6] Based on these studies, we are clearly reaching a point where pharmacologic inhibition of aneurysm growth is feasible.

Designing a clinical trial to target the growth of small AAA requires a precise definition of small AAA, knowledge of the anticipated growth rate in a control group, and establishing a minimum threshold for what one would consider an effective reduction in growth rate. The hypothesis tests whether the drug could reduce the growth rate below this threshold. In addition, the period that the subjects are followed on the study drug must be determined. In order to make a final determination of the sample size required for a prospective randomized trial, an estimate must be made of the anticipated dropout rate, mortality rate, and the proportion of patients expected to require intervention for their aneurysm during the course of the study. In this chapter, we outline the background information for a number of therapies that appear to have the potential for inhibiting AAA and discuss the design of clinical trials to test these therapies.

DEFINING AAA AND EXPECTED AAA GROWTH RATES

Changes in aortic diameter occur with age, and there are gender-based differences in normal aortic diameter. These factors help make the definition of an aortic aneurysm somewhat complicated. Distinguishing between a small AAA and aortic ectasia is important because the expected growth rates would be very different. The standard definition of AAA is a focal dilatation of at least 50% larger than expected normal arterial diameter.[7] In an effort to refine the definition of aortic aneurysm, computed tomography (CT) and ultrasonography has been used to characterize changes in aortic diameter with normal aging. Although the most pronounced increase in aortic diameter occurs during childhood and adolescent growth, there is also a 25% increase in aortic diameter between ages 25 and 75. This increase is greater for males than females, but there is no significant difference between the sexes when data are normalized to body surface area.[8] The findings of these studies indicate that at age 75, the normal infrarenal diameter can range from 12.4 mm in a small woman to 27.6 mm in a large man. A number of measures of aortic diameter relative to other structures such as adjacent normal aorta have been proposed. Because an infrarenal aortic diameter in excess of 29 mm is above the upper limit of normal regardless of age, sex, and body surface area, Lederle et al.[9] suggested simply using 3.0 cm as a practical cutoff for AAA. Indeed, using this definition to screen patients enrolled in a large health survey, Alcorn et al.[10] reported the incidence of AAA to be as high as 9% in a nonselected population of men over the age of 65.

CT scan has shown less variability in the measurement of aortic diameter compared to ultrasound. The attraction of ultrasound is that it is less expensive and the variability can be overcome by obtaining more frequent studies. However, standardizing ultrasound images obtained from multiple centers is an onerous task. This requires uniform protocols and technician training as well as verification of reliability and reproducibility at each center. The increased number of studies along with travel and time for training and validation more than offset the cost savings of ultrasound, making CT the preferred method of imaging in a large, multicenter trial. Pearce and colleagues[8] looked extensively at normal and aneurysmal aortic diameter with magnified CT images. In a recent study, they were able to detect a 1.2-mm increase over time in the diameter of the distal neck of the aneurysm after endografting.[11] This small increase was statistically significant ($P < 0.01$), with 24 patients studied. The interobserver variability was 93%. This study and others show that standard contrast CT scan can reliably detect changes of less than 1 mm and also show that the observations are highly reproducible.

Using serial ultrasounds or CT scans, the growth rates of small AAAs have been tracked. Results from several of these studies are shown in Table 13–1. The largest study

TABLE 13–1. AAA GROWTH RATES

Author	Patient Number	3.0–3.9	4.0–4.9	5.0–5.9	Total
Bernstein	110	0.47	0.42	0.51	0.44
Nevitt	103	0.31	0.55	—	0.38
Limet	114	0.63	0.83	—	—
Kremer	35	0.23	0.22	—	0.20
Delin	35	0.65	0.56	0.56	0.62
Brown	460	0.37	0.63	—	0.50
Bernstein	49	0.31	0.61	—	0.46
Total	**906**	**0.42**	**0.55**	**0.54**	**0.43**

Modified from Wilson et al.[12]

assessing growth of AAA was reported by Brown and colleagues.[13] They followed 460 patients by serial CT scan and found that the mean growth rate of aneurysms of 3.5 to 4.9 cm was 5.4 mm/yr, with a standard deviation of 6.1 mm/yr. This standard deviation demonstrates the large variability in this mean growth. It reflects the fact that 20% of small AAA do not grow during observation, whereas a few (among the 80% that do grow) enlarge more than 10 mm/yr. This variability is consistent across each of the studies described previously. Based on these data, it is possible to develop a hypothesis that tests the idea that an intervention would reduce AAA growth by a specific amount. Furthermore, CT provides the accuracy to measure small differences in growth rate.

FACTORS ASSOCIATED WITH ANEURYSM EXPANSION

A number of investigators have performed retrospective analysis after following patients with AAA to determine factors associated with AAA growth. Although these risk factors have some overlap with the risk factors associated with AAA rupture, they are not the same. The best medical management for small asymptomatic AAA is generally undefined. In addition to "watchful waiting," current treatment for such patients includes control of hypertension and attempts to get the patient to stop smoking. Three standard risk factors for atherosclerosis (hypertension, smoking, and hypercholesterolemia) are also risk factors for development of AAA.[14] Both uncontrolled hypertension and continued smoking are associated with increased expansion rates of AAA. It is unclear that lowering cholesterol will affect the growth rate of AAA.[13,15] Advanced age, a history of CVA, and a large amount of thrombus in the aneurysm have also been shown in retrospective analysis to be associated with increased AAA growth.[16] Obviously, age and history of cardiovascular events are recorded as part of any clinical trial of AAA. Determining the extent of thrombus is dependent on the imaging modality used.

Treatment of hypertension may include beta blockers and/or ACE inhibitors, drugs that could have an impact on aneurysm growth rates independent of their effects on hypertension per se. Recording antihypertensive medications used by patients during the trial is important for covariant analysis of their impact when the study is completed. If the drug being tested in a trial to inhibit AAA growth affects blood pressure, then achieving equivalent blood pressure control in the treatment and placebo group is critical. This is much less of an issue when the drug under study does not have cardiovascular effects because management of hypertension, cholesterol, and assisting with smoking cessation are all within the scope of general health care for this patient population. It is not yet known what impact implementing a rigorous standard of best medical management might have on aneurysm growth rate.

THERAPIES THAT MAY INHIBIT AAA GROWTH

The development of novel therapeutic strategies for inhibiting AAA is dependent on increased efforts to understand the basic pathophysiology of aneurysmal degeneration. As the cellular and molecular events underlying the destruction of aortic wall connective tissue proteins have become better elucidated in recent years, it is anticipated that rational therapeutic targets can now be identified that could suppress the gradual progression of aneurysm disease. If successful, this approach would establish the need to develop population-based screening programs. Moreover, it might eventually limit the number of patients who would require operation, reduce the number of unexpected deaths from aneurysm rupture, and lower the overall costs associated with this condition. Therefore, efforts to solve this problem are expected to meet the unfulfilled therapeutic opportunities that exist for treating patients with small asymptomatic AAA and, ultimately, to help eliminate unnecessary deaths from ruptured aneurysms.

Anti-Inflammatory Agents

The fact that inflammation plays a key role in AAA is abundantly clear. The descriptive analysis of AAA tissue shows the clear association between AAA and dense inflammatory infiltrates, including macrophages and lymphocytes.[17] Animal models of AAA have demonstrated a causal role in experimental aneurysm induction. The dilatation in both the elastase infusion model and the calcium chloride model of aneurysm occur only after the inflammatory response.[18,19] Furthermore, blocking this response with antibodies to these inflammatory cells[6] or with indomethacin[20] attenuates the dilatation. The difficulty of testing this hypothesis in a clinical trial is that anti-inflammatory medication (aspirin) is the current standard of care to most patients with AAA because of their cardiovascular risk factors. This makes it very difficult in practice to design a trial because the only options are stopping a medication that is protective against cardiovascular events in some of the patients or adding an additional anti-inflammatory agent. This second approach would be expected to have only an incremental effect, which means a very large sample size would be required. Thus, in practical terms, setting up and funding a clinical trial testing a general anti-inflammatory compound in AAA would be difficult.

Beta-Blockers

There are several lines of evidence supporting the hypothesis that aneurysm growth can be suppressed *in vivo.* Observational and retrospective clinical studies have revealed differences in the rate and extent of aneurysm growth that appear to depend on various clinical features, including initial aneurysm size, the extent of mural thrombus, uncontrolled hypertension, and active cigarette smoking. Propranolol received considerable interest, initially, because of its beneficial effects on patients with Marfan syndrome. Two retrospective clinical studies[21,22] examined expansion and rupture rates in AAA patients taking beta-blockers. These studies suggest that lower rates of aneurysm expansion are associated with propranolol treatment. Several animal studies have also indicated that propranolol might have beneficial effects in models of aneurysm disease. These studies employed a turkey model of spontaneous aortic dissection and rupture[23] as well as the "blotchy" mouse.[5] This murine model is based on a genetic defect in copper metabolism. Copper is an essential cofactor in the processing and maturation of the aortic matrix. These mice die prematurely of aortic dissection/rupture. Neither of these models appear to reproduce human AAA with a high degree of accuracy.

Propranolol was initially proposed to act through modulation of hemodynamic stress on the compromised aortic wall. It may, however, have other favorable biochemical effects. Indeed, some investigators suggest that the predominant influence of this agent may be through an effect on the stability of cross-linked connective tissue proteins rather than its effect on cardiovascular hemodynamics. More recent studies using the elastase-induced rat model of AAA indicate that propranolol suppresses aneurysm development in rats with spontaneous hypertension, but not in their normotensive counterparts. The exact mechanisms by which propranolol might exert such an effect remains unresolved and controversial. Nonetheless, these studies have led to the initiation of prospective randomized clinical trials in Canada, Great Britain, and Denmark to evaluate the effect of propranolol on the growth of small asymptomatic AAA. At this time, the only results available are from the Danish study.[24] This trial was discontinued after 2 yr because the majority of patients in the propranolol group dropped out because of side effects. Although growth rates did not differ statistically, the relative risk of growth was 2.44 in the patients continuing on propranolol and 1.17 in the placebo group. The conclusion of the trial is that only a small proportion (22%) of patients with small AAA was able to remain on propranolol for 2 yr. Furthermore, in the small group that completed the 2 yr, there was no trend toward reduced AAA growth. Although we await the data from the other trials, the Danish study suggests that propranolol will not inhibit AAA growth and will not likely be an important confounding variable in trial testing other therapies.

Protease Inhibitors

Through numerous studies conducted throughout the 1990s, a pathophysiologic concept has emerged that proteolytic degradation of medial elastin and adventitial collagen is responsible for aneurysm rupture. Because elastin is one of the most durable structural proteins of the extracellular matrix, the dissolution of elastic fibers is thought to require the presence of specific proteinases. Abundant evidence now suggests that members of the matrix metalloproteinase (MMP) family mediate the elastin and collagen degradation in aneurysm tissue in large part. The MMPs implicated in human aneurysm disease, MMP-2,[25] MMP-9,[26] and MMP-12,[27] attracted particular interest because they have activity against insoluble elastin fibers. MMP-9 is the most abundant elastolytic proteinase produced by human AAA tissues *in vitro.* It is abundantly expressed *in situ* by aneurysm-infiltrating macrophages located at the site of tissue damage and is synthesized in AAA tissue in a manner correlating with increased aneurysm diameter. Recent work from Curci et al.[28] demonstrated that macrophage MMP-9 is required for experimental aneurysm induction. Whereas MMP-2 is found in close association with the extracellular matrix in aneurysm tissue,[25] MMP-9 is elevated in the circulating plasma of patients with AAA.[29] MMP-12 is also thought to play a critical role in aneurysm development, because it is selectively expressed by macrophages within the elastic media of AAA tissue and, unlike other MMPs produced in the degenerating aortic wall, it is specifically localized to elastin fiber fragments by immunohistochemistry.[27] These observations have fostered the notion that MMP-2, MMP-9, MMP-12, and possibly other metalloproteinases provide useful biologic markers of aortic aneurysm disease as well as potential targets for pharmacologic therapy.

There are a large number of very potent hydroxamate inhibitors of MMPs in development, and trials involving a number of neoplastic and inflammatory diseases. One of these inhibitors has been shown to block experimental aneurysm formation in a rat model.[30] The tetracyclines may offer some important advantages over the hydromata inhibitors, even though they are less-potent MMP inhibitors. During studies on the mechanisms of periodontitis in diabetic rats, Golub and colleagues made the initial discovery that tetracyclines have substantial metalloproteinase-inhibiting effects.[31] They subsequently reported that like naturally occurring tissue inhibitors of metalloproteinases (TIMPs), tetracyclines directly inhibit MMP activity. Subsequent work has shown that there may be several mechanisms involved in their MMP inhibiting capacity. Non-antibiotic chemically modified tetracyclines (CMTs) have similar efficacy as MMP inhibitors, demonstrating that the MMP-inhibiting property of tetracyclines is unrelated to their antimicrobial activity. Any new hydromate inhibitor would have to undergo extensive testing for safety. Because of the potency of these drugs, fibrosis is a major concern. However, the tetracyclines are inexpensive and readily available.

Tetracyclines prevent matrix degradation in many animal models of disease. Their appeal for a clinical trial relates to their having been used since the early 1960s with a remarkable safety profile. More recently, they have been tested successfully in several conditions associated with elevated MMP activity and connective tissue destruction (i.e., rheumatoid arthritis, osteoarthritis, and periodontal disease). Although this indicates that tetracyclines might have similar utility as other metalloproteinase inhibitors in patients with AAA, it has only recently been demonstrated that these agents can effectively penetrate and suppress MMPs in the complex tissue environment of degenerative human aortic aneurysms[32] (Figure 13–2).

Enhancing the Reparative Response

There is evidence that aneurysmal degeneration is accompanied by an active process of connective tissue repair, as suggested by the expression of tropoelastin and procollagen mRNA in human aneurysm tissue and elevated levels of serum aminoterminal procollagen peptides in patients with AAA.[33,34] Endogenous mechanisms of connective tissue repair are further implied by the reduction in aneurysm size following successful endovascular repair of AAA, a form of treatment in which the aneurysmal wall is left intact. Despite these observations, little is known regarding the functional significance of

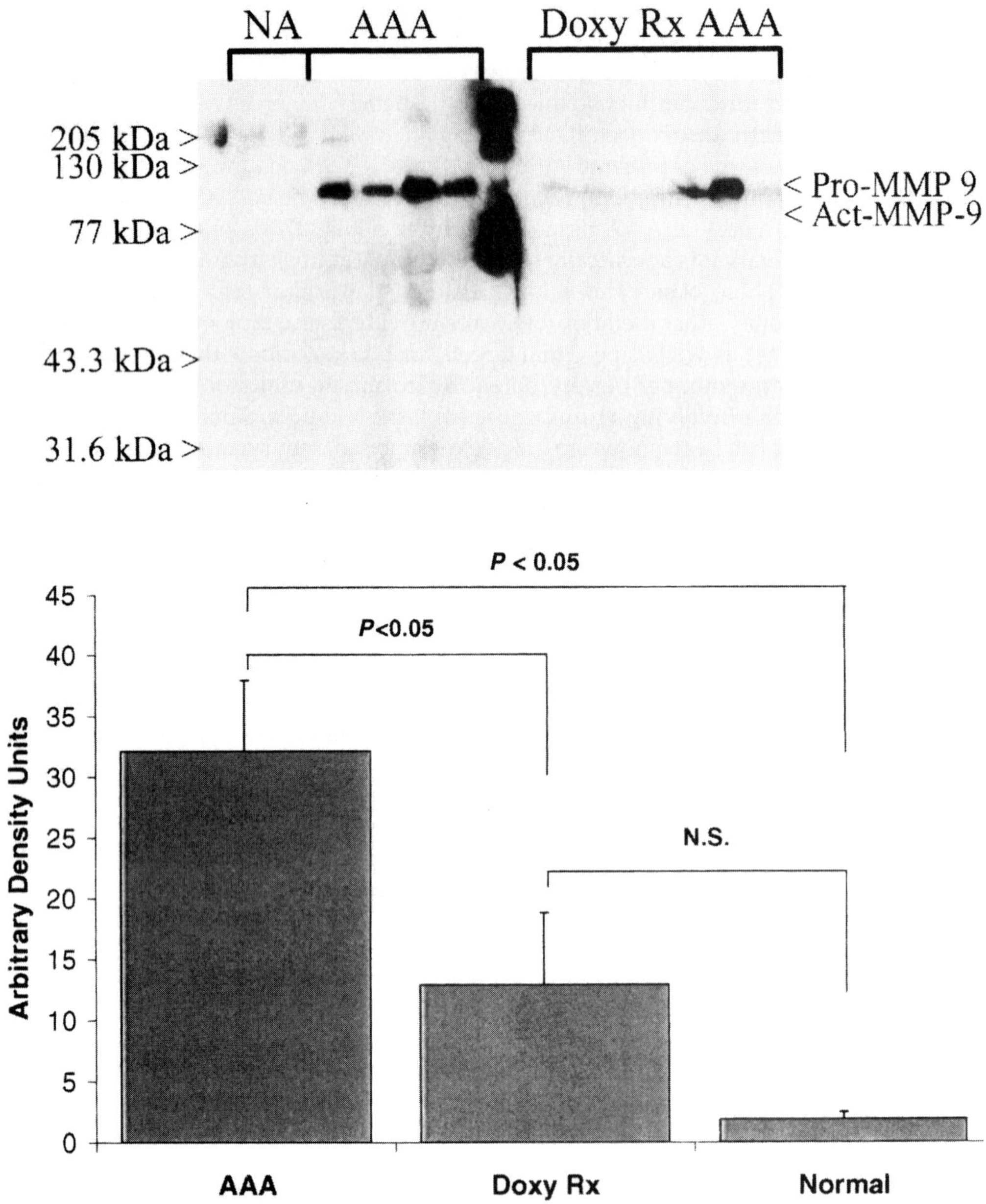

Figure 13–2. Suppression of aortic aneurysm MMP-9 by preoperative treatment with doxycycline. The upper panel shows tissue MMP-9 levels determined by Western immunoblot analysis. The lower panel shows significant suppression of MMP-9 in AAA patients treated with doxycycline. *(Curci JA, Mao D, Bohner DG, et al. Preoperative treatment with doxycycline reduces aortic wall expression and activation of matrix metalloproteinases in patients with abdominal aortic aneurysms. J Vasc Surg. 2000;31:325–342.)*

connective tissue repair during aneurysmal degeneration or the molecular mechanisms that act to promote or limit this reparative response. It is also not known if strategies designed to foster an increase in structural connective tissue proteins have the potential to promote stabilization of an established aneurysm.

PUTTING TOGETHER A CLINICAL TRIAL FOR AAA

Defining a testable hypothesis is the first step in designing a clinical trial to determine if doxycycline or other inhibitors will prevent AAA expansion. In a prospective clinical trial that is now being planned, we will test the hypothesis that doxycycline will reduce the growth rate of AAA by one-third during a 3-yr follow-up period. Ideally, an inhibitor should at least double the time from detection of a small (3.5 cm) AAA to its reaching a size where intervention would be considered (5.5 cm). This would require a 50% reduction in growth rate. A lower threshold (such as 33%) would, however, show that inhibition could be achieved. This would lead to refinement and further testing of other inhibitors. Furthermore, this degree of reduction would be considered very significant to a group of patients now relegated to "watchful waiting" with no alternative medical therapy. The risk of setting the threshold too high (50–75%) in a large clinical trial is that a lesser degree of inhibition may not be detected. A reduction of greater than 50% would provide definitive therapy for most patients (Figure 13–1). Because the all-cause death rate in this group of patients is relatively high (6–7%) based on their age and cardiovascular risk factors, the majority of patients would die with their aneurysm rather than from it during this time. Thus, the need for intervention would be averted in many patients.

After determining the expected reduction in expansion rate, a calculation can be made of the number of patients required to complete the trial to have a high degree of certainty (90% power to detect difference) that a 33% reduction in growth rate could be detected. Because this is the number that must complete the trial, an estimate of the expected attrition during the trial must be made. Reasons for attrition include: (1) failure to tolerate the medication or placebo; (2) death from all causes, including AAA rupture; and (3) aneurysm growth or development of symptoms requiring repair. This estimate must be added to the number required to finish in order to determine the enrollment needed to provide an adequate sample size at the completion of the trial. The anticipated drug-related problems from tetracyclines include GI distress, photosensitivity, vertigo, and secondary fungal infection. In order to assess the incidence of these problems in the elderly population affected by AAA, a 6-mo pilot trial has been conducted. Although follow-up is just now being completed, preliminary analysis suggests the drug is well tolerated in this group.

The second issue, attrition from death related to all causes, is reported to be 6–7% per annum. This was corroborated by the results of the recently published United Kingdom trial comparing early surgery to observation for small AAA. They found the 5-yr mortality was 30% (7%/yr compounding) from deaths unrelated to the aneurysmal disease. The most common causes of death—myocardial infarction, stroke, and cancer—were consistent with previous observations. The United Kingdom small aneurysm trial also provides some information regarding expected rates of crossover to surgery. This randomized trial compared ultrasound observation to immediate surgery for aneurysms between 4 and 5.5 cm in diameter. Their indications for surgery were (1) growth in excess of 10 mm/yr, (2) diameter exceeding 5.5 cm, or (3) development of symptoms. Their was a high rate of crossover from observation to surgery in this trial (17%/yr compounding). This is, perhaps, not surprising because aneurysms in the 5.1 to 5.5 mm-size range would need minimal growth (1–5 mm) to exceed the 5.5 cm threshold for surgery. In fact, based on average growth, most patients in this size would be expected to reach 5.5 cm within the first year of observation. By selecting aneurysms between 3.5 and 5.0 cm, at least 0.6 cm of growth must occur before the 5.5-cm threshold for surgery is exceeded. This would result in a much lower crossover rate. Summing all causes of expected attrition, at least half of the patients will be lost during the 3 yr of follow-up in the trial. The effect of this will be a significant increase in the sample size.

CONCLUSIONS

The 1990s saw significant strides in defining the pathogenesis of abdominal aortic aneurysm as the expertise of researchers from a broad range of scientific backgrounds has been brought to bear on the disease. Enhanced by the convergence of matrix biochemistry, cell biology, and immunology, this work is providing important new insight into how matrix metabolism is regulated in the diseased aorta. As we learned from the evolution in treatment of other pathologic processes, such as peptic ulcer disease, the most effective pharmacologic therapies are designed from a thorough understanding of the pathophysiology of the disease. We are quickly developing that understanding as we move from the descriptive research of the 1990s to the current work defining the various complex interactions that result in the formation of aortic aneurysm. Given the progress of the 1990s, clinical trials are in progress or being initiated. Developing a medical therapy to inhibit AAA growth will have great benefit, including psychological benefit, to the patient with small AAA.

ACKNOWLEDGMENTS

Supported by grants NIH RO1-HL53409 and an American Heart Association Established Investigator Award (BTB) and RO1-HL56701, 64332, 643302 (RWT).

REFERENCES

1. Ernst C. Abdominal aortic aneurysms. *N Engl J Med.* 1993;328:1167–1172.
2. Bickerstaff LK, Hollier LH, Van Peenen HJ, Melton LJ, Pairolero PC, and Cherry KJ. Abdominal aortic aneurysm repair combined with a second surgical procedure—morbidity and mortality. *Surgery.* 1984;95:487–491.
3. Katz DJ, Stanley JC, and Zelenock GB. Operative mortality rates for intact and ruptured abdominal aortic. *J Vasc Surg.* 1994;19:804–815.

4. Allaire E, Forough R, Clowes M, Starcher B, and Clowes AW. Local overexpression of TIMP-1 prevents aortic aneurysm degeneration and rupture in a rat model. *J Clin Invest.* 1998; 102:1413–1420.
5. Brophy CM, Tilson JE, and Tilson MD. Propranolol stimulates the crosslinking of matrix components in skin from the aneurysm-prone blotchy mouse. *J Surg Res.* 1989;46:330–332.
6. Ricci MA, Strindberg G, Slaiby JM, et al. Anti-CD 18 monoclonal antibody slows experimental aortic aneurysm expansion. *J Vasc Surg.* 1996;23:301–307.
7. Johnston KW, Rutherford RB, Tilson MD, Shah DM, Hollier L, and Stanley JC. Suggested standards for reporting on arterial aneurysms. Subcommittee on Reporting Standards for Arterial Aneurysms, Ad Hoc Committee on Reporting Standards, Society for Vascular Surgery and North American Chapter, International Society for Cardiovascular Surgery [see comments]. *J Vasc Surg.* 1991;13:452–458.
8. Pearce WH, Slaughter MS, LeMaire S, et al. Aortic diameter as a function of age, gender, and body surface area [see comments]. *Surgery.* 1993;114:691–697.
9. Lederle FA, Johnson GR, Wilson SE, et al. Prevalence and associations of abdominal aortic aneurysm detected through screening. Aneurysm Detection and Management (ADAM) Veterans Affairs Cooperative Study Group. *Ann Intern Med.* 1997;126:441–449.
10. Alcorn HG, Wolfson SK, Jr., Sutton-Tyrrell K, Kuller LH, and O'Leary D. Risk factors for abdominal aortic aneurysms in older adults enrolled in the Cardiovascular Health Study. *Arterioscler Thromb Vasc Biol.* 1996;16:963–970.
11. Matsumura JS, Pearce WH, McCarthy WJ, and Yao JS. Reduction in aortic aneurysm size: early results after endovascular graft placement. EVT Investigators. *J Vasc Surg.* 1997;25:113–123.
12. Wilson KA, Woodburn KR, Ruckley CV, and Fowkes FG. Expansion rates of abdominal aortic aneurysm: current limitations in evaluation. *Eur J Vasc Endovasc Surg.* 1997;13:521–526.
13. Brown PM, Pattenden R, Vernooy C, et al. Selective management of abdominal aortic aneurysms in a prospective measurement program. *J Vasc Surg.* 1996;23:213–222.
14. Burchfiel CM, Laws A, Benfante R, et al. Combined effects of HDL cholesterol, triglyceride, and total cholesterol concentrations on 18-year risk of atherosclerotic disease. *Circulation.* 1995;92:1430–1436.
15. Chang J, Stein T, Liu J, et al. Risk factors associated with rapid growth of small abdominal aortic aneurysms. *Surgery.* 1997;121:117.
16. Krupski WC, Bass A, Thurston DW, Dilley RB, and Bernstein EF. Utility of computed tomography for surveillance of small abdominal aortic aneurysms. Preliminary report. *Arch Surg.* 1990;125:1345–1349; discussion, 1349–1350.
17. Koch AE, Haines GK, Rizzo RJ, Radosevich JA, Pope RM, and Robinson PG. Human abdominal aortic aneurysms: immunophenotypic analysis suggesting an immune-mediate response. *Am J Pathol.* 1990;137:1199–1213.
18. Anidjar S, Dobrin P, Eichorst M, Graham G, and Chejfec G. Correlation of inflammatory infiltrate with the enlargement of experimental aortic aneurysms. *J Vasc Surg.* 1992;16:139–147.
19. Gertz SD, Kurgan A, and Eisenberg D. Aneurysm of the rabbit common carotid artery induced by periarterial application of calcium chloride *in vivo*. *J Clin Invest.* 1988;81:649–656.
20. Holmes DR, Petrinec D, Wester W, Thompson RW, and Reilly JM. Indomethacin prevents elastase-induced abdominal aortic aneurysms in the rat. *J Surg Res.* 1996;63:305–309.
21. Leach S, Toole A, Stern H, et al. Effect of beta-adrenergic blockage on the growth rate of abdominal aortic aneurysms. *Arch Surg.* 1988;123:606.
22. Gadowski G, Pilcher D, and Ricci, MA. Abdominal aortic aneurysm expansion rate: effect of size and beta-adrenergic blockade. *J Vasc Surg.* 1994;19:727.
23. Boucek R, Gunja-Smith Z, Noble N, and Simpson C. Modulation by propranolol of the lysyl

cross-links in aortic elastin and collagen of the aneurysm-prone turkey. *Biochem Pharmacol.* 1983;32:275–280.

24. Lindholt JS, Henneberg EW, Juul S, and Fasting H. Impaired results of a randomised double blinded clinical trial of propranolol versus placebo on the expansion rate of small abdominal aortic aneurysms. *Int Angiol.* 1999;18:52–57.
25. Davis V, Persidskaia R, Baca-Regen L, et al. Matrix metalloproteinase-2 production and its binding to the matrix are increased in abdominal aortic aneurysms. *Arterioscler Thromb Vasc Biol.* 1998;18:1625–1633.
26. Thompson RW, Holmes DR, Mertens RA, et al. Production and localization of 92-kilodalton gelatinase in abdominal aortic aneurysms. An elastolytic metalloproteinase expressed by aneurysm-infiltrating macrophages. *J Clin Invest.* 1995;96:318–326.
27. Curci JA, Liao S, Huffman MD, Shapiro SD, and Thompson RW. Expression and localization of macrophage elastase (matrix metalloproteinase-12) in abdominal aortic aneurysms. *J Clin Invest.* 1998;102:1900–1910.
28. Pyo R, Lee JK, Shipley JM, et al. Targeted gene disruption of matrix metalloproteinase-9 (gelatinase B) suppresses development of experimental abdominal aortic aneurysms [in Process Citation]. *J Clin Invest.* 2000;105:1641–1649.
29. McMillan WD, Tamarina NA, Cipollone M, Johnson DA, Parker MA, and Pearce WH. Size matters: the relationship between MMP-9 expression and aortic diameter [see comments]. *Circulation.* 1997;96:2228–2232.
30. Bigatel DA, Elmore JR, Carey DJ, Cizmeci-Smith G, Franklin DP, and Youkey JR. The matrix metalloproteinase inhibitor BB-94 limits expansion of experimental abdominal aortic aneurysms. *J Vasc Surg.* 1999;29:130–138; discussion, 138–139.
31. Golub LM, McNamara TF, D'Angelo G, et al. A non-antibiotic chemically-modified tetracycline inhibits mammalian collagenase activity. *J Dental Research* 1987;66:1310–1314.
32. Curci JA, Mao D, Bohner DG, et al. Preoperative treatment with doxycycline reduces aortic wall expression and activation of matrix metalloproteinases in patients with abdominal aortic aneurysms. *J Vasc Surg.* 2000;31:325–342.
33. Ghorpade A and Baxter BT. Biochemistry and molecular regulation of matrix macromolecules in abdominal aortic aneurysms. In Tilson MD, Boyd CD, eds. *The Abdominal Aortic Aneurysm: Genetics, Pathophysiology, and Molecular Biology.* New York: Annals of the New York Academy of Sciences 1996;800:138–150.
34. Satta J, Haukipuro K, Kairaluoma MI, and Juvonen T. Aminoterminal propeptide of type III procollagen in the follow-up of patients with abdominal aortic aneurysms. *J Vasc Surg.* 1997;25:909–915.

14

Surgical Management of Recurrent Aortic and Iliac Aneurysms

James L. Ebaugh, MD, and Jon S. Matsumura, MD

INTRODUCTION

Operations on recurrent aortic and iliac aneurysms are becoming more frequent because patients are living longer after successful treatment of aortic aneurysms. Recurrent aneurysms occur both for technical reasons and also from the generalized nature of aneurysmal disease. Pseudoaneurysms used to be predominant in early years, especially prior to 1967, when degradable materials such as silk were used for many aortic reconstructions.[1] Since then, with improved techniques, suture material, and graft materials, true aneurysms have surpassed pseudoaneurysms as the most common reason for reoperation.

The complex nature of these problems requires an up-to-date review of new endovascular techniques as well as a summary of the well-established conventional surgical techniques of reoperative surgery. Regardless of the cause of the recurrent problem, the operative approaches are similar and depend on the anatomy and clinical presentation.

This chapter describes the distribution and etiology of these aneurysms, ways to monitor for recurrence, and management of these problems in the operating room.

DEFINITION

A proximal or distal aortic or iliac diameter more than or equal to 1.5 times the diameter of the original prosthesis has been used to define recurrent aortoiliac aneurysms[2] (Figures 14–1 and 14–2). Alternatively, diameters of 4.0 cm and 3.0 cm for infrarenal aortic and iliac arteries, respectively, define primary as well as recurrent aneurysms in the average 70-kg individual.[3] A suprarenal aneurysm larger than 5.5 cm has been sug-

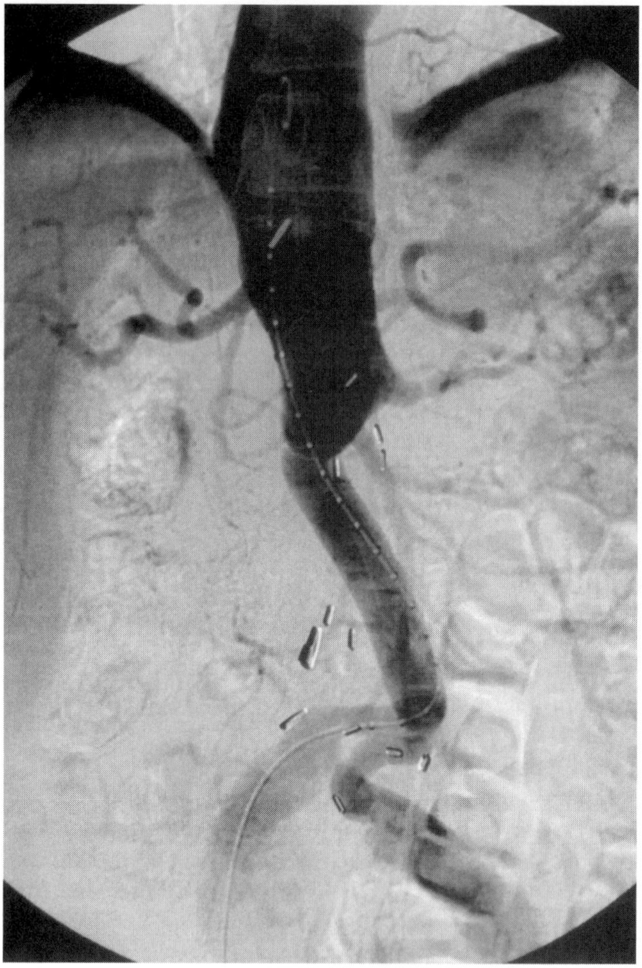

Figure 14–1. Arteriogram reveals diffuse aortic dilation proximal to previous AAA repair. Bilateral iliac aneurysms are also evident.

gested as an arbitrary cutoff for elective replacement by some authors.[4,5] We use the same threshold for operative intervention, with individualization based on patient comorbidities, similar to evaluation for primary aneurysm repair.

ETIOLOGY

True aneurysms of the native arteries represent the cause of the majority of subsequent aneurysms in the Northwestern series (73%)[6] (Figure 14–3). The other 27% were anastomotic pseudoaneurysms or midgraft aneurysms. Preoperative imaging, operative reports detailing the proximity of a previous anastomosis, and history of extensive endarterectomy are important in determining the etiology of subsequent aneurysms.[1] Other factors, such as suture failure, graft dilation, or infection, suggest pseudoaneurysm formation as the cause.

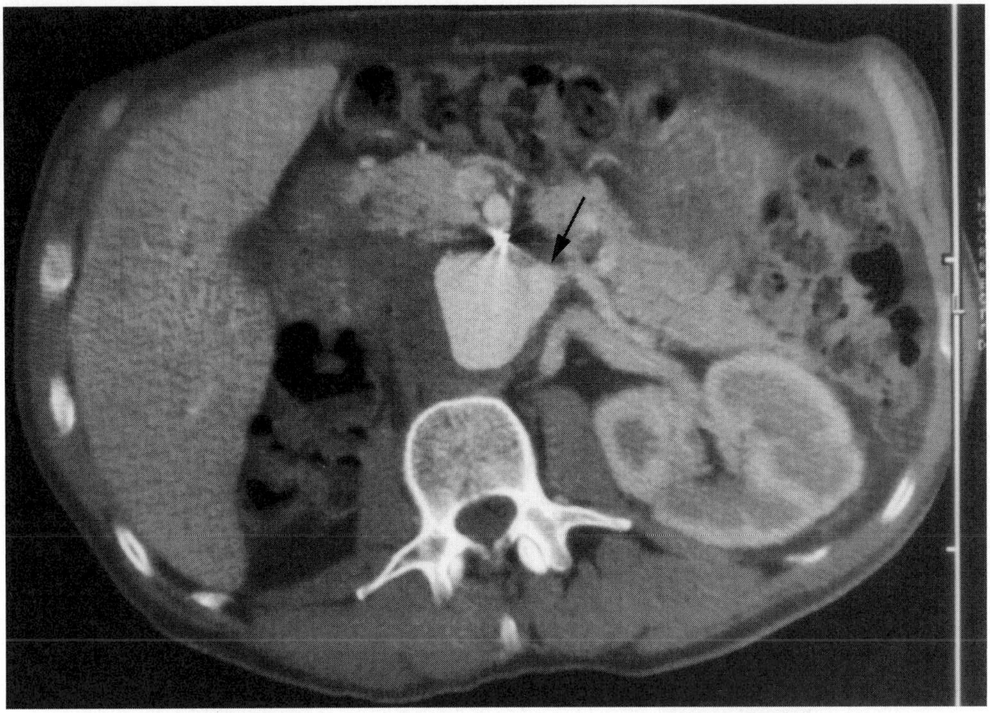

Figure 14–2. Note the significant amount of mural thrombus at the level of the solitary left renal artery (*arrow*) in CT scan of the aneurysm from Figure 14–3. Also, the left renal vein has a large lumbar collateral branch.

Subsequent extension of aneurysmal disease has been documented in several other studies. Hallett et al.[7] showed subsequent proximal neck growth in 13% of patients following conventional open repair with a mean follow-up of 5.8 yr in a population-based study. Coselli et al.[4] reported a range of 3–8% recurrence of aneurysmal disease proximal to previous infrarenal aortic aneurysm surgery (Figures 14–4 and 14–5). Plate et al.[8] reported a 5.4% complication rate at 5 yr due to recurrent aneurysms after abdominal aortic aneurysm (AAA) repair, with true aneurysms also predominating. It is interesting to note that primary endovascular repairs have been associated with proximal and distal aortic neck expansion rates of approximately 0.7 and 1.7 mm per year, respectively.[9] Clearly, intrinsic aortic disease is responsible for the development of many subsequent aortic aneurysms.

Synchronous or retained aneurysms represent the third category of aortic aneurysms that require a second operation. Crawford and Cohen[10] reported a retrospective series of more than 1500 aortic aneurysm patients, of which 12.6% had synchronous aneurysms at their initial presentation. This number may be high due to referral patterns but underlines the need for at least cursory screening for thoracic and thoracoabdominal aneurysms on initial workup of a patient with an AAA.

Retained aneurysms may be more frequent in the case of a ruptured aneurysm repair, and earlier surveillance should be performed in these cases. Retained aneurysms

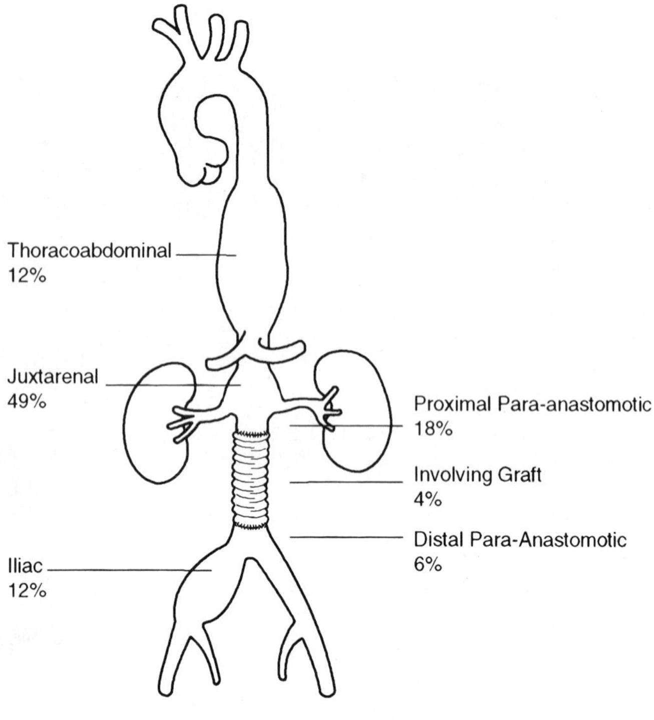

Figure 14–3. Distribution of more than 90 subsequent aneurysms in the Northwestern series. (Adapted from Matsumura et al. *J Cardiovasc Surg* 1999;7:614–621.)

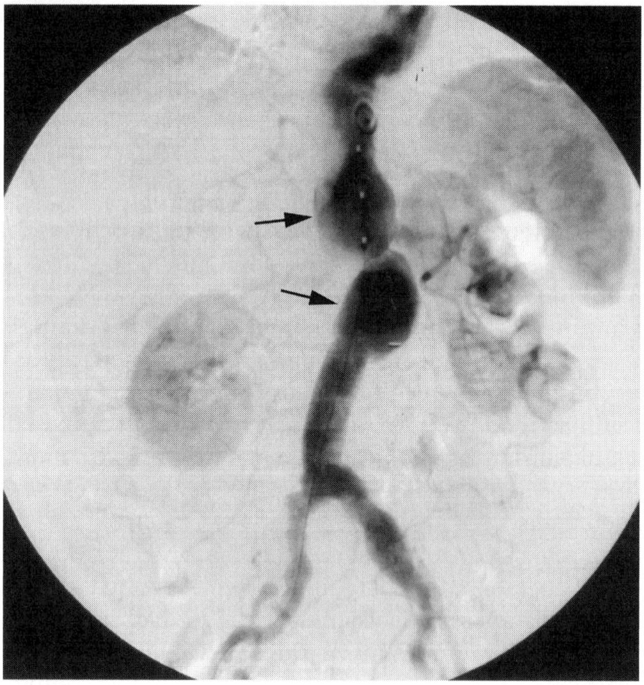

Figure 14–4. Angiogram depicts two distinct recurrent true aneurysms (*arrows*) superior to previous tube graft repair.

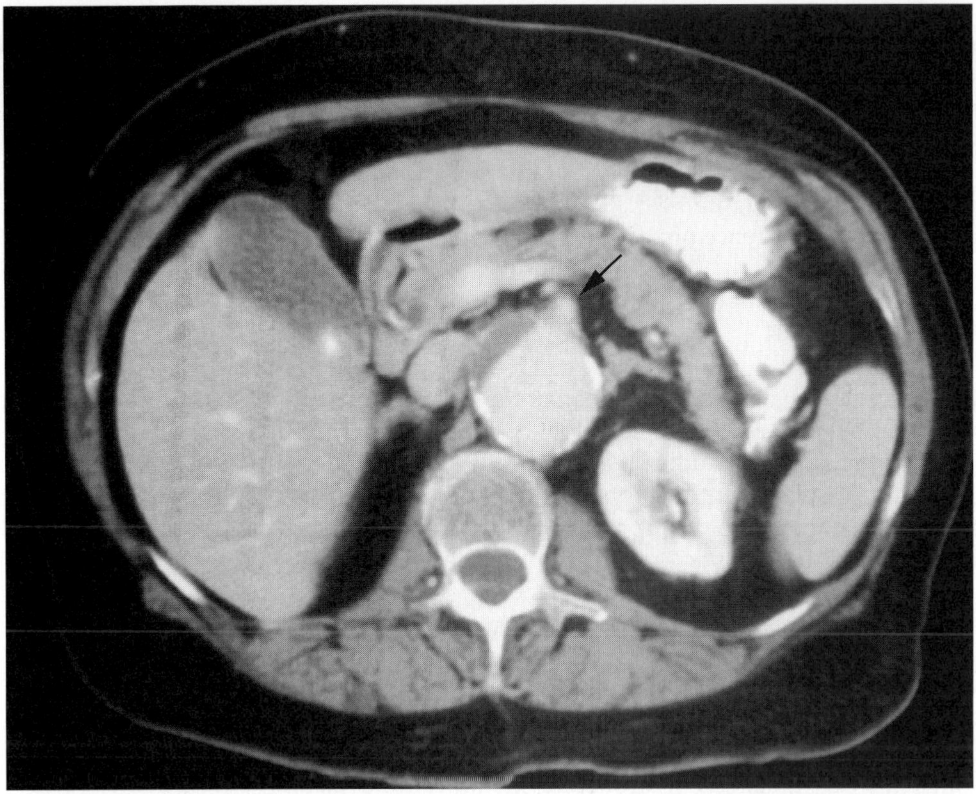

Figure 14–5. CT scan of the proximal aneurysm from Figure 14–4 involving the origins of the celiac and superior mesenteric (*arrow*) arteries necessitated control of the aorta superior to the diaphragm through a thoracoabdominal incision.

should be a rare entity in the elective setting with the modern techniques used to treat juxtarenal aneurysms.

RISK FACTORS AND LOCATION

Aortic surgery is usually quite durable, and identification of risk factors could highlight the need for more frequent clinical and radiologic screening in selected patients. Hypertension, implicated in some studies[4,8] as a marker for aneurysm recurrence, was not a risk factor in other reports. Gender, diabetes, smoking, graft material, type of graft, and pararenal anastomosis were also not independent risk factors for future aneurysm development.[6]

Younger age at initial operation was confirmed as a risk factor for subsequent aneurysms. Patients needing a second operation had a mean age of 58 ± 11 yr at their primary operation and 68 ± 11 yr at reoperation. These patients are an average of 8 yr younger than their counterparts who only require one aortic operation.

End-to-side anastomoses performed at the initial operation also predisposed to para-anastomotic aneurysms. Most of these were not pseudoaneurysms but dilation of the native aorta near the original anastomosis with intraluminal thrombus. We minimize the use of the end-to-side configuration unless significant inferior pole renal arteries, pelvic, or visceral perfusion would be compromised.

The distribution of more than 90 secondary aneurysms in the Northwestern series is summarized by Figure 14–5. Of note, all patients with more than one aneurysm had an aneurysm recurrence proximal to the original graft.

PRESENTATION

Most secondary aneurysms are deep in the pelvis or under the ribs and evade clinical detection. Routine radiographic follow-up is necessary to detect subsequent aneurysms and prevent rupture. Studies that used radiographic follow-up[2,3,11] detected a higher incidence of subsequent aneurysms, approximately 9–15%. Incidental diagnosis of a nonpalpable aneurysm during unrelated medical evaluations shows that without routine imaging, diagnosis is largely left to chance.[12]

Associated clinical findings warrant radiologic evaluation of the entire prosthesis as well as the retained iliac and abdominal aorta.[6] A femoral pseudoaneurysm can hint at the presence of a more proximal pseudoaneurysm. Graft limb occlusion, hydronephrosis, and unexplained abdominal pain should also prompt CT scanning. Proximal aortic aneurysms may also present with microembolization, chest or upper back pain, and acute graft limb occlusion. Iliac aneurysms often present with compressive symptoms, such as unilateral hydronephrosis, bowel and bladder problems from sacral plexus impingement, or lower extremity edema from iliac vein compression.[1]

Even in large patients, a reliable and thorough radiologic assessment may be accomplished with contrast-enhanced CT. Helical CT gives superior images and is particularly advantageous in the deep pelvis and visceral aorta for depicting vascular anatomic relationships.

Recommendations for surveillance are based on the average interval preceding secondary aneurysm repair. This interval averages between 6 and 10 yr.[6,13,14] In the Northwestern study, no patient was known to have rupture within 10 yr of the first operation. It is reasonable to obtain a screening CT every 5 yr, balancing adequate early warning and cost-effectiveness. Earlier surveillance may be indicated for patients who present initially with rupture, a scenario for which tube grafts are likely used, thereby occasionally leaving residual iliac or suprarenal disease.

MANAGEMENT

The standard operative repair of recurrent aneurysms requires generous exposure, common and alternative methods of vascular control, and familiarity with grafting techniques in a reoperative field. Endovascular treatment for these complex problems has been reported and can avoid many of the difficulties encountered in reoperative aortic surgery.

One technique that we have found useful for subsequent iliac aneurysm repair is the use of ureteral stents. They provide palpable landmarks when dissecting scarred lower abdominal and pelvic structures. Stents are placed in the operating room with a flexible cystoscope just prior to making the incision, and are removed immediately postoperatively unless a ureteral injury or gross hematuria occurs during the procedure.

The choice of incision is customized to the location of the recurrent aneurysm. A generous midline incision is used for most scenarios involving simultaneous pararenal and iliac recurrences. For aneurysms extending above the visceral arteries, we prefer a thoracoabdominal approach. A retroperitoneal exposure is useful when a transperitoneal approach was taken at the initial vascular operation, because a previously undissected plane can be developed.

When performing an anterior approach, there are three tactics to improve exposure of the pararenal aorta. One is to mobilize the left renal vein by dividing the adrenal, gonadal, and lumbar branches. This excludes the second option, which is to divide the left renal vein near the vena cava. Division usually provides for adequate left kidney venous drainage via the lumbar, adrenal, inferior phrenic, and gonadal veins. Left renal vein division has been implicated in cases of postoperative azotemia,[15,16] with one study[17] recommending that this not be performed unless absolutely necessary if the left renal vein stump pressure exceeds 50–60 cm of water or in the presence of right kidney dysfunction. If it is essential to preserve marginal kidney function, the left renal vein can be divided and reanastomosed following aortic repair, although the benefit of this maneuver is unknown.

The third tactic is to obtain proximal control of a juxtarenal aneurysm with supraceliac clamping, which is then moved onto the graft after expeditious completion of the proximal anastomosis. This approach is technically easier than clamping above one of the renal arteries or between the superior mesenteric artery (SMA) and both of the renal arteries. These other methods may be associated with a paradoxically higher rate of complications, such as pancreatitis and renal insufficiency.[18] Supraceliac control has been elegantly detailed by May et al.[19] The left lobe of the liver is retracted to the right, the esophagus is retracted to the left, and the gastrohepatic ligament is divided transversely. An incision is then made into the fleshy part of the right crus, superior to the median arcuate ligament and well away from the variable arrangement of the celiac and inferior phrenic arteries. The muscle fibers are split apart with scissors and the aorta straddled with the middle and index fingers of the right hand, which then guide the tips of a vascular clamp posteriorly to the vertebral column.

We prefer supraceliac clamping for most emergent and elective complex aortic operations. Having the aortic clamp out of the immediate field facilitates addressing complex tasks such as converting an end-to-side anastomosis to an end-to-end configuration. Untoward effects of this technique are a transient rise in serum bilirubin and mild perioperative coagulopathy with fibrinolysis even when occlusion times are kept to a minimum. One study with a mean supraceliac aortic cross-clamp time of only 25 ± 6 min[18] highlights the importance of clamping no longer than necessary to complete the proximal anastomoses.

Although the proximal anastomosis is often conducted in a fresh field, the distal anastomosis presents other difficulties. Distal control can be obtained with balloon occlusion catheters in order to avoid treacherous and time-consuming dissection in scarred tissue.[20] Often, the new graft is anastomosed to the old graft, occasionally presenting a size mismatch problem. Fashioning a taper in the new graft or spatulating the old graft (if there is adequate length) provides excellent hemostasis.

Residual iliac aneurysms may occur following tube graft repair of ruptured aneurysms, and iliac pseudoaneurysms comprise 5.5–14.8% of all reported pseudoaneurysms.[1] True iliac aneurysms, however, are rare following elective AAA repair.[6] Endovascular repair of these recurrent or residual iliac artery aneurysms is feasible (Figure 14–6).[21] This option can also be used for recurrent proximal aortic aneurysms when there is an adequate infrarenal neck to seal with the endograft. Currently, no endovascular grafts are approved for this use in the United States.

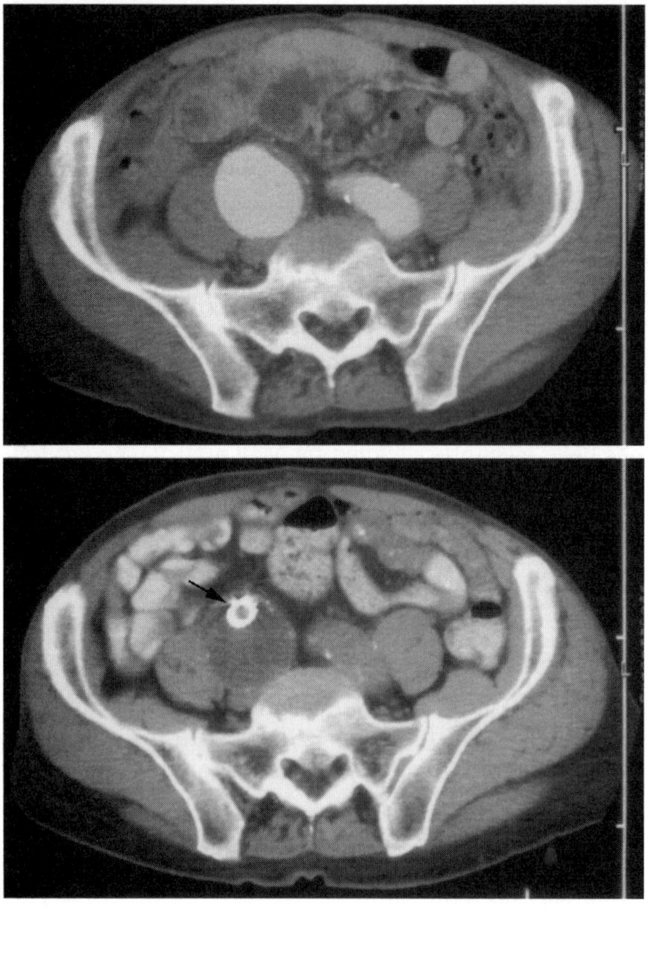

Figure 14–6. Off-label use of an endovascular graft (*arrow*) to exclude a right iliac aneurysm in a patient who had undergone previous ruptured AAA repair, before (*top*) and after (*bottom*) endovascular repair.

RESULTS

Postoperative mortality after operations for recurrent aortic and iliac aneurysms ranges from 5% to 28.6%.[4,6,8,20,22] Similar to emergent primary aortic surgery, mortality after rupture of these subsequent aneurysms is extremely high, ranging from 67% to 100% in several series.[6,8,14,20,22] This profound difference suggests that surveillance may be useful. Limited recurrent proximal disease has also been associated with better survival[22]; there is a significantly lower mortality for infrarenal repair (9%) compared with those requiring reattachment of the renal and/or visceral vessels (28%).

Postoperative paraplegia or paraparesis is associated with proximal thoracoabdominal repairs[4] but is rare after isolated clamping of the supraceliac aorta. Avoiding extensive mobilization of the supraceliac aorta with extensive division of intercostal and lumbar arteries and minimizing clamp time helps prevent this complication.

The incidence of renal failure ranges from 11.4% to 14.3%[4,20,22] in recurrent aortic aneurysm surgery. Oliguric renal failure has a stronger association with perioperative hypotension as opposed to nonoliguric renal failure, which had a correlation with longer aortic cross-clamp times.[4]

Of note, 2 of 65 patients in the Northwestern series experienced recurrence of a third aneurysm several years after their second operation. Both underwent tertiary operations without incident.

CONCLUSION

Subsequent aortic and iliac aneurysms are likely to be more common as the general population ages, use of cardiac revascularization increases, and primary perioperative surgical and anesthetic techniques improve.[23] Patients should undergo periodic monitoring after aortic operations. Principles of reoperative aortic surgery can be applied successfully to patients who need repair of recurrent aortic and iliac aneurysms.

REFERENCES

1. Clark ET, Gewertz BL. Pseudoaneurysms. In: Rutherford RB, ed. *Vascular surgery*, 4th ed. Philadelphia, PA. WB Saunders Co., 1995:1153–1161.
2. Sieswerda C, Skotnicki SH, Barentsz JO, Heystraten FMJ. Anastomotic aneurysms—an underdiagnosed complication after aorto-iliac reconstructions. *Eur J Vasc Surg*. 1989;3:233–238.
3. Edwards JM, Teefey SA, Zierler RE, Kohler TR. Intraabdominal paraanastomotic aneurysms after aortic bypass grafting. *J Vasc Surg*. 1992;15:344–353.
4. Coselli JS, LeMaire SA, Buket S, Berzin E. Subsequent proximal aortic operations in 123 patients with previous infrarenal abdominal aortic aneurysm surgery. *J Vasc Surg*. 1995;22:59–67.
5. Pearce WH, Slaughter MS, LeMaire S, et al. Aortic diameter as a function of age, gender, and body surface area. *Surgery*. 1993;114:691–697.
6. Matsumura JS, Pearce WH, Cabellon A, McCarthy WJ, Yao JST. Reoperative aortic surgery. *Cardiovasc Surg*. 1999;7:614–621.

7. Hallett JW, Marshall DM, Petterson TM, et al. Graft-related complications after abdominal aortic aneurysm repair: reassurance from a 36-year population-based experience. *J Vasc Surg.* 1997;25:277–286.
8. Plate G, Hollier LA, O'Brien P, et al. Recurrent aneurysms and late vascular complications following repair of abdominal aortic aneurysms. *Arch Surg.* 1985;120:590–594.
9. Matsumura JS, Chaikof EL, for the EVT Investigators. Continued expansion of aortic necks after endovascular repair of abdominal aneurysms. *J Vasc Surg.* 1998;28:422–431.
10. Crawford ES, Cohen ES. Aortic aneurysm: a multifocal disease. *Arch Surg.* 1982;117:1393–1400.
11. Berman SS, Hunter GC, Smyth SH, et al. Application of computed tomography for surveillance of aortic grafts. *Surgery.* 1995;118:8–15.
12. Hagino RT, Taylor SM, Fujitani RM, et al. Proximal anastomotic failure following infrarenal aortic reconstruction: late development of true aneurysms, pseudoaneurysms, and occlusive disease. *Ann Vasc Surg.* 1993;7:8–13.
13. Dennis JW, Littooy FN, Greisler HP, Baker WH. Anastomotic pseudoaneurysms: a continuing late complication of vascular reconstructive procedures. *Arch Surg.* 1986;121:314–317.
14. Treiman GS, Weaver FA, Cossman DV, et al. Anastomotic false aneurysms of the abdominal aorta and the iliac arteries. *J Vasc Surg.* 1988;8:268–273.
15. Huber D, Harris JP, Walker PJ, et al. Does division of the left renal vein during aortic surgery adversely affect renal function? *Ann Vasc Surg.* 1991;5:74–79.
16. Anderson JC, Sjolin SU, Holstein P. Ligation of the renal vein during resection of abdominal aortic aneurysm. *J Cardiovasc Surg.* 1986;27:454–456.
17. Calligaro KD, Savarese RP, McCombs PR, DeLaurentis DA. Division of the left renal vein during aortic surgery. *Am J Surg.* 1990;160:192–196.
18. Hines GL, Chorost M. Supraceliac aortic occlusion: a safe approach to pararenal aortic aneurysms. *Ann Vasc Surg.* 1998;12:335–340.
19. May J, Patrick W, Harris J. Transabdominal exposure of the thoracic aorta. *Surg Gynecol Obstet.* 1980;151:427–428.
20. Fox AD, Berkowitz HD. Thoracoabdominal aneurysm resection after previous infrarenal abdominal aortic aneurysmectomy. *Am J Surg.* 1991;162:142–144.
21. Panayiotopoulos YP, Sandison AJ, Reidy JF, et al. Endovascular repair of residual iliac artery aneurysms following surgery for ruptured abdominal aortic aneurysm. *Eur J Vasc Endovasc Surg.* 1996;12:482–486.
22. Curl GR, Faggioli GL, Stella A, et al. Aneurysmal change at or above the proximal anastomosis after infrarenal aortic grafting. *J Vasc Surg.* 1992;16:855–860.
23. O'Hara PJ, Hertzer NH, Krajewski LP, et al. Ten-year experience with abdominal aortic aneurysm repair in octogenarians: early results and late complications. *J Vasc Surg.* 1995;21:830–838.

15

Descending Thoracic Aorta for Mesenteric and Lower Extremity Revascularization

Mark A. Farber, MD, and Blair A. Keagy, MD

The use of the descending thoracic aorta (DTA) as inflow was introduced by Stevenson et al.[1] and Blaisdell[2] in 1961. Since that time, it has usually been reserved for remedial operations involving lower extremity revascularization. It derives its attractiveness from the relative sparing from atherosclerotic disease seen in this portion of the vascular tree. It is, however, unfamiliar territory to many vascular surgeons, and therefore traditionally has not been the approach of choice. More recently, it has been described as an appealing approach to provide antegrade mesenteric revascularization. In the past several years, the indications, surgical techniques, and results of DTA inflow–based procedures have been better defined, and as a result its use is increasing.

INDICATIONS

Lower-Extremity Revascularization

Bypass from the DTA to the iliac or femoral arteries is indicated in situations in which transabdominal aortic reconstruction is inadvisable or impossible. Such compromised conditions include previous failed infrarenal aortic or extra-anatomic grafts or patients requiring removal of an infected aortic prosthesis. DTA to femoral artery bypass is also indicated in selected patients in whom a primary conventional aortofemoral operation is less than optimal. Such situations include patients with severe atherosclerotic disease or complete occlusion of the infrarenal aorta and patients with intra-abdominal conditions precluding a direct aortic approach (i.e., prior intra-abdominal sepsis, multiple abdominal operations, radiation, or colostomy). Other indications for this type of bypass as a primary reconstruction are patients with unusual anatomic constraints, such as horseshoe kidney or hypoplastic abdominal aorta, in whom exposure of the infrarenal aorta may be difficult.

Mesenteric Revascularization

Most mesenteric revascularizations are conducted through a transabdominal approach. When infrarenal aortic based reconstruction becomes unattractive, the DTA may provide a better alternative. Such conditions include the aforementioned "hostile abdominal" situations and patients with multiple episodes of pancreatitis, rendering tunneling of bypasses difficult. In addition, its proximity to the origins of the celiac and superior mesenteric arteries allows for construction of short antegrade bypasses that may have less propensity to kink or thrombose. We therefore have chosen it as our primary reconstructive method for the treatment of chronic mesenteric ischemia.

The use of the descending thoracic aorta as an inflow source for primary aortoiliac and mesenteric reconstruction has a number of advantages over conventional direct aortic repair. First, the descending thoracic aorta typically has less atherosclerotic disease, making it more suitable for proximal anastomosis than the infrarenal aorta.[3] Second, the thoracic approach and use of a partially occluding aortic clamp for the proximal anastomosis maintains spinal cord, mesenteric, and renal blood flow. Third, the retroperitoneal location of the graft avoids unfavorable intra-abdominal conditions. Finally, placement of the proximal anastomosis in the chest further eliminates the potential for aortoenteric fistula.

SURGICAL TECHNIQUE

Thoracobifemoral Bypass

After general anesthesia and placement of a double lumen endotracheal tube, the patient is positioned with the left thorax elevated to a 45° to 60° angle (Figure 15–1). The left arm is elevated to the right and secured to an arm board to avoid left brachial nerve injury. The pelvis is placed flat to allow access to both groins, and pillows are placed under the knees to prevent hyperextension.

Bilateral vertical groin incisions are used to expose the femoral arteries. While the right groin exposure is below the inguinal ligament, the left groin incision is extended cephalad 5 to 10 cm above the inguinal ligament. With division of the internal oblique and transversus muscles parallel to the direction of the muscle fibers, the left retroperitoneal space anterior to the iliac vessels is entered. This space is used for later tunneling of the graft between the left chest and both groins.

A left posterolateral muscle sparing thoracotomy is performed through the eighth or ninth intercostal space. The deflated lung is retracted superiorly, and the inferior pulmonary ligament is divided to the level of the inferior pulmonary vein. To allow exposure of the distal descending thoracic aorta, the diaphragm is retracted inferiorly, avoiding injury to the underlying spleen and visceral organs. The aorta is palpated, and

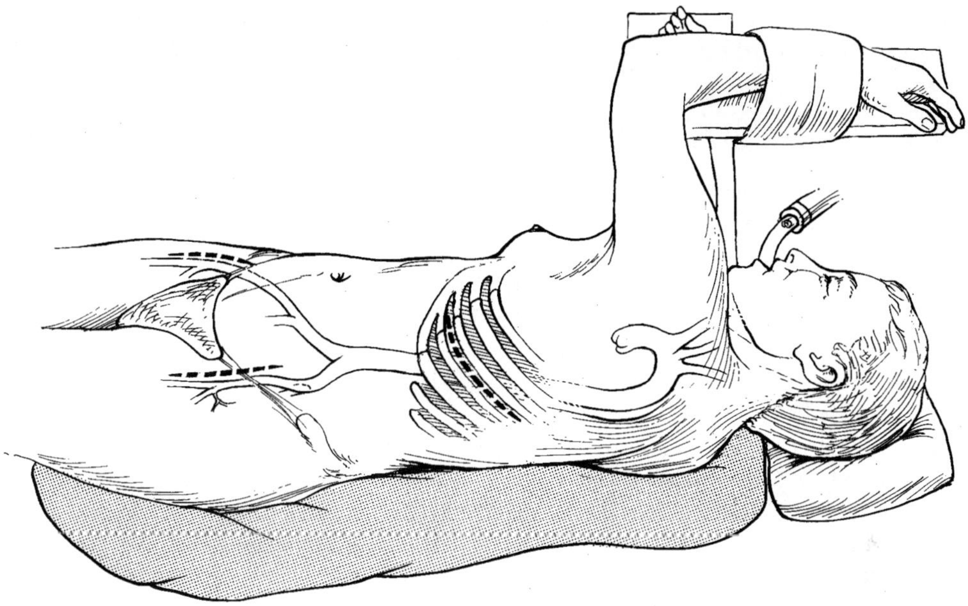

Figure 15–1. Patient positioned with the left hemithorax elevated and pelvis flat prior to descending thoracic aorta (DTA) to femoral artery bypass. Dashed lines show intended location of incisions for posterolateral thoracotomy and bilateral groin exposures. (*From Criado E. Descending thoracic aorta to femoral artery bypass: surgical technique. Ann Vasc Surg. 1997;11(2): 206–215. Used by permission.*)

a site with minimal atherosclerotic disease is selected for proximal anastomosis. The distal descending thoracic aorta is mobilized from the parietal pleura, with careful preservation of the intercostal arterial branches.

The diaphragm is mobilized approximately 5 cm from its posterior attachments. Using blunt finger dissection, a retroperitoneal plane is developed posteriomedial to the spleen, posterior to the kidney, and anterior to the psoas muscle. Simultaneously, using the opposite hand from the left suprainguinal preperitoneal space, blunt dissection is carried upward, crossing over the external iliac vessels onto the anterior surface of the psoas muscle up to the level of the retrorenal space (Figure 15–2). Next, a crossover tunnel is made between the left suprainguinal preperitoneal space and the right groin, posterior to the rectus muscle and anterior and cephalad to the bladder (Figure 15–3). After systemic heparinization, a partially occluding aortic clamp is used for control of the distal descending thoracic aorta, which maintains perfusion to the spinal cord and to the renal and visceral vessels during proximal anastomosis. The proximal end of a bifurcated graft is beveled and anastomosis to the distal descending thoracic aorta is performed.

The graft is tunneled between the left chest and left suprainguinal preperitoneal space as described previously. From this location, the left limb of the graft is tunneled to the left groin over the iliac vessels and under the inguinal ligament, and the right

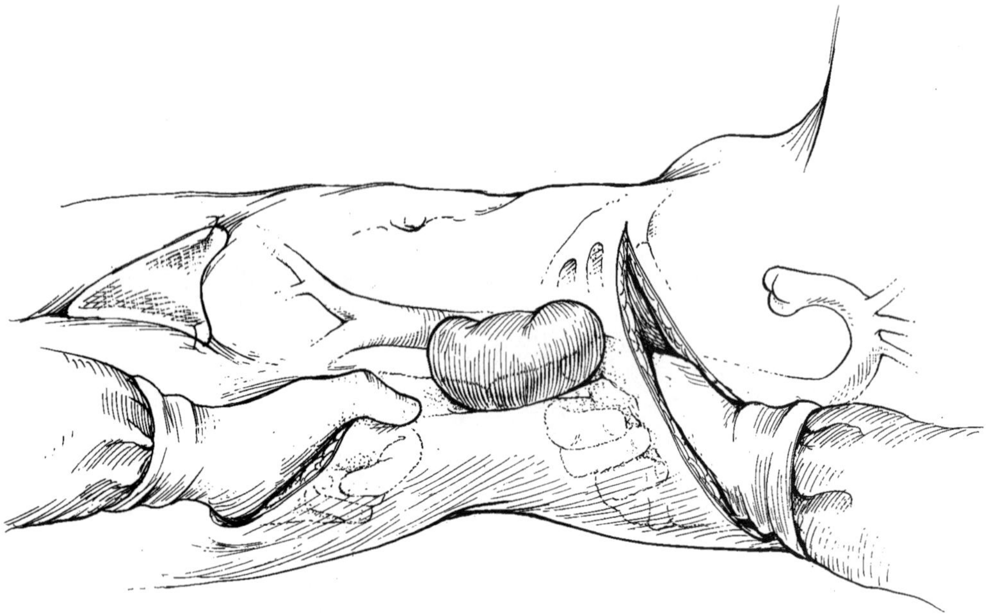

Figure 15–2. Retroperitoneal tunnel formed between left hemithorax and left suprainguinal preperitoneal space, along the psoas muscle, posterior to the spleen and left kidney. (*From Criado E. Descending thoracic aorta to femoral artery bypass: surgical technique. Ann Vasc Surg. 1997;11(2):206–215. Used by permission.*)

limb of the graft is directed to the right groin posterior to the rectus muscles through the previously formed tunnel (Figure 15–4). Distal anastomoses are performed between each limb of the graft and the iliac or femoral arteries. A thoracostomy tube is placed in the left pleural space, and the left lung is reinflated under direct vision. Thoracotomy and groin incisions are closed in a standard fashion.

Thoracomesenteric Bypass

Patients are anesthetized and positioned in an almost identical manner to patients undergoing thoracobifemoral bypass. However, the pelvis is not rotated and the patient is placed in the full lateral decubitus position, unless specific access to the iliac of femoral vessels is required (Figure 15–5). To aid in positioning, a bean bag and axillary roll are routinely required.

A ninth interspace thoracoretroperitoneal incision is used for thoracic and upper abdominal aorta exposure. Mobilization of the peritoneum and its contents from the undersurface of the diaphragm is performed bluntly. The diaphragm is incised in a curvilinear fashion, 2 cm from its costal edge to preserve innervation, using marking stitches to improve reapproximation. The inferior pulmonary ligament is divided, as well as the crus of the diaphragm. Numerous lymphatic vessels are encountered in this

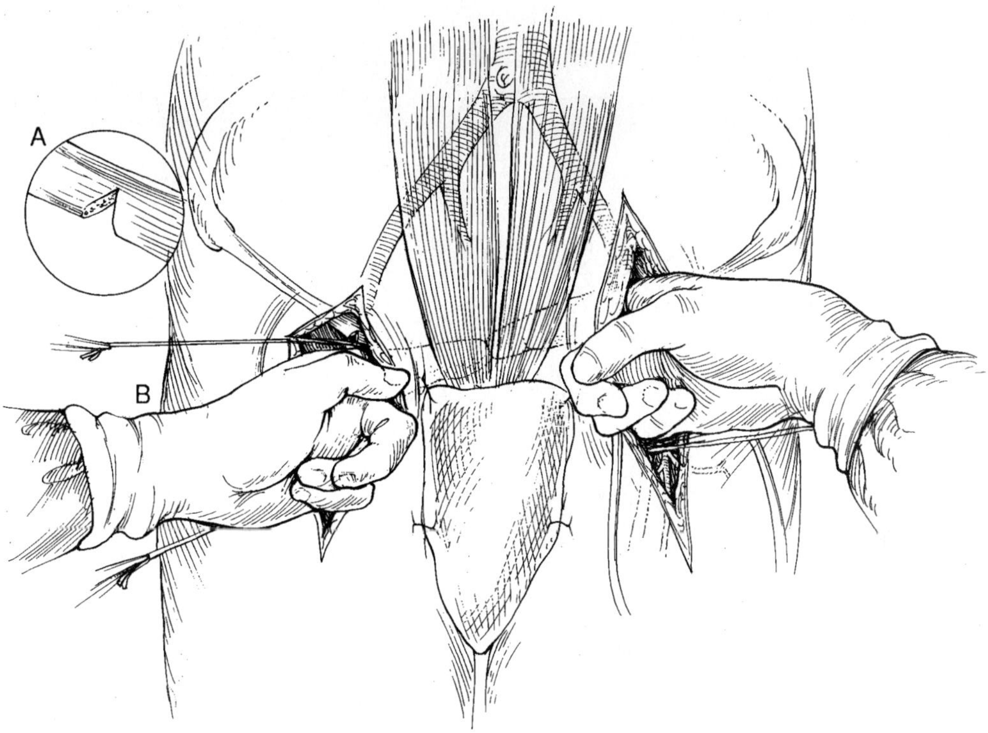

Figure 15–3. Tunnel created from the left suprainguinal space to the right groin, posterior to the rectus muscles, and anterior and cephalad to the bladder. (*From Criado E. Descending thoracic aorta to femoral artery bypass: surgical technique. Ann Vasc Surg. 1997;11(2):206–215. Used by permission.*)

region and require meticulous ligation and division. The celiac and superior mesenteric vessels are exposed until a suitable bypass site is obtained. If required, 8 to 10 cm of vessel can be exposed without significant difficulty. The retroperioneal plane is developed anterior to the left kidney, which is left undisturbed in its native position to facilitate distal exposure of the superior mesenteric artery (SMA). Deflation of the lung may be required to allow for better exposure of the descending thoracic aorta. The DTA is mobilized to allow for secure placement of a clamp with preservation of all intercostal arteries. A partial occlusion clamp technique is used after heparin is administered to maintain distal aortic flow to the kidneys and spinal cord (Figure 15–6). The proximal anastomoses are performed with a single clamp application to minimize repeated trauma to the thoracic aorta. Bifurcation or individual conduit configurations can be used; however, in our experience, individual grafts provide more optimal orientation and alignment. In addition, prosthetic externally supported grafts typically are chosen to reduce the chance of kinking at the haitus. Bypass conduits are routed through the diaphragmatic hiatus to their respective vessels in an end-to-side fashion, thereby

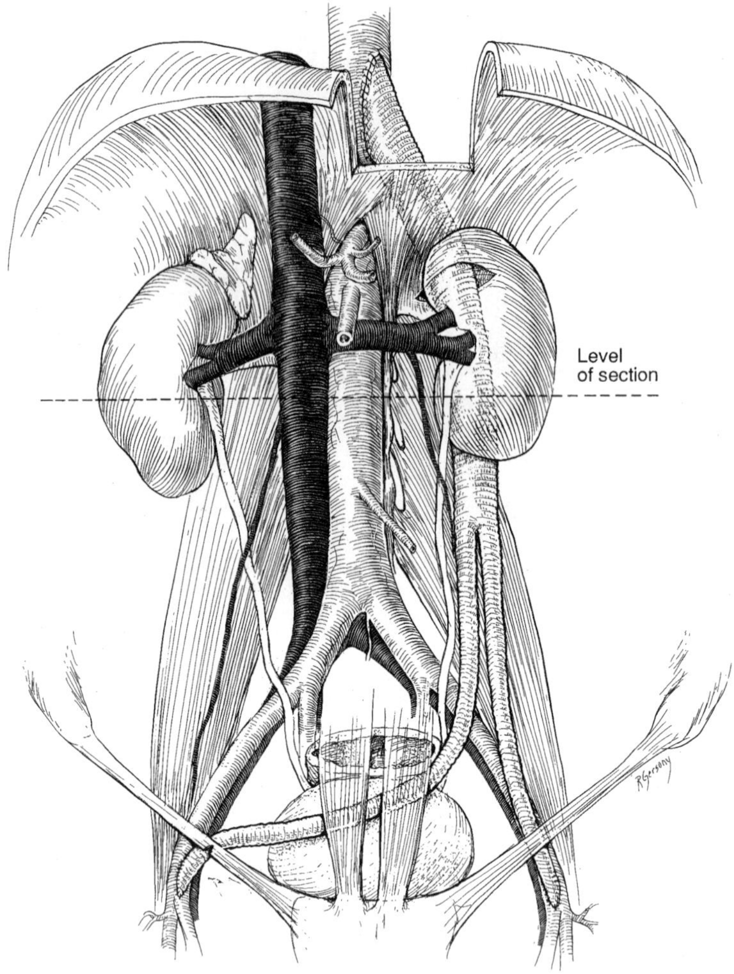

Figure 15–4. Final position of the DTA to femoral artery bypass graft in the retroperitoneal space posterior to the left kidney and spleen, overlying the psoas muscle. The right limb of the graft curves gently posterior to the rectus muscle and cephald to the bladder.

establishing antegrade flow (Figure 15–7). If necessary, the diaphragm can be left intact and a posterior window created if preservation of diaphragmatic function is of paramount importance. However, this requires additional dissection on the under surface of the diaphragm near the spleen, and adds an additional risk of splenic injury.

After revascularization is complete, the diaphragm is reapproximated. A single thoracostomy tube is placed under direct visualization and the left lung is reinflated. The peritoneal contents are then returned to their natural position and the abdominal wall musculature reapproximated. Closure of the abdominal and thoracic portions of the incision are completed in standard fashion.

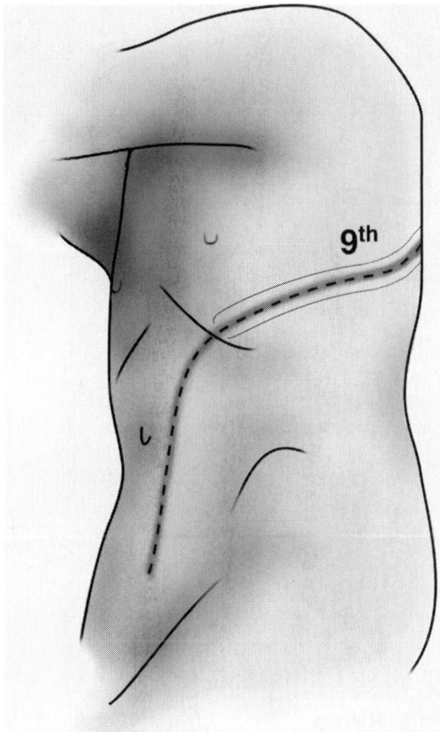

Figure 15–5. Patient positioned decubitus position prior to DTA to mesenteric bypass. Dashed lines show intended location of incisions for thoracoabdominal incision through the nineth interspace.

RESULTS

Thoracobifemoral Bypass

Bypass from the DTA to femoral artery has traditionally been reserved for patients with aortic graft failure or infection. Despite its use as a remedial operation, results have been satisfactory, with patency ranging from 73% to 86% at 5 yr in most published series.[4–11]

Although DTA to femoral artery bypass as a secondary reconstruction is well described, its role as a primary procedure remains controversial. At the University of North Carolina, 50 DTA to femoral artery bypass operations were performed between 1983 and 1997.[11] A primary procedure was performed in 31 patients for severe atherosclerotic disease or complete occlusion of the infrarenal aorta. The indications for 19 secondary revascularizations were prior aortic or extra-anatomic graft failure (17 patients) and aortic graft infection (2 patients). Overall operative mortality was 4%, with a perioperative complication rate of 16%. There was no renal failure or spinal cord ischemia

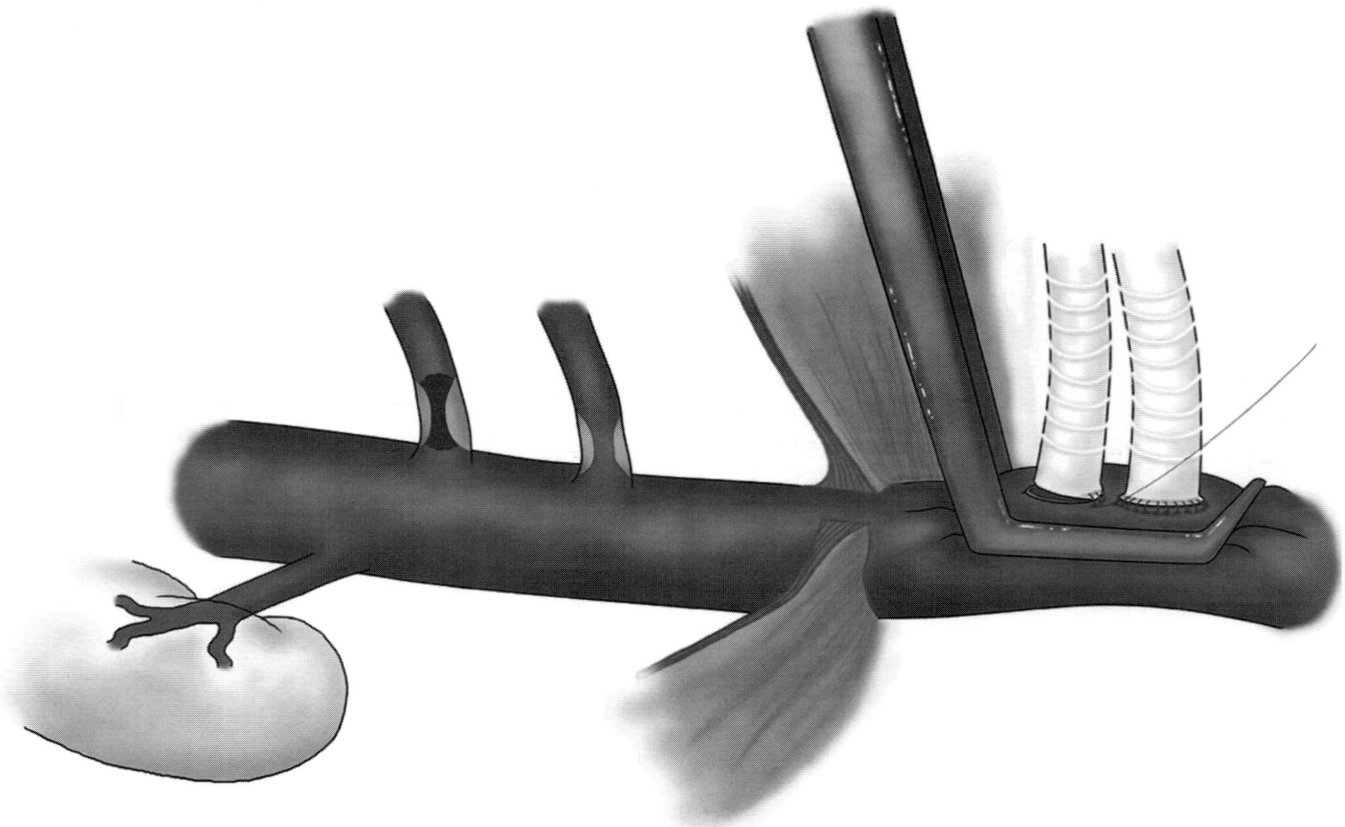

Figure 15–6. Partial occlusion clamp technique to maintain distal aortic flow to the kidneys and spinal cord and allow sequential anastomotic technique.

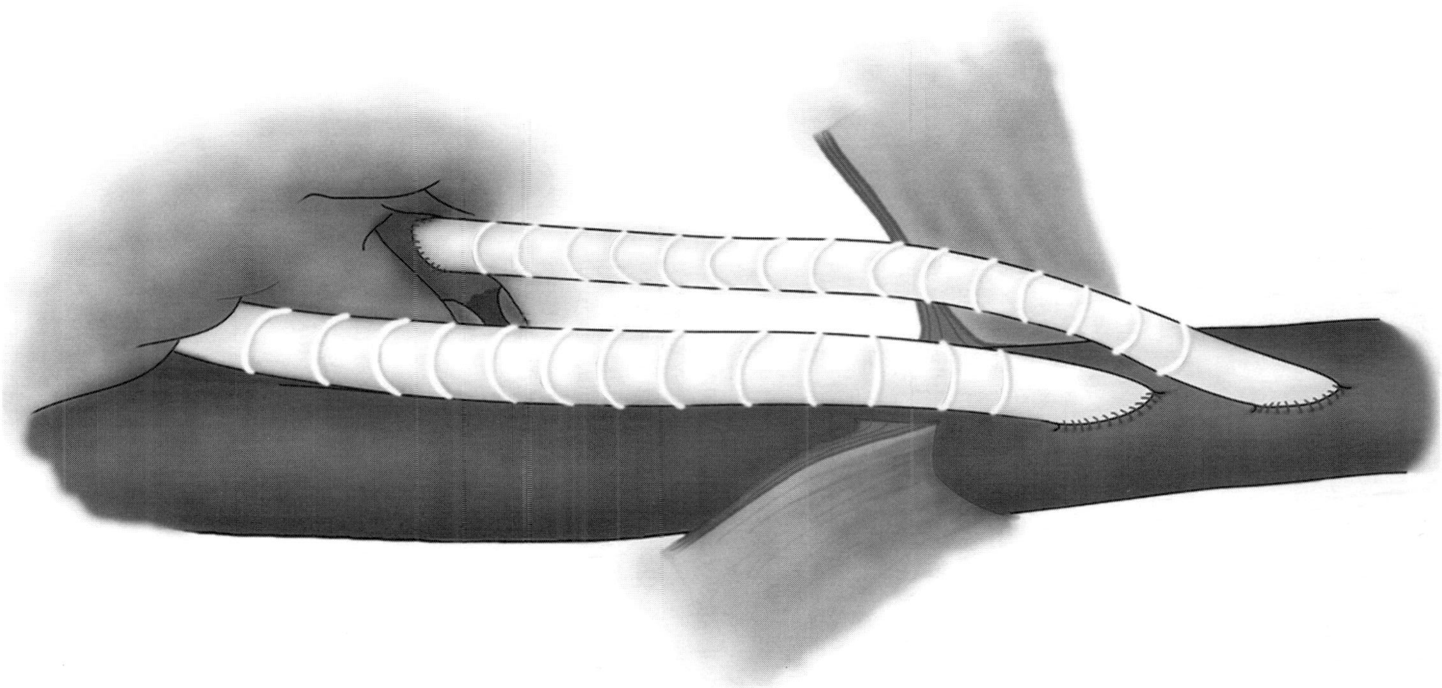

Figure 15–7. Bypass conduits routed through the diaphragmatic hiatus to their respective vessels in an end-to-side fashion, thereby establishing antegrade flow.

associated with the operation. Cumulative life-table 5-yr primary patency, secondary patency, limb salvage, and survival were 79%, 84%, 93%, and 67%, respectively. An improved patency trend was observed for patients operated on for severe claudication compared with limb-threatening ischemia (92% and 69%, respectively). However, there was no difference between primary and secondary operations in patency (81% and 79%, respectively) or survival (72% and 62%, respectively).

Thoracomesenteric Bypass

The use of the descending thoracic aorta as inflow for mesenteric revascularization has rarely been described.[12,13] Much of the hesitancy is related to the perceived mobidity associated with the incision. It is our approach of choice for patients with chronic mesenteric ischemia. During the years 1990 to 1999, we performed reconstruction in 18 patients. All patients were caucasian and presented with abdominal pain and/or weight loss. The pathophysiology involved atherosclerotic occlusive disease in 16 (89%) patients and Takayasu's arteritis in 2 (11%). Two patients required urgent revascularization secondary to acute exacerbation of chronic symptoms. None of the patients had isolated involvement of the celiac (CA) or inferior mesenteric vessels (IMA). Thirty-three vessels were reconstructed, and included CA and SMA reconstruction in 15 patients (83%) and isolated SMA revascularization in 3 (17%). None of the patients had revascularization of their IMA. There was 1 perioperative death (6%) secondary to multisystem organ failure. In this patient, both bypass grafts were patent on postoperative CT imaging. Major complications developed in 3 additional patients (17%), and included 2 myocardial infarctions and 1 respiratory failure requiring short reintubation. Of note, there was no renal failure or spinal cord ischemia. All patients remained clinically asymptomatic and required no additional procedures to assist patency during the mean follow-up of 34.8 mo (range 1 to 97 mo). Objective data was obtained in 13 of the 16 patients surviving longer than 4 months. There were no focal elevations in diastolic graft velocities and all bypass grafts (100%) remain patent. Life-table survival was 89%, 89%, and 75% at 1, 3, and 5 yr respectively.

CONCLUSION

Use of the descending thoracic aorta as inflow for revascularization of the lower extremities provides excellent results with limited morbidity and mortality. DTA to femoral artery bypass grafting has excellent overall long-term results that support its continued use as a secondary procedure for aortic graft failure and graft infection. Although aortofemoral bypass remains the standard treatment for symptomatic aortoiliac occlusive, DTA to femoral artery bypass should be considered an alternative for primary revascularization in selected patients, especially patients who present with severe calcified atherosclerotic disease or complete occlusion of the infrarenal aorta in whom a direct transabdominal aortic approach is less than optimal.

Antegrade mesenteric revascularization using the distal thoracic aorta as inflow is associated with a low mortality and acceptable morbidity. Furthermore, it provides excellent midterm patency and survival results that are not associated with either early or late thrombotic complications. The results do not appear to be influenced by the completeness of revascularization, with the results in life expectancy being limited by other comorbid conditions. It therefore should be considered as a primary approach for reconstruction of patients with chronic mesenteric ischemia.

REFERENCES

1. Stevenson JK, Sauvage LR, Harkins HN. A bypass homograft from thoracic aorta to femoral arteries for occlusive vascular disease. *Am Surg.* 1961;27:632–637.
2. Blaisdell FW. Extraperitoneal thoracic aorta to femoral bypass. *Am J Surg.* 1961;102:83–85.
3. Frazier OH, Oalmann MC, Strong JP, et al. Clinical applications of the supraceliac aorta: anatomic and pathologic observations. *J Thorac Cardiovasc Surg.* 1987;93:631–633.
4. Feldhaus RJ, Sterpetti AV, Shultz RD, et al. Thoracic aorta-femoral bypass: indications, technique, and late results. *Ann Thorac Surg.* 1985;40(6):588–592.
5. Bowes DE, Youkey JR, Pharr WP, et al. Long term follow-up of descending thoracic aorta-iliac/femoral bypass. *J Cardiovasc Surg.* 1990;31:430–437.
6. Criado E, Johnson G Jr, Burnham SJ, et al. Descending thoracic aorta to iliofemoral artery by pass as an alternative to aortoiliac reconstruction. *J Vasc Surg.* 1992;15:550–557.
7. Branchereau A, Magnan PE, Moracchini P, et al. Use of descending thoracic aorta for lower limb revascularization. *Eur J Vasc.* 1992;6:255–262.
8. McCarthy WJ, Mesh CL, McMillan WD, et al. Descending thoracic aorta-to-femoral artery bypass: ten years' experience with a durable procedure. *J Vasc Surg.* 1993;17:336–348.
9. Criado E, Keagy BA. Use of the descending thoracic aorta as an inflow source in aortoiliac reconstruction: indications and long-term results. *Ann Vasc Surg.* 1994;8:38–47.
10. Sapienza P, Mingoli A, Feldhaus RJ, et al. Descending thoracic aorta-to-femoral artery bypass grafts. *Am J Surg.* 1997;174:662–666.
11. Passman MA, Farber MA, Criado E, et al. Descending thoracic aorta to iliofemoral artery bypass: a role for primary revascularization for aortoiliac occlusive disease? *J Vasc Surg.* 1999; 29(2): 249–258.
12. Geroulakos G, Tober JC, Anderson A, et al. Antegrade visceral revascularization via a thoracoabdominal approach for chronic mesenteric ischemia. *Eur J Endovasc Surg.* 1999;17:56–59.
13. Farber MA, Carlin RE, Marston WA, et al. Distal thoracic aorta as inflow for the treatment of chronic mesenteric ischemia. Presented at 2000 Joint Annual Meeting of the NA Chapter of the ISCVS/SVS. June 11, 2000. In press.

16

Treatment of Ruptured Thoracoabdominal Aortic Aneurysms

Joseph S. Coselli, MD, David C. Rice, MB, BCh, and Scott A. LeMaire, MD

Advances in surgical technique have decreased mortality following elective repair of thoracoabdominal aortic aneurysms (TAAAs) to as low as 5% to 15% in some specialist centers.[1–3] The incidence of postoperative morbidity—including paraplegia, paraparesis, renal failure, and cardiopulmonary events—has decreased. Although improved surgical outcome encourages early elective repair of TAAAs, unfortunately, a significant number of patients still present emergently with either impending or complete rupture (between 4% and 33% in published series, see Table 16–1). Successful management of these patients is challenging and requires prompt aggressive surgical management and intensive multispecialty postoperative care. The purpose of this chapter is to review the surgical management of ruptured aneurysms involving the thoracoabdominal aorta. The natural history of untreated TAAAs, risk assessment, and the indications for operative intervention are briefly discussed, followed by a review of management strategies and the senior author's personal experience with ruptured TAAAs.

NATURAL HISTORY

The natural history of TAAAs remains poorly understood due to the relative rarity of the condition and the lack of large population–based studies. Furthermore, because these aneurysms are often asymptomatic, early diagnosis usually depends on the use of computed tomography (CT), transesophageal echocardiography (TEE), or magnetic resonance imaging (MRI), all of which are impractical as screening modalities.

TABLE 16–1. PUBLISHED SURGICAL SERIES OF TAAA/DTAA REPAIR VERSUS MORTALITY

Author (yr)	TAAAs (No.)	Ruptured (No.)	Deaths (No.)	Deaths Nonruptured (No.)	Deaths Ruptured (No.)
Svensson et al., 1993[13]	1509	61 (4%)	123/1509 (8%)	112/1448 (8%)	11/61 (18%)
Coselli et al., 1994[26]	372	38 (10%)	21/372 (6%)	16/334 (5%)	5/38 (13%)
Schepens et al., 1994[29]	88	18 (21%)	5/88 (6%)	2/70 (3%)	3/18 (17%)
Gilling-Smith et al., 1995[14]	130	11 (9%)	—	—	8/11 (73%)
von Segesser et al., 1996[30]	100	33 (33%)	9/100 (9%)	4/53 (8%)	5/33 (15%)
Grabitz et al., 1996[3]	260	38 (15%)	37/260 (15%)	27/222 (12%)	10/38 (26%)
Cambria et al., 1997[2]	160	16 (10%)	15/160 (9%)	10/144 (7%)	5/16 (31%)
Velazquez et al., 1999[31]	110	30 (27%)	14/110 (13%)	10/80 (13%)	4/30 (13%)

Aortic aneurysms are the thirteenth most common cause of death in the United States, and the majority of people who die of aneurysm-related causes die from rupture.[4] Necropsy studies have estimated an incidence of abdominal aortic aneurysms of 43/100,000 for men and 23/100,000 for women; a prevalence of 10.7% has been reported in men older than 74 years of age.[5,6] In contrast, the incidence of thoracic aortic aneurysms has been reported to be as low as 5.9/100,000 person-years, with a male-to-female ratio of 1.1–1.7 : 1.[7,8] Of the 72 patients identified in Bickerstaff and colleagues' report,[9] 27 had aneurysms involving the descending thoracic aorta and only 5 patients had TAAAs. This yields incidences of approximately 2.2 and 0.4 per 100,000 person-years, respectively.[9]

The causes of TAAAs parallel the causes of less extensive aneurysms limited to the descending thoracic aorta. The majority of both descending thoracic aortic aneurysms (DTAAs) and TAAAs are either associated with degeneration of the media or due to chronic dissection. In a review of 260 thoracic aortic aneurysms, Pressler and McNamara[8] reported that the relative frequencies of DTAAs caused by medial degeneration vs dissection were 89% and 11%, respectively. Regardless of the cause, however, ongoing mechanical stress leads to progressive aneurysmal enlargement and ultimately rupture, which is usually fatal without surgical intervention. In the Mayo Clinic study,[7] which spanned the period 1951–1980, 18 (67%) of 27 patients whose aneurysms involved the descending thoracic aorta died from rupture of their aneurysm. The two and 5-yr actuarial survival rates for all patients with thoracic aortic aneurysms were 29% and 13%, respectively. Rupture was fatal in 94% of cases. Crawford and DeNatale[10] followed 94 patients with TAAAs managed nonsurgically for a variety of reasons and reported a similar mortality rate for ruptured TAAAs. There were 64 deaths during the follow-up period, 33 of which were related to aneurysm rupture (52%); aneurysm rupture was fatal in 89% of patients. Salvage surgery was performed in 6 patients with rupture, of whom only 3 survived. Perko and colleagues[11] reported similar rates of rupture. Of 53 patients with TAAAs managed nonoperatively, 31 (58%) died from rupture, with 2- and 5-yr survival rates of 40% and 9%, respectively. Five-year cumulative risk of rupture was higher for aneurysms related to dissection (75%) than for degenerative aneurysms (45%).

FACTORS INFLUENCING RISK OF RUPTURE

Although there is a general consensus that large, symptomatic, or rapidly expanding aneurysms should be repaired,[12] uncertainty remains regarding the appropriate management of patients with asymptomatic, smaller aneurysms. Despite advances in adjunctive operative techniques such as left heart bypass, spinal cord cooling, and cerebrospinal fluid (CSF) drainage, elective surgical repair still carries a mortality between 4% and 15%[3,13] and a risk of paraplegia of 3% to 16%.[13,14] Attempts have therefore been made to better define those patients who are at higher risk of rupture and might benefit from earlier elective surgical intervention. According to LaPlace's Law, aortic wall tension increases as the diameter of the aneurysm increases; therefore, the larger the aneurysm, the greater the risk of rupture. Although this principle has been well established for abdominal aortic aneurysms (AAAs),[15–17] there is a relative paucity of data concerning risk of rupture in thoracoabdominal aneurysms. Perko and colleagues[11] reported outcomes in 170 patients with AAAs, DTAAs, and TAAAs who did not undergo surgical intervention. Regression analysis revealed that aneurysms with a diameter of ≥6 cm were associated with a fivefold increase in cumulative hazard of rupture (1.2 vs 0.24 for smaller aneurysms) and increased 5-yr probability of rupture (66% vs 23%). Multivariable analysis revealed that, in addition to aortic diameter, preoperative renal failure was predictive of rupture. Dapunt and colleagues[18] examined risk factors for rupture in 67 patients with thoracic aortic aneurysms. The study population included 7 patients with TAAAs and 17 patients with DTAAs. In univariate analysis, initial diameter of the aneurysm and a history of smoking significantly effected the expansion rate. In multivariable analysis, however, only an initial diameter of ≥5 cm was an independent predictor of accelerated expansion. In contrast, data reported by Coady and colleagues[19] showed that DTAAs and TAAAs ruptured or dissected at a median size of 7.2 cm, and they recommended surgical intervention when the diameter reached 6.5 cm. The only prospective study to date was performed by Juvonen and colleagues[20] at the Mount Sinai School of Medicine. One hundred two (102) patients with either DTAAs (90 patients) or TAAAs (12 patients) due to medial degenerative disease were prospectively followed with serial CT scans and computerized cross-sectional analysis. Although the sample was somewhat skewed owing to the exclusion of patients who were symptomatic or who had large aneurysms at presentation (>7 cm diameter) and who therefore underwent early repair, the study nevertheless identified useful (and practical) predictors of rupture. In multivariable analysis, increasing age, pain, the presence of chronic obstructive pulmonary disease (COPD), and maximal descending and abdominal aortic diameters were found to be independent risk factors for aneurysm rupture. A mathematical equation was derived to estimate the rate of rupture based on these factors (see Appendix). Smoking, hypertension, diabetes, and the rate of expansion were not found to be statistically significant predictors of rupture (although patients with expansion rates >10 mm per year underwent elective surgery and therefore were censored from analysis). The same investigators later published their experience with TAAAs caused by chronic aortic dissection.[21] A group of 50 patients who had not undergone surgery following their initial dissection was studied. Ten patients underwent elective repair during the median duration of 40 mo follow-up. Older age, COPD, and elevated mean and diastolic blood pressures were significantly associated with rupture. The authors demonstrated that aortic diameter at the time of rupture was greater in patients with dissection compared to patients with degenerative aneurysms (5.8 cm vs 5.4 cm, $p = 0.05$).

CLINICAL PRESENTATION

Most patients with rupture or impending rupture of a TAAA complain of pain involving the chest, back, shoulder, abdomen, or flank. They may present with hemoptysis, hematemesis, or cardiovascular collapse. In patients with free rupture into the pleural or peritoneal cavities, exsanguination occurs rapidly, and survival long enough to permit surgical intervention is unusual (Figure 16–1). In many instances, however, rupture occurs into the mediastinal or retroperitoneal periaortic tissues and is temporarily contained. In the series of ruptured DTAAs and TAAAs reported by Crawford and colleagues,[22] 99 of 117 patients (85%) presented with rupture elsewhere and were

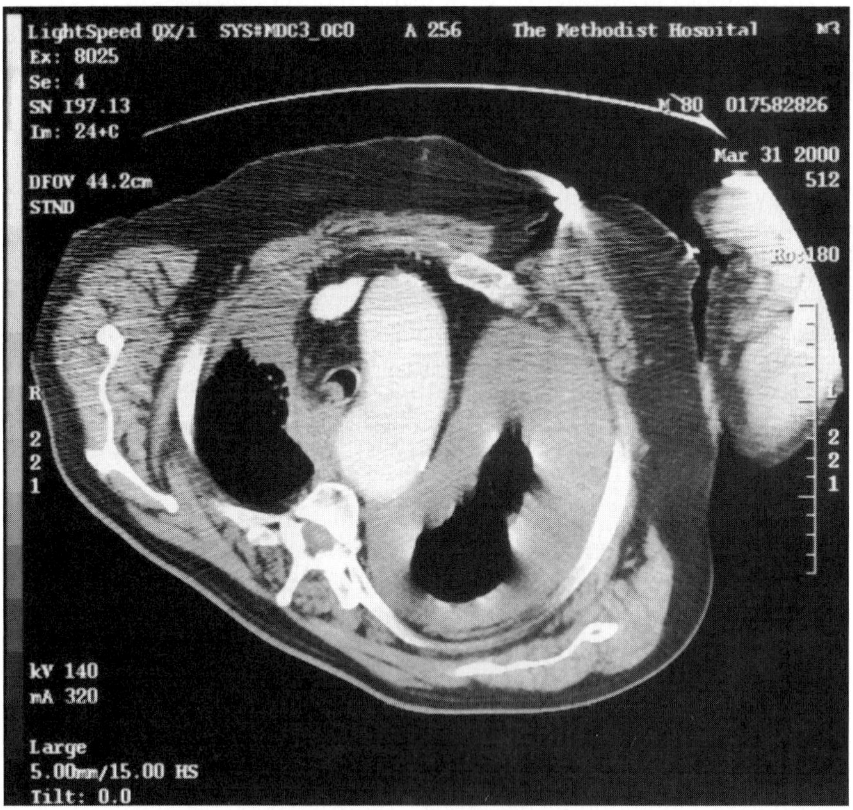

Figure 16–1. Computed tomography (CT) scan demonstrating a thoracoabdominal aortic aneurysm that has ruptured into the left pleural cavity.

sufficiently stable to survive transfer. Of these 99 patients, 29 patients subsequently became hypotensive and 16 suffered cardiac arrest requiring cardiopulmonary resuscitation; 3 patients died before surgery could be performed. Eighteen other patients ruptured between 10 min and 6 hr after admission to the hospital, 4 patients at the time of chest entry or exposure. In this series, 1 patient had an aortotracheobronchial fistula and presented with massive hemoptysis and 3 patients had aortoesophageal fistulae and presented with massive hematemesis.[23,24] Associated comorbidities are frequently present in this high-risk group of patients; in the study reported by Crawford et al.,[22] these included hypertension in 91 patients (78%), COPD in 46 patients (39%), atherosclerotic coronary artery disease in 41 patients (35%), cerebrovascular disease in 22 patients (19%), preoperative renal impairment (creatinine >2 mg/dl) in 25 patients (21%), and diabetes in 9 patients (8%).

PREOPERATIVE ASSESSMENT AND PREPARATION

In approximately 50% of patients presenting with rupture, the presence of an aneurysm has been documented previously by plain radiographs, aortography, TEE, or CT scans. If the patient's condition permits, preoperative chest and abdominal CT scans are performed to define the site of rupture and extent of aneurysmal involvement. The other preoperative evaluations frequently obtained in elective cases—such as pulmonary function tests, carotid ultrasonography, coronary catheterization, and cardiac stress testing—are rarely able to be performed in this emergent setting. Hypertension is controlled with intravenous alpha-antagonists such as nitroprusside or beta-antagonists such as intravenous labetalol. Hypotensive patients are cautiously volume resuscitated with intravenous fluids and blood products. Raising blood pressure excessively may cause extension of dissection or may disrupt a friable periaortic clot and precipitate fatal hemorrhage.[25] Therefore, moderate hypotension (systolic blood pressure 60–90 mmHg) is permitted, and aggressive fluid resuscitation is strictly avoided. For the same reason, vasopressor agents are rarely used.

OPERATIVE TECHNIQUES

The essentials of elective TAAA repair have been reported previously.[1,26,27] Circumstances related to the presentation of ruptured TAAAs mandate flexibility with regard to operative technique. The surgical approach must be tailored to the presenting features of each individual case, and many of these variations are discussed. To optimize outcome, it is essential that the operation be performed in conjunction with an anesthesiologist and a perfusionist who have interest and experience in aortic surgery. A double-lumen endobronchial tube is used to facilitate collapse of the left lung and improve exposure of the aorta. Occasionally—as in patients with an aortobronchial fistula—a single-lumen endotracheal tube may be placed into the right mainstem bronchus and used to preserve right lung ventilation. A pulmonary arterial catheter, large-bore central venous line, right-sided radial arterial line (in case of the need to clamp the left subclavian artery), urinary catheter, esophageal temperature probe, and ECG leads are placed.

Placement of a CSF drain is recommended for hemodynamically stable patients when a Crawford extent I or II aneurysm repair is anticipated (Figure 16–2). In patients with known or suspected cardiac disease, intraoperative TEE is used. A rapid infusion system is primed to allow immediate blood transfusion.

Patients are positioned in a modified right lateral decubitus position with the thorax at about 60° and the hips rotated posteriorly to about 30°. A beanbag underneath the patient helps to maintain this position. The patient is draped to expose the entire left chest, abdomen, and both groins. Both inguinal areas must be accessible because of the potential need to establish femoral access for hypothermic cardiopulmonary bypass or left heart bypass. Our current strategy for spinal cord protection in most cases includes moderate heparinization (1 mg/kg), aggressive reattachment of critical intercostal arteries, and mild permissive hypothermic drift to between 32° and 33°C. Left heart bypass and CSF drainage are used in patients requiring extent I or II repairs. Adjuncts such as naloxone, spinal cord cooling, or intrathecal papaverine are not used routinely.

In patients with aneurysms involving the upper portion of the thoracic aorta (Crawford extents I and II), the thoracotomy incision is made over the superior border of the seventh rib (sixth intercostal space) and extended inferiorly onto the abdomen, ending just to the left of the umbilicus. A portion of the posterior sixth or seventh rib

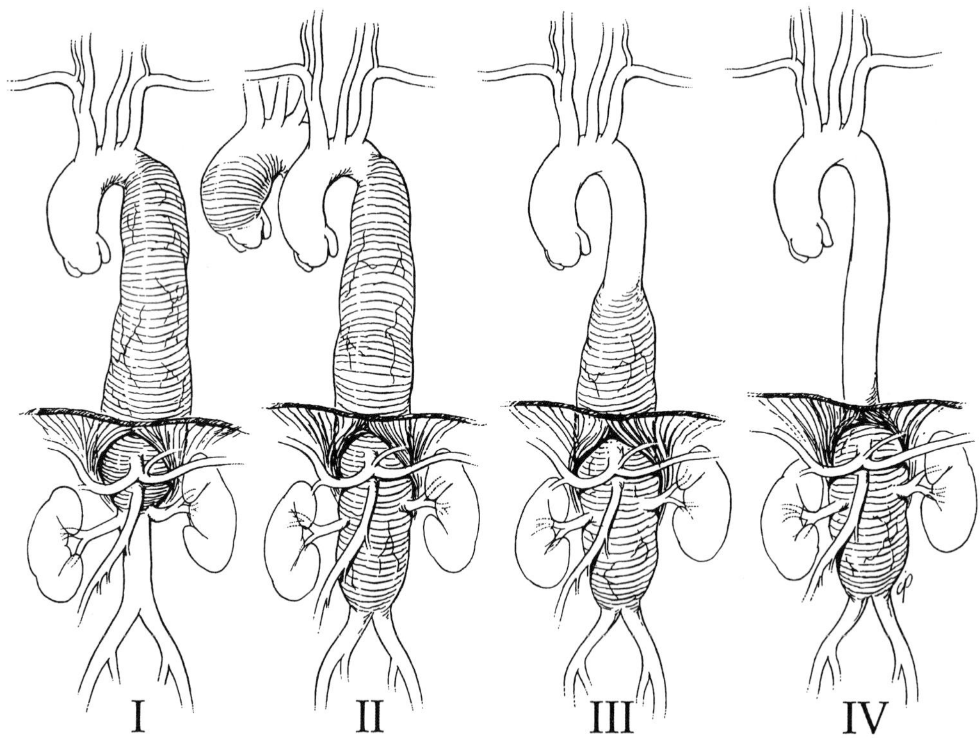

Figure 16–2. The Crawford classification of thoracoabdominal aortic aneurysms based on the extent of aortic involvement.

can be excised as needed to facilitate retraction and exposure. For patients with more distal involvement (extents III and IV) a seventh, eighth, or ninth interspace thoracotomy is used. Although not considered TAAAs, ruptured suprarenal AAAs not involving the celiac and superior mesenteric arteries are also approached through a low thoracoabdominal incision; this allows excellent exposure for supraceliac aortic clamping (often just above the diaphragmatic hiatus) and aortic reconstruction. A transperitoneal abdominal dissection is performed, and the retroperitoneum is entered lateral to the left colon. The benefits of the transperitoneal approach are that it is expeditious and permits direct examination of intra-abdominal visceral perfusion. The diaphragm is divided circumferentially, preserving a 2- to 3-cm cuff of muscle on the chest wall.

While exposing the aorta, areas near the hematoma are carefully avoided. The left crus is divided and the origin of the left renal artery is identified. The proximal extent of the aneurysm is exposed and a clamp site is prepared, taking care to avoid injury to the recurrent laryngeal, vagus, and phrenic nerves.

In patients with extensive aneurysms at high risk for postoperative paraplegia (extents I and II, particularly those with dissection), distal aortic perfusion using left heart bypass is used when feasible. This is achieved by cannulating the left inferior pulmonary vein (the left atrial appendage and superior pulmonary vein are alternatives) and the aorta near the diaphragm (or a common femoral artery). An in-line centrifugal pump is used and flows are adjusted to maintain a distal aortic pressure of 70 mmHg. Core temperature is allowed to drift to between 32° and 33°C without the use of a heat exchanger.

After a proximal clamp is applied, a distal clamp is placed at a suitable position at the T4–T7 level. The aorta is completely transected and an appropriately sized graft sewn in place using a single layer of 3-0 polypropylene, taking full thickness bites on the aorta. In the setting of Marfan syndrome or acute dissection, a 4-0 polypropylene suture is better suited for the fragile aortic tissue. After completing the proximal anastomosis, left heart bypass is stopped, the distal clamp is removed, the remainder of the aneurysm is opened, and balloon perfusion catheters are inserted into the visceral vessels. This allows visceral perfusion to continue while the intercostal arteries are addressed (Figure 16–3). An open distal anastomosis—without a distal aortic clamp—is used to complete the repair.

Because of the emergency nature of the majority of cases of rupture, surgical repair may diverge from the sequence outlined to varying degrees. For instance, cases with cardiac arrest or severe hypotension may require emergency thoracotomy and graft replacement of the aorta using an expedient "clamp-and-sew" technique. In many instances, the graft repair may be accomplished in as little as 15–20 min. Hypothermic circulatory arrest may be used in stable patients in whom uncontrollable hemorrhage is anticipated during exposure of the aneurysm. The femoral artery and vein are cannulated and cardiopulmonary bypass instituted prior to thoracotomy. Core temperature is reduced until the electroencephalogram (EEG) becomes silent. Cardiopulmonary bypass is then discontinued, circulation is arrested, and the aneurysm repaired without a need for proximal clamping. After completing the proximal anastomosis, air is removed from the heart and graft, cardiopulmonary bypass is resumed, and the patient is rewarmed during the remainder of the repair. In certain cases, rupture of the aneurysm may occur prior to initiating cardiopulmonary bypass or achieving adequate cooling. If

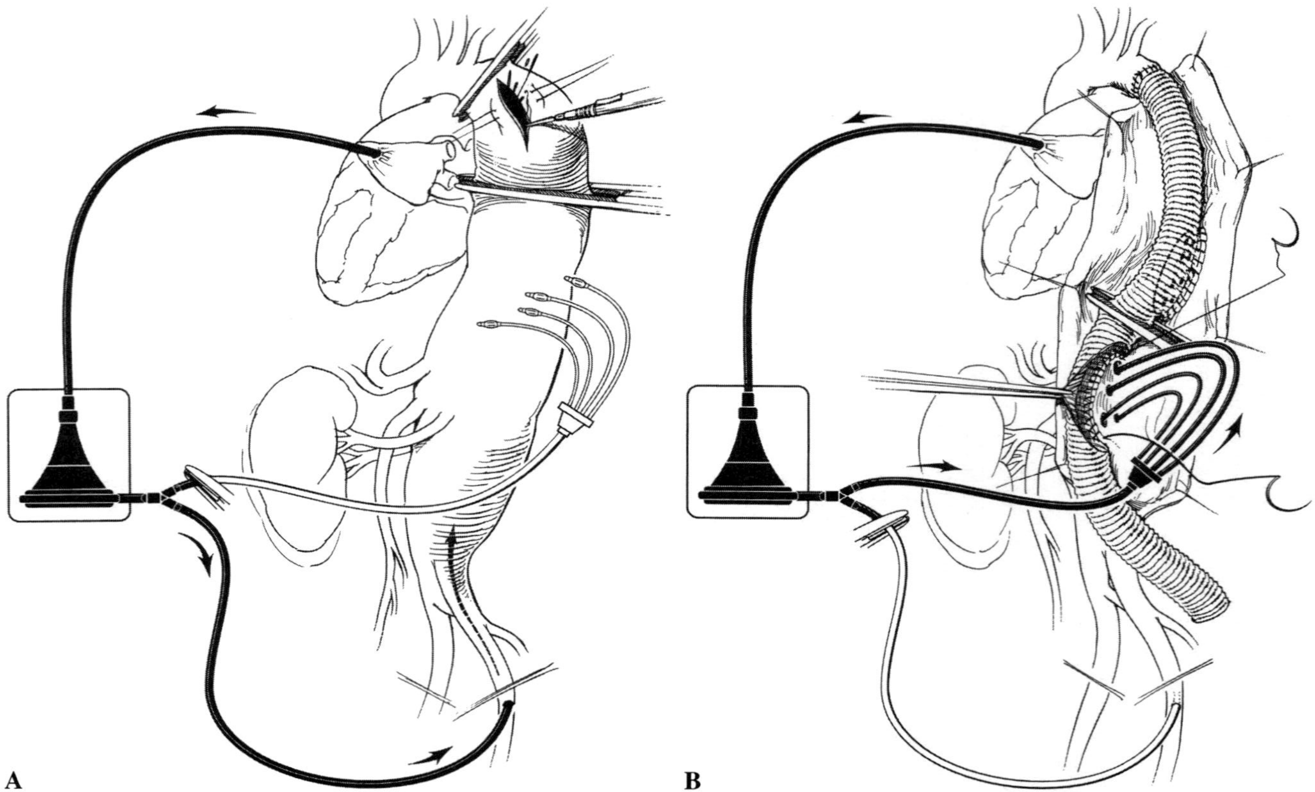

Figure 16–3. Technique of left heart bypass during thoracoabdominal aortic aneurysm repair. (**A**) The aorta beyond the distal clamp is perfused from the circuit during the proximal portion of the repair. After completing the proximal anastomosis, left heart bypass is stopped, the distal clamp is removed, and balloon perfusion catheters are placed into the celiac axis, superior mesenteric artery, and renal arteries to allow selective visceral perfusion while the intercostal arteries are reattached. After the intercostal reattachment is complete (**B**), the clamp can be repositioned below the anastomosis to allow antegrade intercostal perfusion while the visceral reattachment is performed. Selective visceral perfusion is continued until the visceral patch anastomosis is nearly complete; the catheters are then removed and the final stitches are placed. The diagram illustrates use of the left atrial appendage and femoral artery for cannulation sites; we currently prefer to use the left inferior pulmonary vein and distal aorta (near the diaphragm), respectively.

hemorrhage cannot be controlled to allow either proximal clamping or initiation of bypass and completion of cooling, controlled exsanguination with aggressive blood salvage and fibrillatory cardiac arrest may be necessary in order to perform the proximal anastomosis. Once this is completed, the graft is clamped and cannulated with the arterial perfusion cannula, volume is returned to the patient during cardiopulmonary bypass, and the heart is defibrillated. The distal anastomosis may then be performed safely.

SURGICAL RESULTS

As expected, mortality and morbidity following surgical repair of ruptured TAAAs are higher than following elective repair. In larger series, perioperative death has been reported to range from 13% to 72% (Table 16–1); postoperative renal failure and paraplegia rates are generally two to three times higher than nonruptured cases (Table 16–2).

In the senior author's experience with 1220 consecutive surgically treated TAAAs over a 12-yr period, 76 patients underwent surgery for aneurysm rupture. There were 43 (56%) men and 33 (44%) women. The mean age was 70 yr (median, 70 yr) with a range from 45 to 86 yr (Table 16–3). Fifty-eight (58) patients (76%) had medial degenerative fusiform aneurysms, whereas 18 patients had either acute dissection (10 patients, 13%) or chronic dissection (8 patients, 11%). Marfan syndrome was present in only 1 patient. The extent of aortic replacement was categorized based on the Crawford classification and included 32 patients (42%) in extent I, 19 patients (25%) in extent II, 9 patients (12%) in extent III, and 16 patients (21%) in extent IV. Comorbid conditions were frequent and are summarized in Table 16–3.

All patients underwent surgery according to the techniques outlined previously. Intercostal vessels were reattached in 38 cases (50%), with a mean of 2.5 ± 1.3 vessel pairs per patient (range 1–6 pairs). Left heart bypass was used in 14 patients (18%) with a mean pump time of 24.6 ± 7.4 min (range 18–46 min). All patients received blood products with an average of 10.1 ± 6.5 units of cell saver blood returned and 8.1 ± 4.8 units of packed red cells transfused per patient. No patient had CSF drainage.

TABLE 16–2 PUBLISHED SURGICAL SERIES OF TAAA/DTAA REPAIR VERSUS POSTOPERATIVE PARAPLEGIA AND RENAL FAILURE

Author (yr)	Paraplegia Nonruptured	Paraplegia Ruptured	Renal Failure Nonruptured	Renal Failure Ruptured
Svensson et al., 1993[13]	218/1448 (15%)	16/61 (26%)	247/1448 (17%)	22/61 (36%)
Coselli et al., 1994[26]	14/318 (4%)	10/33 (30%)	22/334 (7%)	7/38 (18%)
Schepens et al., 1994[29]	6/70 (9%)	6/18 (33%)	8/67 (12%)	4/18 (22%)
Gilling-Smith et al., 1995[14]	3/110 (3%)	3/20[a] (15%)	21 (19%)	8 (41%)
von Segesser et al., 1996[30]	6/33 (11%)	3/33 (9%)	—	—
Grabitz et al., 1996[3]	35/222 (16%)	4/38 (11%)	13/179 (7%)	13/38 (34%)
Cambria et al., 1997[2]	5/140 (4%)	6/14 (43%)	—	—
Velazquez et al., 1999[31]	3/77 (4%)	2/30 (7%)	5/77 (6%)	5/30 (17%)

[a] Paraparesis rate among threatened/contained rupture or ruptured cases.

TABLE 16–3. DEMOGRAPHIC AND PREOPERATIVE DATA

Variable	Number of Patients (%)
Men	43 (56%)
Women	33 (44%)
Mean age (yr), (±SD)	70 ± 8
Previous aneurysm	26 (34%)
Previous TAAA repair	7 (13%)
Hypertension	61 (80%)
COPD	43 (57%)
Coronary artery disease	31 (41%)
Cerebrovascular disease	8 (11%)
Diabetes	4 (5%)

COPD, chronic obstructive pulmonary disease.

There were 2 intraoperative deaths (3%) and 14 other patients (18%) died either in hospital or within 30 days from the date of surgery, giving an overall perioperative mortality of 21%. Mean follow-up time was 56 ± 8 mo. Median postoperative survival was 5.8 ± 1.1 yr based on Kaplan–Meier analysis (Figure 16–4).

Major postoperative complications occurred in 52 patients (68%). Pulmonary complications—pneumonia, ventilator support >48 hr, reintubation, adult respiratory distress syndrome (ARDS), atelectasis requiring bronchoscopy, and pneumothorax or pleural effusion requiring intervention—were the most common, occurring in 51% of patients (Table 16–4).

Paraplegia and paraparesis occurred in 17% of patients overall; this compares fa-

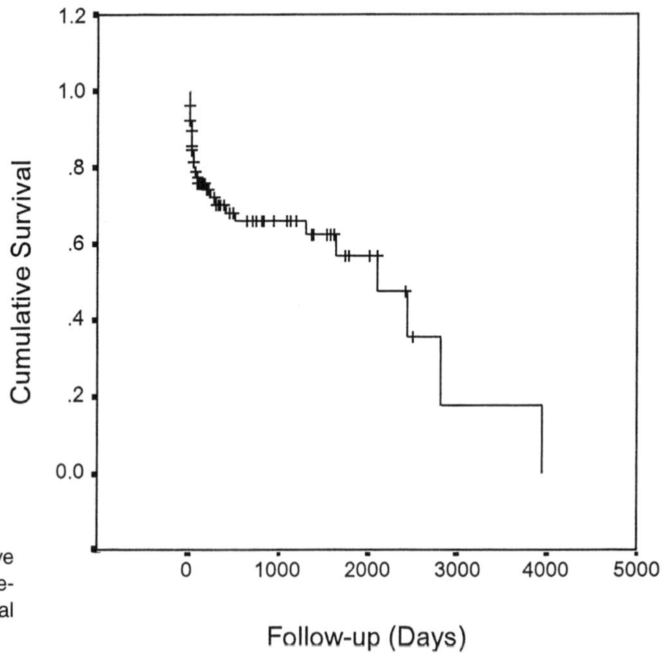

Figure 16–4. Kaplan–Meier curve demonstrating survival following repair of ruptured thoracoabdominal aortic aneurysms.

TABLE 16–4. POSTOPERATIVE COMPLICATIONS FOLLOWING REPAIR OF RUPTURED THORACOABDOMINAL AORTIC ANEURYSMS

Complication	Total n = 76
Pulmonary complications	38 (50%)
Renal insufficiency	22 (29%)
Paraplegia/paraparesis	13 (17%)
Paraplegia	7 (9%)
Paraparesis	6 (8%)
Cardiac complications	11 (14%)
Sepsis	6 (8%)
Gastrointestinal complications	5 (7%)
Postoperative bleeding	3 (4%)
Wound complications	2 (3%)
Stroke	2 (3%)

vorably with other published results, which range from 7% to 42% (Table 16–2). The well-established relationship between the extent of repair and the risk of paraplegia was exaggerated in this series of ruptured TAAAs.[13,28] Ruptured extent II aneurysms had a 42% incidence of neurologic deficit, whereas the risk was only 13% and 6% for extent I and extent IV aneurysms, respectively ($p = 0.03$; Table 16–5).

Postoperative renal failure—defined as a new elevation in serum creatinine beyond 2.0 mg/dL or the need to initiate hemodialysis—occurred in 29% of patients. Dissection did not appear to be a significant risk factor (Table 16–6), but extent of aneurysm repair did appear to correlate with postoperative renal insufficiency (Table 16–5). Patients with extent II repairs had a 50% incidence of renal impairment, and of 13 patients with extent IV aneurysms, 9 (69%) developed postoperative renal impairment, with 5 patients requiring long-term hemodialysis. Patients who underwent left heart bypass had a lower incidence of renal failure (Table 16–7).

The contribution of left heart bypass and intercostal vessel reattachment in this series is difficult to assess because the number of patients is small. No clear difference in the incidence of postoperative paraplegia could be attributed to either the use of left heart bypass or reattachment of intercostal vessels (Tables 16–7 and 16–8). Nevertheless, there does appear to be a trend toward improvement in postoperative renal function and survival when at least one of these modalities was used (Table 16–9).

TABLE 16–5. ANEURYSM EXTENT VERSUS POSTOPERATIVE SURVIVAL, PARAPLEGIA, AND RENAL FAILURE

Crawford Extent	No. Patients	Early Survival	Late Survival	Paraplegia/ Paraparesis	Renal Failure
I	32	26 (81%)	21 (66%)	4 (13%)	4 (13%)
II	19	16 (84%)	12 (63%)	8 (42%)	7 (50%)
III	9	6 (67%)	5 (56%)	0 (0%)	2 (25%)
IV	16	12 (75%)	10 (63%)	1 (6%)	9 (56%)
Total	**76**	**60 (79%)**	**48 (63%)**	**13 (17%)**	**22 (29%)**

TABLE 16–6. ANEURYSM TYPE VERSUS POSTOPERATIVE SURVIVAL, PARAPLEGIA, AND RENAL FAILURE

Cause of Aneurysm	No. Patients	Early Survival	Late Survival	Paraplegia / Paraparesis	Renal Failure
Degenerative aneurysm	58	45 (78%)	35 (60%)	10 (17%)	17 (29%)
Acute dissection	10	10 (100%)	9 (90%)	1 (10%)	3 (30%)
Chronic dissection	8	5 (63%)	4 (50%)	2 (25%)	2 (25%)
Total	**76**	**60 (79%)**	**48 (63%)**	**13 (17%)**	**22 (29%)**

TABLE 16–7. LEFT HEART BYPASS VERSUS POSTOPERATIVE SURVIVAL, PARAPLEGIA, AND RENAL FAILURE

Left Heart Bypass	No. Patients	Early Survival	Late Survival	Paraplegia / Paraparesis	Renal Failure
Yes	14	13 (93%)	11 (79%)	2 (14%)	2 (14%)
No	62	47 (76%)	37 (60%)	11 (19%)	20 (35%)
Total	**76**	**60 (79%)**	**48 (63%)**	**13 (17%)**	**22 (29%)**

TABLE 16–8. REATTACHMENT OF INTERCOSTAL ARTERIES VERSUS POSTOPERATIVE SURVIVAL, PARAPLEGIA, AND RENAL FAILURE

Intercostal Artery Reattachment	No. Patients	Early Survival	Late Survival	Paraplegia / Paraparesis	Renal Failure
Yes	38	31 (82%)	26 (68%)	6 (16%)	7 (18%)[a]
No	38	29 (76%)	22 (58%)	7 (19%)	15 (43%)
Total	**76**	**60 (79%)**	**48 (63%)**	**13 (17%)**	**22 (29%)**

[a] Of patients who underwent intercostal reattachment, 26% also had left heart bypass and distal perfusion.

TABLE 16–9. LEFT HEART BYPASS AND INTERCOSTAL ARTERY REATTACHMENT VERSUS POSTOPERATIVE SURVIVAL, PARAPLEGIA, AND RENAL FAILURE

LHB/INT	No. Patients	Early Survival	Late Survival	Paraplegia/ Paraparesis	Renal Failure
LHB and INT	10	9 (90%)	7 (70%)	1 (10%)	1 (10%)
LHB only	4	4 (100%)	4 (100%)	1 (25%)	1 (25%)
INT only	28	22 (79%)	19 (68%)	5 (18%)	6 (21%)
None	34	25 (74%)	18 (53%)	6 (18%)	14 (45%)
Total	**76**	**60 (79%)**	**48 (63%)**	**13 (17%)**	**22 (29%)**

LHB, left heart bypass; INT, intercostal artery reattachment.

SUMMARY

Ruptured TAAAs continue to have a high mortality rate despite refinements in surgical technique. Nevertheless, their fatal course if left untreated mandates operative intervention. Current morbidity and mortality in specialist centers is two to four times higher than for elective cases, but repair is associated with a reasonable long-term survival. The relatively poor outcome following emergency repair of ruptured TAAAs justifies an aggressive approach to treating these aneurysms at an earlier stage of their development.

APPENDIX

Equation to estimate rate of rupture, λ, after a CT scan[20]:

$$\begin{aligned} \text{Ln}\,\lambda = {} & -21.055 + 0.093\,(\text{age}) + 0.841(\text{pain}) + 18.22(\text{COPD}) \\ & + 0.643(\text{descending thoracic aortic diameter, cm}) \\ & + 0.405(\text{abdominal aortic diameter, cm}) \end{aligned}$$

Pain and COPD = 1 if present and 0 if absent.

Probability of rupture within 1 yr $= 1 - e^{-\lambda(365)}$.

The study population on which this calculation is based excluded patients who were clearly symptomatic at presentation and patients who presented with large aneurysms (>7 cm diameter). The authors acknowledge that the contributions pain and aortic diameter make to the risk of rupture may be underestimated.

REFERENCES

1. Coselli J, LeMaire S. Thoracoabdominal aorta: surgical techniques. *Card Clin N Am.* 1999;17:751–765.
2. Cambria R, Davison J, Zannetti S, L'Italien G, Atamian S. Thoracoabdominal aneurysm repair: Perspectives over a decade with the clamp-and-sew technique. *Ann Surg.* 1997;226:294–305.
3. Grabitz K, Sandmann W, Stuhmeier K, et al. The risk of ischemic spinal cord injury in patients undergoing graft replacement for thoracoabdominal aortic aneurysms. *J Vasc Surg.* 1996;23:230–240.
4. Majumber P, StJean P, Ferrell R. On the inheritance of abdominal aortic aneurysm. *Am J Hum Genet.* 1991;48:164–170.
5. Bengtsson H, Bergqvist D, Sternby N. Increasing prevalence of abdominal aortic aneurysms—a necropsy study. *Eur J Surg.* 1992;158:19–23.
6. Bengtsson H, Bergqvist D, Ekberg O. A population based screening of abdominal aortic aneurysms. *Eur J Vasc Surg.* 1991;5:53–57.
7. Bickerstaff L, Pairolero P, Hollier L, et al. Thoracic aortic aneurysms: a population based study. *Surgery.* 1982;92:1103–1108.
8. Pressler V, McNamara J. Thoracic aortic aneurysm—natural history and treatment. *J Thorac Cardiovasc Surg.* 1980;79:489–498.
9. Panneton J, Hollier L. Non-dissecting thoracoabdominal aortic aneurysms: Part 1. *Ann Vasc Surg.* 1995;9:503–514.

10. Crawford E, DeNatale R. Thoracoabdominal aortic aneurysm: observations regarding the natural course of the disease. *J Vasc Surg.* 1986;3:578–582.
11. Perko M, Norgaard M, Herzog T, Olsen P, Schroeder T, Pettersson G. Unoperated aortic aneurysm: a survey of 170 patients. *Ann Thorac Surg.* 1995;59:1204–1209.
12. Lobato A, Puech-Leao P. Predictive factors for rupture of thoracoabdominal aneurysm. *J Vasc Surg.* 1998;27:446–453.
13. Svensson L, Crawford E, Hess K, Coselli J, Safi H. Experience with 1509 patients undergoing thoracoabdominal aortic operations. *J Vasc Surg.* 1993;17:357–370.
14. Gilling-Smith G, Worswick L, Knight P, Wolfe J, Mansfield A. Surgical repair of thoracoabdominal aneurysm: 10 years' experience. *Br J Surg.* 1995;82:624–629.
15. Cronenwett J, Sargent S, Wall M. Variables that affect the expansion rate and outcome of small aortic aneurysms. *J Vasc Surg.* 1990;11:260–269.
16. Cronenwett J, Murphy T, Zelenock G. Actuarial analysis of variables associated with rupture of small abdominal aortic aneurysms. *Surgery.* 1985;98:472–483.
17. Guirguis E, Barber G. The natural history of abdominal aortic aneurysms. *Am J Surg.* 1991;162:481–483.
18. Dapunt O, Galla J, Sadeghi A, et al. The natural history of thoracic aortic aneurysms. *J Thorac Cardiovasc Surg.* 1994;107:1323–1333.
19. Coady M, Rizzo J, Hammond G, et al. What is the appropriate size criterion for resection of thoracic aortic aneurysms? *J Thorac Cardiovasc Surg.* 1997;113:476–491.
20. Juvonen T, Ergin M, Galla J, et al. Prospective study of the natural history of thoracic aortic aneurysms. *Ann Thorac Surg.* 1997;63:1533–1545.
21. Juvonen T, Ergin M, Lansman S, et al. Risk factors for rupture of chronic type B dissections. *J Thorac Cardiovasc Surg.* 1999;117:776–786.
22. Crawford E, Hess K, Cohen E, Coselli J, Safi H. Ruptured aneurysms of the descending and thoracoabdominal aorta. *Ann Surg.* 1991;213:417–426.
23. Coselli J, Crawford E. Primary aortoesophageal fistula from aortic aneurysm: successful treatment by use of omental pedicle graft. *J Vasc Surg.* 1990;12:269–277.
24. Snyder D, Crawford E. Successful treatment of primary aortoesophageal fistula resulting from aortic aneurysm. *J Thorac Cardiovasc Surg.* 1983;85:457–463.
25. Crawford E. Ruptured abdominal aortic aneurysm: an editorial. *J Vasc Surg.* 1991;13:348–350.
26. Coselli J. Thoracoabdominal aortic aneurysms: experience with 372 patients. *J Card Surg.* 1994;9:638–647.
27. Coselli J. Surgical technique, preoperative and intraoperative management of thoracoabdominal aortic aneurysm. In Yao J, Pearce W, eds. *Arterial Surgery: Management of Clinical Problems.* Stamford, CT: Appleton & Lange; 1996:223–236.
28. Acher C, Wynn M, Hoch J, Popic P, Archibald J, Turnipseed W. Combined use of cerebral spinal fluid drainage and naloxone reduces the risk of paraplegia in thoracoabdominal aneurysm repair. *J Vasc Surg.* 1994;19:236–248.
29. Schepens M, Defauw J, Hamerlijnck R, DeGeest R, Vermeuln F. Surgical treatment of thoracoabdominal aortic aneurysms by simple crossclamping. *J Thorac Cardiovasc Surg.* 1994;107:134–142.
30. von Segesser L, Genoni M, Kunzli A, Lachat M, Niederhauser U, Vogt P, et al. Surgery for ruptured thoracic and thoraco-abdominal aneurysms. *Eur J Cardio-thorac Surg.* 1996;10:996–1002.
31. Velazquez O, Bavaria J, Pochettino A, Carpenter J. Emergency repair of thoracoabdominal aortic aneurysms with immediate presentation. *J Vasc Surg.* 1999;30:996–1003.

17

Surgical Management of Pararenal Aortic Aneurysms Associated with Renal Artery Occlusive Disease

James C. Stanley, MD, Peter K. Henke, MD, and Gilbert R. Upchurch, Jr., MD

Pararenal abdominal aortic aneurysms (AAAs) are an important category of aortic disease.[1–5] Coexistent arteriosclerotic renal artery disease is present in nearly all patients with pararenal AAAs and is severe enough to cause renovascular hypertension or ischemic nephropathy in 10% to 25% of these individuals.[1,4] Simultaneous treatment of AAAs and renal artery disease requires a thorough understanding of their pathophysiology and a carefully planned and executed operation.[6–11]

PARARENAL AORTIC ANEURYSMS

Pararenal AAAs are categorized as juxtarenal (Figure 17–1) or suprarenal lesions (Figure 17–2). By definition, juxtarenal AAAs extend superiorly to just below the renal arteries such that no normal aorta exists between the aneurysm and the renal arteries. Suprarenal AAAs, however, extend superiorly to include the orifices of the renal arteries to one or both kidneys. Juxtarenal AAAs are four times more common than suprarenal AAAs. Pararenal AAAs do not involve the superior mesenteric or celiac arteries, nor do they extend above the diaphragm, as do thoracoabdominal aortic aneurysms.

Pararenal AAAs account for 4% of all AAAs and men are twice as likely as women to have pararenal AAAs. This is in contrast to men having a 3.5 to 4 times greater likelihood of infrarenal AAA compared to women. The relative increase in the number of women having pararenal AAAs compared to infrarenal AAAs may be due

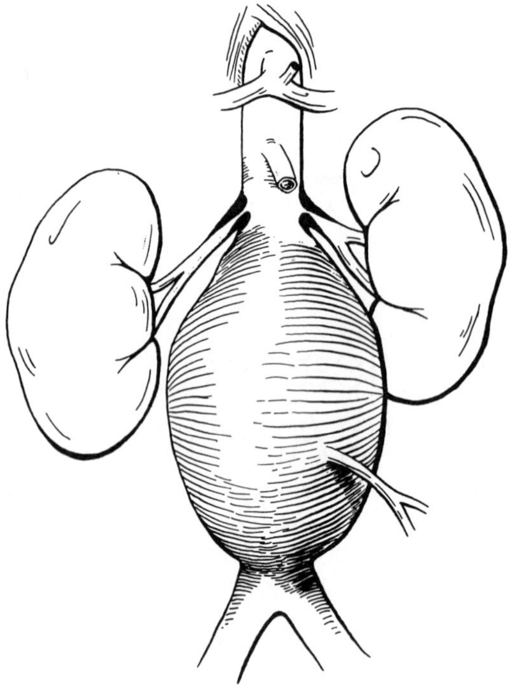

Figure 17–1. Juxtarenal abdominal aortic aneurysm (AAA) abutting renal arteries.

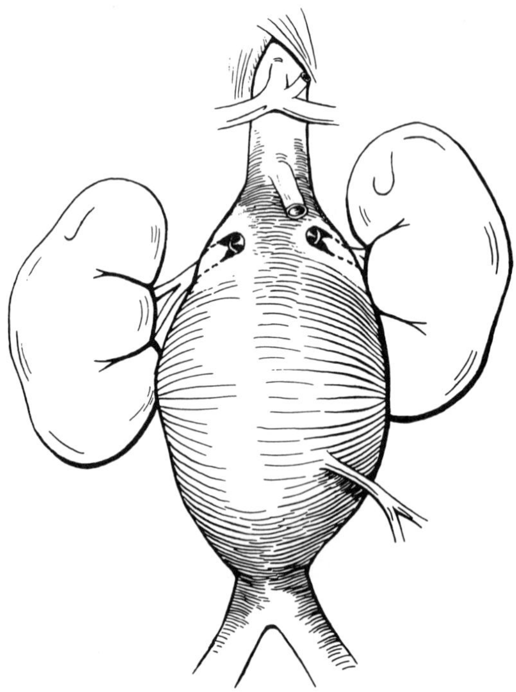

Figure 17–2. Suprarenal AAA involving renal arteries.

to gender-related practice patterns, with more common delays in treating women until their AAAs become larger. This delay may provide a longer time for aneurysmal change to extend to the more cephalic pararenal aorta. However, it is also likely that physiologic changes following menopause are important. Reductions in estrogen levels and a subsequent reduction in elastin and collagen cross-linking may contribute to a generalized form of aortic dilation, such that when infrarenal AAAs evolve in women, the proximal aorta also exhibits aneurysmal changes. Anecdotal experience supports this contention, but definitive data to confirm such an hypothesis have not been forthcoming. Pararenal AAAs are recognized at an average age of 67 yr, and most are larger than infrarenal AAAs when diagnosed.

In contemporary times, the majority of pararenal AAAs are asymptomatic, being discovered during physical examination or during radiologic studies for other illnesses. The primary indication for surgical treatment of asymptomatic pararenal AAAs is the same as for infrarenal AAAs, namely an aneurysm diameter of 5 cm or greater. Rapid increases in transverse diameter, (exceeding 4 mm in 12 mo), severe chronic obstructive pulmonary disease (COPD), and diastolic hypertension place these patients at greater risk for continued AAA expansion and support earlier operative intervention.

RENAL ARTERY STENOTIC DISEASE

Arteriosclerotic renal artery disease is common among patients having pararenal AAAs, and is severe enough itself to justify endovascular or operative intervention in 1 of 10 patients. Aortic spillover arteriosclerosis accounts for nearly 80% of these stenoses,[12] and intrinsic renal artery disease accounts for the remainder. When one renal artery exhibits a hemodynamically significant narrowing of 70% to 80%, the contralateral renal artery is similarly affected in 30% of patients. Although right- and left-sided arteriosclerotic narrowings occur with equal frequency, the left renal artery appears prone to more severe disease.

Surgical treatment of renal artery occlusive lesions in patients with pararenal AAAs is a controversial topic.[13,14] In part, this reflects a lack of clinical data to support three of the four generally stated indications for undertaking simultaneous procedures. These four indications warrant separate discussion.

I. *Evidence of Renovascular Hypertension Secondary to Renal Artery Stenoses*—This is the most accepted reason to treat AAAs and renal artery stenotic disease simultaneously.[12,13] Mortality rates accompanying such combined procedures range from 2% to 7%. A salutary outcome regarding improved hypertension control is expected in 50% to 70% of patients.[5,6] Anatomic evidence of hemodynamically important renal artery stenotic disease (i.e., arteriographic documentation of collaterals, duplex scan data revealing a critical stenosis) or functional studies of relevant disease (i.e., renin hypersecretion, abnormal ACE-nuclide scans) support the diagnosis of renovascular hypertension and justify operative intervention.

II. *Evidence of Ischemic Nephropathy Secondary to Renal Artery Stenoses*—This is a more ethereal indication for concomitant procedures.[7,13] Certain facts deserve attention. First, a flow-reducing critical renal artery stenosis must be present to impair renal function. This usually requires a 70% to 80% stenosis with a 15–40 mmHg pressure gradient across the stenosis.[7,12,13] Confirmation of these hemodynamic changes may be difficult and subject to diagnostic errors. Second, for ischemic nephropathy to exist, with a serum creatinine of at least 1.8–2.0 mg/dL, both kidneys must be affected. If impaired blood flow does not exist to both kidneys, then the contralateral kidney must be affected with parenchymal disease, such as nephrosclerosis.

III. *Prevention of Renal Artery Stenotic Disease Progression*—The natural history of arteriosclerotic renal artery disease remains ill defined, but certain lesions are likely to progress and contribute to both renovascular hypertension and renal insufficiency.[13,15,16] Identification and treatment of such lesions seems justified, if performed with minimal morbidity and mortality.[6] However, this may be a difficult task. Renal artery stenotic disease >50% to 60% is unlikely to progress to occlusion in the immediate future.[15] In these individuals, progression appears to occur at an average rate of 4% to 5% per year. Thus, lesser diseased renal arteries do not mandate immediate and simultaneous treatment at the time of aortic aneurysm surgery. However, renal artery stenoses ranging from 75% to 90% are estimated to carry a 10% to 30% risk of occluding within 2 to 5 yr, and these stenoses warrant operative treatment if such can be done safely at the time of aortic aneurysmectomy. It should be noted that most patients with such critical stenoses have secondary renin-mediated blood pressure elevations, and thus fall into the first indication—category I. Nevertheless, stabilization of renal function to avoid hemodialysis is worthwhile in properly chosen patients, given the high mortality associated with end-stage renal failure and dialysis.

IV. *Presence of a Renal Artery Stenosis Considered to Be a Hazard During Aortic Aneurysmectomy*—Nearly 30% to 40% of patients undergoing treatment of AAAs have a 50% or greater stenosis of their renal arteries.[6] If these patients have a pararenal AAA that originates in close juxtaposition to the renal arteries, the application of an aortic clamp or placement of the aortic suture line near the renal artery orifices may cause plaque disruption or embolization and may compromise blood flow to the kidneys. In such circumstances, concurrent treatment of both the aneurysm and renal artery occlusive disease is appropriate.

A number of general observations regarding simultaneous aortic aneurysmectomy and renal revascularization deserve mention. Bilateral renal revascularizations when both kidneys are ischemic, although associated with increased perioperative hazards, are more likely to improve renal function. Intraoperative duplex ultrasonography often aids in defining whether an otherwise ill-defined renal artery stenosis is at a critical level that would justify simultaneous operative repair.

Small kidney size is an often-cited criteria for operation and is used to decide if a nephrectomy or revascularization should be attempted. If generalized atrophy exists with no evidence of cortical infarction, and a kidney is 5 to 6 cm in length, there will be little functioning parenchyma remaining and nephrectomy may be appropriate. Nevertheless, if the serum creatinine is greater than 3.0 mg/dL, even with areas of infarction, the kidney should be revascularized if the renal artery can be reconstructed technically. However, in these latter circumstances, if the contralateral kidney is of normal size and involved with stenotic disease amenable to correction, then an ipsilateral nephrectomy and contralateral revascularization may be appropriate. Occasionally, preoperative nuclide scans confirm that an ischemic kidney contributes <10% of the total renal function, and in such a setting, a small, contracted kidney is rarely successfully revascularized.

AORTA AND RENAL ARTERY IMAGING

Aortography is useful for assessment of all pararenal AAAs, especially AAAs with associated renal artery disease. Biplanar digital substraction studies usually provide accurate delineation of the pararenal aorta and renal artery. Lateral projections are necessary to define the proximal extent of the aneurysm as well as the presence of arteriosclerotic celiac or superior mesenteric arterial stenoses. Simple computed tomography (CT) does not provide enough detail in most of these patients. However, spiral CT reconstructions provide important information in many patients with complex aortic and renal disease. The nephrotoxic risks of iodinated contrast exposure with conventional aortography and CT studies are considerable in patients with renal insufficiency.[13] Gadolinium (GD) may be an alternative to iodinated contrast for conventional catheter-based intra-arterial studies. Although not currently approved for use by the US Food and Drug Administration, the latter may become an acceptable agent for studying these patients in the future.

Magnetic resonance angiography (MRA), enhanced by intravenous gadolinium and a breath-hold technique, has become a less invasive means of imaging the abdominal aorta and its branches with a high degree of accuracy in identifying significant renal artery stenoses[17] (Figure 17–3). The lack of nephrotoxicity with gadolinium makes MRA an attractive imaging technique in patients with renal insufficiency and pararenal AAAs. MRA defines the proximal AAA extent in all patients and is very sensitive for recognition of stenotic lesions greater than 50% affecting the renal, superior mesenteric, and celiac arteries.

OPERATIVE MANAGEMENT

Surgical risks attending operations for pararenal AAAs with associated renal artery stenoses are considerable. Three factors contribute to these risks. First, cardiac risks are greater due to the increased afterload accompanying more proximal aortic clamp placement. Second, the aortic dissection required for repair of all pararenal AAAs is extensive, and this translates into increased operative risks. Third, renal ischemia due to suprarenal aortic clamping is an inescapable part of these procedures. Whereas one might be selective with preoperative cardiac evaluations for infrarenal AAA repairs, the magnitude of treating pararenal AAAs supports a more comprehensive approach.[3–6] Noninvasive cardiac testing is recommended in all patients with pararenal AAAs, and cardiac catheterization is pursued if significant myocardial ischemia is suspected.

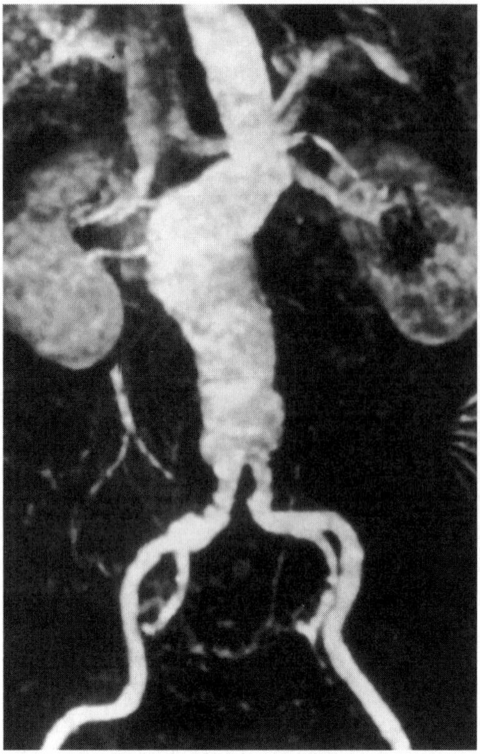

Figure 17–3. Gadolinium-enhanced MRA of pararenal abdominal aortic aneurysm. (*From Prince MR, Narasimham DL, Stanley JC, et al. Gadolinium-enhanced magnetic resonance angiography of abdominal aortic aneurysms. J Vasc Surg 1995;21: 656–669.*)

Aortic Procedures

Adequate pararenal AAA exposure is critical to the successful treatment of these patients. Four basic approaches to pararenal AAAs are (1) transabdominal, (2) retroperitoneal, (3) thoracoretroperitoneal, and (4) thoracoabdominal. At the University of Michigan, a direct abdominal approach through a supraumbilical transverse incision has been favored when treating most pararenal AAAs. Exposure of the pararenal aorta at the base of the mesentery and mesocolon is favored in most patients, although medial visceral rotation is frequently undertaken as an alternative approach, especially in the case of very large pararenal AAAs.[3] Fixed retractors facilitate this exposure, but care with their positioning is important to avoid organ trauma, especially to the pancreas. A retroperitoneal exposure through a flank or thoracoabdominal incision is preferred by some.[4] This later approach may be associated with a reduction in postoperative fluid requirements and a shorter hospital stay, but no differences in morbidity or mortality have been documented. Unfortunately, if a right renal artery reconstruction is required, it is technically more difficult using this later approach, and in such circumstances a second abdominal incision is usually required.

Safe placement of the proximal aortic clamp at the supraceliac, supramesenteric, or suprarenal level is an important issue, especially in the presence of coexisting renal artery disease. Although some clinicians have not observed morbidity or mortality differences with any of the aforenoted three clamp sites, especially in regard to postoperative renal insufficiency or coagulopathy, others have advocated supraceliac clamping as a means of decreasing mortality and postoperative renal failure.[18] Supraceliac aortic exposure involves an easier dissection, and at this level the aorta is relatively spared of severe atherosclerosis. Perhaps most importantly, this site positions the clamp away from the renal artery orifices and the proximal aortic-graft anastomosis. Increases in coagulopathy or cardiac morbidity are not common with routine supraceliac clamp placement.[18,19]

Operative mortality appears greater with aortic clamping between the renal and superior mesenteric arteries and between the superior mesenteric and celiac arteries.[18,19] Clamping below the superior mesenteric artery should only be done if there is at least a 2 to 3 cm distance between the former vessel and the renal arteries, and only if that segment of aorta is free of extensive atherosclerosis and the clamp does not interfere with reconstruction of the renal arteries. It is important to realize that unclamping and repositioning of the aortic clamp to a second site has been associated with atheroembolization, visceral infarction, and death.[1,19] Isolating and occluding the renal and mesenteric arteries with microvascular clamps before proximal aortic clamping should lessen atheroembolic complications affecting the kidneys and intestines, although this benefit has not been studied critically.

Prior to clamping of the aorta and renal arteries, systemic anticoagulation is achieved with intravenous administration of 150 U/kg of heparin. Limiting the dose of heparin may reduce the risk of coagulopathy and some authors use none with proximal aortic clamp placement.[1,19] However, because of a concern for thrombus formation within the kidneys, most surgeons fully anticoagulate patients with heparin before halting blood flow within the renal circulation. Use of a cell-saver during surgery lessens transfusion requirements.[4] Most patients are administered renal-dose dopamine during the procedure. Mannitol, 12.5 g in an average adult, is administered intravenously prior to interrupting blood flow in order to establish or maintain a diuresis. A loop diuretic, such as furosemide, may be necessary in azotemic patients to establish a diuresis.

In treating juxtarenal AAAs, the proximal graft-to-aorta anastomosis is placed at the level of the renal artery orifices in most patients, with the graft being carried posteriorly above the renal arteries in occasional patients when necessary (Figure 17–4). It is important to not leave any aneurysmal aorta within the anastomosis.

Renal Artery Procedures

The specific surgical procedure chosen to restore renal blood flow in patients with pararenal AAAs and renal artery occlusive disease frequently depends on the type of aortic operation being performed.[3,8,10,20] Because the renal arteries are often involved with the aortic aneurysmal disease, percutaneous transluminal angioplasty (PCTA) with stenting is not recommended in these patients. Juxtarenal aneurysmectomy lends itself particularly well to transaortic renal endarterectomy (Figure 17–5).[3,6,9,20] However, in the presence of a suprarenal AAA or markedly diseased infrarenal aorta, an aortorenal bypass from the supraceliac aorta, reimplantation of the renal arteries, or

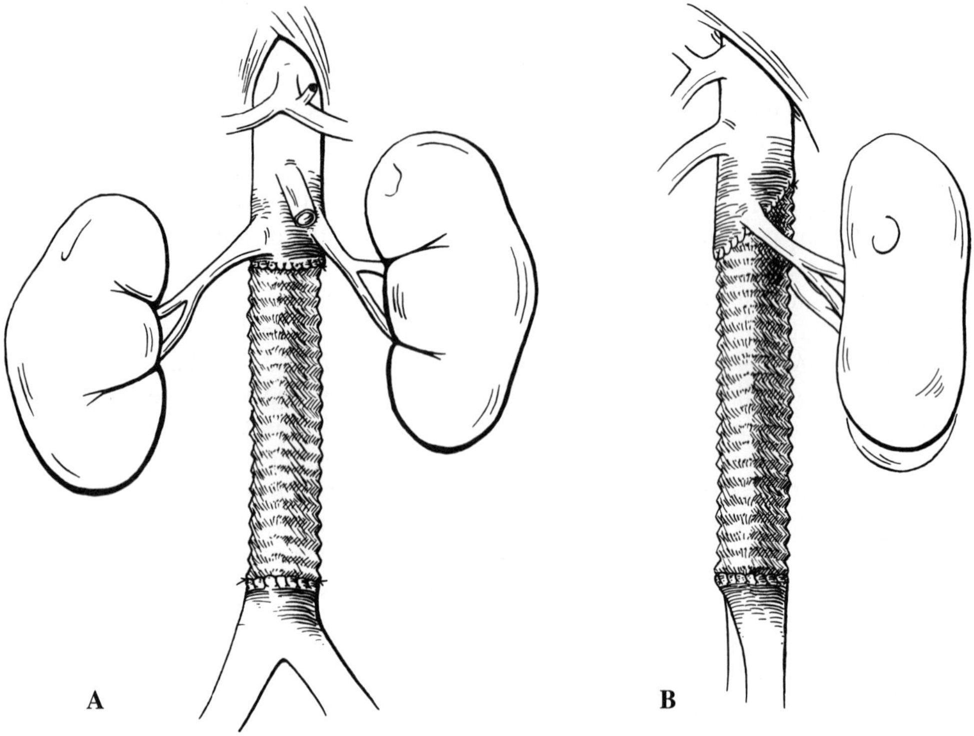

Figure 17–4. Operative options for aortic reconstruction following pararenal aortic aneurysmectomy and transaortic renal endarterectomy. (**A**) aortic graft abutting the renal arteries; (**B**) tapered aortic graft carried posteriorly above the renal arteries. (*From Henke PK, Stanley JC. Surgical treatment of pararenal abdominal aortic aneurysms. In: Ernst CB, Stanley JC, eds. Current Therapy in Vascular Surgery, 4th ed. Philadelphia: Mosby–YearBook, 2000, p. 231, with permission.*)

nonanatomic splenorenal or hepatorenal bypass may be more appropriate (Figure 17–6). In the case of nonanatomic revascularizations involving the hepatic or splenic arteries, lateral aortography must be performed preoperatively to establish the normalcy of the celiac artery because of its common narrowing in these patients.[21] The patient's overall clinical status must be considered when planning these operations, especially when undertaking renal reconstructions for preventative reasons.

Figure 17–5. (A) Transaortic renal artery endarterectomy through the transected aorta, undertaken in association with aortic reconstruction for aneurysmal disease. (**B**) Preoperative aortogram documenting occluded left renal artery and (**C**) postoperative aortogram revealing patent endarterectomized renal artery. (A: *From Stanley JC, Messina LM, Wakefield TW, Zelenock GB. Renal artery reconstruction. In: Bergan JJ, Yao JST, eds. Techniques in Arterial Surgery. Philadelphia: WB Saunders, 1990, p. 247, with permission.*)

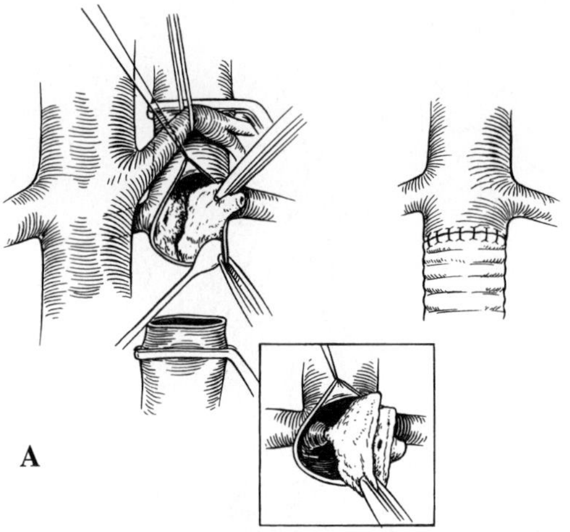

A

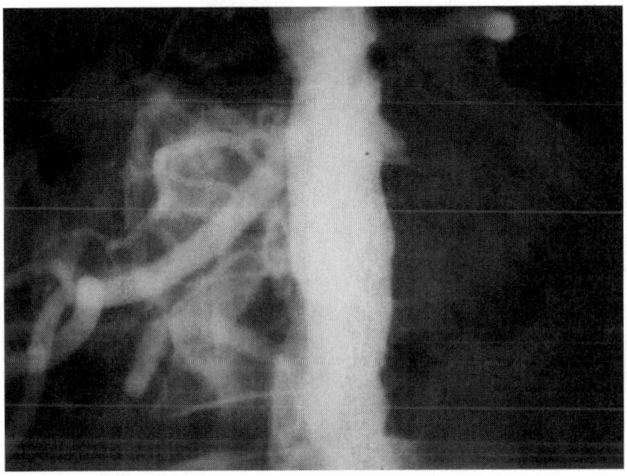

B

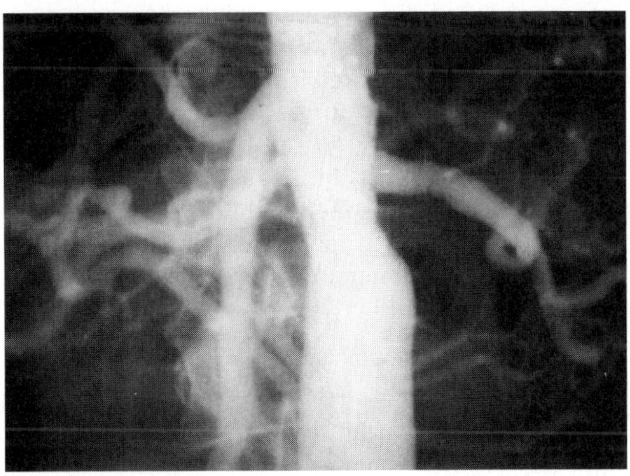

C

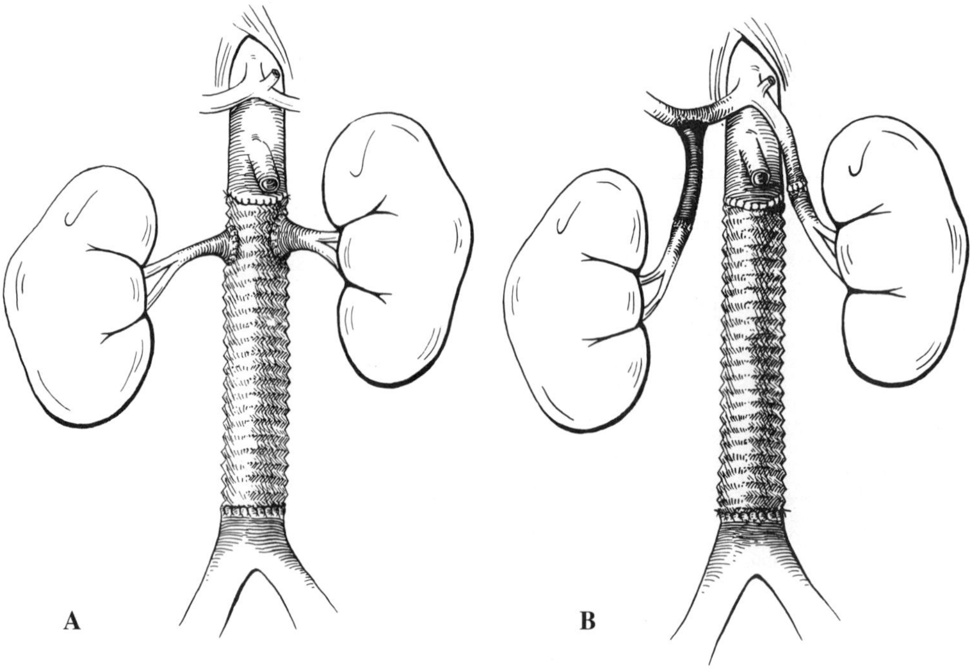

Figure 17–6. Operative options. (**A**) Suprarenal aortic graft with bilateral renal artery implantation; (**B**) suprarenal aortic graft, with right hepatorenal and left splenorenal bypasses. (*From Henke PK, Stanley JC. Surgical treatment of pararenal abdominal aortic aneurysms. In: Ernst CB, Stanley JC, eds. Current Therapy in Vascular Surgery, 4th ed. Philadelphia: Mosby–YearBook, 2000, p. 232, with permission.*)

Transaortic renal artery endarterectomy is the most common reconstructive procedure performed in these patients, and a detailed discussion of this technique is warranted.[20,22] The renal arteries are usually approached anteriorly through the base of the mesocolon and root of the mesentery. Exposure is facilitated by placing a rolled blanket transversely under the lower back so as to accentuate the lumbar lordosis. The small intestines are usually displaced outside the abdominal cavity in a bowel bag, and the transverse colon is retracted into the upper abdomen with the aid of fixed retractors. The ligament of Treitz is divided, and the duodenum is then mobilized. The retroperitoneum over the proximal aortic aneurysm is incised, and the dissection is continued superiorly to the level of the left renal vein, which is mobilized by transecting and ligating its adrenal, gonadal, and lumbar branches.

The renal arteries must be skeletonized from their aortic origin to a point well beyond the distal extent of obvious atherosclerotic plaque. This usually entails a dissection to the first-order branches. Small nonparenchymal branches, such as those to the adrenal gland, must be transected and ligated close to the renal artery. This extensive mobilization is time-consuming but is necessary to facilitate easy eversion of the renal artery during the transaortic endarterectomy.

The aorta is dissected about its circumference to above the superior mesenteric artery (SMA). This requires incision of dense surrounding neural and fibrous tissues and division of the periaortic diaphragmatic crus on both sides of the aorta. The crus is elevated with a right-angle clamp and is transected perpendicular to its fibers with the electrocautery so as to prevent troublesome muscular bleeding. Clamping of the proximal superior mesenteric artery and distal renal arteries prior to aortic occlusion, as previously noted, is done to prevent embolization of atheromatous aortic debris into the intestines and kidneys. This is achieved using low-pressure (30–70 g) microvascular clamps.

The suprarenal aorta is clamped, as are either the iliac arteries or aneurysm neck. The infrarenal aorta is then transected approximately 5 mm below the renal arteries, and a transaortic endarterectomy is performed through the open aorta. The endarterectomy plane is extended to approximately 1 cm above the renal artery orifices, and the plaque is transected transversely. Individual renal endarterectomies are often done after dividing the cylindrical aortic plaque in both the anterior and posterior midline. Endarterectomies are facilitated by everting each renal artery while maintaining gentle traction on the plaque.

The renal endarterectomy as well as the subsequent proximal aortic graft anastomosis are made easier by transposing the transected aorta anterior to the left renal vein. Following the endarterectomy and proximal aortic graft anastomosis, the aorta and graft are repositioned beneath the left renal vein. A soft jaw clamp is placed on the graft, and restoration of renal blood flow occurs with removal of the proximal aortic clamp. Restoring flow to the kidneys must be done with caution. Any aortic debris loosened by the proximal clamp must be flushed out of the aortic graft before restoring renal blood flow. If flushing is not performed, loose material may embolize to the kidneys. One then proceeds with the remainder of the distal aortic reconstruction. An occasional patient requires an eversion endarterectomy of a renal artery arising from the aneurysm, with subsequent direct reimplantation of the artery into the aortic graft (Figure 17–7).

Renal failure is a major cause of morbidity and mortality following combined renal revascularization and pararenal AAA repair. Minimizing ischemia to a kidney not affected with a renal artery stenosis that has not developed a protective collateral circulation is important. Performance of a transaortic renal artery endarterectomy and the proximal aortic anastomosis in <30 min decreases the incidence of postoperative renal insufficiency.[2,5,19] Another technique to minimize renal ischemic injury is to lower the kidney temperature by infusion of chilled (4°C) Ringer's lactate, to which is added 1000 U heparin/L, 12.5 g Mannitol/L, and 44.6 mEq of sodium bicarbonate/L. Approximately 150 mL of this solution is initially infused through each renal artery orifice, with repeated administration if the clamp time is >30 min. This cooling is most important for kidneys without hemodynamically significant stenoses and in patients with preoperative renal insufficiency.[4,18,19] Ice-slurry packing about the kidneys may also lower the core renal temperature, but is less commonly performed. If concern arises postoperatively regarding the anatomic status of the renal circulation in the azotemic patient, one should consider a gadolinium-enhanced MRA to establish the adequacy of the renal revascularization (Figure 17–8).

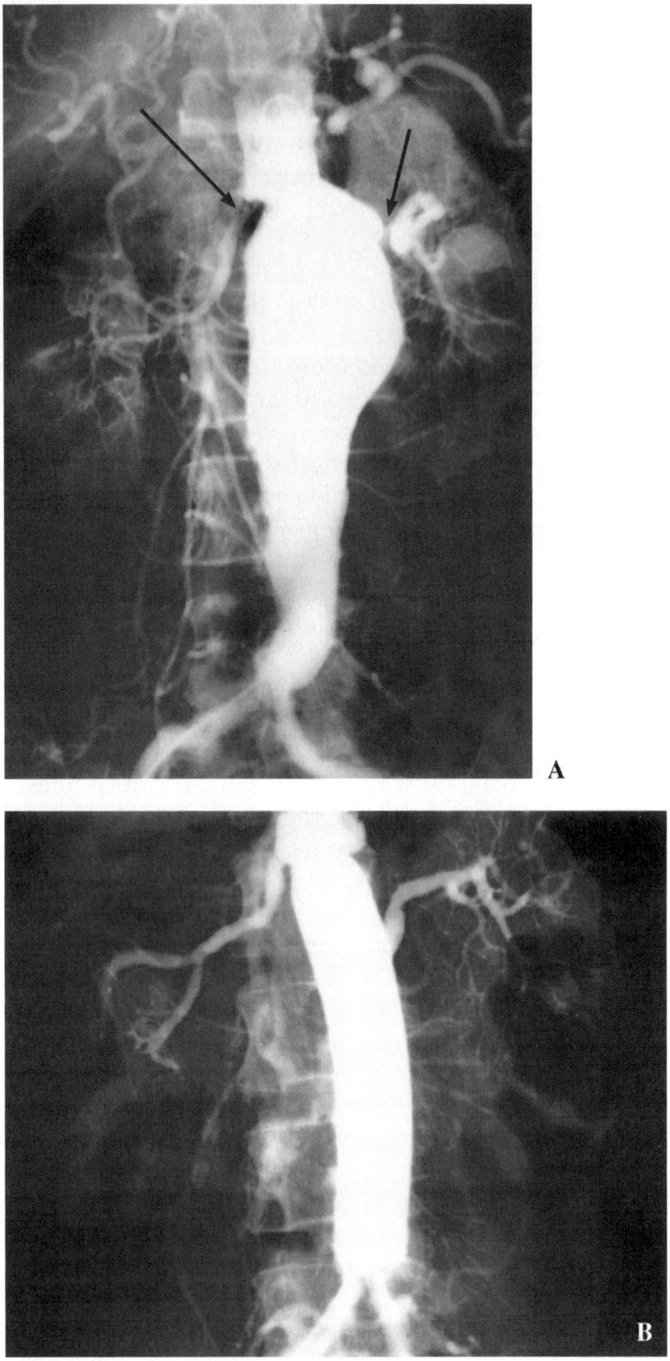

Figure 17–7. (**A**) Pararenal aortic aneurysm with bilateral proximal renal artery stenoses, including the left renal artery arising from the aneurysm. (**B**) Postoperative appearance of interposition aortoaortic graft, after implantation of the endarterectomized left renal artery into the graft, and concomitant transaortic right renal artery endarterectomy. (*From Henke PK, Stanley JC. Surgical treatment of pararenal abdominal aortic aneurysms. In: Ernst CB, Stanley JC, eds. Current Therapy in Vascular Surgery, 4th ed. Philadelphia: Mosby–YearBook, 2000, p. 231, with permission.*)

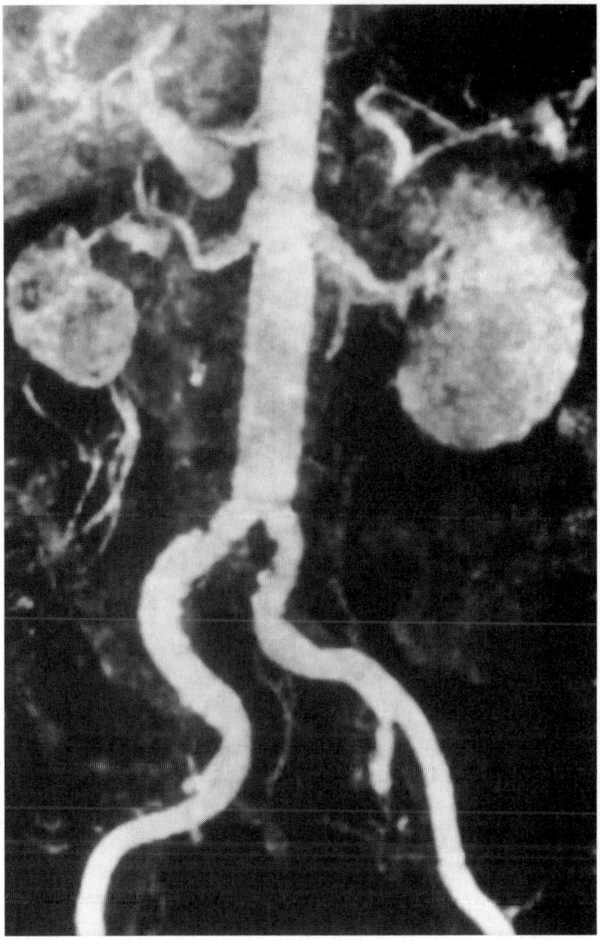

Figure 17–8. Gadolinium-enhanced MRA following bilateral transaortic renal endarterectomy with an aortoaortic graft placement after an abdominal juxtarenal aneurysmectomy.

OPERATIVE RESULTS

Surgical treatment of pararenal AAAs can be undertaken with acceptable morbidity and mortality rates (Table 17–1). In fact, mortality figures are similar to those reported for infrarenal AAA repair.[1–4,23] However, the morbidity associated with the surgical treatment of pararenal AAAs remains high, especially when simultaneous renal artery reconstructions are performed.[2,4,8,24]

The major complication of the operative treatment of pararenal AAAs, and oftentimes the cause of death, is renal failure, accounting for more than half the mortality in several series.[1,2,4,5] Postoperative renal failure is highest among patients with preoperative renal insufficiency and in patients who require concomitant renal artery reconstruction.[1–4,19] Coexistent renal artery disease in patients undergoing pararenal aneurysmectomy, like that affecting patients with nonaneurysmal peripheral arterial occlusive disease,[25] places them at high risk for postoperative complications and death.

TABLE 17–1. OVERALL OPERATIVE OUTCOMES OF TREATING PARARENAL ABDOMINAL AORTIC ANEURYSM[a]

Institution	Number of Patients	Operative Mortality (%)	Postoperative Renal Failure (%)	Postoperative Dialysis (%)
Methodist Hospital, Houston, Texas[2]	101	7	16	7
University of California, San Francisco, San Francisco, California[5]	77	1.2	23	2.5
Washington University, St. Louis, Missouri[1]	65	1.5	12	3
Henry Ford Hospital, Detroit, Michigan[4]	53	3.7	23	5.6
Red Cross Hospital, Athens, Greece[23]	38	5.2	24	2
University of Michigan, Ann Arbor, Michigan	84	3.5	10	2.4

[a] Reports included differing numbers of juxtarenal and suprarenal aneurysms as well as differing numbers of patients subjected to concomitant renal revascularization procedures. Comparisons of one series to another are therefore invalid.

Intestinal infarction is a second recognized cause of death in these patients.[3] Overall survival at 5 yr following surgical therapy of pararenal AAAs is approximately 75%, with most late deaths due to cardiac causes.[1,2,23] Given the lethal nature of aneurysmal expansion with rupture, operative treatment of most pararenal aortic AAAs with associated renal artery disease is warranted in patients who are otherwise acceptable surgical candidates.

Nearly 70% of nonazotemic patients and 50% of azotemic patients undergoing renal revascularization for renovascular hypertension at the same time of pararenal AAA repair will have improved blood pressure control.[5–7,9,11,24] Only 20% of those benefiting are cured of their hypertension. Patients exhibiting renal insufficiency who are most likely to have a salutary outcome are those with serum creatinines <3.0 mg/dL and whose azotemia is of relatively rapid onset, in contrast to those with longstanding renal insufficiency.[7,9] Although benefits can accrue to those with serum creatinines >3.0 mg/dL,[10] good outcomes are much less predictable, and 20% to 30% of these patients are likely to become dialysis dependent within 3 yr.[7] Nevertheless, 30% to 50% of azotemic patients have improved renal function when treated simultaneously for a pararenal AAA and critical renal artery stenoses.[5–7]

REFERENCES

1. Allen BT, Anderson CB, Rubin BG, Flye MW, Baumann DS, Sicard GA. Preservation of renal function in juxtarenal and suprarenal abdominal aortic aneurysm repair. *J Vasc Surg.* 1993;17:948–959.
2. Crawford ES, Beckett WC, Greer MS. Juxtarenal infrarenal abdominal aortic aneurysm. Special diagnostic and therapeutic considerations. *Ann Surg.* 1986;203:661–670.

3. Jean-Claude JM, Reilly LM, Stoney RJ, Messina LM. Pararenal aortic aneurysms: the future of open aortic repair. *J Vasc Surg.* 1999;29:902–912.
4. Nypaver TJ, Shepard AD, Reddy DJ, Elliot JP, Smith RF, Ernst CB. Repair of pararenal abdominal aortic aneurysms. An analysis of operative management. *Arch Surg.* 1993;128:803–813.
5. Qvarfordt PG, Stoney RJ, Reilly LM, Skioldebrand CG, Goldstone J, Ehrenfeld WK. Management of pararenal aneurysms of the abdominal aorta. *J Vasc Surg.* 1986;3:84–93.
6. Cambria RP, Brewster DC, L'Italien G, et al. Simultaneous aortic and renal artery reconstruction: evolution of an eighteen-year experience. *J Vasc Surg.* 1995;21:916–925.
7. Chaikof EL, Smith RB III, Salam AA, et al. Ischemic nephropathy and concomitant aortic disease: a ten-year experience. *J Vasc Surg.* 1994;19:135–148.
8. Dean RH, Keyser JE, Dupont WD, Nadeau JH, Meacham PW. Aortic and renal vascular disease: factors affecting the value of combined procedures. *Ann Surg.* 1984;200:336–344.
9. McNeil JW, String ST, Pfeiffer RB Jr. Concomitant renal endarterectomy and aortic reconstruction. *J Vasc Surg.* 1994;20:331–337.
10. O'Mara CS, Maples MD, Kilgore TL Jr, et al. Simultaneous aortic reconstruction and bilateral renal revascularization. Is this a safe and effective procedure? *J Vasc Surg.* 1988;8:357–366.
11. Stewart MT, Smith RB III, Fulenwider JT, Perdue GD, Wells JO. Concomitant renal revascularization in patients undergoing aortic surgery. *J Vasc Surg.* 1985;2:400–405.
12. Stanley JC. Surgical treatment of renovascular hypertension. *Am J Surg.* 1997;174:102–110.
13. Jacobson HR. Ischemic renal disease: an overlooked clinical entity? *Kid Int.* 1988;34:729–743.
14. Williamson WK, Abou-Zamzam AM Jr, Moneta GL, et al. Prophylactic repair of renal artery stenosis is not justified in patients who require infrarenal aortic reconstruction. *J Vasc Surg.* 1998;28:14–22.
15. Tollefson DF, Ernst CB. Natural history of atherosclerotic renal artery stenosis associated with aortic disease. *J Vasc Surg.* 1991;14:327–331.
16. Zierler RE, Bergelin RO, Isaacson JA, Strandness DE. Natural history of atherosclerotic renal artery stenosis: a prospective study with duplex ultrasound. *J Vasc Surg.* 1994;19:250–258.
17. Prince MR, Schoenberg SO, Ward JS, Londy FJ, Wakefield TW, Stanley JC. Hemodynamically significant atherosclerotic renal artery stenosis: MR angiographic features. *Radiology.* 1997;205:128–136.
18. Green RM, Ricotta JJ, Ouriel K, DeWeese JA. Results of supraceliac aortic clamping in the difficult elective resection of infrarenal abdominal aortic aneurysm. *J Vasc Surg.* 1989;9:125–134.
19. Nypaver TJ, Shepard AD, Reddy DJ, Elliot JP, Ernst CB. Supraceliac aortic cross clamping: determinants of outcome in elective abdominal aortic reconstruction. *J Vasc Surg.* 1993;17:868–876.
20. Stanley JC, Messina LM, Wakefield TW, Zelenock GB. Renal artery reconstruction. In: Bergan JJ, Yao JST, eds. *Techniques in Arterial Surgery,* Philadelphia: WB Saunders, 1990:247–263.
21. Valentine RJ, Martin JD, Myers SI, Rossi MB, Clagett GP. Asymptomatic celiac and superior mesenteric artery stenoses are more prevalent among patients with unsuspected renal artery stenoses. *J Vasc Surg.* 1991;14:195–199.
22. Stoney RJ, Messina LM, Goldstone J, Reilly LM. Renal endarterectomy through the transected aorta: a new technique for combined aortorenal atherosclerosis. A preliminary report. *J Vasc Surg.* 1989;9:224–233.
23. Poulias GE, Doundoulakis N, Skoutas B, et al. Juxtarenal abdominal aneurysmectomy. *J Cardiovasc Surg.* 1992;33:324–330.
24. Benjamin ME, Hansen KJ, Craven TE, et al. Combined aortic and renal artery surgery. A contemporary experience. *Ann Surg.* 1996;223:555–567.
25. Missouris CG, Buckenham T, Cappuccio FP, MacGregor GA. Renal artery stenosis: a common and important problem in patients with peripheral vascular disease. *Am J Med.* 1994;96:10–14.

18

The Use of Stent–Grafts in the Treatment of Isolated Iliac Artery Aneurysms

Osvaldo J. Yano, MD, Michael Marin, MD, and Larry H. Hollier, MD

Although the aortoiliac region is frequently affected by atherosclerotic disease, isolated iliac artery aneurysms are rare and account for only between 2% and 5% of atherosclerotic aneurysms in the aortoiliac segment.[1–4] Because of their location, iliac artery aneurysms are difficult to diagnose, and the majority of isolated iliac artery aneurysms are asymptomatic. However, as they grow they have the potential to rupture, embolize, thrombose, or produce extrinsic compression on adjacent anatomic structures.

As with abdominal aortic aneurysms (AAAs), which can extend into iliac artery segments in as many as 21% of all patients with aortic aneurysms,[5] the maximum transverse diameter of the aneurysm sac appears to be the main predictor of whether intervention is warranted to avoid significant clinical sequelae.[6] Currently, the gold standard treatment for isolated iliac artery aneurysms is anatomic conventional repair. However, in emergent cases following rupture, the mortality rates can reach as high as 33%.[7]

Alternative surgical therapies for iliac artery aneurysms can range from simple aneurysm ligation to coil embolization and implantation of bare stents in an attempt to exclude aneurysms. However, subsequent aneurysm expansion and rupture have been reported when these alternative techniques have been used.[8–12]

Endovascular stent–graft devices have been used in limited series of patients with satisfactory midterm results. This chapter explores the potential benefits and limitations of using stent–grafts as a therapeutic option in patients with isolated iliac artery aneurysms.

DEFINITION AND BACKGROUND

Somewhat surprisingly, there is no firm consensus in the literature as to how to define iliac artery aneurysms and what maximum transverse diameter constitutes an aneurysm.[5] Conceptually, there are two different methods that can be used to define the pathology. The first is to compare the dilated portion of the iliac artery to the normal caliber adjacent vessel diameter. This concept can be used for local lesions but it is not feasible when the entire artery is dilated. The second method depends on measurements of arterial morphology that are based on the average reported in studies of large population groups. Once this information is known, two standard deviations from the mean can be categorized as an abnormal dilatation or an aneurysm. However, this approach is limited because of the considerable variations in age as well as the regions in which the data were collected. To illustrate the possible discrepancies, the results of a prior study on males between the ages of 60 and 80 yr that were based on CT scan measurements of a US-based population group showed a mean common iliac diameter of 1.17 to 1.30 cm according to the age group.[13] Conversely, another study carried out in Europe that was based on a large group of male subjects over the age of 50 yr revealed an average common iliac diameter of 1.1 cm.[14] The question is how to determine what diameter common iliac artery constitutes an aneurysm. In a population-based study, Armon and colleagues[5] reviewed the incidence of concomitant iliac artery aneurysms in patients with AAAs. They concluded that normal variation of the Gauss bimodal curve occurs in patients with iliac artery aneurysms that are 2.4 cm in diameter. Once the iliac artery becomes larger, a bimodal curve is no longer seen, indicating that the normal distribution pattern no longer exists and suggesting an abnormal behavior similar to that occurring in AAAs.

Once a diagnosis is established, a second question concerns how these isolated iliac artery aneurysms behave. Santilli and colleagues[6] studied the expansion of 321 iliac artery aneurysms in 189 patients over a period of 9 yr with a mean follow-up of 31 mo. These authors concluded that small iliac artery aneurysms with diameters <3.0 cm grow slowly, at a rate of 1 mm per year. Conversely, for aneurysms >3 cm in diameter, the growth rate was >2.5 mm annually. High rates of rupture based on small numbers of subjects have been reported in the literature, thus raising the statistical validity of these conclusions.[7,15] Santilli and coworkers[6] reported the largest number of subjects studied in a longitudinal fashion, and their 4-yr life-table survival rate (Kaplan–Meyer curve) was 78.4% with no deaths being attributed to the aneurysms. Iliac artery aneurysm rupture occurred in 6 of their 189 patients (3.1%), all of whom had aneurysms >4.0 cm in diameter. The authors concluded that elective repair should be considered in patients with aneurysms >3.5 cm because of the likelihood of growth and before the aneurysm reaches the critical size of 4 cm in diameter.

CONFIGURING DEVICES ACCORDING TO THE ANATOMY

Iliac artery aneurysms with adequate proximal and distal necks within the common iliac artery and no involvement of the orifice of the internal iliac artery are extraordinarily rare (Figure 18–1). This finding was seen only twice in our series of more than 400 en-

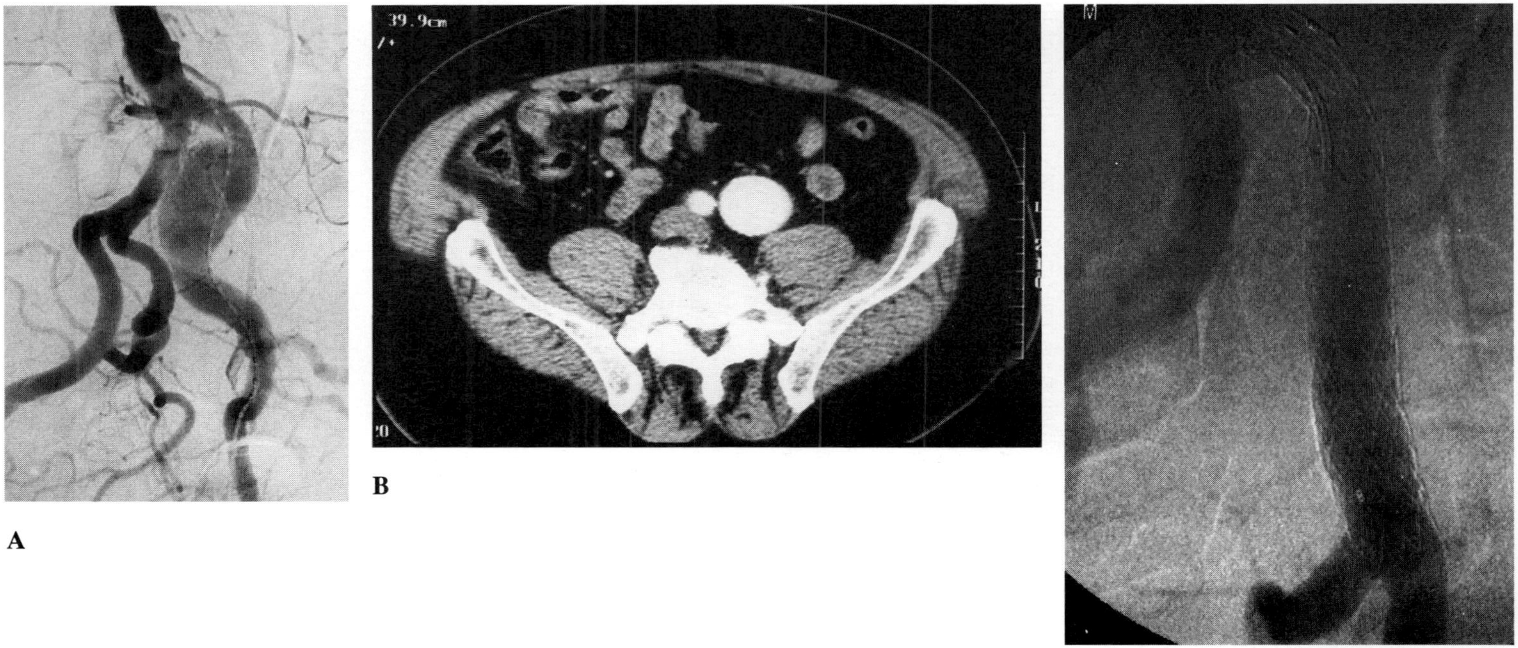

A B C

Figure 18–1. Preintervention angiogram (**A**) and CT scan (**B**) of an isolated common iliac artery aneurysm with sufficient proximal and distal necks to allow stent–graft anchorage to achieve durable repair. (**C**) The completion angiogram immediately following stent–graft deployment demonstrating complete angiographic exclusion of the common iliac artery aneurysm and preservation of the internal iliac artery orifice.

dovascular stent–graft repairs of aortoiliac aneurysms.[16] In the majority of isolated iliac artery aneurysms, the orifice of the internal iliac artery arises from the aneurysm sac (Figure 18–2). In these instances, the major limiting factor in accomplishing full exclusion of the aneurysm by the stent–graft is the involvement of the orifice of the internal iliac artery that originates from the aneurysm sac. Two main adjunctive techniques that deal with the internal iliac artery when common iliac artery aneurysms are present can be used to circumvent this problem. Parodi and Ferreira[17] described direct revascularization of the internal iliac artery, followed by proximal ligation and transection of the vessel (Figure 18–3) to allow the distal anchoring site to a more distant site (external iliac artery). A second alternative is to simply occlude the internal iliac artery by using catheter-based technology (Figure 18–4). The opponents of this approach to endovascular management of common iliac artery aneurysms argue that there may be major undesired consequences related to the occlusion of one or both patent internal iliac arteries following AAA repair or iliac aneurysm repair, including colonic and pelvic ischemia. To address this controversy, our group conducted a study based on the preoperative angiographic pelvic anatomy of patients who required internal iliac artery embolization and correlated specific vascular patterns with postoperative clinical outcome related to pelvic ischemia.[18] We found that in the majority of patients, the intricate network of collateral pelvic vessels usually compensated for the sacrifice of one of the internal iliac arteries. If an aggressive approach is planned to treat complex iliac and aortoiliac aneurysms, careful preoperative imaging tests are recommended for assess-

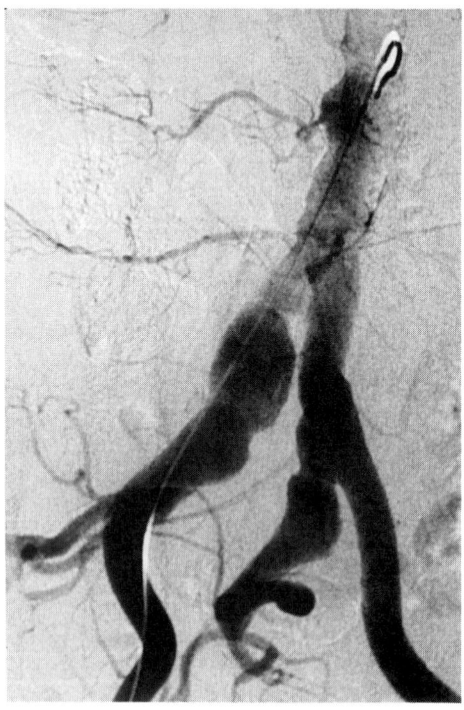

Figure 18–2. Angiogram of bilateral iliac artery aneurysms involving both internal iliac artery orifices.

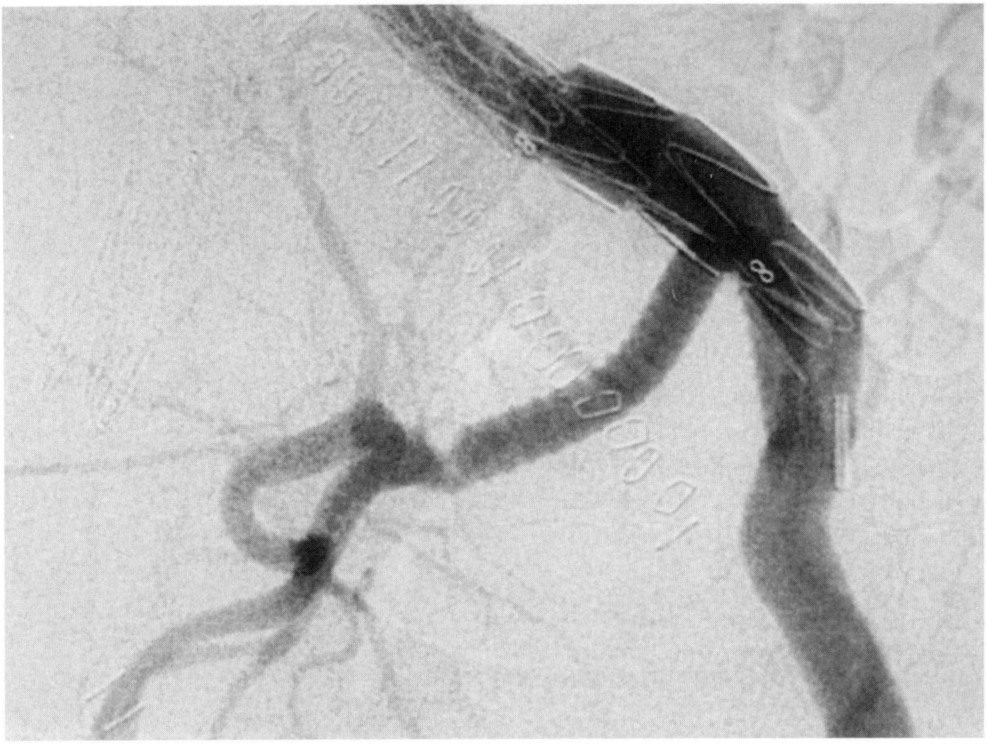

Figure 18–3. Transposition of the internal iliac artery by disconnection and construction of a direct bypass conduit from the external iliac artery.

ing all possible sources of collateral vessels that can be recruited to provide perfusion to the pelvis from visceral, pelvic, and upper thigh circulations following sacrifice of one or both of the internal iliac arteries.

Because atherosclerosis in the pelvic circulation appears to impede the development of new collaterals and promotes the underdevelopment of the ipsilateral femoral circulation, based on the findings of our study, we recommend that caution and good clinical judgment be exercised prior to intentional occlusion of one or both of the internal iliac arteries.

The results of our study suggested that despite the complexity of the pelvic arterial circulation, careful preoperative evaluation of the visceral, pelvic, and upper thigh circulations should be performed using bilateral delayed angiograms of the internal iliac arteries and deep femoral branches prior to intentional embolization to search for signs of chronic pelvic ischemia. When occlusion of both internal iliac arteries is planned, both deep femoral arteries must be studied and should be reconstructed if stenosis is present to maximize the inflow to the ascending collateral vessels to the pelvis. However, to virtually eliminate the probability of pelvic ischemia in patients with bilateral internal iliac artery occlusions, an iliac artery relocation or bypass should be performed to preserve blood flow to the pelvis. In the presence of normal superior

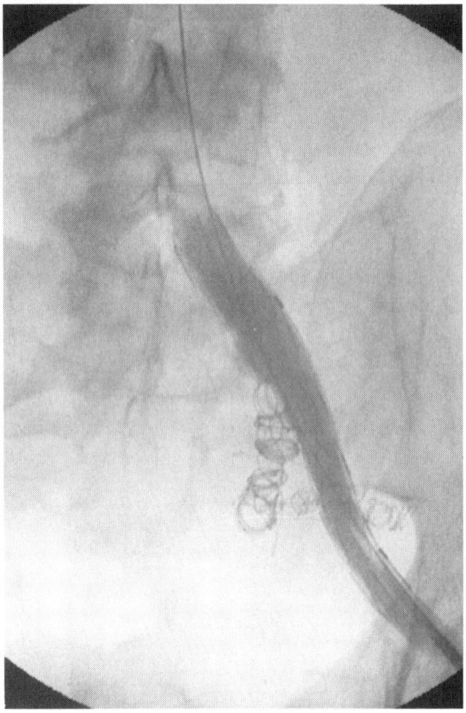

Figure 18–4. Complete exclusion of a common iliac artery aneurysm by a stent–graft following coil embolization of the internal iliac artery to allow extension of the distal attachment site to a normal caliber external iliac artery.

mesenteric and celiac artery anatomy, sacrifice of one internal iliac artery appears to be safe and does not represent a significant risk factor for ischemia of the colon. When the previously mentioned guidelines are used, intentional internal iliac artery occlusion can be performed safely as an adjuvant intervention to endovascular exclusion of aortoiliac aneurysms.

ENDOVASCULAR SERIES

Parsons and colleagues[16] recently reported the various endovascular strategies they used in 28 iliac artery aneurysms with different anatomic configurations. All intended endovascular repairs were accomplished. There was one type I endoleak without further growth of the aneurysm sac. The overall 3-yr survival rate was 86%. Four procedure-related complications (12%) occurred in this series, including one distal embolization, two wound infections, and one mild episode of colonic mucosal ischemia.

Sanchez and colleagues[19] reported a series that included pseudoaneurysms as well as atherosclerotic lesions of the iliac artery. Their results were equally satisfactory, with all intended procedures successfully accomplished. Their 4-yr cumulative patency rate was 95%, the complication rate was 8%, and the perioperative mortality rate was 2.5%, which occurred as the result of a ruptured aneurysm. They observed only one endoleak in their entire series. It is noteworthy to mention that the mean isolated iliac artery aneurysm diameter in both studies was >4.0 cm. These authors' conclusions were based on the minimal invasiveness of this relatively safe and efficacious treatment of patients with coexistent medical problems. However, caution was recommended because of the lack of long-term results of endovascular repair of the iliac arteries.

FUTURE APPLICATIONS

Iliac artery dilatations or aneurysms most frequently present in association with AAAs. New generation stent–grafts that are constructed to repair AAAs have iliac artery extensions that are tapered to anchor at moderately dilated iliac arteries (transverse diameters of approximately 24 mm). The Zenith stent–graft (Cook Inc., Bloomington IN) and the Talent stent–graft (World Medical Co., Fort Lauderdale, FL) are two that have these features.

There are also new branched devices that are potentially capable of repairing common iliac artery aneurysms even when the orifice of the internal iliac artery is involved in the sac. However, these devices are currently still experimental and are being tested in animal models only.

REFERENCES

1. Lowry SF, Kraft RO. Isolated aneurysms of the iliac artery. *Arch Surg*. 1978;113:1289–1293.
2. McCready RA, Pairolero PC, Gilmore JC, Kazmier FJ, Cherry KJ, Hollier LH. Isolated iliac artery aneurysms. *Surgery*. 1983;93:688–693.
3. Nachbur BH, Inderbitzi RG, Bar W. Isolated iliac artery aneurysm. *Eur J Vasc Surg*. 1991;5:375–381.
4. Sachs NPM, Huddy SPJ, Wagner T, Geldings AEB. Management of solitary iliac aneurysm. *J Cardiovasc Surg*. 1992;33:679–683.
5. Armon MP, Wenham PW, Whitaker SC, Gregson RHS, Hopkinson BR. Common iliac artery aneurysms in patients with abdominal aortic aneurysms. *Eur J Vasc Endovasc Surg*. 1998;15:255–257.
6. Santilli SM, Wernsing SE, Lee ES. Expansion rates and outcomes for iliac artery aneurysms. *J Vasc Surg*. 2000;31:114–121.
7. Richardson JW, Greenfield LJ. Natural history and management of iliac aneurysms. *J. Vasc Surg*. 1988;8:165–171.
8. Krupski WC, Selzman CH, Floridia R, Strecker PK, Nechler MR, Whitehill TA. Contemporary management of isolated iliac artery aneurysms. *J Vasc Surg*. 1998;28:1–13.
9. Deb B, Benjamin M, Comerota AJ. Delayed rupture of an internal iliac artery aneurysm following proximal ligation for abdominal aortic aneurysm repair. *Ann Vasc Surg*. 1992;6:537–540.
10. Kwaan JHM, Dahl RK. Fatal rupture after successful surgical thrombosed abdominal aortic aneurysm. *Surgery*. 1984;95:235–237.
11. Schanzer H, Papa MC, Miller CM. Rupture of surgically thrombosed abdominal aortic aneurysm. *J Vasc Surg*. 1985;2:278–280.
12. Cho SI, Johnson WC, Bush HL, Widrich WC, Huse JB, Nebseth DC. Lethal complications associated with nonresective treatment of abdominal aortic aneurysms. *Arch Surg*. 1982; 117:1214–1217.

13. Horejs D, Gilbert PM, Bustein S, Vogelzang RL. Normal aortoiliac diameters by CT. *J. Comp Assist Tomogr.* 1988;12:602–603.
14. Pederson OM, Aslaksen A, Vik-Mo H. Ultrasound measurement of luminal diameter of abdominal aorta and iliac arteries in patients without vascular disease. *J Vasc Surg.* 1993;17:596–601.
15. Brunkwall J, Hauksson H, Bengtsson H, Bergquist D, Takolander R, Bergentz SE. Solitary aneurysms of the iliac arterial system: an estimate of their frequency of occurrence. *J Vasc Surg.* 1989;10:381–384.
16. Parsons RE, Marin ML, Veith FJ, Parsons RB, Hollier LH. Midterm results of endovascular stented grafts for the treatment of isolated iliac artery aneurysms. *J Vasc Surg.* 1999;30:915–921.
17. Parodi JC, Ferreira M. Relocation of the iliac artery bifucation to facilitate endoluminal treatment of abdominal aortic aneurysms. *J Endovasc Surg.* 1999;6:342–347.
18. Yano OJ, Morrisey N, Eisen L, et al. Intentional internal iliac artery occlusion to facilitate endovascular repair of aortoiliac aneurysms. *J Vasc Surg.* (in press).
19. Sanchez LA, Patel AV, Ohki T, et al. Midterm experience with endovascular treatment of isolated iliac aneurysms. *J Vasc Surg.* 1999;30:907–914.

19

Endovascular Therapy for Arteriovenous Malformation

Wayne F. Yakes, MD

Vascular malformations constitute some of the most difficult diagnostic and therapeutic enigmas that can be encountered in the practice of medicine. The clinical presentations are extremely protean and can range from an asymptomatic birthmark to fulminating life-threatening congestive heart failure. Attributing any of these extremely varied symptoms that a patient may present with to a vascular malformation can be challenging to even the most experienced clinician. Compounding this problem is the extreme rarity of these lesions. If a clinician sees one patient every several years it is extremely difficult to gain a learning curve to diagnose and to determine how to manage them optimally. Typically, these patients bounce from clinician to clinician, only to experience disappointing outcomes, complications, and recurrence or worsening of their presenting symptoms.

Based on the landmark research of Mulliken et al.,[1–4] a rational classification of pediatric hemangioma and vascular malformations has evolved that should be incorporated into every clinician's modern clinical practice. This classification system, based on endothelial cell characteristics, has removed much of the confusion in terminology present in the literature today. Once all clinicians understand and use this important classification system, ambiguity and confusion will be removed and all clinicians will speak a common language.

Vascular malformations are lesions that present at birth and grow commensurately as the child grows. Trauma, surgery, hormonal influences caused by birth control pills, puberty, and pregnancy may cause the lesion to expand and grow hemodynamically. Vascular malformations at the histologic level demonstrate no endothelial cell proliferation, contain large vascular channels lined by flat endothelium, have a unilamellar basement membrane, do not incorporate tritiated thymidine into endothelial cells, and have normal mast cell counts. They may be formed from any combination of arterial, capillary, venous, or lymphatic elements with or without direct arterial venous shunts.

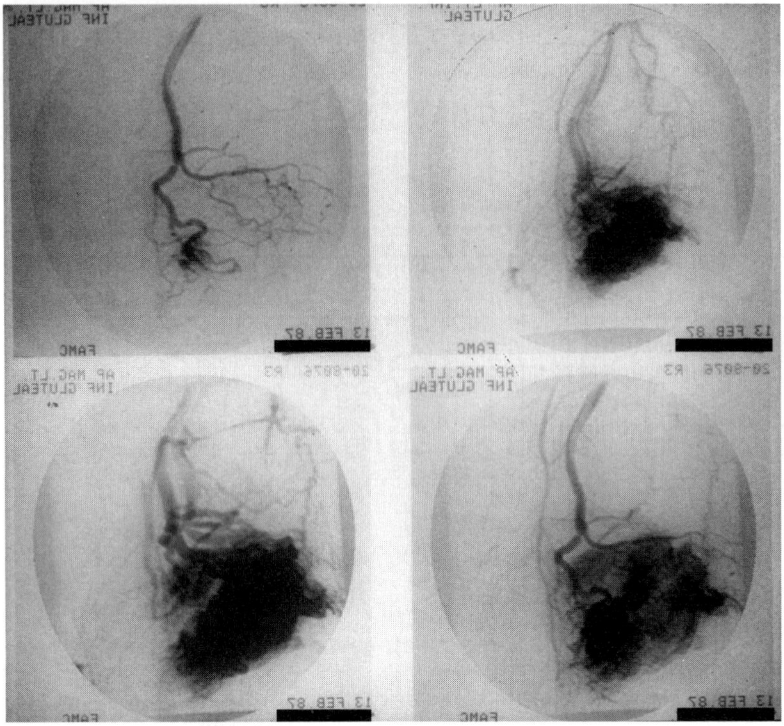

A

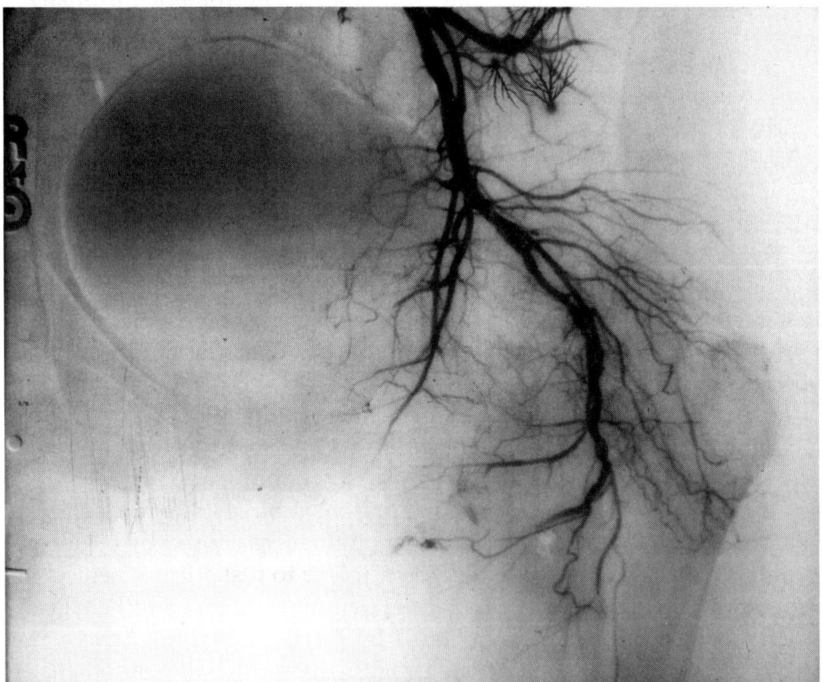

B

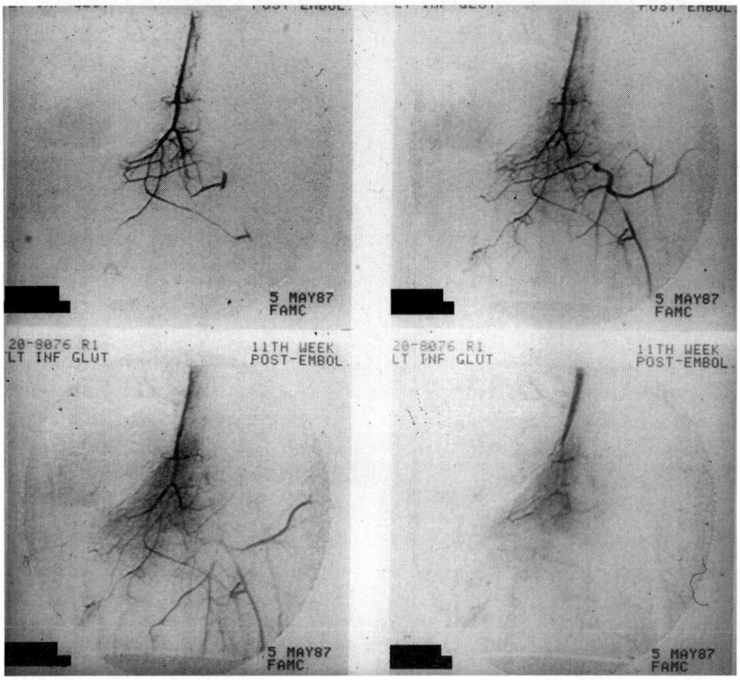

C

Figure 19–1. (**A**) Left internal pudendal arteriogram documenting position for embolization of arteriovenous malformation (AVM) in the left perineum. (**B**) Left internal iliac arteriogram postembolization documenting absence of arteriovenal (AV) shunting and thrombosis of AVM. (**C**) Left internal pudendal arteriogram 11 weeks posttherapy documenting cure of AVM.

Vascular malformations are true structural anomalies resulting from incomplete resorption of primitive blood vessels.

Work-up of a vascular malformation includes a thorough physical examination with history. Appropriate issues are the time of occurrence of the initial symptoms and whether it was present at birth are essential. Were there issues with regard to hormonal influences? Does the patient have a positive Nicoladoni–Branham test (whether reflex bradycardia occurs with an inflow arterial occlusion)? Color Doppler imaging is an essential tool in the work-up of vascular malformations, particularly with high-flow lesions. Color Doppler imaging is also an important noninvasive method for following patients undergoing treatment. Magnetic resonance imaging (MRI) has proved to be invaluable in the initial diagnosis and the follow-up management of patients with vascular malformations in all anatomic locations. It is able to distinguish between high-flow and low-flow lesions. Furthermore, it is able to determine the efficacy of therapy at long-term follow-up.

High-flow lesions include congenital arteriovenous malformations (AVMs), arteriovenous fistula, and acquired vascular lesions; low-flow lesions include venous malformations, lymphatic malformations, capillary venous malformations, and mixed lesions.

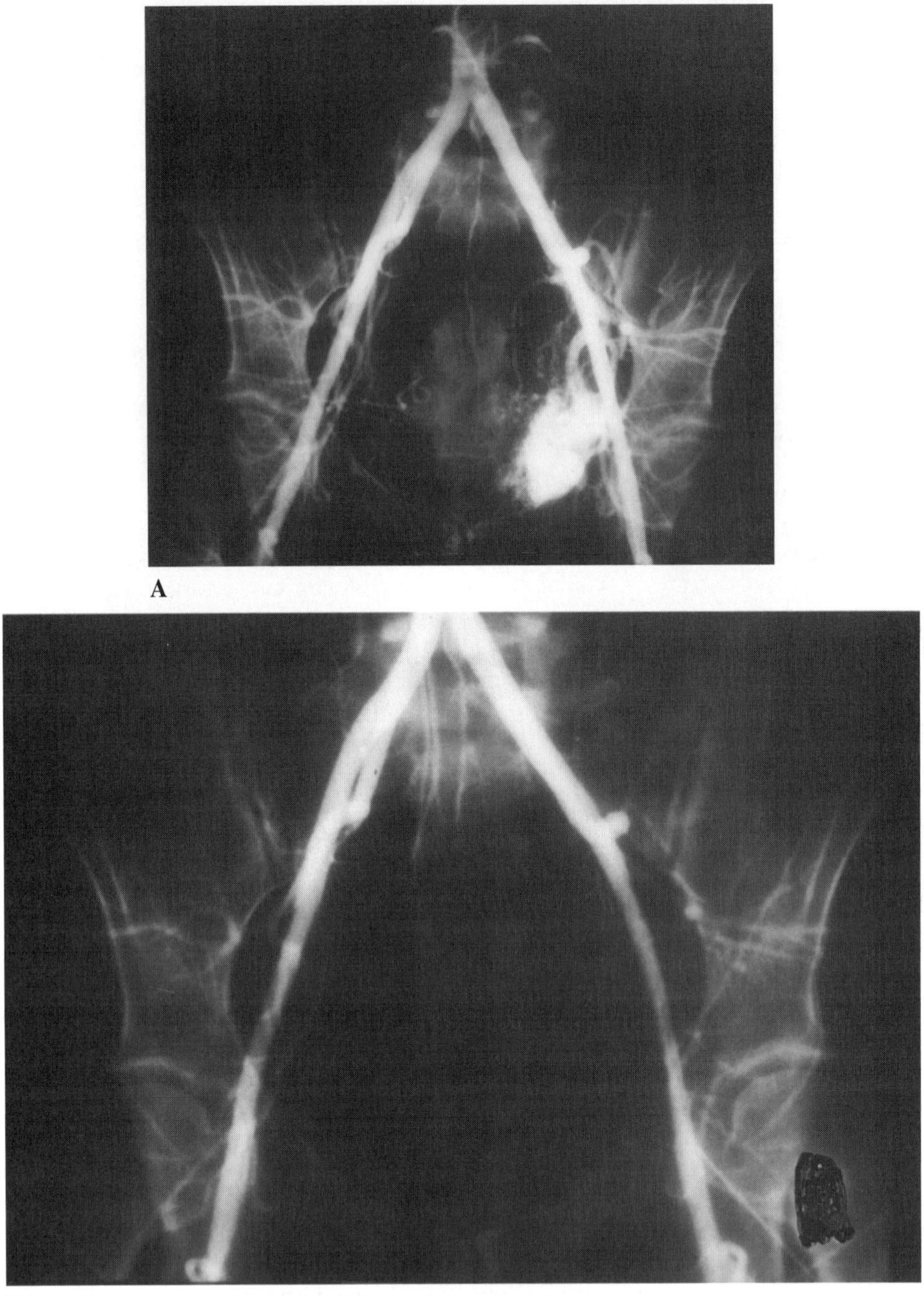

A

B

Figure 19–2. (**A**) Pelvic arteriogram documenting left pelvic arteriovenous malformation. Three months prior to this arteriogram, the anterior division of the left internal iliac artery had been ligated surgically. It must be reinforced that proximal arterial ligation is not only futile, but it also hinders endovascular approaches dramatically. (**B**) AP pelvis arteriogram 3 yr posttherapy documenting permanent cure of AVM. Despite the proximal arterial ligation hindering endovascular approaches, ultimately, success was achieved.

After the diagnosis is established, the next hurdle is to determine whether therapy is warranted. A vascular malformation team should be in place, even though the interventional radiologist does primarily plan and direct patient's care. According to D. Emerick Szilagyi, MD,[5] former editor for the *Journal of Vascular Surgery*,

> . . . with few exceptions, their [vascular malformations] cure by surgical means is impossible. We intuitively thought that the only answer of a surgeon to the problem of disfiguring, often noisome, and occasionally disabling blemishes and masses, prone to cause bleeding, pain, or other unpleasantness, was to attack them with vigor and with the determination of eradicating them. The results of this attempt at radical treatment were disappointing.

Indeed, of 82 patients seen in this patient series, only 18 were even deemed operable, with no therapy offered to the remaining patients. Of the 18 patients operated upon, 10 improved, 2 remained unchanged, and 6 were worse at follow-up. This patient series points to the enormity of the problem posed by vascular malformations. They are best treated in centers where these patients are seen regularly. The interventional radiologist who occasionally evaluates a patient every year or so will have difficulty gaining a significant learning curve or have enough experience to manage these challenging lesions. All too frequently, it is ultimately the patient who pays for the interventional radiologist's initial enthusiasm, inexperience, folly, and lack of necessary clinical back up. For optimal treatment, a vascular malformation team should be in place. Headed by the interventional radiologist, the various surgical and medical specialties function together much like a tumor board team of specialists. When patients are seen and treated regularly, then experience can be gained, rational decisions can be made, and patient care is optimized. It cannot be emphasized enough that, as a group, vascular malformations pose one of the most difficult challenges in the practice of medicine. A cavalier approach always leads to significant complications and dismal patient outcomes.

In our treatment of more than 400 patients, the vast majority of our patients undergo general anesthesia. In addition, in selected cases, additional Swan–Ganz line monitoring and arterial line may be necessary. Pulmonary artery pressures are constantly monitored during the injection of absolute ethanol. During a procedure, we rarely treat patients with >0.5 mL/kg body weight total dose. Depending on how to access the nidus of the high-flow or low-flow lesion determines if transvascular approaches or direct percutaneous puncture approaches is used.

In our practice, patients are treated with 98% ethyl alcohol as the embolic agent. This is our preferred agent of choice. As has been published by several authors, the use of Ethibloc, glue, coils, PVA, and so on is "palliative at best."[6] In fact, many authors have reported not only an incomplete treatment, but also recanalization at follow-up.[6–9]

Our approach is to treat AVMs in a curative fashion, not a palliative fashion. The main reason recanalizations and neovascular recruitment phenomenon occur in AVM management is that all embolic agents do not completely destroy the endothelial cells of the AVM. Only sclerosants, in particular the sclerosant ethanol, does it the best. The endothelial cell, when it is intact during thrombosis, senses decreased oxygen tension and sends out an angiogenesis factor that stimulates neovascular formation. Furthermore, it sends out chemotactic factors that cause a cellular infiltration to carry debris from the thrombosed vascular channels. Once this occurs, the endothelial cell reendothelializes and recanalization occurs. With the use of ethanol, the endothelial cell is denuded from the vascular wall, its protoplasm is precipitated, and there is a fracture in the vascular wall to the level of the internal elastic lamina. Because of this destruction of the endothelial cell, the permanence encountered by ethanol in treating vascular malformations is almost routine.[10–23] In more than 400 patients, we have been able to cure peripheral AVMs at long-term follow-up in excess of 2 yr and >80% of the time. In arteriovenous fistulae that are congenital and not traumatic, the cure rate at the same mean follow-up is 100%. We are able to cure approximately 90% of acquired arteriovenous fistula at 2-yr mean follow-up. The low-flow lesions also demonstrate permanent occlusion at long-term follow-up. In the world's published literature the cure rate for brain AVM with endovascular approaches is <5%, and of those that are cured, it is almost always in the Spetzler–Martin grading scale of 1–2. The higher-grade lesions, grades 3–5, are almost never cured by endovascular means and require additional radiosurgery or surgical extraction to achieve cure. In the series of Frizzel and Frazier,[24] who did a review of the years from 1960 to 1996 of all embolization papers published concerning brain AVM, a cure rate of 5% was noted. In our first paper using ethanol as the embolic agent to treat brain AVM, our cure rate was 47%.[25] Currently, our rate is >60% in patients with brain AVM grades 3, 4, and 5.

Thus we conclude that at long-term follow-up, cure of vascular malformations is a distinct possibility. Acceptable complication rates can occur with the use of ethanol. Patients are best treated in centers that manage these patients regularly. In the endovascular management of vascular malformations, ethanol demonstrates a level of permanence that is seldom encountered by other agents.

REFERENCES

1. Mulliken JB, Glowacki J. Hemangiomas and vascular malformations in infants and children: a classification based on endothelial characteristics. *Plast Reconstr Surg.* 1982;69:412–420.
2. Mulliken JB, Zetter BR, Folkman J. *In vitro* characteristics of endothelium from hemangiomas and vascular malformations. *Surgery.* 1982;92:348–353.
3. Glowacki J, Mulliken JB. Mast cells in hemangiomas and vascular malformations. *Pediatrics.* 1982;70:48–51.
4. Finn MC, Glowacki J, Mulliken JB. Congenital vascular lesions: clinical application of a new classification. *J Pediatr Surg.* 1983;18:894–900.
5. Szilagyi DE, Smith RF, Elliott JP, Hageman JH. Congenital arteriovenous anomalies of the limbs. *Arch Surg.* 1976;111:423–429.
6. Widlus DM, Murray RR, White RI Jr., et al. Congenital arteriovenous malformations: tailored embolotherapy. *Radiology.* 1988;169:511–516.
7. Rao VRK, Mandalan KR, Gupta AK, et al. Dissolution of isobutyl 2-cyanoacrylate on long-term follow-up. *AJNR.* 1989;10:135–141.
8. Vinter HV, Lundie MJ, Kaufmann JCE. Long-term pathological follow-up of cerebral arteriovenous malformations treated by embolizations with bucrylate. *N Engl J Med.* 1986;314:477–483.
9. Brothers MF, Kaufmann JCE, Fox AJ, Deveikis JP. *N*-butyl-2-cyanoacrylate substitute for IBCA in interventional radiology: histopathologic and polymerization times studies. *AJR.* 1988;10:777–786.

10. Takebayaski S, Hosaka M, et al. Arteriovenous malformations of the kidneys: ablation with alcohol. *AJR*. 1988;150:587–590.
11. Vinson AM, Rohrer DB, Willcox CW, et al. Absolute ethanol embolization for peripheral arteriovenous malformation: report of two cures. *South Med J*. 1988;1:1052–1055.
12. Yakes WF, Pevsner PH, Reed MD, Donohue HJ, Ghaed M. Serial embolizations of an extremity arteriovenous malformation with alcohol via direct percutaneous puncture. *AJR*. 1986; 146:1038–1040.
13. Yakes WF, Haas DK, Parker SH, et al. Symptomatic vascular malformations: ethanol embolotherapy. *Radiology*. 1989;170:1059–1066.
14. Rak KM, Yakes WF, Ray RL, et al. MR imaging of symptomatic peripheral vascular malformations. *AJR*. 1992;159:107–112.
15. Yakes WF, Parker SH, Gibson MD, et al. Alcohol embolotherapy of vascular malformations. *Semin Intervent Radiol*. 1989;6:146–161.
16. Yakes WF, Luethke JM, Parker SH, et al. Ethanol embolization of vascular malformations. *RadioGraphics*. 1990;10:787–796.
17. Yakes WF, Luethke JM, Merland JJ, et al. Ethanol embolization of arteriovenous fistulas: a primary mode of therapy. *JVIR*. 1990;1:89–96.
18. Yakes WF, Rossi P, Odink H. How I do it: arteriovenous malformation management: *CVIR*. 1996;19:65–71.
19. Yakes WF. Discussion of sclerotherapy of head and neck venous malformations. *Plast Reconstr Surg*. 1999;104:12–15.
20. Berenguer B, Burrows PE, Zurakowski D, Mulliken JB. Sclerotherapy of craniofacial venous malformations: complications and results. *Plast Reconstr Surg*. 1999;104:1–11.
21. Berthelsen B, Fogdestam I, Svendsen P. Venous malformation in the face and neck: radiologic diagnosis and treatment with absolute ethanol. *Acta Radiol Diag (Stockh.)*. 1986;27:149–155.
22. Svendsen P, Wikholm G, et al. Installation of alcohol into venous malformations of the head and neck. *Scand J Plast Reconstr Surg Hand Surg*. 1994;28:279–283.
23. Mourao GS, Hodes JE, Gobin YP, Casasco A, Aymard A, Merland JJ. Curative treatment of scalp arteriovenous fistulas by direct puncture and embolization with absolute alcohol. *J Neurosurg*. 1991;75:634–637.
24. Frizzel RT, Fisher WS. Cure, morbidity, and mortality associated with embolization of brain AVMs: a review of 1246 in 32 series over a 35-year period. *Neurosurgery*. 1995;37:1031–1040.
25. Yakes, WF, Krauth L, Ecklund J, et al. Ethanol endovascular management of brain AVMs; initial results. *Neurosurgery*. 1997;40:1145–1154

20

Renal Artery Angioplasty and Stenting

Srinivas Tummala, MD, Chet Rees, MD, and Gary J. Becker, MD, FSCVIR, FACR, FACC

The prevalence of atherosclerotic renovascular disease (ASRVD) is increasing as the demographics shift progressively toward a more elderly population. This increase as well as the extensive accumulation of knowledge and experience in revascularization techniques has led to increased use and broadening of the role of percutaneous revascularization. The following is an update and expansion of a comprehensive review on renal revascularization published by one of the present authors, CR Rees, in the *Journal of Vascular & Interventional Radiology* in 1999.[1] This update provides additional published data, new illustrative case material, some new discussion, and very similar conclusions.

In general, ASRVD and renovascular hypertension must be distinguished. ASRVD refers to atherosclerotic changes in the renal vasculature with or without coexistent hypertension. Because essential hypertension is extremely prevalent in the overall population, the coexistence of renal artery stenosis and hypertension in the same patient does not necessarily imply a cause and effect relationship. For example, in a series of 295 autopsies, 81% of the patients with moderate to severe renal artery stenosis were normotensive during their lifetime, whereas 77% of the hypertensive patients and 49% of the normotensive patients had renal artery stenosis.[2] In another series of 821 angiograms performed for numerous indications, all of which included visualization of the renal arteries, 50% of the patients had renal artery stenosis. Of these patients, 62% were hypertensive and 38% were normotensive.[3] Renovascular hypertension, however, implies a cause-and-effect relationship between the renal artery stenosis and hypertension. Although the majority of renal artery lesions receiving therapy are atherosclerotic in nature, fibromuscular disease is an important etiology of renovascular hypertension (Figures 20–1 and 20–2). Fibromuscular disease causes hypertension in a younger and healthier overall group of patients than ASRVD. These patients are much less likely to

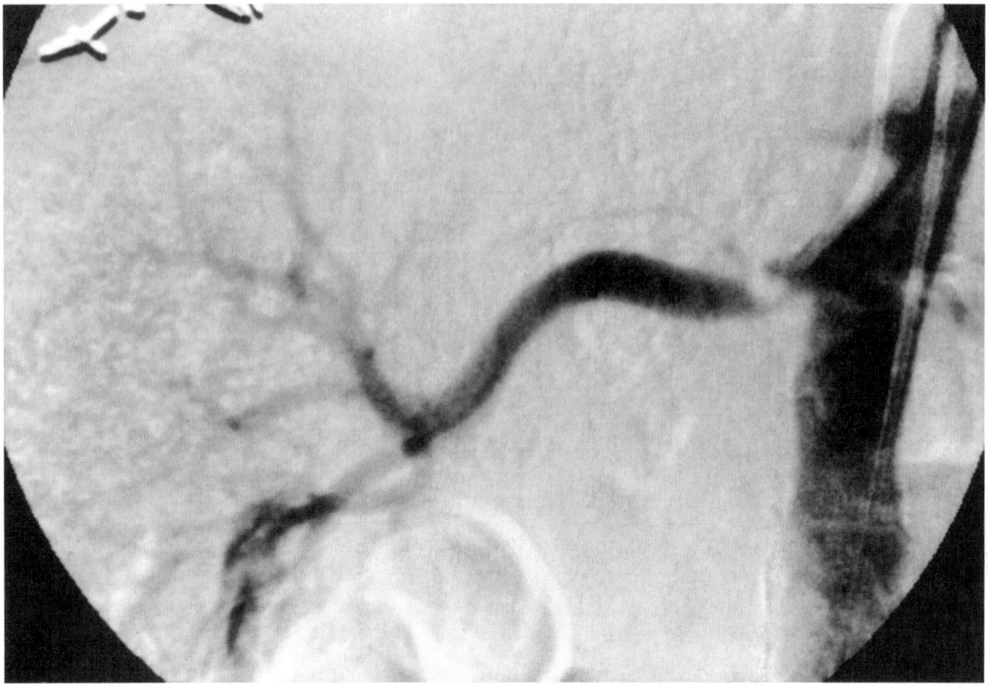

Figure 20–1. Eccentric atherosclerotic renal artery stenosis.

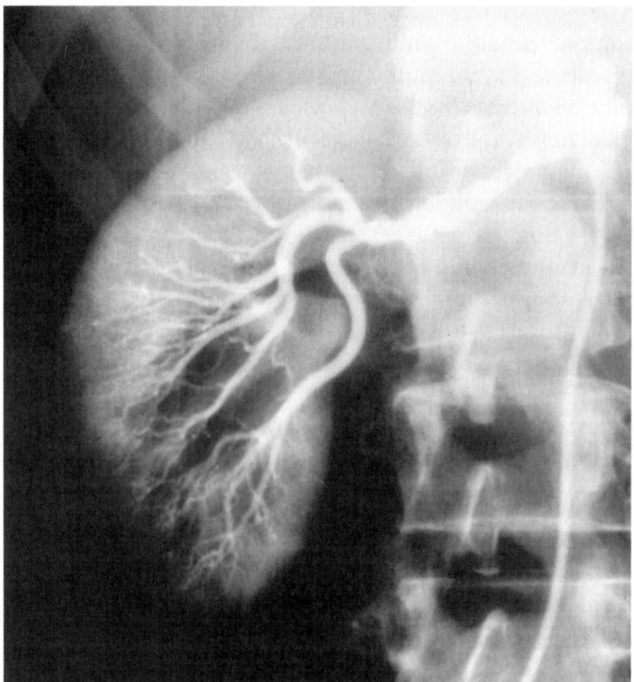

Figure 20–2. Fibromuscular renovascular disease.

develop renal failure as a result of their stenosis and are more apt to respond beneficially to percutaneous transluminal renal angioplasty (pTRA). Numerous studies have shown very high success rates, with cure of hypertension in 41% of patients and significant improvement of hypertension or cure in 87% of patients with fibromuscular disease.[4–16]

Other rare causes of hypertension that are not related to renal artery stenosis include pheochromocytoma and aldosteronoma, which should be ruled out before any form of revascularization is undertaken.

NATURAL HISTORY OF ATHEROSCLEROTIC RENOVASCULAR DISEASE

Unfortunately, patients with ASRVD have relatively poor survival as demonstrated by Scobel et al.[17] In this study, 60 patients were followed and divided into "intervention" and "nonintervention" groups. Without intervention, 3-yr survival was only 56%. With intervention (angioplasty or surgery), 3-yr survival was 78%. Although this study does not provide an adequate comparison of intervention and nonintervention groups because it was not randomized or controlled, it does clearly underscore the relatively dismal fate of this population when treated with medical management alone. Their poor survival stems not only from the direct and indirect effects of the renal artery stenosis but is also related to their elderly status, the coexistence of atherosclerotic disease in the coronary and cerebral vasculature, and the coexistence of malignancy.

The morphologic natural history of ASRVD was best described by Schreiber et al.[18] in 1984. In their study, serial angiography performed in 85 patients with ASRVD showed progression of stenosis in 44% of cases over a 5-yr timespan. Of these patients, 46% had progression of disease within the first 2 yr of angiographic follow-up. Furthermore, progression to occlusion occurred in 16% of patients, and high-grade lesions progressed to occlusion in 39% of cases over 2–3 yr. This progression of stenosis was noted to correlate with deterioration in kidney size and renal function as determined by serum creatinine levels. Interestingly, these findings contrast sharply with fibromuscular disease of the renal vasculature. In these patients, 0 of 66 cases progressed to occlusion, and only very minimal elevation in serum creatinine levels was noted. In another study by Dean et al.,[19] 41 patients treated with medical therapy alone had angiographic progression to occlusion in 12% of 35 patients at 6 and 12 mo. In this group, 41% also had a >25% fall in their glomerular filtration rate despite good blood pressure control. These studies indicate the strong need for effective revascularization in patients with atherosclerotic renovascular disease. In contrast, a study by Leertouwer et al.[40] demonstrated that over an 8- to 10-yr follow-up period, patients with incidental renal artery stenosis, discovered during angiographic evaluation for ischemic peripheral vascular disease, did not develop end-stage renal failure.[4] In this study, 126 patients had incidental renal artery stenoses, whereas the control group consisted of 126 randomly selected patients (matched for age and gender) without renal artery stenoses. Renal artery stenosis was unilateral in 88 patients and bilateral in 32 patients. In addition, 6 patients had a single functioning kidney, and on average the cohort of patients evaluated had a lower Cockroft serum creatinine clearance than the control group. Five patients returned with symptomatic renal artery stenosis requiring revascularization, and one patient in the control group progressed to end-stage renal failure necessitating hemodialysis. A more recent study reported by Van Jaarsveld et al.[41] in the *New England Journal of Medicine* came to the conclusion that angioplasty had little advantage over anti-hypertensive drug therapy in patients with hypertension and atherosclerotic renal artery stenosis.[4] This study, however, had several shortcomings. First, the study was not really a "long-term" evaluation, as renal function was only assessed for 12 mo. Second, approximately 50% of the patients who were assigned to receive anti-hypertensive drug therapy alone eventually underwent renal artery angioplasty. Third, renal artery stent placement, which more accurately reflects modern practice in ASRVD, was not evaluated. Although this study evaluated a large number of patients, its weaknesses prevent it from being conclusive. Unfortunately, a good randomized prospective trial comparing medically treated patients with patients treated percutaneously or surgically still has not been completed. As a result, the indications for renal revascularization should be based on the improvements in blood pressure control and renal function that have been achieved in numerous other studies.

RENAL FAILURE

Renal failure is a condition being treated increasingly by renal revascularization. This is due to the recognition of the high prevalence of renovascular disease in the elderly renal failure population as well as the documented benefit that may be achieved in many patients with percutaneous and surgical techniques. Renal failure is usually multifactorial and rarely due to the hemodynamic effect of the stenoses alone. Kidneys without parenchymal disease have considerable reserve and provide adequate function even in the presence of relatively severe renovascular disease. In the great majority of patients with renal failure, the current hemodynamic condition is only one factor, complicated by loss of renal mass due to other entities such as benign nephrosclerosis from long-standing hypertension, diabetic nephropathy, or ischemic nephropathy. Nevertheless, revascularization may improve or stabilize renal function and may have an important effect on the quality and even the duration of life.

An understanding of the natural history of renal failure is required by any individual who treats renovascular disease. In their textbook, Maroni and Mitch[20] stated, "Patients with established renal failure rarely recover. They continue to lose renal function even when the disease process that initially damaged the kidneys is no longer active. The rate of loss of renal function with time is constant in the majority of patients although the rate of decline can vary widely between individuals with the same disease." When the inverse of serum creatinine is plotted over time, a straight line function is usually observed. Thus, any intervention that reduces the slope of this curve has had a favorable impact on the natural history of renal failure. Recognition of this concept has led to the widespread acceptance of "stabilization" as an indicator of success in the management of renal failure. Thus the results of revascularization for renal failure described as follows are listed in terms of (1) *improvement,* which implies a lower value of serum creatinine on long-term follow-up relative to preintervention; or

TABLE 20–1. EFFECT OF pTRA ON RENAL FAILURE IN 431 PATIENTS

Researchers	*N*	Improved (%)	Stable (%)
Giroux et al.[43]	?	38	34
Tykarski[47]	16	69	—
Weibull et al.[23]	37	50	39
Pickering[48]	55	47	—
Pattison[49]	60	45	45
Martin et al.[11]	79	43	—
Madias[50]	11	42	25
O'Donavan[51]	17	41	24
Bell et al.[8]	20	30	59
Lossino et al.[46]	60	27	67
Luft[52]	12	25	33
Martinez-Amenos et al.[15]	24	21	—
Pattnama[53]	40	—	—
Mean		**40**	**42**

Reprinted with permission from Rees CR. Stents for atherosclerotic renovascular disease. *JVIR* 1999;10:689–705.

(2) *stabilization,* which refers to a lack of significant decline in renal function at follow-up, with serum creatinine levels within 15%–20% relative to preintervention values.

The results of pTRA and stent placement on renal failure are shown in Tables 20–1 and 20–2. The results of renal stenting on renal failure are illustrated in an excellent manner by Harden et al.[21] They graphically plotted the reciprocal of serum creatinine over time before and after renal stent placement. The slope values corresponding to preintervention and postintervention were compared. An upward change in slope value clearly indicates beneficial impact on the natural history of the disease in 18 of 32 patients. The effect was most favorable in patients with mild renal failure, with prestent serum creatinine values of <400 micromoles/L (4.5 mg/dL) where 17 of 19 patients (89%) had a favorable decline in rate of progression. Five patients showed acceleration of progression of renal failure after stent insertion. An explanation for progression of deterioration in some patients was not provided. It is possible that this acceleration was

TABLE 20–2. EFFECT OF STENTS ON RENAL FAILURE IN 241 PATIENTS

Researchers	*N*	Improved (%)	Stable (%)
Giroux et al.[43]	?	38	35
Leertouwer[42]	26	35	—
US Multicenter Trial[24]	124	37	37
Dorros et al.[27]	30	28	28
Boisclair[54]	17	41	35
Harden et al.[21]	32	34	34
Hennequin 1994[55]	6	17	50
Joffre et al.[28]	6	50	33
Mean		**35**	**35**

Reprinted with permission from Rees CR. Stents for atherosclerotic renovascular disease. *JVIR* 1999;10:689–705.

not related to the intervention; however, the possibility of injury to the kidneys by cholesterol embolization must be considered. Another important finding of this study was the poor survival of these patients; approximately 40% at 2 yr, with death due to ischemic heart disease, peripheral arterial disease, cerebrovascular disease, colon carcinoma, bleeding, and uremia (in decreasing order of frequency). Such poor survival has also been demonstrated in the natural history of similar populations. Relatively few reports of renal revascularization for atherosclerotic disease report survival, and at this point demonstration of an improved survival has not been made definitively.

None of these studies are comparative between pTRA and renal stents. In addition, comparison is fraught with the same problems as described previously for hypertension. Percutaneous transluminal renal angioplasty has been very effective in the treatment of renal failure in a large proportion of patients, and the use of stents in patients who technically have failed angioplasty has also shown very good results. Thus it appears that stents have provided a great benefit in patients with technical failures of angioplasty who would have been expected to experience a low likelihood of improvement of renal function.

APPROACHES TO THE ATHEROSCLEROTIC LESION

The approach to an atherosclerotic renovascular lesion (Figure 20–1) depends on one's knowledge of indications and results of angioplasty and stents as well as vascular surgical repair. Many issues are still controversial due to the lack of conclusive studies that provide the information necessary for optimum treatment in each patient. The approach also depends on the skills and attitudes of the physicians caring for the patient, including the medical doctor, the interventionalist, and the surgeon. What follows is an attempt to consider all factors and construct a rational approach using the current state of experience and knowledge.

For the purpose of this discussion, it is assumed that the patient is already known to have a hemodynamically significant atherosclerotic renal artery stenosis as determined by intra-arterial angiography. Hemodynamic significance implies a stenosis causing ≤50% diameter reduction relative to the normal reference vessel diameter and a significant pressure gradient across the lesion. Most operators do not measure pressure gradients routinely when a severe lesion is present on the angiogram; however, in the presence of a borderline stenosis, such as a stenosis in the 50% range, pressure gradients can be very useful for determination of lesion significance. At this point, careful consideration of the medical indications for revascularization must be considered. Renal artery lesions are often diagnosed incidentally during catheterizations for other reasons, sometimes leading to a tendency to perform an intervention "on the way out," even in the absence of a clear-cut medical indication. Avoiding this tendency can prevent the occurrence of rare but catastrophic complications such as cholesterol embolization, reduce cost, and restore the balance of the risk–benefit ratio.

Poorly controlled hypertension is the most common indication for revascularization. This includes patients who are not responding to their antihypertensive medication regimen despite careful implementation, patients whose blood pressures cannot be maintained within a normal range on the medication regimens that have been tried, and patients whose medication regimens are difficult to adjust due to extreme lability of their blood pressure. Also in this group are patients who suffer deterioration in renal function on administration of antihypertensive medication (e.g., a patient with bilateral renal artery stenosis who requires ACE inhibitors to control hypertension, with a resultant decline in renal function).

Patients with abnormal renal function determined by serum creatinine level or other means are candidates for revascularization in order to improve or prevent the relentless decline in renal function.

Other less common indications that have been described in the recent literature include episodic flash pulmonary edema, congestive heart failure, and unstable angina. Preliminary small reports have demonstrated that these entities may be ameliorated by correction of significant renovascular disease.

In the absence of the previously mentioned medical indications, revascularization is recommended if the stenosis is severe and therefore considered to be preocclusive in its nature. This is especially true in the presence of a solitary kidney or when very severe lesions are present bilaterally. The results of progression to complete occlusion are unpredictable. Some patients rapidly lose a substantial amount of renal mass, whereas others may sustain renal mass, which on revascularization with surgical bypass can result in recovery of renal function and improvement in hypertension.

Once it has been determined that revascularization is indicated due to the presence of a hemodynamically significant lesion and strong medical indications, then the decision between percutaneous and surgical techniques must be made. This decision requires careful consideration of surgical risk factors and discussion among medical physicians, interventionalists, and surgeons. Most atherosclerotic renovascular lesions are relatively focal in nature and are therefore amenable to angioplasty or stent placement. Unusually long lesions are often treated surgically. Completely occluded renal arteries may be successfully recanalized percutaneously in some cases, however, bypass surgery is usually recommended. In patients about to undergo vascular surgery for other problems (e.g., treatment of abdominal aortic aneurysm, renovascular disease) may be best corrected simultaneously. However, the morbidity and mortality of aortic surgery are thereby increased. Some patients with very difficult to control hypertension may be better treated by percutaneous renal revascularization prior to or following surgery. Although the presence of risk factors usually weighs in favor of percutaneous treatment, some risks may favor surgery. At some institutions, solitary kidneys are revascularized surgically to reduce the risk of kidney loss. Other institutions with experienced interventionalists may elect to treat such patients percutaneously. Very severe, widespread, diffuse atherosclerotic disease in the aorta and other access vessels may place the patient at undue risk for cholesterol embolization during percutaneous treatment. Some of these patients may be better served with surgery.

In a prospective randomized trial of pTRA vs surgery, the results supported the use of pTRA as the primary treatment for atherosclerotic lesions $\leq$1 cm from the aorta, with surgery for failed pTRA or second restenosis after repeat pTRA.[22] This algorithm may be further modified by the use of stents for pTRA failures. This study is particularly valuable because, to our knowledge, it represents the only randomized prospective comparison of pTRA to surgery. In this study, 58 patients with 58 stenoses were randomized between pTRA and surgery. In the 29 patients undergoing pTRA, technical success was achieved in 24 (83%), and restenosis occurred in 6 lesions. Of the 6 restenoses, 5 had long-term patency after repeat pTRA and did not require surgery, and 1 patient experienced a second restenosis that required surgery. Lesions were followed carefully over 2 yr with serial angiography. The secondary patency rate was 90%. Thus, surgery was required in 6 patients: in 5 patients due to immediate technical failure, and only in 1 patient due to restenosis. The surgical group had only one failure initially due to thrombosis, and two pTRA procedures were required to maintain a secondary long-term patency of 97%. Thus, long-term secondary patencies between the two groups were roughly similar, and in the pTRA group, 23 of 29 patients were spared surgery. The authors concluded that ostial atherosclerotic lesions should be treated first with angioplasty, restenosis lesions should be treated with repeat angioplasty, and surgery should be reserved for initial technical failure or second restenosis. Although a similar study with stents would be very useful, it may never be performed due to the complexity of randomizing between percutaneous intervention and surgery. It would, however, be expected that the 5 technical failures of angioplasty in that study could have been treated effectively with stent placement, thus significantly reducing the need for surgery even in that group of more refractory patients because surgery for second restenosis was very uncommon.

Once percutaneous treatment has been selected, the most common treatment algorithm involves the performance of pTRA, with the addition of a stent in the event of technical failure, which is usually defined as elastic recoil or dissection with significant luminal compromise, or a transstenotic mean pressure gradient of >5 mmHg (Figure 20–3). The definition of an angiographically significant stenosis is variable. Classically, a 50% residual stenosis is considered significant; however, the more widespread use of vascular stents in recent years has resulted in a lowering of the threshold to the approximate level of 30% diameter reduction stenosis. Although pressure gradients are helpful in determining the severity of a lesion, their correlation with eventual outcome is poorly established in the literature.

APPROACH TO POST-pTRA RESTENOSIS

The approach to post-pTRA restenosis lesions is not well established. Restenosis of lesions treated with pTRA is often managed effectively by repeat angioplasty with excellent secondary patency rates as demonstrated by Weibull et al.[23] and other studies (see Approach to Atherosclerotic Lesion). In this study, 5 of 6 restenosis lesions had long-term angiographic patency after repeat pTRA (Figure 20–4).

In the United States Multicenter Trial, the long-term patency and clinical results of stent placement for post-pTRA restenosis were equivalent to the results for stenting of *de novo* lesions. Many operators deploy stents in post-pTRA restenosis lesions with the presumption that long-term patency will likely be superior to a technically successful angioplasty of the restenosis lesion. This hypothesis is unproved at present. However, it is compelling because of the tendency for the patient and interventionalist to want to proceed to a new treatment after the first-line treatment has failed. At some institutions, surgery is performed after restenosis of pTRA or restenosis after stenting. Surgery has a very high long-term patency rate, and when performed by an experienced surgeon, it eliminates the need for further intervention in the great majority of patients. A good study of the most effective management of restenosis lesions will be quite difficult to obtain due to the difficulty in accruing a large number of such patients and the long duration of study that would be necessary. At our institution, restenosis lesions are usually treated with either a stent or surgery, depending on patient risk factors and preferences, and also depending on the evaluations of the referring physician, interventionalist, and surgeon.

RATIONALE FOR THE USE OF STENTS FOR ATHEROSCLEROTIC DISEASE OF THE RENAL ARTERIES

The rationale for the use of stents stems from the inconsistent results that are achieved with conventional pTRA for atherosclerotic renovascular lesions. Immediate technical results vary widely, as shown in Table 20–3. This is attributable to numerous factors, including different types of patient populations with differing risk factors, different techniques, as well as advances in patient selection and technique that have occurred over time. Perhaps most importantly, definitions of technical success as well as methodology of reporting results vary widely and oftentimes are poorly described in studies. Nevertheless, it is clear on review of the literature and to any experienced operator that although the overall results of angioplasty for renovascular lesions are good, they are not reliable, and there is a definite need for improvement of the initial technical results and maintenance of long-term patency. At this time, renal stents have represented the only advancement in this area that have proved helpful and gained widespread acceptance. As described later in this chapter, rates for technically successful renal artery stent placement are consistently reported in the 98%–100% range for atherosclerotic lesions (including ostial lesions) even by the strictest reporting standards.

The technical goal of percutaneous revascularization is long-term patency, which is a function of the rates of initial technical success and restenosis. Long-term patency rate = (initial technical success rate) (1-restenosis rate). As described later, the rate of restenosis with renal stents appears to be slightly lower than that for pTRA. This improvement may be due to advances in patient selection and technical considerations. Therefore, stents provide markedly superior initial technical success rates relative to pTRA, and may provide an additional benefit with regard to restenosis. Currently, treatment of technical failures of pTRA with stents is clearly indicated (Figure 20–5). Treatment of lesions after technically successful angioplasty, with the intention of reducing the risk of restenosis is more controversial. Similarly, primary stenting of ostial lesions is based on the premise that overall results must be superior to those of pTRA. This is as yet unproved but deserves strong consideration owing to the inconsistent results of pTRA for such lesions. A randomized comparison of primary stenting vs pTRA

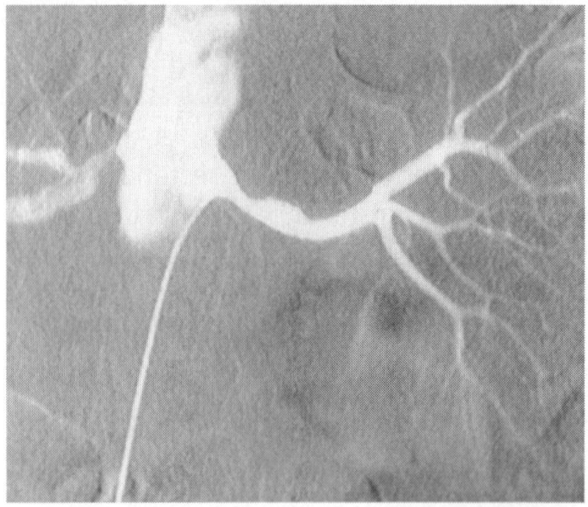

A

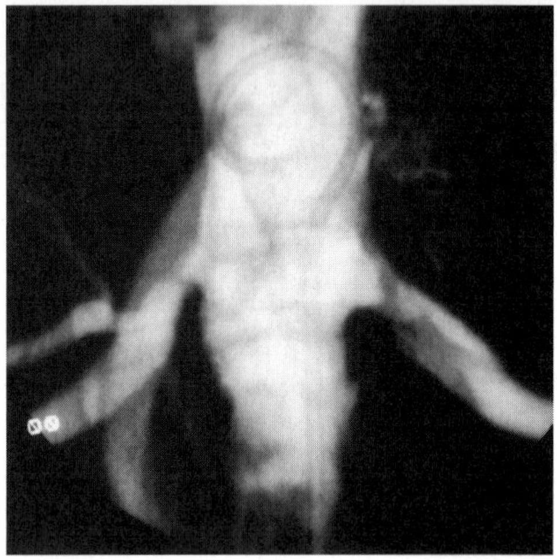

B

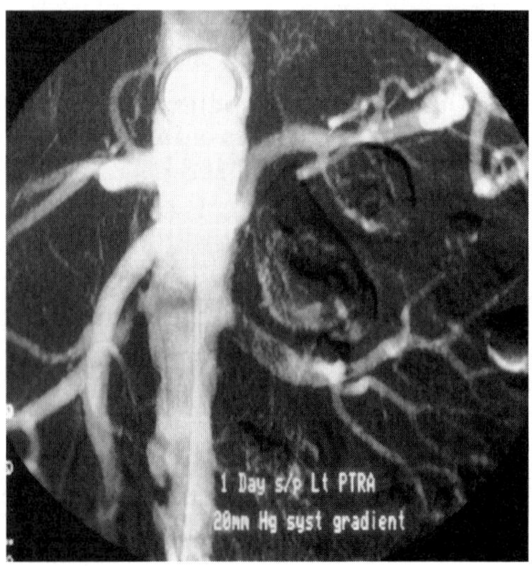

C

Figure 20–3. **(A)** Left atherosclerotic renal artery stenosis. **(B)** Post-pTRA dissection was nonflow limiting with a mean pressure gradient of 4 mmHg. Therefore, no further intervention was performed. **(C)** The following day, the dissection had worsened, resulting in a flow-limiting lesion with a mean pressure gradient of 20 mmHg. **(D,E)** After stent placement, no residual pressure gradient remained.

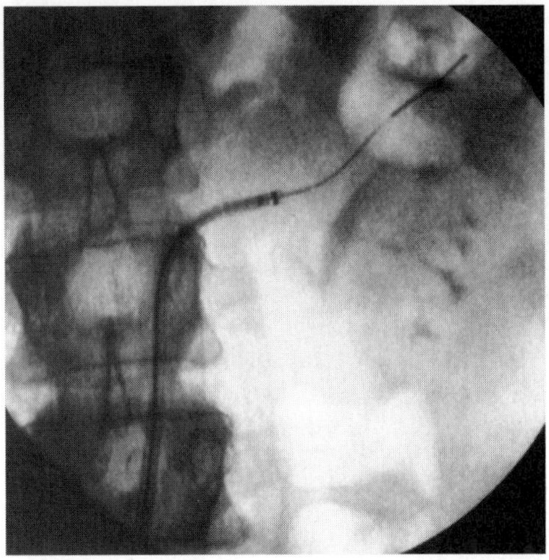

D

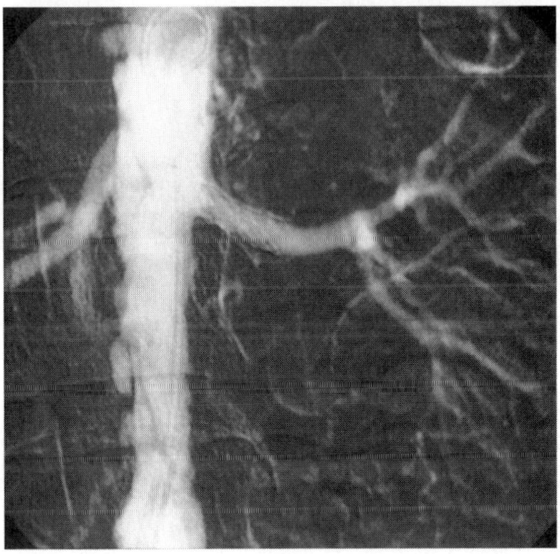

E

Figure 20–3. *(Continued)*

for ostial lesions is in early stages and may provide useful information; however, justification for primary stenting of all ostial lesions would require not only demonstration of its superiority in such a trial, but also in a trial that compares primary stenting to selective stenting of pTRA failures, similar in design to a study for iliac stenoses described by Tetteroo et al.[25] This study showed equivalence of long-term patencies and clinical outcomes for primary iliac stenting vs selective stenting of PTA failures, with significantly lower costs for the latter. Such an outcome could also possibly occur for renal stents. In the absence of such information, consideration of the results of angioplasty

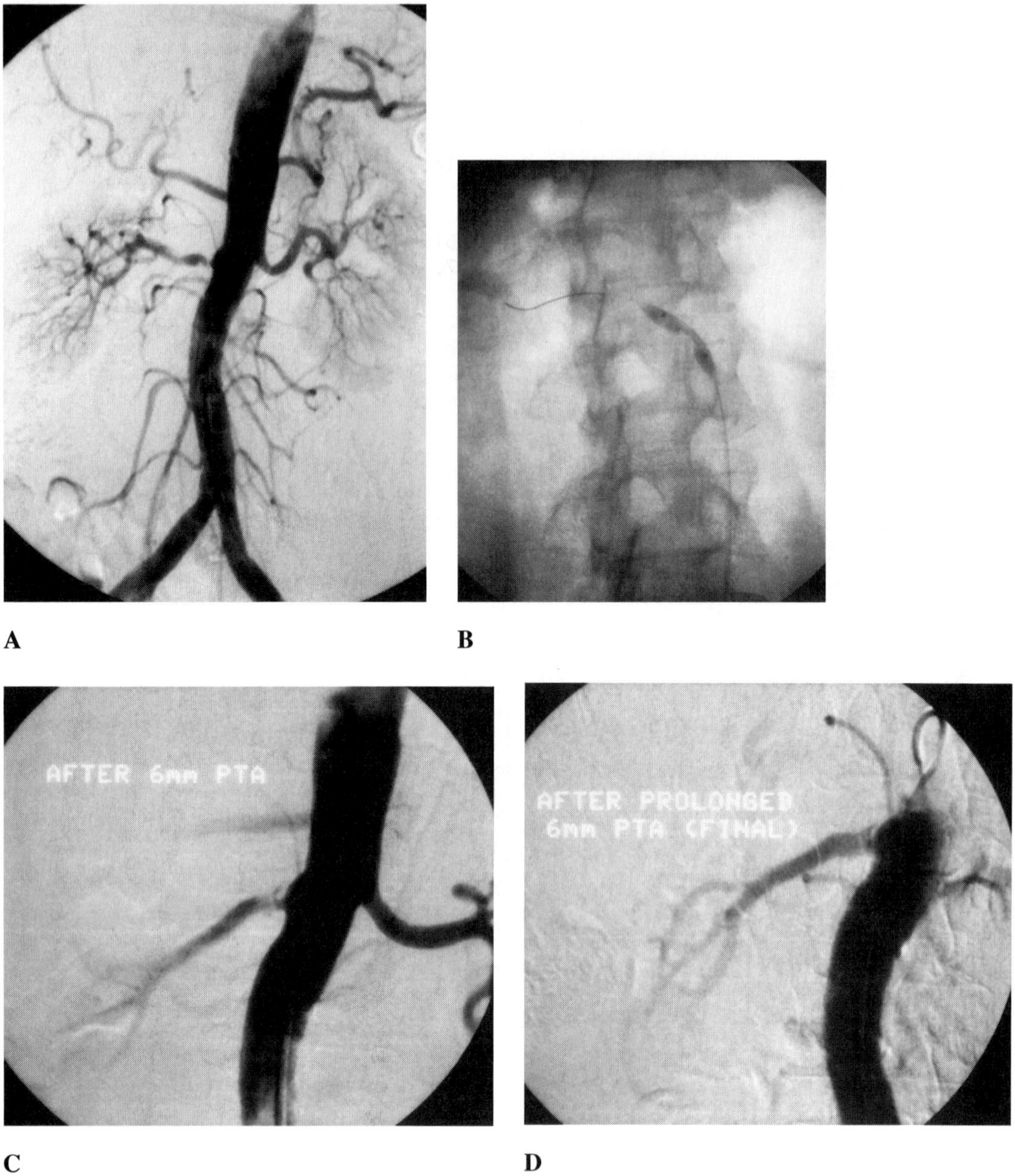

Figure 20–4. (A) Right ostial atherosclerotic renal artery stenosis. **(B)** 6 mm pTRA was performed. **(C)** 60% residual stenosis postangioplasty. **(D)** Repeat prolonged 6 mm pTRA was performed, resulting in an excellent angiographic result.

TABLE 20–3. TECHNICAL SUCCESS OF TRANSLUMINAL ANGIOPLASTY IN 1372 ARTERIES WITH ATHEROSCLEROTIC DISEASE

Reference	*N* (Patients)	Success (%)
Giroux et al.[43]	33	95
Bell et al.[8]	25	92
O'Donovan 1992[51]	17	89[a]
Plouin 1993[56]	59	88[a]
Miller et al.[4]	46	87
Calapinto 1982[57]	51	86
Julien et al.[30]	70	86[a]
Weibull et al.[23]	65	86[b]
Baert et al.[13]	165	83[a]
Weibull et al.[22]	29	83[c]
Pattison 1992[49]	60	82
Sos 1991[58]	55	82
Rodriguez-Perez et al.[6]	37	78[a]
Klinge et al.[10]	134	77[d]
Canzanello 1989[59]	125	68[a]
Flechner 1982[60]	27	63
Sos et al.[12]	72	53[a]
Martin 1992[61]	110	35[e]
Eldrup-Jorgensen 1995[62]	51	38[a]
Jensen 1995[63]	147	85[f]
Knorring 1996[64]	27	90
Mean		**77**

Difficult to calculate because specific numbers not provided.
[a] <50% residual diameter.
[b] "Total elimination of stenosis."
[c] 4–9 mm.
[d] <60% residual and ≥15% improvement.
[e] <50% residual and <10 mmHg gradient.
[f] "Wider lumen."
Reprinted with permission from Rees CR. Stents for atherosclerotic renovascular disease. *JVIR.* 1999;10:689–705.

and stents and of the various risk factors and technical considerations is therefore necessary in order to provide the optimum treatment in each patient.

BACKGROUND AND RESULTS OF RENAL REVASCULARIZATION

Currently, no stents are approved for use in the renal arteries in the United States outside of research studies. The first renal artery stent procedure in the United States was performed in 1987 using a coronary version of the Palmaz stent (Cordis, Division of Johnson & Johnson, Warren, NJ) as part of the United States Multicenter Trial.[24,26] Prior to this, there had been very limited use of the Palmaz and Wallstent endoprostheses. The Palmaz stent satisfied the important criteria for renal artery stenting, including low thrombogenicity, ability for highly accurate positioning, and strong hoop strength. Hoop strength must be adequate throughout the length of the stent, including the edge

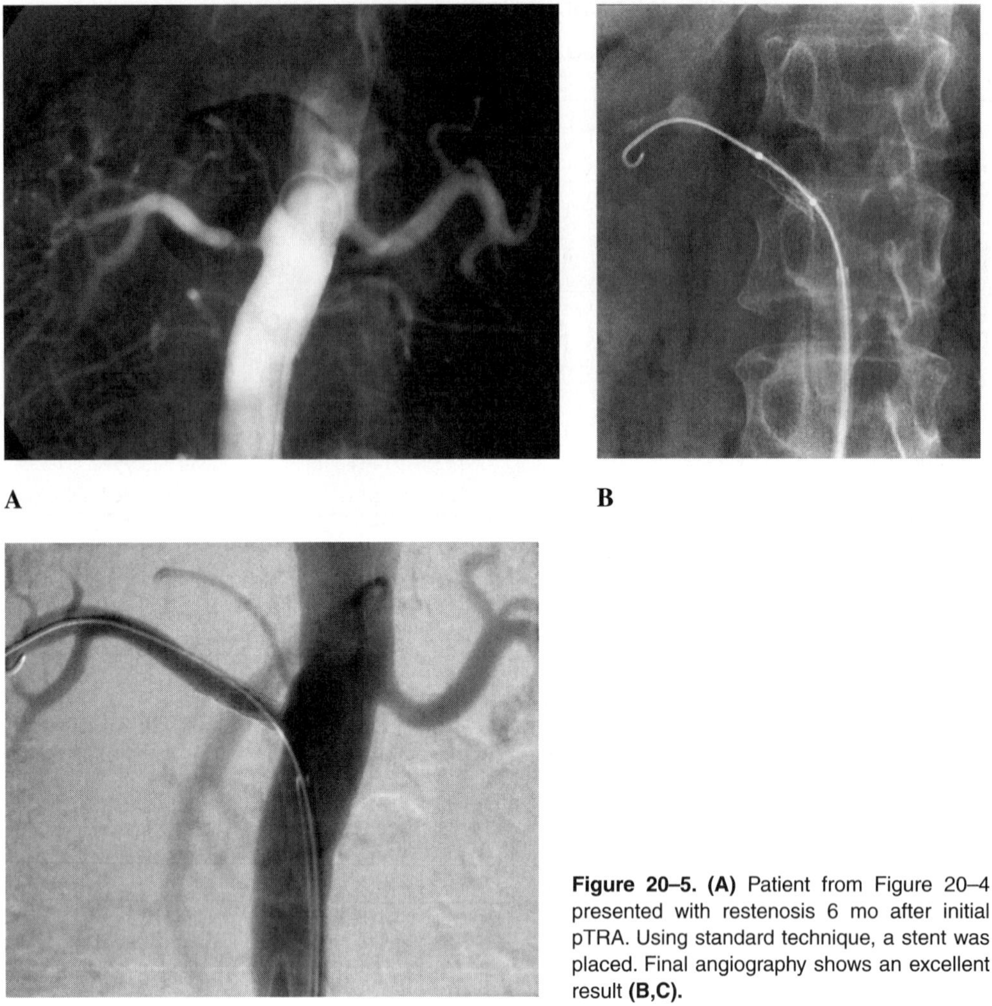

A B C

Figure 20–5. (A) Patient from Figure 20–4 presented with restenosis 6 mo after initial pTRA. Using standard technique, a stent was placed. Final angiography shows an excellent result **(B,C).**

that protrudes minimally into the aorta, in order to resist the strong compressive forces of heavily calcified ostial plaques.

An overview of published series on results of renal stents is seen in Tables 20–2, 20–4, and 20–5. The vast majority of stents have been placed in atherosclerotic lesions. Technical success, usually defined as a residual stenosis of ≤30%, is seen in a mean of 99% and is 100% in most series (Table 20–4). Lower success rates were achieved with stents other than the Palmaz stent, presumably due to lesser hoop strength and difficulty in accurate positioning. Patency by angiographic follow up ranging from 6 mo to 2 yr and usually defined as <50% stenosis relative to normal reference vessel diameter, was present in a mean of 77% of lesions (Table 20–6). This represents an average

TABLE 20–4. TECHNICAL SUCCESS OF RENAL STENTS IN 1128 ARTERIES

Reference	*N* (Patients)	Success (%)	Definition (%)[a]
Giroux et al.[43]	30	95	
Leertouwer[42]	40	100	<20
US Multicenter Trial[24]	296	98	≤30
Dorros 1995[27]	202	99	<50
Tuttle 1998[65]	148	98	<30
White 1997[66]	133	99	<30
Blum et al.[36]	82	100	<50
Henry et al.[37]	64	100	<20
Boisclair 1997[54]	35	100	<30
MacLeod et al.[38]	32	100	<30
Harden et al.[21]	32	100	<10
van de Ven 1995[67]	28	100	<10
Hennequin 1994[55]	21	100[b]	
Raynaud 1994[68]	18	100[b]	<20
Joffre et al.[28]	16	100[b]	
Kuhn 1991[69]	10	80[c]	<20
Wilms 1991[70]	11	80[b]	<20
Mean		**99**	

[a] Residual diameter stenosis after stent placement.
[b] Wallstent.
[c] Strecker stent; all others Palmaz stent.
Reprinted with permission from Rees CR. Stents for atherosclerotic renovascular disease. *JVIR.* 1999;10:689–705.

restenosis rate of 23%. Hypertension was cured (normotensive off medication) in 6% and improved in 55%, with a sum of cure or improvement in 61% of patients at the latest follow-up interval. In patients with renal failure, 35% showed long-term improvement of function, with stabilization in another 35%.

TABLE 20–5. EFFECT OF RENAL STENTS ON HYPERTENSION IN 845 PATIENTS

Reference	*N*	Cure (%)	Improved (%)	Benefit (%)	Follow-up (mo)
Giroux et el.[43]	?	6	48	54	
US Multicenter Trial[24]	263	3		61	12 (Life table)
Dorros 1998[27]	163	1	42	43	24
Tuttle 1998[65]	129	0	55	55	6–12
Blum et al.[36]	75	16	62	78	3–84
Henry et al.[37]	54	18	57	75	1–42
Boisclair 1997[54]	33	6	61	67	1–34
MacLeod et al.[38]	29	0	44	44	1–32
van de Ven 1995[67]	24	0	73	3	6–35
Hennequin 1994[55]	21	14	86	100	12–60
Raynaud 1994[68]	18	6	45	50	6
Joffre et al.[28]	16	31	69	100	6–36
Kuhn 1991[69]	10	23	34	56	6–12
Wilms 1991[70]	10	40	40	80	6.7
Mean		**6**	**55**	**61**	

Reprinted with permission from Rees CR. Stents for atherosclerotic renovascular disease. *JVIR.* 1999;10:689–705.

TABLE 20–6. ANGIOGRAPHIC PATENCY OF RENAL STENTS IN 563 ARTERIES

Study Group	Location	*N*	Patency (%)	Follow-up (mo)
Rees et al.[24]	US Multicenter	150	67	4–32
White 1997[66]	New Orleans	80	81	≤6[a]
Dorros et al.[27]	Milwaukee	56	75	6
Henry et al.[37]	France	54	79	4–6
Tuttle 1998[65]	USA	49	86	2–24
Blum et al.[36]	Germany	48	85	12
MacLeod et al.[38]	Scotland	24	84	7
Harden et al.[21]	Scotland	24	88	6
van de Ven 1995[67]	Netherlands	23	87	6
Hennequein 1994[55]	France	20	77	12–60
Raynaud 1994[68]	France	16	81	6–36
Wilms 1991[70]	Belgium	11	29	9
Kuhn 1991[69]	Germany	8	75	6–12
Mean			**77**	**7.9**

[a] Assigned a mean of 5 months for purposes of weighted mean calculation.

Reprinted with permission from Rees CR. Stents for atherosclerotic renovascular disease. *JVIR.* 1999;10:689–705.

The majority of the patients in the renal stent literature suffered from failure of conventional pTRA prior to stent placement. The most common cause of failure was immediate elastic recoil, with a significant dissection as the second most common cause. Post-pTRA restenosis was also a common indication for stents. The practice of placement of the stent without prior angioplasty or predilatation or without regard for the result of prestent balloon dilatation is no longer uncommon; however, it is minimally reported in peer-reviewed manuscript form. Of note, the study by Dorros et al.[27] was heavily weighted toward primary stenting but yielded similar results to the other studies outlined in Tables 20–1, 20–4, 20–5, and 20–6, which are composed primarily of failed angioplasty patients.

Comparison of the results of renal angioplasty to renal stenting is difficult at this time for several reasons. The predominance of pTRA failures in the stent reports creates a selection bias with the potential for skew in the direction of poorer results. In addition, the angioplasty literature is generally older with less-stringent reporting standards. Whereas in the angioplasty literature, technical success was often never defined, or loosely defined, the stent literature contains clear definitions of success, which are usually quite stringent relative to pTRA reports. Most stent series define success as ≤30% diameter reduction postprocedure compared to normal reference vessel diameter, whereas the most-stringent definitions in the pTRA literature used 50% as the cutoff. Criteria for cure or improvement of hypertension have changed little since the early 1990s and are quite similar between the angioplasty and stent literature. The same is also true for those involving revascularization for treatment of renal failure. Review of Tables 20–4 and 20–7 shows relatively similar overall results for pTRA and stenting on hypertension, with a mean benefit ratio (cure or improvement) in 66% of patients having pTRA and in 61% of patients having renal stent placement. The benefit of stents is probably underestimated by the 5% overall difference because most of the patients in these stent series had suffered technical failure of angioplasty and would have been expected to suffer clinical failure. Therefore, clinical success in 61% of stent patients rep-

TABLE 20–7. ATHEROSCLEROSIS: EFFECT OF TRANSLUMINAL ANGIOPLASTY ON HYPERTENSION IN 1095 PATIENTS WITH ATHEROSCLEROTIC DISEASE

Reference	*N* (Patients)	Cure (%)[a]	Total (%)[b]
Giroux et al.[43]	26	6	54
Tegtmeyer 1984[71]	65	23	94
Weibull et al.[23]	65	15	90
Weibull et al.[22]	29	12	83
Rodriguez-Perez et al.[6]	37	0	81
Julien et al.[30]	53	9	79
Klinge et al.[10]	134	10	78
Greminger et al.[9]	48	23	77
Mahler 1982[72]	8	12	75
Bell et al.[8]	22	14	73
Marshall 1990[73]	39	8	72
Martin L. 1992[61]	94 (Nonostial)	22	68
Martin et al.[14]	13	22	66
Martin et al.[11]	60	15	65
Miller et al.[4]	34	15	64
Martinez-Amenos et al.[15]	42	9	61
Martin L. 1992	110 (Ostial)	10	58
Flechner 1982[60]	27	7	48
Canzanello 1989[59]	100	4	43
Sos et al.[12]	51	14	34
Beebe et al.[7]	38	11	34
Mean		**13**	**66**

[a] Normotensive without medication

[b] Cured patients, plus those with significantly improved blood pressure control.

Reprinted with permission from Rees CR. Stents for atherosclerotic renovascular disease. *JVIR.* 1999,10.689–705.

resents a high rate of salvage of angioplasty failures. If stents are demonstrated to reduce the incidence of restenosis after technically successful angioplasty, then primary stenting would be indicated in the majority of atherosclerotic lesions of the renal artery. Post-pTRA restenosis occurred in 30% of 518 patients with angiographic follow-up and in 23% of patients with stents (Table 20–6).[28–35] More recent studies of stents showed improved restenosis rates in the range of 15%–20% or less. This is likely due to the accumulation of knowledge regarding patient selection and techniques as learned in several studies, including the U.S. Multicenter Study (see Effects of Variables on Percutaneous Revascularization).[21,24,36–38]

Of interest is the frequent reports of healing and improvement in luminal caliber after technical failure of angioplasty, when this occurred in association with plaque fracture without extensive elastic recoil. This phenomenon has been described in 20%–40% of angioplasty failures, and reported as high as 53%.[29,31–33] This phenomenon will probably become of increasingly lower significance as renal stents are more increasingly used because technical failures of angioplasty are managed with stents and the natural history of post-pTRA plaque remodeling will not be studied further. Instead, the final status of the vessel lumen depends on the degree of late loss due to tissue deposition over and between the stent struts. When using Palmaz stents, mechanical recoil over time is poorly quantitated thus far, but appears to be ≤15%.

POST-STENT RESTENOSIS

Restenosis lesions after stent placement are usually amenable to pTRA (Figures 20–6, 20–10, and 20–11). There can sometimes be some difficulty in crossing the lesion due to wire passage through stent–strut interstices. However, success is achieved in most instances. Immediate technical results are usually very good. Little is known about the long-term results of redilatation of these lesions.

COMPLICATIONS OF RENAL STENTS

The types of complications that may occur with renal stent placement are very similar to those of conventional renal angioplasty, with the addition of stent delivery problems, which may result in malpositioning. Access site complications are slightly more common with renal stents due to the larger sheaths that are most often used. Severe flow-limiting dissection of the renal artery is less common with stent placement than with renal angioplasty alone, since stents effectively ameliorate this problem (Figure 20–3). Renal stents result in the use of more contrast material relative to pTRA; however, us-

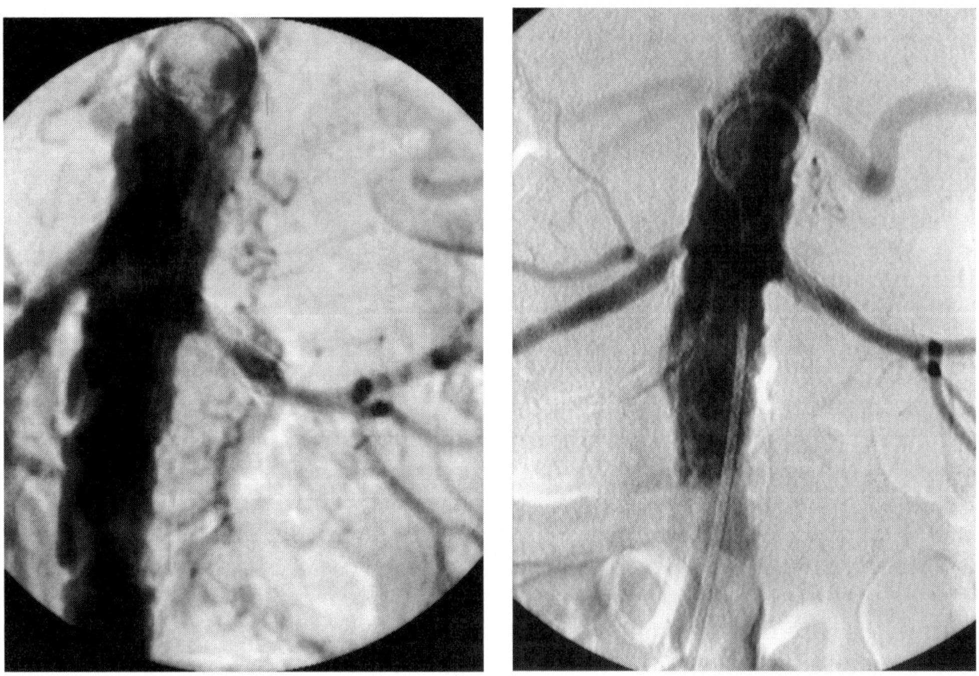

A B

Figure 20–6. (A) Poststent deployment restenosis secondary to intimal hyperplasia. **(B)** After repeat pTRA, there is an excellent angiographic result with no residual mean pressure gradient.

ing the techniques outlined in this chapter, additional contrast dose can be minimized. Stent infection is rare but has been reported, and can cause severe morbidity or mortality. Bleeding complications other than at the access site should not be any higher for stents than for renal angioplasty, especially if the guidelines in this chapter regarding anticoagulation are followed.

Thirty-day mortality after renal stent placement occurred in 2.7% of patients in the United States Multicenter Trial with causes including cholesterol embolization, sepsis, renal failure, aortic dissection, GI bleeding, and cardiopulmonary failure.[24] Access site complications are the same for renal revascularization as for all endovascular procedures. This includes the occurrence and frequency of pseudoaneurysms and arteriovenous fistulae, major procedure–related hematomas, thrombosis, or infection. Thrombosis of the renal artery has been very rare with Palmaz stents, occurring in approximately 1% of patients studied in the United States Multicenter Trial.[24] In this study, thrombosis occurred in three patients and was attributable to an obvious mechanical or technical problem in each instance.[24] The incidence of renal artery thrombosis after technically successful Palmaz renal stent placement is difficult to determine accurately due to its extreme rarity, but it can be stated to be <1%. Thus far, the use of oral anticoagulation with warfarin after renal stent placement has failed to demonstrate benefit with regard to reduction of renal artery thrombosis or the incidence of restenosis and increases the risk of bleeding complications. Currently, we prescribe aspirin indefinitely and clopidogrel 75 mg PO qd for 1 mo.

Other complications reported after renal stent placement include clot or plaque embolization, pseudoaneurysm of the renal artery due to overdilatation with the balloon and not secondary to stent placement, thrombosis of renal artery branch vessels due to guidewire trauma, and renal failure due to contrast nephrotoxicity or, more uncommonly, due to cholesterol embolization.

In a review by Beek et al.,[39] complications of severe or minor clinical significance were seen in 19.2% of 263 renal stent patients and in 14.9% of 719 pTRA patients. Wide variation between services is noted due to different reporting methods and patient populations. Beek et al.[39] noted cholesterol emboli in 5 of 50 patients receiving stents, but severe clinical consequences in only 3 of these patients. Such findings suggest the possibility that the risk of cholesterol embolization may be higher with stents due to the bulkier apparatus and extra manipulations necessary compared to those of pTRA alone with use of modern low-profile balloon catheters.

Once an operator is very experienced with renal stents, the complication rates of stent placement probably approach those of conventional pTRA. Operators who are inexperienced with renal stents or with stents in other vascular territories should probably expect higher complication rates in their early experience relative to conventional pTRA. Knowledge of these facts may influence one's threshold for renal stent placement because inexperienced operators may apply a conservative approach, using stents only in the event of the most clearcut angioplasty failures.

Using techniques described later in this chapter, the need for emergency surgery postprocedure is extremely rare. Before stents, severe postangioplasty dissection was the major cause for emergency surgery (Figure 20–3). However, this is successfully treated by stents in most situations. Perforation of the renal artery requiring surgery has also decreased in frequency, owing to improved technology such as roadmapping, rapid imaging with digital subtraction angiography, lower profile balloons and catheters with less rigid shafts, the availability of more delicate and sensitive guidewires, and the accumulation of knowledge regarding techniques. Another reason that the risk of perforation has decreased is the fact that aggressive overdilatation of a severe stenosis to achieve adequate results is no longer necessary, owing to the satisfactory treatment of such lesions with stents.

EFFECTS OF VARIABLES ON PERCUTANEOUS REVASCULARIZATION

Although pTRA and stenting of renal artery stenoses have been shown to be technically feasible and successful, predicting which patients will have an improvement in blood pressure or renal function postintervention has been difficult.

The earliest experience regarding this topic was the United States Multicenter Trial, which involved 263 patients enrolled from 1988 to 1992.[24] It provided important information about the effects of various clinical and morphologic variables on the outcome of renal stenting with regard to blood pressure, renal function, and restenosis that has been used effectively to improve patency and clinical results through improved patient selection and technical considerations. The patients were generally elderly (mean age = 66 yr) with extensive atherosclerotic disease including coronary artery disease in 68%, peripheral vascular disease in 62%, diabetes in 27%, and hypertension in 98%. The lesions were atherosclerotic in 98% and ostial in 80%. Lesions with stents that were dilated to 4 or 5 mm were 1.9 times more likely to develop restenosis than those dilated to 6, 7, or 8 mm ($p = 0.029$). Females were 1.7 times as likely to develop restenosis as males ($p = 0.044$). These risk factors were independent of each other, and were both statistically significant. The lowest risk group was men with normal reference vessel diameters of 6 mm or greater. They had a restenosis rate of 10.5%. Currently, in some practices, a male with a large renal artery will receive a stent even if there is a very minimal residual stenosis postangioplasty. In a female, however, with a small normal reference vessel diameter, a more significant residual stenosis (e.g., in the range of 35%–50% diameter) may be accepted without stent placement. The great majority of vessels with ≥50% residual stenosis after angioplasty receives a stent. However, a vessel that is ≤4 mm in its normal reference vessel diameter will not receive a stent unless the postangioplasty residual stenosis is in the range of ≥65% or there is a significant dissection.

In the United States Multicenter Trial, vessel caliber also had an important effect on clinical outcome.[24] Kaplan–Meier analysis showed that patients whose stents were dilated to ≥6 mm had a cumulative rate of improvement or cure in hypertension in 66% of cases at 1 yr vs 48% for patients with smaller caliber dilatations. Currently, it is advisable to dilate stents as large as safely possible in order to minimize restenosis due to tissue deposition or intimal hyperplasia. The US Multicenter Trial also showed that patients with larger normal reference vessel diameters experienced a greater benefit with regard to renal function compared to patients with smaller vessel diameters.[24] The trial showed a 41% improvement for those with reference vessel diameters of ≥6 mm, compared to a 20% improvement for patients with smaller vessels.

Smoking history was associated with a twofold risk of restenosis but did not appear to have an impact on blood pressure or renal function outcome. The presence of small vessel intrarenal disease on angiography had an adverse effect on blood pressure and renal function response, although it did not appear to have an impact on patency of treated vessels. Age beyond 65 yr also adversely affected blood pressure and renal function outcome without affecting vessel patency.

Interestingly, ostial location had no effect on long-term patency but did have a non-statistically significant effect on blood pressure response, with cumulative benefit by Kaplan–Meier analysis in 52% of patients vs 79% of patients with nonostial disease. The absence of effect of ostial location on long-term patency is not surprising because the technical success rate is 98% regardless of ostial versus nonostial location. Also for ostial and nonostial lesions, the stent is essentially in the same location, and the intimal hyperplastic response that may subsequently ensue can occur at any location along the length of the stent. Usually, this occurs in the portion of the vessel that was not diseased prior to stent placement.

A less common but increasingly used approach includes the use of stents in all ostial atherosclerotic lesions. Stents are either applied primarily without predilatation or are applied after predilatation without regard for the technical results of this initial dilatation. (The theory and rationale of this technique are discussed in the background section.) Support for the rationale of this approach is based on the presumption that the long-term results with renal stents will be superior to those of technically successful angioplasty, although this has not been demonstrated as yet. At the current time, such use of renal stents should be considered investigational and limited to experienced operators. This technique may have the result of shortening overall procedure times; however, this minor advantage must be weighed against the disadvantages of increased cost, increased access size, and risks of stent delivery failure or other complications that may not occur with basic pTRA. This is especially true with operators whose renal stent experience is limited.

In a study by Leertouwer,[42] pretreatment parameters that may predict 1-yr clinical success after renal artery stent placement were evaluated. In this study, 40 patients with hypertension and/or renal failure and a $\geq$50% angiographically proven renal artery stenosis were treated with stent placement. Anatomic parameters obtained from angiography and intravascular ultrasound as well as functional parameters obtained from renal scintigraphy and renal vein renin sampling were evaluated.[42]

Overall, the study showed that patients treated for hypertension had a better clinical success at 1-yr follow-up (85%) than patients with impaired renal function (35%). These results are in agreement with prior studies in the literature (Tables 20–1, 20–2, 20–4, and 20–7). Interestingly, clinical success for hypertension was not influenced by the coexistence of impaired renal function, but clinical success for renal failure was influenced by the coexistence of hypertension ($p = 0.002$). In addition, patients with a focal stenosis without plaque accumulation, as determined by intravascular ultrasound, did better than patients with an accumulation of atherosclerotic plaque at their stenosis site ($p = 0.07$).

Regarding impaired renal function, patients with a lower baseline serum creatinine and a higher glomerular filtration rate had a better clinical response after renal artery stenting at follow-up. Consequently, this may suggest the need to intervene on patients with renal artery stenosis before their renal function becomes severely impaired.[42]

Of particular interest was that lateralization of the renal scintigram prior to stent placement was a highly significant predictor of clinical success in patients treated for hypertension or renal function impairment. Patients with this finding were 15 times more likely to have clinical success at 1 yr.

A study by Giroux et al.[43] also found that a shorter duration of hypertension, higher diastolic blood pressure, and fibromuscular renovascular disease were predictive of a favorable clinical outcome after percutaneous revascularization.[43–46] In addition, patients with less atheromatous aortic disease and a more severe angiographic stenosis were also more likely to have a favorable clinical response with a strong association in hypertensive patients and a weak association in renal insufficiency patients. However, diabetes had a negative impact on clinical outcome in patients with renal insufficiency, but no impact on patients with hypertension.

With regards to Doppler evaluation, Giroux et al.[43] found that quantitative Doppler analysis was not useful as a prognostic parameter. However, morphologic analysis of the Doppler waveform was useful for predicting clinical success of renal insufficiency patients after percutaneous therapy. Giroux and colleagues[43] explained that this abnormal intrarenal Doppler waveform morphology reflected the hemodynamic significance of a proximal renal artery stenosis and therefore related to renal function more directly than to the complex mechanisms involved in renovascular hypertension.

TECHNIQUE

Numerous techniques for pTRA and renal stent placement have been described. The major differences between various techniques are in regard to axillary, brachial, or radial vs femoral approach; predilatation vs no predilatation; and preloading the balloon–stent assembly in a guiding catheter vs advancing the balloon–stent assembly through the guide catheter or sheath after it is already in position across the renal artery stenosis. Next, the most common techniques are described in detail. Because pTRA is an extension of angioplasty in other vessel territories, the following discussion focuses on stent placement for renal artery stenosis. The techniques described here are a variation of the original techniques used for placement of Palmaz stents. They have the advantage of being time tested and very reliable with a minimization of delivery problems.

FEMORAL ACCESS, PRELOADED GUIDING CATHETER TECHNIQUE

Percutaneous transluminal renal angioplasty is performed in the usual manner as a predilatation prior to stent placement. The fluoroscopy tube is then positioned in order to profile the renal artery origin for accurate stent placement. A relatively stiff 0.035-in. guidewire is left across the renal artery stenosis, with the tip of this wire located as far distally as safely possible without causing injury to a branch vessel (Figure 20–7). We

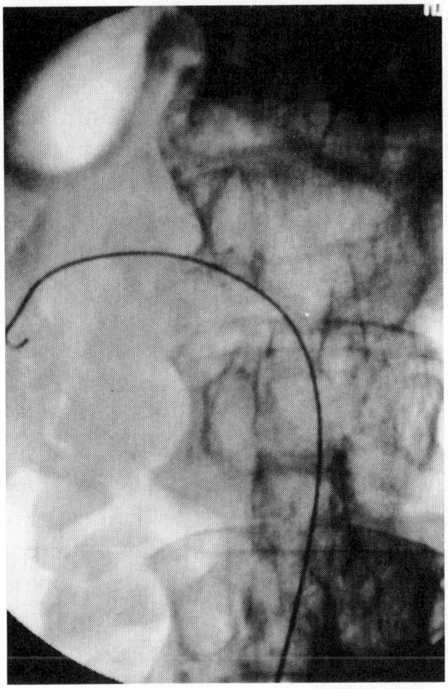

Figure 20–7. A .035-in. guidewire is across the right renal artery stenosis. The guidewire tip is placed as far distally as safely possible without causing perforation of the renal capsule or injury to a branch vessel.

prefer to use a TAD II wire, which has a tip that tapers to 0.018 in. This mandril wire offers the advantage of fewer exchanges because it has a tip soft enough to be placed through the stenosis at the beginning of the pTRA procedure, however, inexperienced interventionalists may find tracking of the guiding catheter and stent assembly to be superior over 0.035-in. wires. Other guidewires that have been used with success include the New York wire, which has a straight leading end and a relatively short taper similar to the Rosen wire, (without the J tip, of course). Then, on the procedure tray, a 2-cm long balloon of the desired diameter is passed through a 5.5–8 French sheath or a 45- to 55-cm long guiding catheter. Alternative, currently available techniques allow for smaller access sheaths and the use of guiding catheters of 6–7 Fr, coupled with low-profile PTA balloon catheters (4–5 F) and 0.018 steerable guidewires with floppy, platinum radiopaque tips for improved visualization. The balloon used should be a relatively low-profile balloon made of scratch-resistant material that minimizes the risk of balloon rupture before complete stent deployment. With the stent mounted and manually crimped onto the balloon surface, the leading balloon tip is advanced within the guide catheter until its tip, but not the leading stent edge, protrudes beyond the tip of the guiding catheter. Balloon-expandable stents are used almost exclusively in the renal arteries rather than self-expanding stents. The most commonly used balloon-expandable stent has been the Palmaz 154 (Cordis, Warren, NJ), but more recently, other balloon-expandable stents by Guidant Corporation, Medtronic Corporation, Intratherapeutics, and other companies are being used.

For deployment, approximate positioning of the stent, still within the guiding catheter, is accomplished using bony landmarks. The guiding catheter is then withdrawn slightly so that it still partially covers the stent and a test injection is performed, usually with approximately 5 cc of contrast material injected at 3 cc/sec. Position of the stent is finely adjusted. When it appears to be in satisfactory position, the guiding catheter is pulled back until the stent is completely exposed. At this point, contrast is again administered using digital subtraction angiography in multiple projections, and final precise positioning of the stent is performed (Figure 20–8). The stent is positioned so that on deployment, 1 mm protrudes into the aortic lumen. Consideration is given to slight shortening of the stent on full expansion. The balloon is then slowly inflated using dilute contrast material or saline. Undiluted contrast material may result in delayed opening of the leading end of the balloon, which could potentially alter the stent position. It may also result in delayed or even incomplete balloon deflation. After deployment and deflation, completion angiography is performed through the guiding catheter, whose tip is still directed at the origin of the renal artery, with the guidewire still in place (Figure 20–9).

As stated previously, the long-term patency appears to correlate with stent diameter. For this reason, the stent is dilated to the largest size considered safe. The balloon tip is not advanced beyond the distal end of the stent to prevent perforation or dissection distal to the stent. High-pressure inflation is used to help form good apposition of the stent against the wall of the vessel. These efforts to improve long-term patency are performed even when the initial stent deployment diameter is adequate to provide

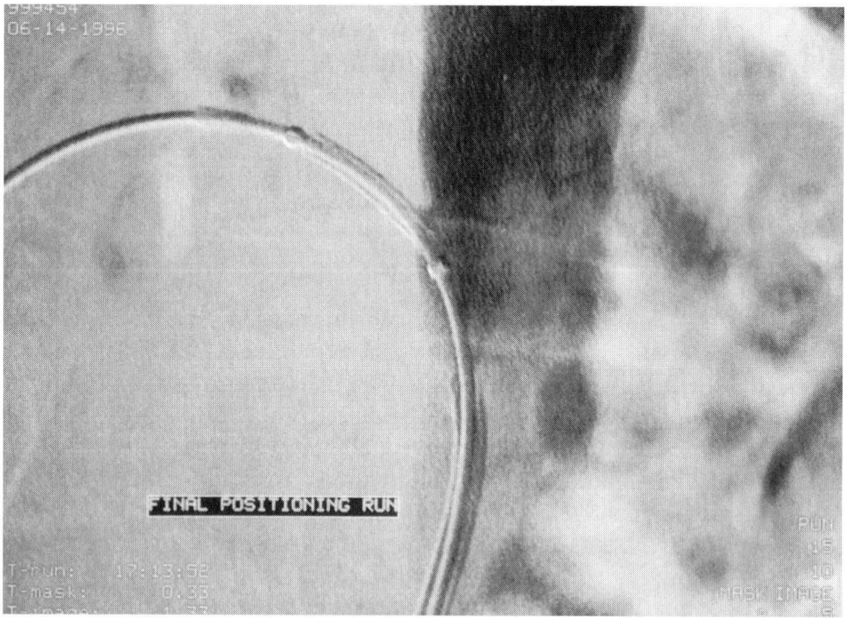

Figure 20–8. The position of the stent is finely adjusted using bony landmarks so that the proximal end of the stent protrudes 1 mm into the aorta. The guiding catheter is then pulled back, exposing the stent, and a final contrast injection is performed. In this profile view, the stent is ideally positioned.

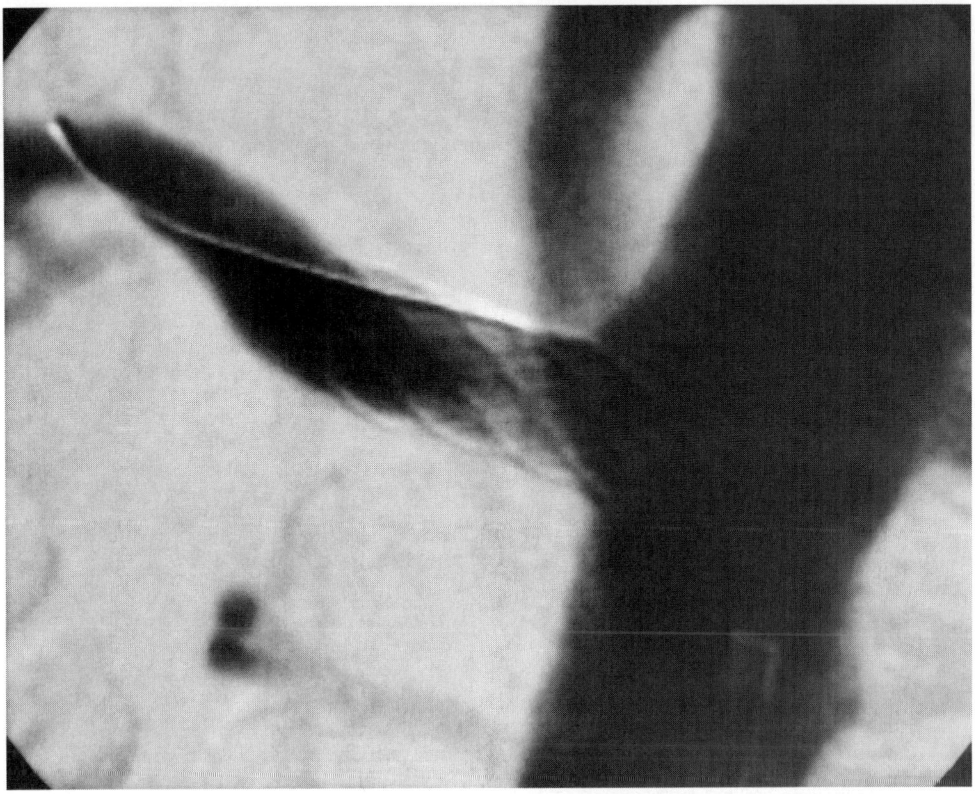

Figure 20–9. The stent is deployed with balloon expansion. Once the balloon is deflated, completion angiography is performed through the guiding catheter. The stent is dilated to the largest size considered safe.

minimal residual stenosis and complete obliteration of the pressure gradient. Deposition of a thin layer of neointima is inevitable (Figures 20–6, 20–10, and 20–11). Restenosis results if initial stent diameter is not optimized at the time of placement.

This technique is associated with a very low likelihood of balloon rupture on stent implantation because the balloon–stent assembly is not forced through a long sheath or guiding catheter that can sometimes result in scratching or puncturing of the balloon.

MODIFIED APPROACHES

Some operators prefer the axillary, brachial, or radial approach because they claim a more favorable angle of approach to the renal artery. Although this approach may make the procedure technically easier in some patients, the axillary and brachial approach carry the disadvantage of a higher likelihood of access complications, including brachial plexus injury or arterial thrombosis. As a result, this approach usually is not

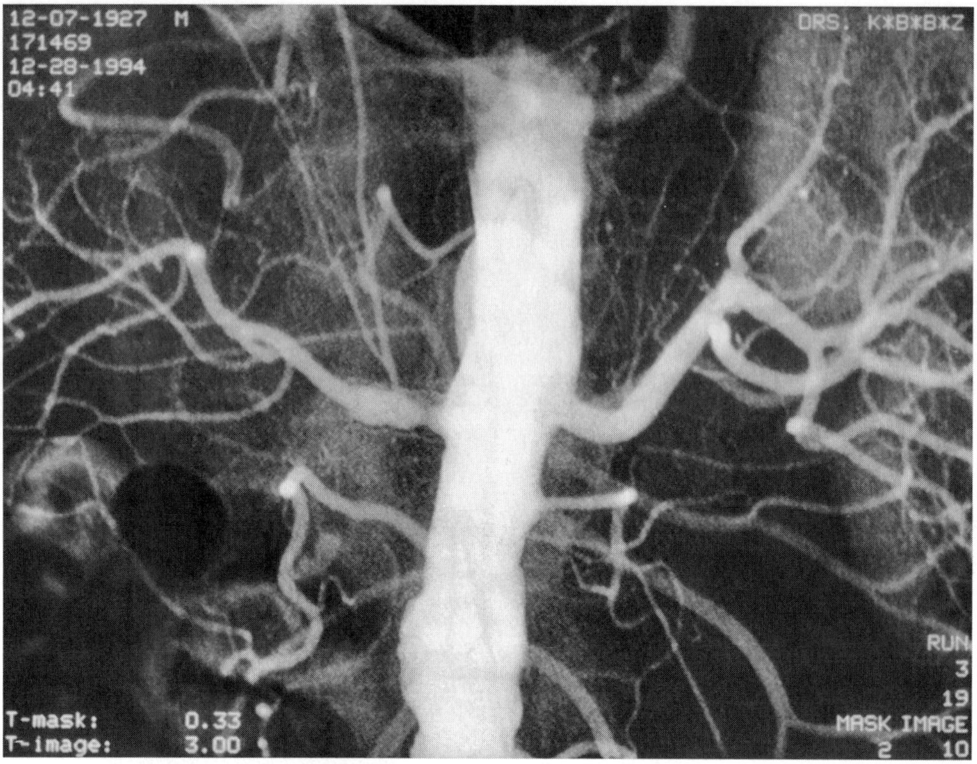

Figure 20–10. Six months after stent placement, a thin layer of neointima is present.

preferred by operators with extensive experience with catheterization of down-going vessels with precurved catheters from the femoral access, and in fact, our experience indicates that the need for an upper extremity approach arises in <1% of cases. One theoretical advantage to the upper extremity approach is a minimization of catheter manipulation in severely atherosclerotic infrarenal aortas. However, even this problem can be addressed from below with use of a long transfemoral sheath that reaches or nearly reaches the renal artery origins.

Prior to the pTRA or stent procedure, most operators give a bolus of heparin. The vascular sheath is then removed when the ACT value is within acceptable limits (<180 sec).

SUMMARY

In summary, comparative studies between pTRA and renal stents have not been performed. There is, however, extensive documentation of excellent clinical results with renal stents in technically failed angioplasties. These same patients might have been expected to otherwise have a high likelihood of clinical failure. In addition, the technical

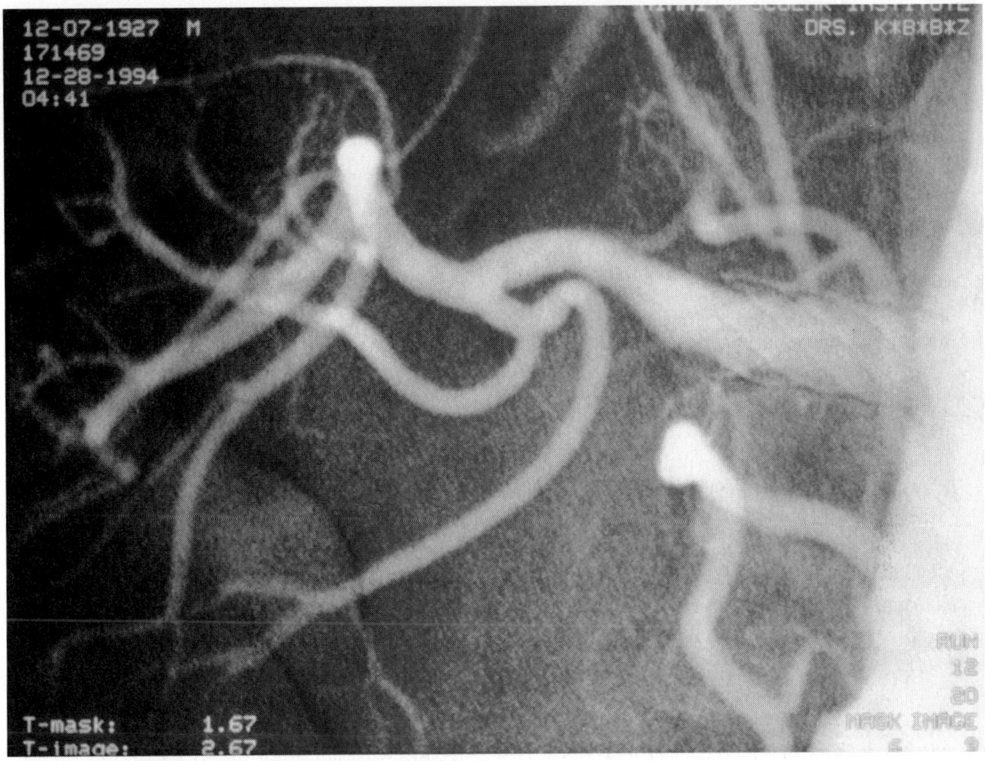

Figure 20–11. After intimal hyperplasia is treated with repeat pTRA, completion angiography shows an excellent angiographic result.

success of renal artery stents is vastly superior to conventional angioplasty in ASRVD, and restenosis rates appear to be roughly equivalent or perhaps even lower in recent trials, as far as can be determined without good comparative studies. Poststent restenosis appears to have declined to approximately 15%–20% in more recent series, perhaps due to the accumulation of knowledge regarding patient selection and techniques. Therefore, it is clear that the use of stents to treat technical failures of angioplasty results in overall improved patency. Nevertheless, it remains to be determined whether stents should be placed routinely to prevent restenosis, even in the presence of technically successful angioplasty. Such a determination may require comparative study that is more complicated than a simple randomized comparison of pTRA vs stents.

REFERENCES

1. Rees CR. Stents for atherosclerotic renovascular disease. *JVIR*. 1999;10:689–705.
2. Holley KE, Hunt JC, Brownal JR, Kincaid OW, Sheps SG. Renal artery stenosis, a clinical–pathologic study in normotensive and hypertensive patients. *Am J Med*. 1964;37:14–22.

3. Van Velzer DA. Atherosclerotic narrowing of renal arteries associated with hypertension. *Am J Roent.* 1961;86:807–818.
4. Miller GA, Ford KK, Braun SD, et al. Percutaneous transluminal angioplasty vs. surgery for renovascular hypertension. *Am J Roent.* 1985;144:447–450.
5. Tegtmeyer CJ, Selby JB, Hartwell GD, Ayers C, Tegtmeyer VT. Results and complications of angioplasty in fibromuscular disease. *Circulation.* 1991;83(Suppl):I155–I161.
6. Rodriguez-Perez JC, Plaza C, Reyes R, et al. Treatment of renovascular hypertension with percutaneous transluminal angioplasty: experience in Spain. *JVIR.* 1994;5:101–109.
7. Beebe HG, Chesebro K, Merchant F, Bush W. Results of renal artery balloon angioplasty limit its indications. *J Vasc Surg.* 1988;8:300–306.
8. Bell GM, Reid J, Buist TA. Percutaneous transluminal angioplasty improves blood pressure and renal function in renovascular hypertension. *Quart J Med.* 1987;241:393–403.
9. Greminger P, Steiner A, Schneider E, et al. Cure and improvement of renovascular hypertension after percutaneous transluminal angioplasty of renal artery stenosis. *Nephron.* 1989;51:362–366.
10. Klinge J, Mali WPTM, Puijleart CBAJ, Geyskes G, Becking W, Feldberg M. Percutaneous transluminal angioplasty: initial and long-term results. *Radiology.* 1989;171:501–506.
11. Martin LG, Price RB, Casarella WJ, et al. Percutaneous angioplasty in clinical management of renovascular hypertension: initial and long-term results. *Radiology.* 1985;155:629–633.
12. Sos TA, Pickering TG, Sniderman K, et al. Percutaneous transluminal renal angioplasty in renovascular hypertension due to atheroma or fibromuscular dysplasia. *N Engl J Med.* 1983;309:274–279.
13. Baert AL, Wilms G, Amery A, Vermylen J, Suy R. Percutaneous transluminal renal angioplasty: initial results and long-term follow-up in 202 patients. *Cardiovasc Interven Radiol.* 1990;13:22–28.
14. Martin E, Mattern R, Baer L, Fankuchen E, Casarella W. Renal angioplasty for hypertension: predictive factors for long-term success. *AJR.* 1981;137:921–924.
15. Martinez-Amenos A, Rama H, Sarrias X, Galceran J, Alsina J, Montanya X. Percutaneous transluminal angioplasty in the treatment of renovascular hypertension. *J Hum Hyperten.* 1991;5:97–100.
16. Simunic S, Winter-Fuduric I, Radanovic B, et al. Percutaneous transluminal renal angioplasty (pTRA) as a method of therapy for renovascular hypertension in children. *Eur J Radiol.* 1990;10:143–146.
17. Scobel JE, Sweny P, Stansby G, Hamilton G. Patients with atherosclerotic renovascular disease presenting to a renal unit: an audit of outcome. *Postgrad Med J.* 1993;69:461–465.
18. Schreiber MJ, Pohl MA, Novick AC. The natural history of atherosclerotic and fibrous renal artery disease. *Urol Clin North Am.* 1984;11(3):383–392.
19. Dean RH, Kieffer RW, Smith BM, et al. Renovascular hypertension: anatomic and renal function changes during drug therapy. *Arch Surg.* 1981;116:1408–1415.
20. Maroni BJ, Mitch WE. In: Seldin DW, Giebisch G, eds. *Nutritional Therapy in Renal Failure in the Kidney: Physiology and Pathophysiology,* 2nd ed. New York: Raven Press, Ltd. 1992:3471–3495.
21. Harden PN, MacLeod MJ, Rodger RSC, et al. Effect of renal artery stenting on progression of renovascular failure. *Lancet.* 1997;349:1133–1136.
22. Weibull H, Bergvist D, Bergentz SE, Johsson K, Hulthen L, Manhem P. Percutaneous transluminal renal angioplasty versus surgical reconstruction of atherosclerotic of renal artery stenosis: a prospective randomized study. *J Vasc Surg.* 1993;18:841–852.
23. Weibull H, Bergvist D, Jonsson K, Hulthen L, Manhem P, Bergentz SE. Long-term results after percutaneous transluminal angioplasty of atherosclerotic renal artery stenosis—the importance of intensive follow-up. *Eur J Renovasc Surg.* 1991;5:291–301.

24. Rees CR, Snead D. Results of United States Multicenter Trial of stents in renal arteries. *Abs Cardiovasc Intervent Radiol.* 1994;17(Suppl)2:S1–145.
25. Tetteroo E, van Engelen AD, Spithoven JH, et al. Stent placement after iliac angioplasty: comparison of hemodynamic and angiographic criteria. *Radiology.* 1996;201:155–159.
26. Rees CR, Palmaz JC, Becker GJ, et al. Palmaz stent in atherosclerotic stenoses involving the ostia of the renal arteries: preliminary report of a multicenter study. *Radiology.* 1991;181:507–514.
27. Dorros G, Jaff M, Jain A, Dufek C, Mathiak L. Follow-up of primary Palmaz–Schatz stent placement for atherosclerotic renal artery stenosis. *Am J Cardiol.* 1995;75(15):1051–1055.
28. Joffre F, Rousseau H, Bernadet P, et al. Midterm results of renal artery stenting. *Cardiovasc Intervent Radiol.* 1992;15:313–318.
29. Wilms GE, Baert AL, Amery AK, Staessen JA, Vermylen JG. Short-term morphologic results of percutaneous transluminal renal angioplasty as determined with angiography. *Radiology.* 1989;170:1019–1021.
30. Julien J, Jeunemaitre X, Raynaud A, et al. Influence of age on the outcome of percutaneous angioplasty in atheromatous renovascular disease. *J Hyperten.* 1989;7(Suppl 6):S188–S189.
31. Schwarten DE. Percutaneous transluminal angioplasty of the renal arteries: intravenous digital subtraction angiography for follow-up. *Radiology.* 1984;150:369–373.
32. Ingrisch H, Hegele T, Frey KW. Angiographic control of renal artery stenoses 6 months following percutaneous transluminal angioplasty. *Cardiovasc Intervent Radiol.* 1982;5:249–256.
33. Kuiper KJ, de Jong PE, de Zeeuw D, Schuur KH, van der Hem GK. *Proc Eur Dial Transplant Assoc.* 1983;20:538–545.
34. Grim CE. Percutaneous transluminal dilatation: the treatment of choice for renal artery stenosis causing hypertension. *Am J Kidney Dis.* 1981;1:186–187.
35. Tegtmeyer CJ, Dyer R, Teates CD, et al. Percutaneous transluminal dilatation of the renal arteries. *Radiology.* 1980;135:589–599.
36. Blum U, Krumme B, Flugel P, et al. Treatment of ostial renal artery stenoses with vascular endoprostheses after unsuccessful balloon angioplasty. *N Engl J Med.* 1997;336:459–465.
37. Henry M, Amor M, Henry I, et al. Stent placement in the renal artery: three year experience with the Palmaz stent. *JVIR.* 1996;7:343–350.
38. MacLeod M, Taylor AD, Baxter G, et al. Renal artery stenosis managed by Palmaz stent insertion: technical and clinical outcome. *J Hyperten.* 1995;13:1791–1795.
39. Beek FA, Kaatee R, Beutler JJ, van de Ven PJ, Mali WM. Complications during renal artery stent placement for atherosclerotic ostial stenosis. *Cardiovasc Intervent Radiol.* 1997;20:184–190.
40. Leertouwer TC, Pattynama PMT, Van den Berg-Huysmans A. Ten Year follow-up of untreated incidental renal artery stenosis in peripheral vascular disease: a case for treatment? RSNA 1999. *Radiology.* 1999;213:348. [Abstract]
41. Van Jaarsveld BC, Krijnen P, Pieterman H, et al. The effect of balloon angioplasty on hypertension in atherosclerotic renal artery stenosis. *N Engl J Med.* 2000;342:1007–1014.
42. Leertouwer TC. *Stent Placement for Renal Artery Stenosis (Functional Aspects and Morphologic Intravascular Ultrasound Parameters that Define Clinical Success).* Chapter 10: Predictors for clinical success at one year following renal artery stent placement. Ridderprint BV 2000:107–115.
43. Giroux MF, Soulez G, Therasse, E, et al. Percutaneous revascularization of the renal arteries: predictors of outcome. *JVIR.* 2000;11:713–720.
44. Barri YM, Davidson RA, Senler S, et al. Prediction of cure of hypertension in atherosclerotic renal artery stenosis. *South Med J.* 1996;89:679–683.
45. Davidson RA, Barri Y, Wilcox CS. Predictors of cure of hypertension in fibromuscular renovascular disease. *Am J Kidney Dis.* 1996;28:334–338.
46. Losinno F, Zuccala A, Busato F, Zucchelli P. Renal artery angioplasty for renovascular hypertension and preservation of renal function: long-term angiographic and clinical follow-up. *AJR.* 1994;162:853–857.

47. Tykarski A, Edwards R, Dominiczak AF, Reid JL. Percutaneous transluminal renal angioplasty in the management of hypertension and renal failure in patients with renal artery stenosis. *J Human Hyperten* 1993;7:491–496.
48. Pickering TG, Devereux RB, James GD, Silane M, Herman L, Sotelo J, Sos T, Laragh J. Recurrent pulmonary edema in hypertension due to bilateral renal artery stenosis: treatment by angioplasty or surgical revascularization. *The Lancet* 1988;551–552.
49. Pattison JM, Reidy JF, Rafferty MJ, Ogg CS, Cameron JS, Sacks SH, Williams DG. Percutaneous transluminal renal angioplasty in patients with renal failure. *Quarterly Journal of Medicine* 1992;85:883–888.
50. Madias NE, Kwon OJ, Millan VG. Percutaneous transluminal renal angioplasty: a potentially effective treatment for preservation of renal function. *Arch Intern Med* 1982;195:693.
51. O'Donovan RM, Gutierrez OH, Izzo JL. Preservation of renal function by percutaneous renal angioplasty in high risk elderly patients: short-term outcome. *Nephron* 1992;60:187–189,
52. Luft FC, Grim CE, Weinberger MH. Intervention in patients with renovascular hypertension and renal insufficiency. *J of Urology* 1983;130:654-656.
53. Pattynama PM, Becker GJ, Brown J, Zemel G, Benenati JF, Katzen BT. Percutaneous angioplasty for atherosclerotic renal artery disease: effect on renal function in azotemic patients. *Cardiovascular and Interventional Radiology* 1994 May–Jun; 17(3):143–146.
54. Boisclair C, Therasse F, Oliva VL, et al. Treatment of renal angioplasty failure by percutaneous renal stenting with palmaz stents: midterm technical and clinical results. *AJR* 1997;168:245–251.
55. Hennequin LM, Joffre FG, Rousseau HP, Aziza R, Tregant P, Bernadet P, Salvador M, Chamontin B. Renal artery stent placement: long-term results with the Wallstent endoprosthesis. *Radiology* 1991 Jun; 191(3):713–719.
56. Plouin PF, Darne B, Chatellier G, Pannier I, Battaglia C, Raynaud A, Azizi M. Restenosis after a first percutaneous transluminal renal angioplasty. *Hypertension* 1993;21:89–96,
57. Colapinto F, Stronell R, Harries-Jones E, Gildiner M, Hobbs BB, Farrow GA, Wilson DR, Morrow JD, Logan AG, Bilch SJ. Percutaneous transluminal dilatation of the renal artery: follow-up studies on renovascular hypertension. *AJR* 1982;139:727–732.
58. Sos TA. Angioplasty for the treatment of azotemia and renovascular hypertension in atherosclerotic renal artery disease. *Circ.* 1991;83 (Supplement):162–166.
59. Canzanello VJ, Millan VG, Spiegel JE, Ponce SP, Kopelman RI, Madias NE. Percutaneous transluminal renal angioplasty in management of atherosclerotic renovascular hypertension: results in 100 patients. *Hypertension* 1989;13:163–172.
60. Flechner S, Novick A, Vidt D, Buonocorc E, Meaney T. The use of percutaneous transluminal angioplasty for renal artery stenosis in patients with generalized atherosclerosis. The *Journal of Urology* 1982;127:1072–1075.
61. Martin LG, Cork RD, Kaufman SL. Long-term results on angioplasty in 110 patients with renal artery stenosis. *JVIR* 1992;3:619–626.
62. Eldrup-Jorgensen J, Harvey MR, Sampson LN, Amberson SM, Bredenberg CE. Should percutaneous transluminal renal artery angioplasty be applied to ostial renal artery atherosclerosis? *J Vasc Surg* 199;21:909–915.
63. Jensen G, Zachrisson BF, Delin K, Volkmann R, Aurell M. Treatment of renovascular hypertension: one year results of renal angioplasty. *Kidney Int* 1995;48:1936–1945.
64. Knorring J, Edgren J, Lepantalo M. Long-term results of percutaneous transluminal angioplasty in renovascular hypertension. *Acta Radiologica* 1996;37:36–40.
65. Tuttle KR, Chouinard RF, Webber JT, et al. Treatment of athersclerotic ostial renal artery stenosis with the intravascular stent. *Am J Kidney Dis* 1998;32:611–622.
66. White CJ, Ramee SR, Collins TJ, Jenkins JS, Escobar A. Renal artery stent placement: utility in lesions difficult to treat with balloon angioplasty. *J Am Coll Cardiol* 1997;30:1445–1450.

67. Van de Ven PG, Beutler JJ, Kaatee R, Beck F, Mali W, Geyskes G, Koomans H. Transluminal vascular stent for ostial atherosclerotic renal artery stenosis. *Lancet* 1995;346:672–674.
68. Raynaud AC, Beyssen BM, Turmel-Rodrigues LE, Pagny JY, Sapoval MR, Gaux JC, Plouin PF. Renal artery stent placement: immediate and midterm technical and clinical results. *JVIR* 1994 Nov–Dec;5(6):849–858.
69. Kuhn FP, Kutkuhn B, Torsello G, Modder U. Renal artery stenosis: preliminary results with the Strecker stent. *Radiology* 1991;180:367–372.
70. Wilms G, Peene P, Baert A, Nevelsteen A, Suy R, Vergacgne R, Wermylen J, Fagerd R. Renal artery stent placement with use of Wallstent endoprosthesis. *Radiology* 1991;179:457–462.
71. Tegtmeyer CJ, Kellum CD, Ayers C. Percutaneous transluminal angioplasty of the renal artery. *Radiology* 1984;153:77–84.
72. Mahler F, Probst P, Heartel M, Weidmann P, Kmeta A. Lasting improvement of renovascular hypertension by transluminal dilatation of atherosclerotic and non-atherosclerotic renal artery stenoses. *Circulation* 1982;65:611–617.
73. Marshall FI, Hagen S, Mahaffy RG, Petrie JC, Roy-Chaudhyury P, Russell IT, Webster J. Percutaneous transluminal angioplasty for atheromatous renal artery stenosis-blood pressure response and discriminate analysis of outcome predictors. *Quarterly J Med* 1990;75,277: 483–489.

ADDITIONAL READINGS

Tetteroo E, van der Graaf Y, Bosch JL, et al. Randomized comparison of primary stent placement versus angioplasty with selective stent placement in patients with iliac artery obstructive disease. In: Tetteroo E, ed. *The Dutch Iliac Stent Trial: Results from a Randomized Multicenter Study.* Utrecht, The Netherlands: FEBO Druk B.V. Enschede, 1997;69–89.

Whalen E. Palmaz stents in the renal arteries: results of US multicenter trial. *Am J Roent.* 1992;159(3):639–645. [Abstract]

21

Endovascular Approaches for Aortoiliac Occlusive Disease

Peter H. Lin, MD, and Alan B. Lumsden, MD

INTRODUCTION

The first report of percutaneous transluminal dilatation of vascular occlusion by Dotter and Judkins[1] in 1964 represents the beginning of a new era in the endovascular management of aortoiliac occlusive disease. Early studies of transluminal angioplasty used a series of sequential dilators introduced over a guidewire to expand the intraluminal space.[2] This technique was met with limited success due to the inability to maintain luminal patency. The introduction of an angioplasty balloon made of polyvinyl chloride (PVC) in 1976 by Gruntzig and Hopff[3] followed by the subsequent rigid balloons composed of polyethylene and polyethylene terephthalate (PET) marked a significant advance in endovascular therapy, as the latter angioplasty balloons displayed a low compliance and high radial force in a fully inflated condition. Since the early 1980s, transluminal balloon angioplasty has evolved into an important treatment modality in the treatment of peripheral vascular disease.

Despite numerous studies that demonstrate the short-term clinical success of transluminal angioplasty, it has several limitations due in part to the architectural variation of atherosclerotic lesions. Early restenosis or occlusion following angioplasty may occur due to either elastic recoil of the arterial wall or intimal dissection.[4] Vessels that are heavily calcified, completely occluded, or contain ulcerated plaques may not be amenable to balloon angioplasty. Moreover, residual luminal irregularities following angioplasty may occasionally trigger mural thrombus formation, leading to thrombotic occlusion.[5,6] Late restenosis following angioplasty may occur as a result of intimal hyperplasia or atherosclerotic progression.[7,8] In an effort to deal with these limitations of transluminal angioplasty, the intravascular stent was developed as a means of maintaining vessel patency against the restenotic process as well as improving the clinical outcome of balloon angioplasty. In certain selective situations, intraluminal stenting is a highly effective modality in overcoming elastic recoil of the arterial wall, stabilizing intimal dissection at the site of angioplasty, and maintaining luminal patency of arteries with calcified and eccentric atherosclerotic plaques.

GENERAL PRINCIPLES OF INTRAVASCULAR STENTS

Because stenting provides a mechanical scaffold within a stenotic vessel to maintain luminal patency, certain characteristics are desirable in an intravascular stent. The stent should be flexible and durable, with a simple deployment mechanism. The stent device should have a relatively small profile before deployment, along with the capacity to expand to a larger profile once fully deployed. Moreover, the stent should have noticeable radiographic opacity to facilitate visualization. The structural material used in the stent construction should have a low thrombogenic nature and a high radial force on expansion. Finally, the ideal stent should be biocompatible to promote endothelialization without causing intimal hyperplasia.

The physical property of intravascular stents can be separated based on two distinct design concepts: self-expanding stents and balloon-expandable stents. Within each of these categories, there are numerous stents with different structural materials, deployment devices, and biocompatible characteristics. Although many of these stents are currently under clinical trials, only the Wallstent (Schneider Inc., Minneapolis, MN)) and the Palmaz stent (Cordis Corp, Warren, NJ) have been approved by the Food and Drug Administration (FDA) for iliac artery placement. The characteristics of these two stents, therefore, are discussed in this chapter.

Self-Expanding Stents

Self-expanding stents are generally manufactured with stents constrained within a delivery sheath. The stent device is placed intravascularly through an introducer sheath and over a guidewire for deployment. The deployment is achieved by withdrawing the constraining sheath while keeping the stent in position, which permits the stent to self-expand and anchor to the vessel lumen. These stents are generally noted for their ease of deployment with a high degree of flexibility. Compared to the balloon-expandable stents, however, they may have lower hoop strength, which is the resistance to radial compression. Most delivery systems of self-expanding stents have a smaller diameter as compared to balloon-expandable stents. Examples of self-expanding stents include the Wallstent, the Gianturco-Z stent (Cook, Inc., Bloomington, IN), and the Mass double helix stent (Medinvent, Switzerland).

Another type of self-expanding stent is the nitinol stent, which consists of a nickel–titanium alloy. This is known as the *nitinol*, which has a unique temperature-associated memory property. The nitinol wires can be shaped into a coil spring configuration to serve as a stent when heated at 500°C temperature. As it cools down to 0°C temperature, the nitinol coil straightens into a linear alignment that can be constrained into a delivery catheter for stent deployment. The exposure to warm body temperature following deployment causes the nitinol stent to resume its original coil spring shape. Although the nitinol stents are not presently approved by the FDA for intravascular application, numerous clinical studies have demonstrated the early clinical efficacy of the nitinol stents in iliac lesions.[9–11] Common examples of nitinol stents include the Symphony stent (Boston Scientific Vascular, Waterstown, MA), Cragg stent (Mintech, French), Rabkin stent (National research Center of Surgery, Russia), Smart stent (Cordis Corp, Miami, FL), and Memotherm stent (Bard/Angiomed, Karlsruhe, Germany).

The Wallstent

The Wallstent, which is the most commonly used self-expanding stent in the United States, was approved by the FDA in 1996 for its 6- through 10-mm diameter stent size in iliac artery placements. It is composed of 16 to 20 thin, stainless steel alloy filaments braided into a flexible cylindrical tube. Because the attaching wires are not soldered to each other, the stent expands spontaneously by a spring mechanism and exerts a flexible movement in all directions. The flexible nature of the Wallstent contributes to its major advantage as it conforms to the tortuosity or angulation along the vessel course. Moreover, the Wallstent can be deployed in the iliac artery from a contralateral approach. Such flexibility, however, also created a disadvantage of this device, as significant shortening can occur once the stent is fully expanded. The tissue response to the Wallstent is similar to all stainless steel devices, which can induce intimal hyperplasia resulting in a varying degree of luminal wall thickening.[12,13] Because the stainless steel wires have a low radiopacity, the stent is more difficult to visualize under fluoroscopy than the Palmaz stent.[14,15]

Commonly used Wallstents for iliac artery application range from 8-, 10-, to 12-mm in diameter in a fully deployed state. Wallstents are available in various lengths, ranging from 50 to 150 cm. The flexible nature of such a stent allows it to be introduced into the arterial lumen using a relatively small introducer sheath. A 7F sheath is used for stents >10 mm in diameter, and a 9F sheath is needed for stents 12 mm in diameter. Because the deployment is achieved by withdrawing the constraining sheath to allow stent expansion, the final diameter is influenced by the stent flexibility and the elastic recoil of the stenotic vessel. If a residual stenosis remains following the stent deployment, additional expansion by balloon angioplasty may be performed to gain increased luminal diameter. The patency of side branches crossed by Wallstents varies in clinical series. Sapoval et al.[15] noted that the occlusion rate of stent-bridged side branches such as the internal iliac artery was 40% at 2 yr. In a study by Rousseau et al.,[16] in contrast, 90% of the bridged femoral collateral remained patent 2 yr following stent placement.

Balloon-Expandable Stents

The balloon-expandable stent is first mounted and compressed onto an angioplasty balloon. Once the stent is positioned intraluminally, it is deployed by inflating the balloon to expand the stent. Unlike a self-expanding stent, the balloon-expandable stent can be expanded further by a larger angioplasty balloon catheter beyond their predetermined diameter. Most of balloon-expandable stents are characterized by an excellent hoop strength due to the stent rigidity once deployed, which can be advantageous in treating stenotic vessels containing calcified plaques. The rigid property of such a stent, however, may create a technical challenge when treating lesions in tortuous vessels. Moreover, it does not permit a contralateral approach for iliac artery stenting. Common examples of balloon-expandable stents include the Palmaz stent (Johnson & Johnson Interventional Systems, Warren, NJ), Strecker stent (Boston Scientific Vascular, Waterstown, AIA), Gianturco–Roubin stent (Cook, Bloomington, IN), AVE stent (Arterial Vascular Engineering, Santa Rosa, CA), Wiktor Stent (Medtronic, San Diego, CA), and IntraStent (IntraTherapeutic, Minneapolis, MN).

The Palmaz Stent

The Palmaz stent is the most widely used balloon-expandable stent in the United States. It is made of stainless steel arranged in staggered rows of rectangular slots, with a wall thickness of 0.12 mm. Although it is available in various sizes, the FDA has currently approved the Palmaz P308 stent for the iliac artery placement. This is 3 cm in predilated length and can be expanded from 8 to 12 mm in diameter following expansion. The Palmaz stent is packaged from the manufacturer either premounted on an angioplasty balloon or alone, and can be mounted on a balloon catheter separately by the physician.

The deployment of the Palmaz stent requires a balloon angioplasty catheter 8 to 12 mm in diameter, a 7F to 10F introducer, and an introducer tube. A crimping tool may be used to crimp the stent on the balloon. The placement of an introducer tube enables the mounted catheter stent device to advance through the hemostatic valve and deliver to the lesion site. Once the fluoroscopy confirms the stent device is positioned within the stenotic lesion, the introducer sheath is slowly withdrawn, followed by balloon inflation to deploy the stent.

The rigid wire structure provides the Palmaz stent with an excellent radial strength against external compression, which minimizes elastic recoil from the vessel wall.[17,18] The rigidity of the stent keeps the wire mesh embedded within the vessel wall, which may facilitate endothelialization. The foreshortening of the Palmaz stent is minimal due in part to its inflexibility, which allows relatively precise deployment at the stenotic site. Short segmental iliac lesions are ideal for this type of stent. The diameter of the Palmaz stent can be adjusted based on the size of the balloon catheter. For instance, following the deployment of a P308 Palmaz stent using an 8 mm angioplasty balloon, it can be dilated to 12 mm in diameter using a larger balloon without stent recoil. However, stent distortion may occur as a result of overdilatation. The placement of the Palmaz stent in tortuous vessels can pose difficulty due to its inflexibility. The rigidity of the Palmaz stent is associated with the risk of stent collapse if external compression, such as vascular clamping, is applied to the deployment site of the vessel. Because of its rigid nature, stent placement across articular joints such as the shoulder or knee is generally discouraged.

INDICATIONS FOR STENT PLACEMENT

Indications approved by the FDA for iliac stent placement include (1) stenotic or occlusive atherosclerotic lesions, and (2) failed or inadequate balloon angioplasty in the iliac artery. The latter condition can be assessed by either angiographic or hemodynamic means. Angiographic detection of residual stenosis of ≥30%, unstable intimal flaps or dissection along the subintimal or medial layers are considered inadequate angioplasty

TABLE 21–1. COMMONLY ACCEPTED INDICATIONS FOR ILIAC ARTERY STENTING

Insufficient hemodynamic result of balloon angioplasty due to elastic recoil based on residual pressure gradient (>5 mm Hg in resting pressure gradient or >10 mm Hg in postvasodilatation pressure gradient)
Massive or lumen-obstructing dissection
Treatment of chronic occlusions
Iliac artery ulceration associated with symptoms
Restenoses after previously performed balloon angioplasty (>30% residual stenosis)
Complex lesions for which primary stenting may give more satisfactory results

results that warrant intraluminal stent placement. A transstenotic pressure gradient of >5 mm Hg or postvasodilatation pressure gradient of >10 mm Hg following angioplasty is also considered an indication for iliac stent placement.

In addition to the FDA-approved indications for iliac artery stenting, certain conditions may also be considered reasonable for stent placement. Early restenosis following balloon angioplasty is suitable for stent placement. The patency of the iliac artery following angioplasty ranged from 65% to 81% in 2 yr and is affected by numerous factors, such as the degree of stenosis, the length of narrowing, and the distal vessel patency.[4,8] Restenosis of the iliac artery frequently occurs at the original angioplasty site,[7,8] which can be caused by neointimal hyperplasia or rapid atherosclerotic progression. Iliac artery stenting in such a condition may delay the restenotic process.

Primary stent placement, as opposed to stenting following inadequate angioplasty, has been used more frequently in the treatment of otherwise difficult iliac lesions. Nearly or totally occluded iliac arteries may be appropriate for primary stenting because angioplasty alone in these situations generally yields poor long-term patency rates.[8,19,20] Stenotic iliac vessels with ulcerative plaques may cause distal embolization when treated with balloon angioplasty. It is appropriate to perform primary stent placement in such a condition to prevent plaque dislodgment. Moreover, primary stenting may be used as an adjunctive procedure to improve iliac inflow when combined with a planned infrainguinal bypass operation.[21] Commonly accepted indications for iliac artery stenting are listed in Table 21–1.

RECOMMENDED GUIDELINES FOR ILIAC STENTING BASED ON MORPHOLOGIC STRATIFICATION

Recommended guidelines for iliac stenting was published by the TASC (TransAtlantic Inter-Society Consensus) working group in 2000,[22] based on the morphologic stratification of iliac lesions, which are listed in Table 21–2. The stratification was based on the length, location, focal involvement, and degree of stenosis of the iliac vessels. The recommended treatment of choice for type A aortoiliac lesion, which contains a single stenosis <3 cm in the common or external iliac artery, is either balloon angioplasty or stent placement. Surgical intervention, rather than endovascular treatment, was recommended for the type D lesion, which includes either iliac occlusion or diffuse multiple

TABLE 21–2. MORPHOLOGIC STRATIFICATION OF ILIAC LESIONS FOR ENDOVASCULAR THERAPY

Type A iliac lesions	
	Single stenosis <3 cm of the common iliac artery (CIA) or external iliac artery (EIA) (unilateral/bilateral)
Type B iliac lesions	
	Single stenosis 3–10 cm in length, not extending into the common femoral artery (CFA)
	Total of two stenosis <5 cm long in the CIA and/or EIA and not extending into the CFA
	Unilateral CIA occlusion
Type C iliac lesions	
	Bilateral 5- to 10-cm long stenosis of the CIA and/or EIA, not extending into the CFA
	Unilateral EIA occlusion not extending into the CFA
	Unilateral EIA stenosis extending into the CFA
	Bilateral CIA occlusion
Type D iliac lesions	
	Diffuse, multiple unilateral stenoses involving the CIA, EIA, and CFA (usually >10 cm)
	Unilateral occlusion involving both the CIA and EIA
	Bilateral EIA occlusions
	Diffuse disease involving the aorta and both iliac arteries
	Iliac stenoses in a patient with an abdominal aortic aneurysm or other lesion requiring aortic or iliac surgery

(Developed by the TASC Working Group)[22]

stenotic iliac lesions. Although endovascular treatment is more commonly used in type B lesion and surgical revascularization is more commonly performed in type C lesion, currently available clinical studies are insufficient to provide a definitive treatment recommendation for these two lesion types.

CONTRAINDICATIONS TO STENT PLACEMENT

Table 21–3 summarizes the contraindications to intravascular stent placement. Arterial perforation as a result of balloon angioplasty, as evidenced by contrast extravasation, is considered a contraindication to intra-arterial stent placement. Stent placement in such a condition may lead to severe hemorrhagic complications or pseudoaneurysm formation. Stent placement should also be avoided in aneurysmal arteries, as persistent blood flow around the stent may lead to further aneurysm expansion. In addition, patients with hypercoagulable disorders should not undergo intra-arterial placement. In these patients, an intra-arterial stent may trigger the coagulation cascade resulting in early thrombosis in the stented regions.[10,23,24] Because balloon-expandable stents such as the Palmaz stents are relatively rigid in structure, these stents are less ideal in tortuous vessels. Self-expanding stents, such as the Wallstents, have greater flexibility and are more appropriate in vessels with marked tortuosity. Severely calcified arteries often are not amenable to balloon angioplasty; similarly, stent placement should not be expected to

TABLE 21–3. CONTRAINDICATIONS TO INTRAVASCULAR STENT PLACEMENT

Arterial perforation with contrast extravasation in the target vessel
Severely calcified vessels
Marked vessel tortuosity (not a contraindication for the Wallstent placement)
Target lesions cross areas of flexion, such as the inguinal ligament, knee, or shoulder
Coexistent aneurysmal disease requiring surgical intervention
Successful balloon angioplasty
Presence of hypercoagulable disorder
Long-standing arterial occlusion
Target vessels that may serve as the proximal or distal site of a bypass grafting procedure

restore the normal vessel lumen because stent deployment requires the basic techniques in balloon angioplasty. Long-standing arterial occlusion is considered a relative contraindication to stent placement. In this condition, the risk of plaque embolization resulting from stent expansion may outweigh the potential benefit of arterial recanalization. Finally, stent deployment should be avoided in arteries that may serve as either the proximal or distal site of a bypass grafting procedure. Application of vascular clamps in a stented artery may not only cause significant damage to the arterial wall, but also crush the stent so severely that further stent expansion may not be possible. If vascular control is needed in a stented artery, intraluminal occlusion balloon catheter should be used rather than vascular clamps.

COMPLICATIONS OF INTRALUMINAL STENT PLACEMENT

Because the deployment of a Palmaz stent requires the physical mounting of the stent on a balloon catheter, accidental dislodgment of the Palmaz stent from the catheter delivery system has been reported.[25] Moreover, a larger introducer sheath is needed for Palmaz stent placement, complications related to the puncture sites including hematoma,[24–29] arterial dissection,[25,28] and rupture of the artery[25,28] have been reported. Unlike the self-expanding stents, which constantly exert an outward radial force, external compression on the Palmaz stents due to vascular clamping injury can result in permanent stent deformity.[28] Although short-term failure of the Palmaz stent is mainly thrombosis in the stented vessel, the long-term patency can be adversely affected by restenosis induced by intimal hyperplasia. Several studies reported factors associated with stented artery thrombosis, which include iliac artery occlusion, multiple stent deployment, and hypercoagulable disorders.[14,28] Stent placement in an occluded iliac artery is particularly prone to restenosis, due in part the lack of an endothelial lining in the occluded vessel. Deployment of the Palmaz stent may further denude the intimal lining, thereby reducing the protective antithrombotic function of endothelium. Moreover, intimal hyperplasia may be induced by either under- or overdeployment of the Palmaz stent, presumably due in part to flow disturbance or endothelial injury.[25,28] Although flow abnormalities may occur at the proximal and distal stented segment, restenosis typically occurs at the initial vessel narrowing or occlusion sites.

TABLE 21–4. COMPLICATIONS ASSOCIATED WITH INTRAVASCULAR STENT PLACEMENT

Local complications
Hematoma
Pseudoaneurysm
AV fistula
Plaque distal embolization
Stent dislodgment in the delivery system
Stent migration and embolization
Stent misplacement
Contrast allergic reaction
Vessel perforation
Side-branch occlusion
Accelerated intimal hyperplasia
Extrinsic compression of the stent
Stent infection

Complications associated with the Wallstent in the treatment of iliac occlusive disease have also been reported. The incidence of distal embolization following the stent placement ranged from 2.4% to 7.8%.[30,31] The flexibility of the Wallstent is associated with foreshortening during deployment, which may lead to stent misplacement. Similar to the Palmaz stent, acute thrombosis and late restenosis also occur in the Wallstent. The regions of restenosis in the Wallstent generally occur in either the proximal, middle, or distal portion of the stented segment, rather than the entire stented lesion.[30]

As with all radiographic intervention, transient contrast-induced renal failures can develop following stent placement. Moreover, postprocedural mortality secondary to myocardial or cerebral infarction have also been reported.[25,28] A study by Palmaz and colleagues[25] reported two deaths related to contrast reaction. Several studies noted a 30-day mortality rate following iliac stenting ranging from 1.2% to 1.9%.[25,28] Table 21–4 summarizes the possible complications associated with intravascular stent placement.

CLINICAL SERIES

Palmaz Stents

Although iliac artery occlusive disease responds favorably to percutaneous balloon angioplasty, with 2-yr patency rates exceeding 80% in most series,[4,8,31–34] the 5-yr results are less satisfactory, and range from 20% to 76%.[8,32] Numerous factors, including distal vessel runoff, occlusion versus stenosis, and vessel restenosis, can affect the outcome of the intervention. The majority of long-term failure results from neointimal hyperplasia or atherosclerotic progression.[4,7,8,19,32] Several series have examined the intraluminal stent placement in the treatment of aortoiliac occlusive disease to improve long-term patency.

Since the FDA issued its approval of the Palmaz stent for the adjunctive use on iliac artery angioplasty, numerous studies have shown excellent clinical success. The indications include suboptimal results of iliac angioplasty based on intraluminal pressure gradient, restenosis, intimal flap or dissection, and stenotic or occlusive iliac disease. The results of most series generally are not separated by these indications but rather are combined to demonstrate the overall clinical outcomes. Palmaz and colleagues[25] presented the largest series using the Palmaz stents in the iliac artery in 486 patients who underwent 587 iliac artery stenting procedures in 17 institutions. Seventy percent (70%) of patients in this series presented with intermittent claudication with short iliac lesions (<3 cm), and the remaining patients had tissue loss or rest pain. Follow-up at 12, 24, and 43 mo showed patency rates of 90.9%, 84.1%, and 68.6%, respectively. Although these results demonstrated the benefit of iliac stenting in improving early clinical outcome when compared to balloon angioplasty alone,[5,8] several issues must be considered when interpreting these data. The mean follow-up was relatively short (13.3 mo), due in part to the infrequent patient entry during the early phase of the trial. Moreover, 75% of the participants had follow-up of 12 mo or less, and approximately 20% of all patients underwent postprocedural angiogram ranging from 1 to 35 mo following the stent placement. Follow-up angiogram demonstrated a mean loss of luminal diameter of 15% and a restenosis rate of 3.3% (<50% of original stent diameter). Two-thirds of the patients received one iliac stent placement, whereas the remaining patients received two or more Palmaz stents in the iliac artery. Finally, the overall complication rate was 10%, with the majority of complications related to the access site. Acute thrombosis and pseudoaneurysm formation occurred at the access site in 5 and 2 patients, respectively. The 30 day mortality rate was 1.9%.

Henry and colleagues[24] reported the Palmaz stent application in 184 patients who received 230 iliac stent placements. Mean follow-up was 35 mo and consisted of angiography at 4 to 6 mo following stent placement (in 98% of patients) and serial duplex scan studies. Similar to the study reported by Palmaz et al.,[25] the majority of patients (89%) included in this series were treated for claudication. Immediate clinical improvement was achieved in 91% of patients. The primary patency rates at 1, 2, and 3 yr were 94%, 91%, and 86%, respectively, which were superior to those of balloon angioplasty.[8,35] More than 70% of patients received one stent placement, whereas the remaining patients had two or more Palmaz stents in the iliac artery. The restenosis rate in the iliac artery was 0.5% at 6 mo. The authors reported predictors for success in iliac artery stenting, which included lesion length of <3 cm, artery diameter >6 cm, and absence of secondary arterial lesions.

Cikrit and colleagues[36] reported their experience with Palmaz stent application in iliac artery disease with long-term follow-up. In 39 iliac occlusive lesions, the placement of the Palmaz stent significantly decreased the intraluminal pressure gradient from 32 mm Hg to 1 mm Hg. Similar improvement of ankle/brachial pressure index was also noted following stent deployment, which increased from 0.53 to 0.8. Life-table analysis showed cumulative patency rates of 1, 3, and 5 yr at 91%, 91%, and 86%, respectively.

Although iliac stent placement is traditionally reserved for situations of suboptimal or failed angioplasty results, the potential benefits of primary treatment of iliac lesions using the Palmaz stents have also been investigated. Early report by Bonn and colleagues[37] noted that primary stenting using the Palmaz stents for iliac lesions had early technical success without incurring any additional complications compared to angioplasty alone. A similar finding was also reported by Williams and colleagues,[27] who found that 73 patients underwent a primary stenting procedure for aortoiliac lesions, with an overall complication rate of 13%. They also demonstrated an initial cost savings of 25% to 66% compared with surgical interventions.

A prospective randomized multicenter trial comparing the results of primary Palmaz stenting versus angioplasty alone for iliac lesions was reported by Richter and colleagues.[38] Patients in both groups had similar mean transstenotic pressure gradients prior to the treatment. However, patients who were treated with primary Palmaz stenting had significantly less pressure gradients following the stent placement. At the 2-yr follow-up, the restenosis rates in the angioplasty group and the stent group were 27% and 14%, respectively. Twenty-eight percent (28%) of the angioplasty group required additional intervention for iliac restenosis at 3 yr, in contrast to 2% of the stent group who required reintervention. The improved patency rates and clinical outcomes of primary stent placement using the Palmaz stents have been further validated by other studies, including primary stenting of the infrarenal aorta.[27,39–42]

A study reported by Sullivan and colleagues[18] examined the outcome of 424 limbs in 288 patients treated with balloon angioplasty and primary stenting for occlusive iliac lesions. Palmaz stents were used in 86% of cases, whereas Wallstents were used in the remaining 14% of cases. Angiographic patency at 1 and 2 yr were 88% and 75%, respectively. The authors noted factors that affected clinical outcomes favorably, including younger age, higher degree of initial iliac stenosis, and patent ipsilateral superficial femoral artery.

Wallstents

The Wallstents has been studied extensively throughout Europe during the 1990s, due in part to the collaborative effort of the European Wallstent Peripheral Artery Implant Study. In the initial series by Gunther and colleagues,[43] 31 patients with iliac artery disease (including 16 iliac occlusions) underwent Wallstent placement based on inadequate iliac angioplasty. Restenosis with stent occlusion occurred in 1 patient after 6 mo. The benefit of stent placement in improving poor angioplasty results was highlighted by the authors. In the subsequent update study, the same authors[23] reported the results of 100 occlusive iliac lesions treated with the Wallstent. Stent placement was based on poor balloon angioplasty results, which included residual stenosis, iliac occlusion, and dissection. Ninety percent (90%) of the patients had claudication. Technical success was achieved in 97% of cases. The reduction of the iliac stenosis ranged from 30% to 50% following the stent placement. Follow-up angiography was performed on all symptomatic patients. The authors defined an angiographic stenosis as a >20% decrease from the original poststenting luminal diameter. The prevalence of clinically relevant stenosis was 5% and the angiographic prevalence of restenosis was 16% at 1 yr.

Martin and colleagues[44] reported results of a multicenter trial of the Wallstent in the 140 patients with iliac occlusive lesions. The average length of iliac lesions was <10 cm. The 6-mo angiographic patency was 93%. The results using the Wallstent were similar to those with the Palmaz stent in the treatment of iliac lesions. The primary patency rates at 1 and 2 yr were 81% and 71%, respectively; and secondary patency rates were 91% and 86%, respectively.

Murphy and colleagues[45] reported their finding of using the Wallstent in treating 94 iliac artery lesions. Indications for therapy included diffuse stenoses (>3 cm in length), chronic occlusions, failed angioplasty procedures, and dissections of the iliac arteries. Approximately half of the patients had claudication, and the remaining half had limb-threatening ischemia. Initial technical success was achieved in 91% of patients. Overall complication rate was 9%, which included iliac artery rupture, distal embolization, and groin hematoma. Primary patency rates at 1 and 2 yr were 78% and 53%, respectively. Secondary patency rates were 86% and 82%, respectively. The limb salvage rate for patients with limb-threatening ischemia was 98% at a mean follow-up of 14 mo. In a study that reported the long-term patency of Wallstent in treating iliac lesions, Sapoval and colleagues[15] included 101 occlusive iliac arteries. More than 95% of the lesions were treated for claudication. The primary and secondary patency rates at 4 yr were 80% and 61%, respectively. The authors reported factors associated with long-term angiographic failure, which included superficial femoral artery occlusion, a stent diameter <8 mm, two or more stents implanted, and continued tobacco consumption.

The application of the Wallstent as the primary treatment of iliac lesions was also examined. Vorwerk and Gunther[31] used the Wallstent as the primary treatment in 125 patients with a wide array of complex iliac lesions, which include iliac occlusion, long-segmental stenosis, aneurysm, ulcerated plaques, proximal iliac ostial lesions, eccentric stenosis, and acute complications of balloon angioplasty. Mechanical passage of the guidewire across the iliac occlusion was attempted prior to primary stent placement, which was successful in 63 of 85 patients. The cumulative patency rates at 6 and 24 mo were 100% and 89.4%, respectively. Although the overall complication rate was 4%, the major complications that required either percutaneous or surgical intervention occurred in 1.6% of patients. Iliac artery reocclusion as a result of lesion within or adjacent to the stented segment occurred in 6.5% of cases, and typically occurred >6 mo following the Wallstent deployment. Embolic complications following treatment of complete iliac artery occlusion continued during the course of this study, with an incidence of 4.7% during the follow-up period.

Vorwerk and colleagues[30] also studied the results of primary stenting using the Wallstent in the treatment of 103 patients with chronic iliac artery occlusions. No predilation of the iliac lesions was performed prior to stent placement. The duration of iliac artery occlusions was >3 mo in all patients, with an average occlusion length of 5.1 cm. All patients had symptoms that included claudication, rest pain, or trophic changes. Nearly all patients (99%) showed clinical improvement following the Wallstent placement. Initial success rate was 81%. Primary patency rates after 1, 2, and 4 yr were 87%, 83%, and 78%, respectively. Secondary patency rates after 1, 2, and 4 yr were 94%, 90%, and 88%, respectively. In another report by the same investigators,[46] primary stenting using the Wallstents was studied in 118 patients with iliac artery stenosis. The average length of the stenotic segment was 3 cm. More than 97% of patients showed clinical improvement, with an increase of mean ankle/brachial index from 0.58 to 0.92 following the stent placement. Primary patency rates after 1, 2, and 4 yr were 95%, 88%, and 82%, respectively. Secondary patency rates after 1, 2, and 4 yr were 96%, 93%, and 91%, respectively.

CONCLUSIONS

Intravascular stent placement has proved to be an invaluable tool in both the treatment of iliac occlusive disease and the management of complications of balloon angioplasty. Clinical application of iliac stents has also extended to treatment of patients with total iliac occlusion and restenosis. Although balloon angioplasty has met with limited success in treating totally occluded iliac arteries, the use of intravascular stents has improved the success rate to approximately 80% at 3 yr, with a late occlusion rate similar to that of stenotic lesions.[31,47] The benefit of primary stenting the iliac artery has been demonstrated in several series with a favorable 5-yr patency rate of >90%, which is comparable to conventional surgical reconstruction.[48,49] The main shortcoming of intravascular stenting is the induction of intimal hyperplasia leading to restenosis. The incidence of restenosis, as occurred within 1 yr following the stent placement, has been shown to occur in >20% of cases in most series.[12,43,50] A review by Palmaz[51] addressed several areas of research to improve the outcome of intravascular stenting. Development of new coating material for the stent surface can potentially minimize unwanted cellular proliferation and inherent stent thrombogenicity, particularly in small-caliber vessels.[52] Application of biodegradable or removable stents also constitutes promising alternatives to improve clinical results.[52–55] Adjunctive pharmacologic therapy, including new antithrombotic, antiplatelet, and anti-inflammatory agents, may provide a significant benefit in improving the clinical outcome of intravascular stenting.[56,57]

REFERENCES

1. Dotter CT, Judkins MP. Transluminal treatment of arteriosclerotic obstruction: description of a new technique and a preliminary report of its application. *Circulation.* 1964;30:654.
2. Porstman W. Ein neuer Korseh-Balloon katheter zur transluminalen Rekanalizationnach Dotter unter Besondeur Barucksichtigung von obliterationen an den Beckenarterien. *Radiol Diagn (Berl).* 1973;2:239.
3. Gruntzig A, Hopff M. Perkutane Rekanalisation chronischer arterieller Verschlussen-dt einem neuen Dilatationskatheter: modifikation der Dotter-Technik. *Dtsch Med Wochenschr.* 1974;99: 2502–2510.
4. Wilson SE, Wolf GL, Cross AP. Percutaneous transluminal angioplasty versus operation for peripheral arteriosclerosis. *J Vasc Surg.* 1989;9:1–9.
5. Becker G, Palmaz J, Rees C, et al. Angioplasty-induced dissections in human iliac arteries: Management with Palmaz balloon-expandable intraluminal stents. *Radiology.* 1990;176:31.
6. Gardiner G, Moyerovitz M, Strokes K, et al. Complications of transluminal angioplasty. *Radiology.* 1986;159:201.
7. Glover JL, Bendick PJ, Dilley RS et al. Efficacy of balloon catheter dilation for lower extremity atherosclerosis. *Surgery.* 1982;91:560–565.
8. Johnston KW, Rae M, Hogg-Johnston SA, et al. Five-year results of a prospective study of percutaneous transluminal angioplasty. *Ann Surg.* 1987;206:403–413.
9. Henry M, Amor M, Beyar R, et al. Clinical experience with a new Nitinol self-expanding stent in peripheral arteries. *J Endovasc Surg.* 1996;3:369–374.

10. Raza Z, Shaw JW, Stonebridge PA, McCollum PT. Management of iliac occlusions with a new self-expanding endovascular stent. *Eur J Vas Endovasc Surg.* 1998;15:439–443.
11. Hausegger KA, Cragg AH, Lammerj, et al. Iliac artery stent placement: clinical experience with nitinol stent. *Radiology.* 1994;190:199–202.
12. Rousseau H, Joffre F, Raillat C, et al. Self-expanding endovascular stent in experimental atherosclerosis. *Radiology.* 1989;170:773–778.
13. Vorwek D, Redha F, Neuerburg J, et al. Neointima formation following arterial placement of self-expanding stents of different radial force: experimental results. *Cardiovasc Intervent Radiol.* 1994;17:27–32.
14. Long A, Page P, Raynaud A, et al. Percutaneous iliac artery stent. Angiographic long-term follow-up. *Radiology.* 1991;180:771.
15. Sapoval M, Chatellier G, Long A, et al. Self-expandable stents for the treatment of iliac artery obstructive lesions: long-term success and prognostic factors. *Am J Roentgenol.* 1996;166:1173–1178.
16. Rousseau HP, Raillat CR, Joffre FG et al. Treatment of femoropopliteal stenoses by means of self-expandable endoprostheses: midterm results. *Radiology.* 1989;172:961–964.
17. Palmaz JC, Garcia O, Schatz RA, et al. Placement of balloon expandable stents in iliac arteries: first 171 patients. *Radiology.* 1990;174:969–975.
18. Sullivan TM, Childs MB, Bacharach JM, et al. Percutaneous transluminal angioplasty and primary stenting of the iliac arteries in 288 patients. *J Vasc Surg.* 1997;25:829–838.
19. Cambria RP, Faust G, Gusberg R, et al. Percutaneous angioplasty for peripheral arterial occlusive disease. *Arch Surg.* 1987;122:238–287.
20. Colapinto RF, Stronell RD, Johnston WK. Transluminal angioplasty of complete iliac obstruction. *AJR.* 1986;146:859–862.
21. Andros G. Interventional technology: intraoperative strategies and techniques. In Yao JST, Pearce WH, eds. *Technologies in vascular surgery,* Philadelphia: WB Saunders. 1992.
22. Management of Peripheral Arterial Disease (PAD) by TransAtlantic Inter-Society Consensus (TASC) Working Group. *J Vasc Surg.* 2000;31:S1–S296.
23. Gunther RW, Vorwerk D, Antonucci F, et al. Iliac artery stenosis or obstruction after unsuccessful balloon angioplasty: treatment with a self-expandable stent. *AJR.* 1991;156:389–393.
24. Henry M, Amor M, Ethevenot G, et al. Palmaz stent placement in iliac and femoropopliteal arteries: primary and secondary patency in 310 patients with 2–4 year follow-up. *Radiology.* 1995;197:167–174.
25. Palmaz JC, Laborde JC, Rivera FJ, et al. Stenting of the iliac arteries with the Palmaz stent: experience from a multicenter trial. *Cardiovasc Intervent Radiol.* 1992;15:291–297.
26. Cikrit DF, Becker GJ, Dalsing MC, et al. Early experience with the Palmaz expandable intraluminal stent in iliac artery stenosis. *Ann Vasc Surg.* 1991;5:150–155.
27. Williams JB, Watts PW, Nguyen VA, Peterson CL. Balloon angioplasty with intraluminal stenting as the initial treatment modality in aortoiliac occlusive disease. *Am J Surg.* 1994; 168:202–204.
28. Murphy KD, Encarnacion CE, Le VA, Palmaz JC. Iliac artery stent placement with the Palmaz stent: follow-up study. *J Visc Intervent Radiol.* 1995;6:321–329.
29. Bergeron B, Pinot JJ, Poyen V, et al. Long term results with the Palmaz stent in the superficial femoral artery. *J Endovasc Surg.* 1995;2:161–167.
30. Vorwerk D, Gunther RW, Schurmann WG, et al. Primary stent placement for chronic iliac artery occlusions: follow-up results in 103 patients. *Radiology.* 1995;194:745–749.
31. Vorwerk D, Gunther RW. Stent placement in iliac arterial lesions: three years of clinical experience with the Wallstent. *Cardiovasc Intervent Radiol.* 1992;15:285–290.

32. Stokes KR, Strunk HM, Campbel DR, et al. Five-year results of iliac and femoropopliteal angioplasty in diabetic patients. *Radiology.* 1990;174:977–982.
33. Kadir S, White RI, Kaufman SL, et al. Long-term results of aortoiliac angioplasty. *Surgery.* 1983;94:10–14.
34. Walden R, Siegel Y, Rubinstein ZJ, et al. Percutaneous transluminal angioplasty. *J Vasc Surg.* 1986;3:583–590.
35. Stanley B, Teague B, Raptis S, et al. Efficacy of balloon angioplasty of the superficial femoral artery and popliteal artery in the relief of leg ischemia. *J Vasc Surg.* 1996;23:679–685.
36. Cikrit DF, Gustafson PA, Dalsing MC, et al. Long-term follow-up of the Palmaz stent for iliac occlusive disease. *Surgery.* 1995;118:608–613.
37. Bonn J, Gardiner GA Jr, Shapiro MJ, et al. Palmaz vascular stent: initial clinical experience. *Radiology.* 1990;174:741–745.
38. Richter GM, Roeren T, Noeldge G, et al. Initial long-term results of a randomized 5-year study: iliac stent implantation versus PTA. *Vasa* 1992;35:192–193.
39. Diethrich EB, Santiago O, Gustafson G, et al.: Preliminary observations on the use of the Palmaz stent in the distal portion of the abdominal aorta. *Am Heart J* 1993;125:490–493.
40. Long A: Infrarenal aortic stents: initial clinical experience and angiographic follow up. *Cardiovasc Intervent Radiol.* 1993;16:203–206.
41. El Ashmaoui A: Angioplasty of the terminal aorta: follow up of 20 patients treated by PTA or PTA with stents. *Eur J Radiol.* 1991;13:113–116.
42. Roeren T: Stent angioplasty of the infrarenal aorta and aortic bifurcation. Clinical and angiographical results of a prospective study. *Radiology.* 1994;34:504–508.
43. Gunther RW, Vorwerk D, Bohndorf K, et al. Iliac and femoral artery stenoses and occlusions: treatment with intravascular stents. *Radiology.* 1989;172:725–730.
44. Martin EC, Katzen BT, Benenati JF, et al. Multicenter trial of the Wallstent in the iliac and femoral arteries. *J Vasc Intervent Radiol.* 1995;6:843–849.
45. Murphy TP, Webb MS, Larabiase RE. Percutaneous revascularization of complex iliac artery stenosis and occlusions with use of Wallstents: three-year experience. *J Vasc Intervent Radiol.* 1996;7:21–27.
46. Vorwerk D, Gunther R, Schurmann K, et al. Aortic and iliac stenoses: follow-up results of stent placement after insufficient balloon angioplasty in 118 cases. *Radiology.* 1996;198:45–49.
47. Rees CR, Palmaz JC, Garcia O, et al. Angioplasty and stenting of completely occluded iliac arteries. *Radiology.* 1989;172:953–959.
48. Richter GM, Roeren T, Brado M, et al. Results of randomized trial of PTA vs. primary stenting. Abstract presented at Fifth Annual Symposium on Vascular Diagnosis and Intervention, Heidelberg, Germany. January, 1993.
49. Onal B, Ilgit ET, Yucel C, et al. Primary stenting for complex atherosclerotic plaques in aortic and iliac stenoses. *Cardiovasc Intervent Radiol.* 1998;21:386–392.
50. Zollikofer CL, Antonucci F, Pfyffer M, et al. Arterial stent placement with use of the Wallstent: midterm results of clinical experience. *Radiology.* 1991;179:449–456.
51. Palmaz JC. Intravascular stents: tissue–stent interactions and design considerations. *AJR.* 1993;160:613–618.
52. deJaegere PP, de Feyter PJ. Endovascular stents: preliminary clinical results and future development. *Clin Cardiol.* 1993;16:369–378.
53. Ozaki Y, Violaris AG, Serruys PW. New stent technologies. *Prog Cardiovasc Dis.* 1996; 39:129–140.
54. Bertrand OF, Sipehia R, Mongrain R, et al. Biocompatibility aspects of new stent technology. *J Am Coll Cardiol.* 1998;32:562–571.
55. Tanguay JF, Zidar JP, Phillips HR 3rd, Stack RS. Current status of biodegradable stents. *Cardiol Clin.* 1994;12:699–713.

56. Urban P, Macaya C, Rupprecht HJ, et al. Randomized evaluation of anticoagulation versus antiplatelet therapy after coronary stent implantation in high-risk patients: the multicenter aspirin and ticlopidine trial after intracoronary stenting. *Circulation.* 1998;98:2126–2132.
57. Schömig A, Neumann FJ, Kastrati A, et al. A randomized comparison of antiplatelet and anticoagulant therapy after the placement of coronary-artery stents. *N Engl J Med.* 1996;334: 1084.

22

Current Consensus on Carotid Bifurcation Angioplasty and Stenting

*Frank J. Veith, MD, Max Amor, MD, Takao Ohki, MD, and The Consensus Conference Participants**

Carotid bifurcation angioplasty and stenting (CBAS) represents a relatively new and controversial treatment for carotid bifurcation arteriosclerotic lesions. Several single center results have been promising.[1] However, others have observed an unacceptably high incidence of periprocedural embolic strokes,[2] and angioplasty and stenting of carotid bifurcation lesions in an *ex vivo* model have been shown to generate a large amount of intraluminal particulate debris.[3]

Recommendations regarding the current role of CBAS vary widely. On one extreme are clinicians who advocate near-universal replacement of carotid endarterectomy (CEA) by CBAS and widespread use of carotid stenting, even by clinicians with little or no experience in the management of patients with carotid disease. On the other extreme are clinicians who condemn CBAS as a dangerous and unproved treatment that rarely, if ever, should be used to replace CEA.

To resolve this controversy and these conflicting recommendations, it was decided to hold a consensus conference on this topic. The organizers of this conference (Frank J. Veith and Max Amor) elected to hold this conference at the time of the annual Montefiore–Einstein Vascular Surgery Symposium, when many leaders in the CBAS field would be in New York. These leaders, along with several other experts representing the disciplines of vascular surgery, interventional radiology, interventional cardiology, and neurosurgery, agreed to participate in the conference and answer before the conference a list of key questions about the present role of CBAS. These questions and their answers would serve as a focus for discussion at the conference.

* These experts are listed in Table 22–1.

TABLE 22–1. PARTICIPANTS

Radiologists	Cardiologists	Surgeons
Amman Bolia, UK	Michel Henry, France	Hugh G. Beebe, USA
John J. Connors, USA	Gary S. Roubin, USA	Patrice F. Bergeron, France
Robert D.G. Ferguson, Canada	Sanjay S. Yadav, USA	Peter R.F. Bell, UK
Barry T. Katzen, USA		Edward B. Diethrich, USA
Klaus Matthias, Germany		Robert W. Hobson II, USA
Jacques Theron, France		L. Nelson Hopkins, USA
Mark H. Wholey, USA		Takao Ohki, USA

The conference participants, 17 in number, represented the best and brightest leaders in the field with the widest experience and greatest interest in CBAS (Table 22–1). Participants from five different countries were involved in the consensus effort. They included 7 interventional radiologists, 3 interventional cardiologists, 6 vascular surgeons, and 1 neurosurgeon. All 17 had an endovascular orientation, and all but 3 were major endovascular therapists. All 17 had an interest in CBAS, had performed important clinical or laboratory studies in the field, and had published and lectured widely on this topic.

The goal of the consensus process was to reach agreement on as many crucial questions relating to CBAS as possible. To this end, these 17 participants were asked before the conference to provide answers to 15 key questions regarding CBAS. All 17 participants provided these answers. One participant posed 3 additional questions that were also asked and answered by all 17 participants.

The answers to these 18 questions were collected, analyzed, and summarized for presentation to the participants at the conference. The intent was to discuss both the questions and the answers in an effort to reach agreement or consensus on as many questions and issues related to CBAS as possible. In the course of the conference discussions, 2 of the original questions were modified slightly to facilitate the attainment of consensus. This brought the total number of questions answered to 20.

It was decided that consensus or agreement was reached if 12 or more of the 17 responding participants agreed on the response to a question. If 10 or 11 of the 17 participants agreed on a response, that response was considered to represent near-consensus or prevailing opinion. Near-consensus was also achieved when 9 respondents agreed on a response about which 2 or 3 where uncertain and with which 5 or 6 disagreed. If only 9 or less of the 17 participants agreed on a response to a question, that response was considered an area of divided opinion, disagreement, or uncertainty.

RESULTS

Consensus

Consensus or agreement was reached on the answers to 9 of the original 18 questions and the 2 derivative questions posed at the conference. It was agreed as follows:

1. CBAS should not currently be recommended for widespread practice; that is, the procedure should not become the general standard of care (14 of the 17 participants).
2. Widespread application of CBAS should await the results of randomized prospective trials (12 of the 17 participants).
3. CBAS should not currently be considered appropriate only for low-risk patients (16 of the 17 participants).
4. High-level neuro-rescue skills and techniques must currently be available in the institution in which CBAS is performed (12 of the 17 participants). Several experts commented that these skills could be possessed by individuals other than those performing the CBAS procedure.
5. The optimal stent for use in CBAS has not been defined (13 of the 17 participants).
6. Assuming equivalent results for CBAS and CEA could be shown, CBAS should be offered to patients in some circumstances (14 of the 17 participants).
7. CBAS should not be offered to patients requiring treatment of carotid bifurcation stenosis in *all* circumstances (13 of the 17 participants).
8. Five indications for CBAS were agreed on for patients requiring treatment for carotid bifurcation stenoses. These indications were as follows:
   a. High-risk symptomatic patients
   b. Recurrent stenosis
   c. Previous radical neck dissection or cervical irradiation
   d. High bifurcation or extent of the lesion
   e. Patients with indications for CEA who are unfit for surgery
9. Five contraindications to CBAS were agreed on, as follows:
   a. Intraluminal thrombus
   b. Complex bifurcation lesions (long or multifocal lesions or an angulated internal carotid artery)
   c. Extensive aortic or brachiocephalic trunk plaque or calcification, or severe tortuosity of the aortic arch vessels
   d. Ringlike heavy calcification of the carotid bifurcation
   e. Neurologically unstable patient or a patient who suffered a stroke within 3 weeks of the intended CBAS
10. When cerebral protection devices were available, CBAS should only be performed with some form of such device (all 12 of the participants present at the oral conference).
11. Adequate stents and technology for performing CBAS are currently available, when effective cerebral protection devices become available.

Near-Consensus

Near-consensus was reached on the answers to 6 additional questions. These expressions of prevailing opinion were as follows:

1. Optimal techniques for performing CBAS are not currently defined (11 of the 17 participants).

2. CBAS is currently appropriate only for high-risk patients (11 of 17 participants).
3. CBAS is not currently appropriate for high- and low-risk patients (10 of the 17 participants).
4. CBAS operators with complication rates equivalent to CEA should presently be able to offer some patients a stenting option (11 of the 17 participants).
5. CBAS currently can be performed without a cerebral protection device (because in the United States, no such device is available). (Nine participants held this view and 3 were uncertain; 5 participants felt that CBAS should only be performed with some form of cerebral protection.)
6. Adequate stents and technology for performing CBAS are currently available (10 of the 17 participants).

Divided Opinion

Opinion was divided on the answers to 3 of the 20 questions. These answers reflected disagreement or areas of uncertainty. These areas were as follows:

1. The need for an FDA investigational device exemption (IDE) in the United States, or an equivalent approval elsewhere. The FDA has expressed the opinion that such an IDE is necessary to perform CBAS in the United States.[4] However, only 8 of the 17 participants agreed with this position.
2. The proportion of patients requiring treatment for carotid bifurcation disease that is presently acceptable for CBAS. This varied from <5% to approximately 100%, with a mean of 44%. There were wide ranges within specialties (radiologists: <5%, 6%, 15%, 80%, 9%, ~100%, and uncertain, mean 49%; cardiologists: 40%, 80%, 95%, mean 72%; and surgeons: 5%, 10%, 20%, 20%, 35%, 60%, and uncertain, mean 25%).
3. The proportion of patients requiring treatment for carotid bifurcation disease that is presently best treated by CBAS. This varied from <3% to approximately 100%, with a mean of 34%. Again, there were wide ranges within the three specialties (radiologists: 3%, <5%, 15%, 45%, 90%, ~100%, and uncertain, mean 43%; cardiologists: 25%, 80%, and uncertain, mean 53%; and surgeons: <3%, <5%, 5%, 15%, 20%, 25%, and 50%, mean 18%).

Thus, of the 18 questions originally proposed to the conference participants, consensus or agreement with regard to the answers was attained on 9 questions and near-consensus on 6 questions. The answers to the 3 remaining questions reflected divided opinion or wide ranges of opinion based on conflicting views, uncertainty, or actual disagreement. In addition, 2 derivative questions were posed at the conference, and the answers to both of these modified questions were converted from "prevailing opinion" to consensus. Thus, consensus was reached on 11 of 20 questions, or 55% of the answers to all of these key questions. Near-consensus was reached on 6 of the 20 questions, an additional 30%. Therefore, the consensus process reflected agreement on 85% of the crucial questions posed. This agreement should be helpful to all investigators in the field, and should provide a guide to primary-care physicians and various specialists who are called on to treat patients with carotid stenosis or to advise such patients on how they should view the role of CBAS at the present time and until more accurate scientific information becomes available.

ACKNOWLEDGMENTS

This work was supported by grants from the US Public Health Service (HL 02990-05), the James Hilton Manning and Emma Austin Manning Foundation, the Anna S. Brown Trust, and the New York Institute for Vascular Studies.

NOTE

A more complete resume of this Consensus Conference will be published in the *Journal of Vascular Surgery* and a full description of the Consensus Conference including chapters written by each participant will appear in a book published by Marcel Dekker Inc.

REFERENCES

1. Wholey MH, Wholey M, Bergeron P, et al. Current global status of carotid artery stent placement. *Cathet Cardiovasc Diagn.* 1998;44:1–6.
2. Naylor AR, Bolia A, Abbott RJ, et al. Randomized study of carotid angioplasty and stenting versus carotid endarterectomy: a stopped trial. *J Vasc Surg.* 1998;28:326–334.
3. Ohki T, Marin ML, Lyon RT, et al. *Ex vivo* carotid artery bifurcation stenting: correlation of lesion characteristics with embolic potential. *J Vasc Surg.* 1998;27:463–471.
4. Callahan TJ, Spyker D, Sapirstein W. Concern about safety of carotid angioplasty. *Stroke.* 1996;27:2144–2145.

23

Carotid Angioplasty and Stenting

The Cleveland Clinic Experience

Kenneth Ouriel, MD

The first carotid repair for symptomatic bifurcation atherosclerosis was performed in 1951 by Carrea and coworkers.[1] Three years thereafter, DeBakey first used an endarterectomy technique to treat carotid disease,[2] heralding the era of surgical carotid repair that has culminated in the performance of almost 200,000 carotid endarterectomies annually.

Carotid endarterectomy (CEA) has been investigated with a wide array of well-designed and well-executed clinical trials. In fact, a landmark trial was organized in 1959 to compare the surgical and medical management of carotid disease.[3] This multicenter, randomized study was organized within a decade of Carrea and coworkers'[1] initial report of carotid repair, and the results of 1200 patients appeared in a series of publications in the late 1960s and early 1970s.[4]

Despite the findings of this large trial, enthusiasm for carotid repair waned over the following decade. In the late 1980s, however, a series of clinical trials were instituted, including the North American Symptomatic Carotid Endarterectomy Trial (NASCET)[5] the European Carotid Surgery Trial (ECST), the Veterans Administration (VA) symptomatic endarterectomy trial,[6] the VA asymptomatic carotid endarterectomy trial,[7] and the Asymptomatic Carotid Artery Surgery Trial (ACAS). In spite of questions regarding its efficacy at the commencement of every trial, the final data supported the use of CEA each time.

With the demonstration of the efficacy of coronary angioplasty and stenting, investigators became interested in a percutaneous treatment for carotid disease. The large number of patients with suitable carotid lesions sparked interest on the part of industry, and, despite a national "noncoverage" policy for carotid angioplasty by the Health Care Financing Administration, carotid stenting became one of the most widely discussed and hotly debated topics of recent years. Interventional cardiologists, well versed in percutaneous angioplasty and with nothing to lose and much to gain, were quick to embrace the new technology. Vascular surgeons, by contrast, viewed carotid angioplasty as a rather crude and yet unproved threat to the meticulous procedure of CEA, one of the mainstays of contemporary peripheral vascular surgical practice. With neurologists in the middle, a conflict ensued, the resolution of which could be achieved only through the completion of well-controlled comparisons of the two treatment modalities.

ENDARTERECTOMY AS STANDARD THERAPY FOR CAROTID DISEASE

Carotid endarterectomy is a well-proved intervention for carotid disease. The results of numerous clinical trials have documented its safety and efficacy such that it remains the standard of care for patients with severely stenotic extracranial lesions, regardless of whether the patient is symptomatic. Nevertheless, the excellent results achieved with the procedure appear to be quite dependent on the baseline medical status of the patient. Relatively healthy patients, not unexpectedly, do very well with open surgical repair of carotid lesions. The treatment of medically compromised patients, however, is associated with a much greater risk of complications, as illustrated in a review of more than 3000 patients undergoing CEA at the Cleveland Clinic Foundation between 1988 and 1998 (Figure 23–1). In this analysis of a consecutive series of patients, the risk of the

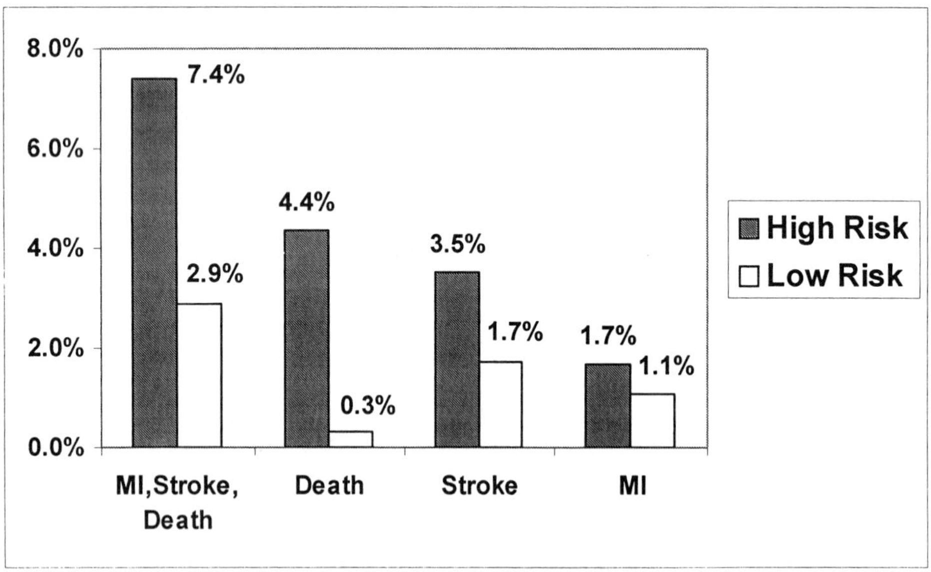

Figure 23–1. The risk of stroke, myocardial infarction (MI), and death, as composite endpoints and separately, in 3061 high- and low-risk patients undergoing carotid endarterectomy (CEA) at the Cleveland Clinic.[5]

composite endpoint stroke, myocardial infarction, or death was quite satisfactory in patients who were medically fit. By contrast, outcome was poorer in patients manifesting one or more baseline comorbidities, including significant coronary artery disease, history of congestive heart failure, chronic obstructive lung disease, and chronic renal insufficiency. The risk of perioperative morbidity and mortality was substantial in these high-risk patients. The risk of perioperative death was elevated by a factor of >5; stroke or myocardial infarction each by a factor of 2; and the composite endpoint of death, stroke, or myocardial infarction by a factor of almost 3.

We have interpreted the Cleveland Clinic data to suggest that, in most cases, CEA is a procedure with an extremely low rate of complications. In studies that specifically exclude high-risk patients from eligibility—for example, the NASCET and ACAS trials—the rate of periprocedural complications can be expected to be extremely low. Casual review of these trials is fraught with the grave error of assuming that the results of CEA are analogous in the unselected patients undergoing carotid repair at the "grass-roots" level. To the contrary, there exist data to suggest that the results of the trials cannot even be generalized to patients undergoing CEA at the hospitals that participated in the studies. In a study of 113,000 Medicare patients who underwent CEA during patient acquisition for the NASCET and ACAS trials (1992–1993), Wennberg and colleagues[8] noted that the perioperative mortality rate was 1.4% in hospitals participating in the trials and 1.7% in hospitals that did not participate in the trials. The rate of perioperative death rose to 2.5% in low-volume non-trial hospitals where <7 CEAs were performed yearly. These relatively high complication rates are in direct contrast to the much lower mortality rates observed in the patients entered into the trials (0.1% in ACAS and 0.6% in NASCET). These findings suggest that eligibility criteria were sufficiently strict that patients in the NASCET and ACAS trials represented a small subset of the total population of patients undergoing CEA, comprising a subgroup with the lowest frequency of baseline comorbid conditions, and likely the lowest rate of perioperative adverse events.

The data from the Cleveland Clinic registry[9] offer an explanation for the findings of Wennberg et al.[8] Patients in the multicenter trials of CEA were similar to the low-risk group of patients undergoing carotid repair at the Cleveland Clinic. In fact, the mortality rate of 0.2% in more than 1500 low-risk asymptomatic patients treated with CEA is remarkably similar to the ACAS mortality rate of 0.1%. Similarly, the mortality rate was 0.5% in 925 symptomatic patients undergoing CEA at the Cleveland Clinic, almost identical to the 0.6% mortality rate observed in the NASCET trial.

These observations have implications in the design of trials aimed at assessing carotid stenting procedures. Periprocedural morbidity is likely to be highest during the relatively early evolution of stent design and stenting treatment paradigms. At a time when the safety and efficacy of carotid stenting remains unproved, investigations seem most appropriately undertaken in the population of patients with less ideal outcomes following the standard therapy of CEA. To evaluate carotid stenting versus CEA in a subgroup known for its low rate of perioperative morbidity jeopardizes successfully demonstrating equivalence between the stenting and CEA, resulting in the premature abandonment of the new technology. It is the author's opinion that the true benefit of carotid stenting is in the reduction of periprocedural myocardial infarction and death, events that are correlated with the invasiveness of the intervention. Given this thesis, the probability of demonstrating equivalence between carotid stenting and CEA is less likely in a patient population with a low rate of perioperative complications, especially if stenting proves to be associated with a slightly higher rate of perioperative stroke.

In addition to baseline comorbidities, there exist a variety of anatomic features that are also associated with poorer outcome. These include such variables as contralateral carotid occlusion,[5] recurrent carotid lesions,[10] and a history of radiation therapy to the neck.[11] These issues may be quite important in determining the outcome with open carotid procedures, with regard to perioperative stroke, myocardial infarction, and death, as well as softer endpoints, such as wound complications and cranial nerve injury. These anatomic features should also be taken into account in the differentiation between high- and low-risk patients. Complications that are associated with the invasive nature of open surgery would be likely to occur at a lower frequency in the stented subgroup. As such, both clinical and anatomic baseline variables should be addressed when delineating a high-risk patient population suitable for an initial investigation of CEA versus stenting.

INDICATIONS FOR CAROTID STENTING

The etiology of carotid bifurcation disease can be categorized into atherosclerotic and nonatherosclerotic processes, the former presenting much more frequently than the latter in clinical practice. The nonatherosclerotic causes of carotid bifurcation disease may be further subdivided into the inflammatory problems, such as Takaysu's arteritis, postendarterectomy intimal hyperplasia, and carotid stenosis occurring as a result of spontaneous dissections.[12] It is attractive to hypothesize that the short-term results of carotid stenting would be best in the nonatherosclerotic disease because the lesions are, by and large, smooth. As such, the potential for embolization is theoretically lower than that associated with complex atherosclerotic lesions. Many of these disease entities produce long, tapered carotid lesions, however, rendering them exceedingly difficult to treat with any modality. In addition, hypercoagulable problems may occur in association with some of the nonatherosclerotic etiologies, raising the risk of early postprocedural thrombosis. Clearly, the treatment of patients with the more esoteric causes of carotid stenosis is complicated, based on little more than anecdotal experience and, as such, should involve consultative input from a broad spectrum of specialists, including rheumatologists, hematologists, and vascular medicine practitioners.

In patients with atherosclerotic disease, the risk of carotid stenting is correlated with the extent of the atherosclerotic process. Patients with diffuse disease involving the aortic arch and common carotid vessels should be viewed with caution, as should patients with significant intracranial disease. The heavily calcified, tortuous vessel is one fraught with difficulty, and the use of alternate treatment modalities should be strongly entertained.

CAROTID STENTING TECHNIQUE

The technique of carotid stenting continues to evolve as a less-invasive alternative to open CEA. Where balloon angioplasty alone was formerly an acceptable option, angioplasty and stenting have emerged as the preferred method. The results, like that of CEA, are directly related to the experience of the operator and the use of meticulous technique to cross the carotid stenosis and deploy the stent.

Pharmacologic adjuvants have played an important role in carotid stenting. Although there are no controlled trials of antiplatelet agents as adjuvants for carotid stenting, their use is almost universal, reasoning that the observations of the randomized trials of ticlopidine for coronary stenting are applicable to the carotid setting. Thus, most patients undergoing carotid stenting receive a loading dose of a theinopyridine derivative, usually 300 mg of clopidogrel (Plavix, Sanofi Winthrop, New York, NY), and aspirin (325 mg), continuing the clopidogrel (75 mg/day) for 2 to 4 wk and the aspirin (325 mg/day) indefinitely.

There exists anecdotal evidence to suggest that the glycoprotein IIb/IIIa platelet antagonists may be of benefit in patients undergoing the placement of a carotid stent. The use of agents such as abciximab (ReoPro, Centocor, Malvern, PA), eptifibitide (Integrilin, Cor Therapeutics, San Francisco, CA), and tirofiban (Agrastat, Merck, West Point, PA) makes theoretic sense given the presumed increase in thrombogenicity of the stented luminal surface. Abciximab is a large Fc fragment with activity against not only the platelet glycoprotein IIb/IIIa receptor, but also the MAC-1 and $\alpha_v\beta_3$ receptor, it has the potential to block leukocyte chemotaxis and smooth muscle cell migration, respectively—two processes that are intimately involved in restenosis. By contrast, the small molecules eptifibitide and tirofiban possess specific activity against the glycoprotein receptors alone, limiting action to platelet-mediated events such as immediate stent thrombosis. There is empiric and somewhat circumstantial evidence from the coronary literature to support this contention. In stented diabetics treated with abciximab, the need for repeat revascularization, a surrogate endpoint for restenosis, was lower than in those not receiving the agent. No such preventative effect was noted in trials of the small molecules eptifibitide and tirofiban, suggesting that their actions are limited to the platelet. In view of these observations, we used abciximab, 0.25 mg/kg bolus loading dose, followed by a 0.125 g/kg/min infusion for 12 hr following the procedure. There exists theoretical advantages to using eptifibitide or tirofiban when an open surgical procedure such as coronary artery bypass is anticipated to be necessary within a few days of carotid stenting, given the longer half-life of abciximab. In practice, abciximab is readily and instantaneously reversible with platelet transfusions, whereas the small molecules are not. In this regard, protracted platelet dysfunction despite platelet transfusion has been, in our experience, almost universally the result of clopidogrel and aspirin rather than the glycoprotein IIb/IIIa inhibitors. In a series of 95 patients undergoing carotid stenting with abciximab, there were no periprocedural neurologic events.[13] A single patient developed a small hemorrhagic conversion within a previous cerebral infarct 4 days after stenting.

The procedure of carotid stenting commences with a high-quality diagnostic arteriographic study of the cerebrovasculature. Failure to detect a carotid bifurcation lesion of the severity suggested by a previous duplex scan should prompt one to obtain as many oblique projections as necessary because contemporary, well-performed duplex studies may be more sensitive than single- or dual-projection contrast arteriography. One should be certain to obtain adequate views of the intracranial vasculature to document any postprocedural changes resulting from iatrogenic embolization.

Following diagnostic arteriography, the patient is heparinized and a 0.035″ Glide wire is advanced through the diagnostic catheter into the external carotid artery. The diagnostic catheter is advanced over the wire and into the external carotid vessel, thereafter exchanging the Glide wire for a 0.038″ superstiff guidewire. The diagnostic catheter is exchanged for a 9F guide catheter, which is placed at the level of the mid-common carotid artery. Once the guiding catheter has been threaded to a level just below the carotid lesion, the lesion is crossed with a fine (e.g., 0.014″) guidewire. Recently, in the presence of friendly anatomy, the guiding catheter has been left at the more proximal common carotid level.

An embolic protection device may be used prior to crossing the lesion or immediately thereafter. There exist at least two devices that can function as the guidewire for subsequent angioplasty and stenting—the AngioGuard (Cordis, Warren, NJ) and MedNova NeuroShield (MedNova, Galway, Ireland) devices, both of which use distal internal carotid artery filters that maintain antegrade flow during the procedure. Other devices use proximal and or distal occluding balloons (e.g., ArteriA, San Francisco, CA; PercuSurge, Sunnyvale, CA) to arrest antegrade blood flow and allow aspiration of debris through a proximal guide catheter or sheath.

Once the lesion has been crossed with a wire, the lesion is predilated with a 3- or 4-mm balloon. Next, a self-expanding stent of an appropriate diameter and length is positioned across the lesion and the sheath is retracted to allow deployment. Postdilation with an appropriate-size balloon (usually 5–7 mm) is usually necessary, followed by completion arteriography with extra- and intracranial views. After a satisfactory clinical and arteriographic result has been achieved (Figure 23–2), the sheath is removed and the femoral access site is sealed with a closure device such as the Perclose system (Perclose, Menlo Park, CA) to limit the risk of bleeding secondary to platelet inhibition.

REGULATORY APPROVAL OF DEVICES

The approval of medical devices by the US Food and Drug Administration (FDA) is governed by comments contained within the Federal Code of Regulations. Devices in use prior to 1976 are excluded from these regulations, and in fact, new devices must be shown to be superior to or at least not inferior to a pre-1976 device. In some cases, the FDA has determined that a "510(k)" pathway is appropriate for approval, usually when the device is deemed "noncritical." In these scenarios, the device is merely shown to be equivalent to a pre-1976 device with clinical or even nonclinical data. Once data has been submitted, the FDA has 60 days in which to notify the marketer whether the device may be sold or, alternatively, the data submitted is inadequate to justify similarity to the comparator device and additional information is necessary. Biliary stents are a

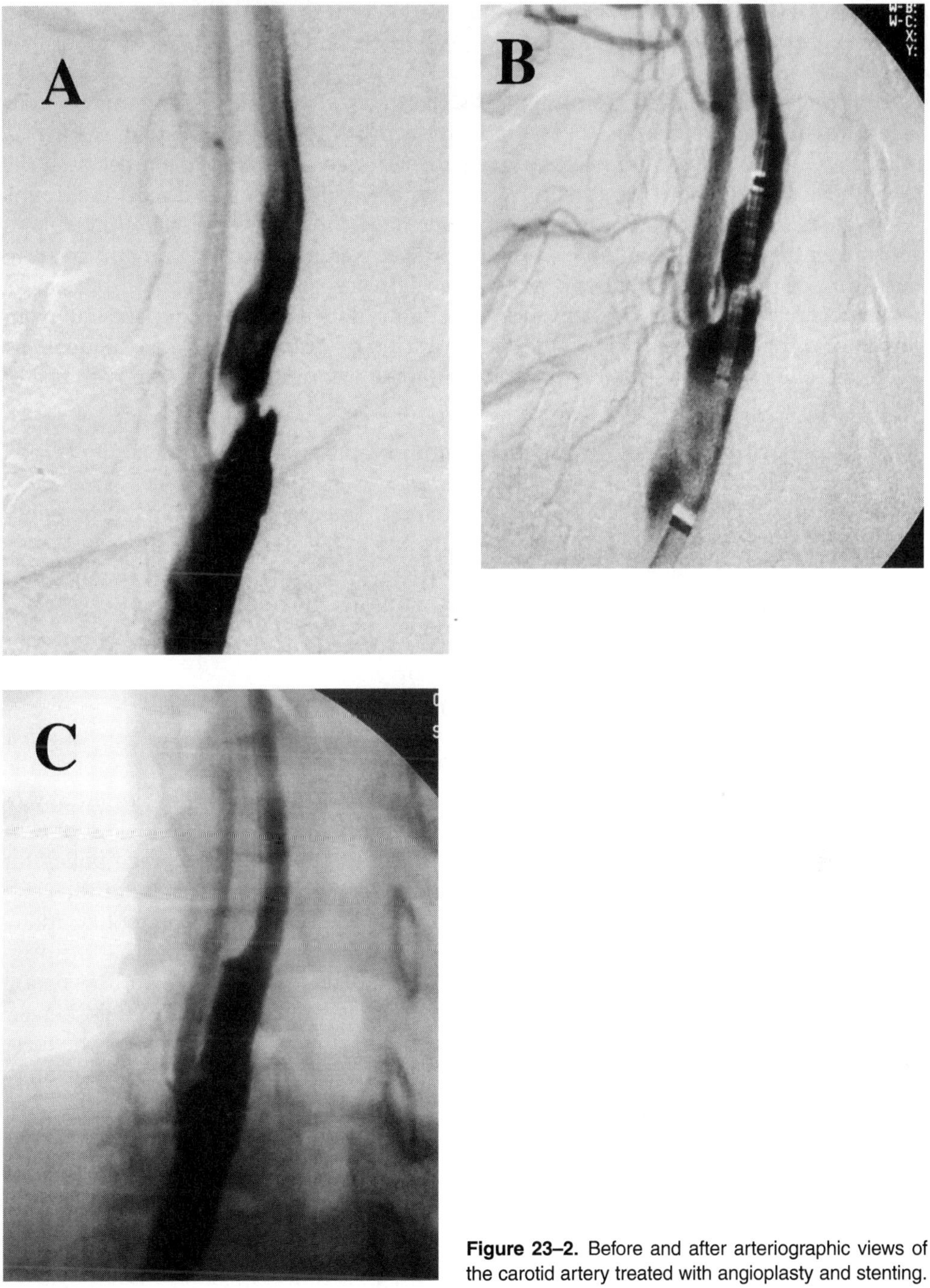

Figure 23–2. Before and after arteriographic views of the carotid artery treated with angioplasty and stenting.

prime example of devices in which a 510(k) pathway was acceptable. Once approved for the biliary indication, the same devices were used off-label in the treatment of iliac or renal disease.

By contrast, dedicated carotid stents, like coronary stents, must follow the premarket approval (PMA) pathway. A PMA strategy is much more complex than the 510(k) pathway. Clinical studies are necessary, usually directed at a comparison between the new device and standard treatment. In the case of carotid stents, standard therapy is CEA. The CREST and SAPPHIRE clinical trials have chosen to randomize patients to carotid stenting or CEA, and at least the latter trial was designed to gain approval for marketing of the carotid stent and adjuvants (delivery system and emboli protection device). Approval of a carotid stent for marketing is dependent on the successful completion of a trial that uses a clinically relevant primary endpoint (e.g., stroke, death or the composite endpoint stroke, myocardial infarction or death) to demonstrate one of the following:

1. superiority of the device over open carotid repair with an α probability (type I error) of $\leq$5%, or
2. noninferiority of the device in comparison to open repair, with an α probability of $\leq$5% or less (95% certainty) that outcome in the stented patients is not more than a predetermined percentage (the delta) worse than standard therapy. The appropriate level for the delta value remains a topic of discussion.

REIMBURSEMENT ISSUES FOR CAROTID ANGIOPLASTY AND STENTING

The US Health Care Financing Administration (HCFA) determined that carotid angioplasty should not be reimbursable to Medicare beneficiaries as a result of a lack of data documenting clinical benefit. As such, in 1988 HCFA issued a noncoverage policy for carotid angioplasty, specifically excluding reimbursement for angioplasty of the cerebrovasculature. In the years that have passed since the issuance of this policy, many HCFA management teams have come and gone. Thus, it is not surprising that the original intent of the policy is ill-defined and we are left to guess whether its authors meant to exclude carotid stenting or merely balloon angioplasty of the carotid vessels. Nevertheless, once a noncoverage policy has been issued, neither the casual use of the technique nor careful clinical investigatory procedures are reimbursable to the physician in the form of Medicare Part B professional fees or to the hospital by way of Medicare Part A remuneration. This dilemma is associated with a "catch-22" phenomenon, whereby percutaneous carotid intervention cannot be reimbursed because of a lack of data documenting medical necessity (benefit), yet scientific studies aimed at evaluation of efficacy cannot be performed unless the treating physician and the hospital are willing to provide services for study patients on a pro-bono basis or the manufacturer is willing to reimburse costs to the health-care providers. The inability to solve reimbursement problems for carotid angioplasty and stenting represents a major impediment to the performance of clinical trials.

REFERENCES

1. Carrea R, Molins M, Murphy G. Surgical treatment of spontaneous thrombosis of the internal carotid artery in the neck. Carotid–carotideal anastomosis. Report of a case. *Acta Neurol Latinoamer.* 1955;1:17.
2. DeBakey ME. Successful carotid endarterectomy for cerebrovascular insufficiency. Nineteen-year follow-up. *JAMA.* 1975;233(10):1083–1085.
3. Fields WS, North RR, Hass WK, et al. Joint study of extracranial arterial occlusion as a cause of stroke. I. Organization of study and survey of patient population. *JAMA.* 1968;203:153–158.
4. Fields WS, Maslenikov V, Meyer JS, Hass WK, Remington RD, Macdonald M. Joint study of extracranial arterial occlusion. V. Progress report of prognosis following surgery or nonsurgical treatment for transient cerebral ischemic attacks and cervical carotid artery lesions. *JAMA.* 1970;211:1993–2003.
5. Barnett HJ, Taylor DW, Eliasziw M, et al. Benefit of carotid endarterectomy in patients with symptomatic moderate or severe stenosis. North American Symptomatic Carotid Endarterectomy Trial Collaborators [see comments]. *N Engl J Med.* 1998;339(20):1415–1425.
6. Mayberg MR, Wilson SE, Yatsu F. Carotid endarterectomy and prevention of cerebral ischemia in symptomatic carotid stenosis. *JAMA.* 1991;266:3289–3294.
7. Hobson RW, Weiss DG, Fields WS. Efficacy of carotid endarterectomy for asymptomatic carotid stenosis. *N Engl J Med.* 1993;328:221–227.
8. Wennberg DE, Lucas FL, Birkmeyer JD, Bredenberg CE, Fisher ES. Variation in carotid endarterectomy mortality in the Medicare population: trial hospitals, volume, and patient characteristics. *JAMA.* 1998;279(16):1278–1281.
9. Ouriel K, Hertzer NR, Beven EG, et al. Pre-procedural risk stratification: identifying an appropriate group in whom to study the role of carotid stenting. *Circulation.* 1999;100:1–67.
10. Rockman CB, Riles TS, Landis R, et al. Redo carotid surgery: an analysis of materials and configurations used in carotid reoperations and their influence on perioperative stroke and subsequent recurrent stenosis. *J Vasc Surg.* 1999;29(1):72–80.
11. Kashyap VS, Moore WS, Quinones-Baldrich WJ. Carotid artery repair for radiation-associated atherosclerosis is a safe and durable procedure. *J Vasc Surg.* 1999;29(1):90–96.
12. Begelman SM, Olin JW. Nonatherosclerotic arterial disease of the extracranial cerebrovasculature. *Semin Vasc Surg.* 2000;13:153–164.
13. Silver MJ, Yadav JS, Wholey MH. Intermediate outcome after carotid stenting: what should we expect? *Semin Vasc Surg.* 2000;13:130–138.

24

When Should Carotid Endarterectomy Be Combined with Any Other Procedure?

Apostolos K. Tassiopoulos, MD,
and William H. Baker, MD, FACS

INTRODUCTION

Since the early 1990s, large multicenter trials have proved the safety and efficacy of carotid endarterectomy (CEA) in the prevention of ischemic stroke.[1–4] The benefit of CEA, however, is established only when the procedure is associated with low perioperative stroke and death rates. A significant percentage of patients presenting with carotid bifurcation disease that requires surgical management have concomitant conditions that may increase the risk for perioperative complications and adversely affect the outcome. Some of these conditions are also amenable to surgical correction, raising the dilemma of managing them by a staged or a combined surgical approach. Unfortunately, large prospective trials studying the different management options in these patients are lacking because the coexistence of these conditions with carotid artery stenosis is relatively rare, the clinical presentation of the patients in some of them is so diverse that makes randomization and overall design of such a study complex, or the number of adverse effects is so low that it makes statistical comparisons difficult. Obviously, in the absence of prospective randomized studies, a clear benefit of one specific treatment option versus another cannot be demonstrated with certainty. Careful review of the existing literature, however, allows for setting some evidence-based guidelines.

CAROTID ENDARTERECTOMY AND CORONARY ARTERY BYPASS: STAGED OR COMBINED SURGICAL APPROACH?

Because atherosclerosis is a systemic disease, it is not surprising that a group of patients have coexisting surgically significant coronary and carotid artery disease. Patients in this group may present initially with either cardiac or neurologic symptoms, and occasionally with a combination of the two. Approximately 35% to 50% of patients presenting for CEA have clinically apparent coronary artery disease in the form of angina, history of previous myocardial infarction (MI), or evidence of myocardial ischemia on electrocardiogram. In addition, approximately 50% of patients with symptomatic or asymptomatic carotid artery disease have abnormal cardiac nuclear scans.[5,6] On the other hand, up to 22% of patients scheduled for coronary artery bypass (CABG) have ≥50% carotid artery stenosis, and up to 12% have ≥80% stenosis when screened by duplex.[7–9] CABG patients with concomitant severe carotid artery disease represent a subgroup with very advanced atherosclerosis with a higher incidence of left main coronary artery disease and reduced ejection fraction compared to patients who have isolated coronary artery disease.[10]

Coronary artery disease has been shown to increase the risk of perioperative morbidity and mortality in CEA patients. In the 1970s, mortality rates as high as 20% were reported during CEA in patients with uncorrected significant coronary artery disease.[11,12] The overall incidence of MI complicating CEA ranges between 1.5% and 5% and it is the leading cause of perioperative and late deaths in these patients.[5,13–15] More specifically, when the entire population undergoing CEA is considered, MI is responsible for 25% to 50% of perioperative mortality, whereas in the subgroup of patients who have symptomatic coronary artery disease, cardiac complications account for up to 75% of all perioperative deaths.[16] However, these statistics are misleading. Most surgeons agree that patients without critical coronary artery disease (e.g., severe left main stenosis or its equivalent, unstable or postinfarction angina, severely depressed left ventricular function, uncontrolled congestive heart failure, malignant ventricular arrhythmia) may undergo CEA safely by maximizing medical treatment for their cardiac disease. This notion is supported by a recent multicenter randomized trial that confirmed the cardioprotective effect of beta-blockade in the perioperative period of peripheral vascular reconstructions.[17]

On the other hand, multiple reports suggest that the presence of significant carotid artery stenosis increases the risk for perioperative stroke in patients undergoing CABG. In a retrospective study of 1179 cardiac surgery patients, Ricotta et al.[7] found that the risk for perioperative stroke increased six-fold in patients with >50% carotid artery stenosis. Brenner et al.[18] noted a 9.2% incidence of stroke and/or TIA during CABG in patients with significant carotid artery stenosis, as compared to 1.9% in patients without carotid disease. Hertzer et al.[19] reported that in 275 CABG patients with angiographically proved severe (≥70%) carotid artery stenosis, the incidence of stroke was 8.9%, significantly higher than the 1.3% institutional stroke rate for CABG in general. Despite the evidence provided by these studies, there is no consensus regarding the significance and, thus, treatment of a carotid lesion in patients scheduled to undergo a CABG procedure. A usual argument is that, in CABG patients who experience cerebrovascular accidents (CVAs) during the procedure, the carotid lesion cannot always be correlated to the neurologic symptomatology. It has been shown that in these patients, potential sources of stroke include atheromatous plaques in the ascending aorta, pump-related air embolism or thromboembolism, cardiogenic embolism, intracranial hemorrhage, and segmental cerebral hypoperfusion related to carotid and/or intracranial occlusive disease combined with low cardiac output (watershed infarcts). Therefore, it is not surprising that in the study by Ricotta et al.,[7] the anatomic distribution of the strokes did not correlate with the side of the carotid lesion in >50% of the patients. Roach et al.[20] found proximal aortic atherosclerosis to be the most significant predictor of postoperative neurologic events in cardiac surgery patients. Obviously, CVA cannot be prevented entirely by surgically correcting an existing significant carotid artery stenosis. It must be emphasized, however, that out of all potential sources of stroke listed previously, extracranial carotid disease is perhaps the only one that can be surgically corrected either prior to or at the time of the CABG procedure.

Several studies since the early 1960s have tried to correlate the risk for perioperative stroke with the severity of the carotid disease. Although the true incidence of perioperative CVA is unknown, it is generally agreed that symptomatic carotid lesions causing >70% stenosis carry an increased risk for stroke. Similarly, patients with an asymptomatic carotid stenosis ≥80% and a contralateral carotid occlusion represent a high-risk group for neurologic complications during CABG surgery.[8] Patients who belong in these two categories may be considered to undergo CEA either prior to or at the time of CABG, depending on the severity of their coronary artery disease. Although multiple studies have reported that combined CABG/CEA procedures in this patient population are associated with a high incidence of perioperative mortality and stroke,[21–23] physicians assume that even higher risks should be expected if an alternative approach is chosen.

The optimal management of less-severe asymptomatic carotid lesions in CABG patients is still debated. Faggioli et al.[24] reported that the incidence of stroke in patients with asymptomatic carotid stenosis ≥75% who underwent CABG without CEA was 14.3%. He estimated that the presence of such carotid lesions increased the risk for perioperative stroke during CABG 9.9-fold. In a more recent study, Schwartz et al.[8] used duplex to screen 582 patients undergoing CABG for carotid disease. He reported that 22% of the patients had carotid stenosis of ≥50%. Perioperative stroke developed in 6.2% of patients, but no patient with a unilateral carotid stenosis between 50% and 79% had a CVA in this series. The authors found that patients with (1) 80% to 99% unilateral carotid artery stenosis, (2) bilateral carotid artery stenosis ≥50%, and (3) unilateral carotid occlusion combined with a contralateral carotid stenosis ≥50% had a higher incidence of perioperative CVA.

The surgical planning for patients with concomitant coronary and carotid artery disease is guided by three assumptions. First, patients with left main coronary artery disease (or its equivalent) are at an increased risk of perioperative MI and death; thus, their treatment plan includes primary coronary revascularization, with or without CEA. Second, patients with bilateral severe and perhaps unilateral severe carotid stenosis may have an increased perioperative stroke rate with CABG. Finally, repair of the carotid stenosis decreases this perioperative CABG stroke rate. Although the first assumption is well accepted and the second assumption sounds reasonable, the last assumption is far from a proven fact. How, then, should surgeons time correction of both carotid and coronary atherosclerosis when both exist in the same patient?

The management options include CEA followed at a later time by CABG (*staged approach*), CABG followed at a later time by CEA (*reversed staged approach*), and simultaneous CEA and CABG (*synchronous approach*). Although there are multiple reports in the literature favoring one approach or the other, there are no prospective randomized trials comparing these three options. In the only study that included partial randomization, Hertzer et al.[19] reported that patients with unstable coronary artery disease and asymptomatic carotid stenosis ≥70% who were randomized to the synchronous approach had a perioperative stroke rate of 2.8%, which was significantly lower compared to the stroke rate seen in the reversed staged group (14%). The stroke rate in the staged group was 4.2% and the mortality rate 0%, but these patients obviously had less severe coronary artery disease. In the synchronous and reversed staged groups, mortality was 4.2% and 6.1%, respectively (no statistically significant difference). A meta-analysis of 56 studies conducted between 1970 and 1992 did not show a distinct outcome advantage for any of the three management options mentioned previously, but it indicated that (1) the staged approach was associated with the lowest perioperative stroke rate, but resulted in higher myocardial infarction and death rates; (2) the reversed staged approach resulted in lower MI and death rates, but was also associated with the highest risk for stroke; and (3) the simultaneous approach resulted in intermediate stroke, MI, and death rates.[25]

From the previously mentioned statistics, the simultaneous approach makes the most sense, especially if this approach is safe. However, mortality rates range between 2% and 12% and stroke rates between 1% and 15% in different reports.[19,21–23,26,27] This significant variation can be attributed, at least partially, to differences in the patient population included. Thus, studies coming from centers that routinely screen CABG patients for carotid disease and offer the synchronous approach in all patients with carotid stenosis ≥60% report the lowest mortality and stroke morbidity rates, which, in some recent reports, are quite impressive. In one of them, Darling et al.[23] reported that in 420 patients who underwent combined CEA and CABG, the perioperative mortality rate was 2.4% and the incidence of permanent neurologic deficit was 1%, whereas 1.7% of patients developed a transient neurologic deficit that improved prior to discharge. However, centers that offer the synchronous approach only to patients with either symptomatic or severe asymptomatic carotid disease (critical bilateral stenoses or critical unilateral stenosis with contralateral occlusion) report significantly higher mortality and perioperative stroke rates. In such studies, Mackey et al.[22] reported that mortality and stroke rates were 8% and 9%, respectively, whereas Coyle et al.[21] reported mortality of 10.8% and stroke rate of 15.4%. Interestingly, in the study by Darling et al.,[23] the mortality rate was 1.5% in patients with asymptomatic carotid stenosis and 5.4% in those with symptomatic lesions. In addition, the perioperative stroke rates were 0.8% for the asymptomatic patients and 2% for those with symptoms, indicating that they represent two different risk groups.

Based on current literature and practice, we believe that certain guidelines can be applied safely when treating patients who require consideration of surgical management for both their coronary disease and carotid artery disease. These principles are designed to minimize the risk for perioperative mortality and stroke morbidity, and are summarized as follows:

1. CABG patients with left main coronary disease or its equivalent
   a. Repair ≥80% asymptomatic carotid artery stenoses or ≥50% symptomatic stenoses synchronously with the CABG procedure. Any other approach results in increased death and/or stroke rates.[1–4] This appears to be the best compromise.
2. CABG patients with less-severe coronary artery disease
   a. Repair ≥80% asymptomatic carotid artery stenoses or ≥50% symptomatic stenoses prior to CABG.[1–4]
   b. Synchronous repair may be considered in those institutions with a proved record of acceptable morbidity and mortality rates.

As stated repeatedly, these guidelines are intended to assist but not dictate patient care. In the absence of a prospective randomized study, the management of these patients should be individualized, taking into consideration the individual patient characteristics and preference, the physician, and institutional capabilities.

When a synchronous approach is selected, the operation is best conducted using some basic principles. The patient is positioned, prepped, and draped for a CABG procedure. The entire neck must be accessible. The cardiac surgeon performs the median sternotomy and prepares to go on bypass. The conduits for CABG are simultaneously harvested. When the cardiac surgeon has completed his initial work in the mediastinum, the carotid artery is exposed. If at any time the patient's heart function significantly deteriorates, the neck operation is aborted, the patient is placed on bypass, and cardiac revascularization is accomplished. If the patient is stable, the CEA is completed as the vein harvest proceeds. The neck is left open until the patient is off bypass and the heparin is reversed.

The role of angioplasty in the management of these patients is still not clearly defined. Coronary angioplasty has been used successfully to treat patients with critical coronary lesions, thus reducing the mortality of a subsequent CEA. In the future, will the reverse be true? That is, will a pre-CABG carotid angioplasty reduce the stroke rate of a subsequent bypass? This scenario depends on several unproved hypotheses:

1. Carotid endarterectomy and angioplasty are equivalent. This unproved tenet is being addressed by the beginning CREST trial.[28]
2. Carotid angioplasty is safer than CEA in the patient with a critical left main coronary artery stenosis. Both procedures can be accomplished using either local or general anesthesia. Angioplasty in general requires less time to perform, although many accomplished vascular surgeons can complete a carotid revascularization procedure within 60–90 min. Neither procedure requires specialized postoperative care, and both may have associated bradycardia.

Thus, although carotid angioplasty on the surface appears to be applicable to this patient population, the authors reserve judgment, pending reports of significant numbers of treated patients.

CONCURRENT STENOSIS OF THE SUPRA-AORTIC TRUNKS AND THE CAROTID BIFURCATION

Stenosing lesions involving the arterial branches of the aortic arch are usually located at the origin of these vessels and often involve more than one artery. These atherosclerotic lesions may be continuous with plaques in the aortic arch, and are very often associated with carotid bifurcation and/or vertebral artery lesions. Although there are no concrete data on the natural history of atherosclerotic lesions involving the supra-aortic trunks, they do indeed cause strokes. Therefore, patients with symptomatic stenosis are always considered for surgical repair. The role of intervention for asymptomatic lesions is yet to be defined, but these authors decry this indication.

The incidence of innominate artery stenosis is low. Innominate artery lesions were found to represent only 1.7% of 1961 operations performed for occlusive lesions of the brachiocephalic vessels, vertebral arteries, and carotid bifurcation at UCSF in 1979.[29] Proximal left common carotid artery stenosis is also uncommon. However, concurrent lesions at the aortic arch and the carotid bifurcation do occur. When ipsilateral tandem lesions are associated with hemispheric neurologic symptoms, it is difficult to assign the symptoms to either lesion, and thus both should be considered for repair.

In patients undergoing CEA, the incidence of proximal disease is 1.5% to 2%.[29,30] However, in patients with proximal arch lesions, the incidence of carotid bifurcation disease is much higher. Kieffer et al.[31] reported 148 patients treated for innominate artery stenosis or occlusion. Carotid bifurcation disease was detected in 108 (73%) patients, and 17 (11%) had radiographically proved stroke. CEA was performed as part of the same procedure in 57 (39%) patients and involved the right carotid artery in 42 patients, the left carotid artery in 12 patients, and both carotid arteries in 3 patients. Nine patients underwent a left CEA prior to surgery for the innominate artery lesion. The incidence of perioperative neurologic events in the series was 5.4% (stroke: 3.4%; TIAs: 2%) and did not differ significantly in the subgroup of patients with combined innominate and carotid bifurcation procedures. The authors strongly advocate synchronous right bifurcation CEA whenever indicated, and they recommend avoiding bilateral carotid reconstructions during the same procedure to avoid cerebral hyperperfusion syndrome postoperatively. In another series, Berguer et al.[32] reported their experience in 100 patients with severe stenosis or occlusion of the proximal CCA and/or the innominate artery. The prevalence of severe (>60%) carotid bifurcation disease in this group was 25%. Twenty-six patients underwent synchronous carotid bifurcation CEA, either as a remote component to the operation or incorporated into the distal anastomosis of the bypass graft. Fourteen patients had CEA after the initial operation. The stroke rates in these two groups are not provided, but the overall perioperative stroke rate in the series was reported to be 10%.

Surgical options for proximal CCA and innominate artery occlusive disease include (1) endarterectomy of the stenotic segment; (2) an axial bypass from the aorta to the affected vessel distal to the occlusion; (3) an extra-anatomic bypass, usually subclavian–carotid artery bypass or carotid–carotid artery bypass; and (4) transposition of the CCA to the ipsilateral subclavian artery. Since the early 1980s, extra-anatomic bypass procedures have become the preferred method for surgical management of proximal lesions. A short innominate artery bypass or endarterectomy cannot be combined with a bifurcation CEA, although both can be performed during the same operation. The distal limb of a longer bypass can be sutured to the bifurcation CEA site as a patch angioplasty, and this is our preference. We believe that ipsilateral carotid bifurcation lesions that require surgical management may undergo endarterectomy combined with the revascularization procedure of the supra-aortic trunks. CEA for significant stenosis of the contralateral carotid bifurcation should be individualized depending on the severity of the lesion and the presence or absence of neurologic symptomatology. Symptomatic and preocclusive asymptomatic lesions should be treated prior to the proximal revascularization procedure.

Although surgical management for severe stenosis of the aortic arch vessels has been proved to have excellent long-term results, these procedures are associated with increased perioperative mortality and significant perioperative stroke rates. In the two large reports mentioned previously, mortality was 5.4% for Kieffer et al.[31] and 8% for Berguer et al.[32] The advent of percutaneous balloon angioplasty has provided the option of correcting the proximal common carotid or innominate artery stenosis by balloon dilatation while avoiding the mortality associated with the open procedure. The approach to these lesions may be antegrade (via groin access) or retrograde (open neck incision with carotid control). Queral and Criado[33,34] and Levien et al.[35] prefer the retrograde method. The initial success rate is between 95% and 100%, and the authors report no mortality or stroke. In the study by Levien et al.,[35] a Palmaz stent was not used routinely and a recurrent stenosis of 9% was reported. In the study by Queral and Criado,[34] with routine stenting there were no recurrences. Obviously, a synchronous bifurcation CEA could be added to this neck procedure with anticipated excellent results.[35]

The simultaneous occurrence of arch and bifurcation atherosclerosis in a symptomatic patient is uncommon. Our preference is an extra-anatomic bypass, with the distal limb anastomosed as a patch angioplasty over the endarterectomized carotid bifurcation. Retrograde innominate or common carotid angioplasty and concomitant CEA has yielded excellent results. Anterograde arch vessel angioplasty has been reported less often, but almost assuredly will be performed more often. Combined arch and bifurcation angioplasty should not be contemplated until good results have been reported by multiple investigators.

CONCURRENT CAROTID BIFURCATION AND VERTEBRAL ARTERY STENOSIS

Atherosclerotic lesions of the vertebral artery are most commonly seen at the artery's origin from the subclavian artery, and the second most common location is the segment of the vessel that traverses through the cervical vertebrae. Occlusions of the vertebral artery usually involve most of its cervical segment but frequently the artery reconstitutes at or immediately below the level of the C2 vertebra. For many years, these lesions were considered to have only hemodynamic significance; however, the advent of magnetic resonance imaging (MRI) has clearly shown that they can be the source of emboli to the brain stem and other areas of the brain supplied by the posterior circulation, occasionally with detrimental consequences.[36] Vertebrobasilar ischemia may result from either hemodynamic or embolic mechanisms. Proximal lesions are less often associated with embolic events. In recent years, the following indications for vertebral artery reconstructions have been established:

1. Symptoms of vertebrobasilar insufficiency associated with a significant (>80%) stenosis of the vertebral artery (with or without radiographic evidence of embolization to the distribution of the posterior circulation) in the absence of conditions that may cause similar neurologic symptomatology (cardiac arrhythmias, seizures, orthostatic hypotension, etc.).
2. Unilateral or bilateral symptomatic stenosis of the vertebral artery associated with bilateral internal carotid artery occlusion.
3. Asymptomatic significant (>80%) stenosis of a dominant vertebral associated with bilateral internal carotid artery occlusion.

The only difficult decision is in the patient with vertebrobasilar insufficiency symptoms, a tight carotid stenosis, and a tight vertebral artery stenosis. Many, if not most, of these patients have symptomatic relief with CEA alone, ignoring the vertebral artery lesion. This is our preferred treatment plan. However, a few patients remain symptomatic if CEA alone is performed. Thus, if the lesions are ipsilateral, proximal vertebral reconstruction (reimplantation or bypass) are combined with CEA.[37] Distal reconstruction of the vertebral artery above the level of the C2 vertebra usually requires a vein graft from the carotid artery. A concomitant CEA may be necessary in order to establish adequate inflow in selected patients.[36] The distal anastomosis is always performed end-to-end. Other options include transposition of the C0–C2 segment of the vertebral artery to the ipsilateral internal carotid artery or transposition of the ipsilateral external carotid artery or its occipital branch to the C0–C2 segment of the vertebral artery. Occasionally, vein patch angioplasty of a favorable stenotic lesion can be used.[36,37]

In the largest series reported in the literature,[36] the perioperative mortality was 4% (2% only in the most recent group of patients) and all deaths were associated with a stroke. The incidence of nonfatal stroke was 1%. Concomitant bifurcation CEA was performed in 18% of the patients without a perioperative neurologic event. A study by Sottiurai et al.[37] reported on 49 symptomatic patients with concomitant carotid bifurcation and severe proximal vertebral artery stenosis. Twenty-one patients had an occluded internal carotid artery and underwent common/external CEA and vertebral–carotid transposition or bypass, and the rest had synchronous bifurcation CEA and vertebral reconstructions. There were no perioperative deaths, strokes, or other neurologic deficits in this series.

MANAGEMENT OF SEVERE CAROTID ARTERY STENOSIS IN PATIENTS REQUIRING INFRARENAL AORTIC RECONSTRUCTION OR LOWER EXTREMITY BYPASS

Stroke is a rare but devastating complication of abdominal aortic reconstructions. A study that used routine duplex ultrasound screening reported significant (≥50%) carotid stenosis in approximately 40% of patients undergoing aortic reconstruction for aortoiliac occlusive disease and in 17% of those treated for an abdominal aortic aneurysm (AAA). Severe (70–99%) stenosis was found in 9.9% of patients in the first group versus 3.6% of patients in the latter.[38] Gerraty et al.[9] reported a significant risk for perioperative stroke in patients with symptomatic severe (≥80%) carotid stenosis or with symptomatic carotid occlusion undergoing peripheral arterial reconstructions. A report by Deville et al.[39] recommends routine duplex carotid screening for all patients scheduled for elective aortic reconstruction and surgical treatment for all surgically significant carotid lesions prior to the aortic procedure. The perioperative stroke rate in this series was 0%.

Although stroke may indeed complicate distal vascular repairs, there is no evidence that a prophylactic CEA is required prior to these reconstructions. Certainly, concomitant operations should be rare—indeed, and confined to patients with dual symptomatic progressive lesions. In general, patients scheduled for elective distal vascular repairs have a prophylactic CEA performed prior to the repair when indicated. Patients facing emergent distal reconstructions have their associated carotid lesion repaired at a later date.

NECK DISSECTION WITH SIMULTANEOUS CAROTID ENDARTERECTOMY

Patients with metastatic neck disease from upper aerodigestive tract carcinomas are typically males with an extensive history of alcohol and tobacco abuse. These patients have a high incidence of peripheral vascular and coronary artery disease. Treatment options for head and neck carcinomas include surgical resection of the lesion and/or neck dissection (modified or complete) and radiation therapy to the neck. The presence in the operative field of a symptomatic severe carotid artery stenosis or of an asymptomatic stenosis that is likely to progress under the influence of pre- or postoperative radiation therapy raises the dilemma for a synchronous CEA. Violation of the aerodigestive tract, however, may be associated with a spit fistula and wound infection. These complications may in turn lead to carotid blowout, even without CEA. Thus, enthusiasm for combined operations must be tempered.

Our policy is to defer CEA whenever possible. Although the incidence of stroke is reported to be elevated following head and neck operations[40] and successful combined procedures have been reported,[41] we have but meager experience in this area. We are not hesitant to combine CEA with neck dissection when the aerodigestive tract is not violated, coverage of the carotid artery is adequate and the risk for wound infection is low. Even in these patients, however, Dacron or PTFE patches are avoided. As the risks for wound infection increase, our inclination for synchronous CEA decreases. We strongly recommend erring on the side of caution in these difficult patients.

REFERENCES

1. North American Symptomatic Carotid Endarterectomy Trial Collaborators. Beneficial effects of carotid endarterectomy in symptomatic patients with high-grade stenosis. *N Engl J Med.* 1991;325:445–453.

2. European Carotid Surgery Trialist's Group. MRC European Carotid Surgery Trial. Interim results for symptomatic patients with severe (70–99%) or with mild (0–29%) carotid stenosis. *Lancet.* 1991;337:1235–1243.
3. Hobson RW, Weiss, Fields WS, et al. Efficacy of carotid endarterectomy for asymptomatic carotid artery stenosis. *N Engl J Med.* 1993;328:221–227.
4. Executive Committee for the Asymptomatic Carotid Atherosclerosis Study. Endarterectomy for asymptomatic carotid artery stenosis. *JAMA.* 1995;273:1421–1428.
5. Mackey WC, O'Donnell TF, Callow AD. Cardiac risk in patients undergoing carotid endarterectomy: impact on perioperative and long-term mortality. *J Vasc Surg.* 1990;11:226–234.
6. Love BB, Grover-McKay M, Biller J, et al. Coronary artery disease and cardiac events with asymptomatic and symptomatic cerebrovascular disease. *Stroke.* 1995;26:188–201.
7. Ricotta JJ, Faggioli GJ, Castilone A, et al. Risk factors for stroke after cardiac surgery. *J Vasc Surg.* 1995;21:359–364.
8. Schwartz LB, Bridgman AH, Kieffer RW, et al. Asymptomatic carotid artery stenosis and stroke in patients undergoing cardiopulmonary bypass. *J Vasc Surg.* 1995;21:146–153.
9. Gerraty RP, Gates PC, Doyle JC. Carotid stenosis and perioperative stroke risk in symptomatic and asymptomatic patients undergoing vascular or coronary surgery. *Stroke.* 1993; 24:1115–1118.
10. Lazar HL, Menzoian JO. Coronary artery bypass grafting in patients with cerebrovascular disease. *Ann Thor Surg.* 1998;66:968–974.
11. Bernhard VM, Johnson WD, Peterson JJ. Carotid artery stenosis: association with surgery for coronary artery disease. *Arch Surg.* 1972;105:837–840.
12. Enuex CL Jr, Laurie GM, Morris GC Jr, et al. Improved results of carotid endarterectomy in patients with symptomatic coronary artery disease. An analysis of 1546 consecutive carotid operations. *Stroke.* 1979;10:122–125.
13. Burke PA, Callow AD, O'Donnell TF, et al. Prophylactic carotid endarterectomy for asymptomatic bruits: a look at cardiac risk. *Arch Surg.* 1982;117:1222–1227.
14. Barnes RW, Liebman PR, Marszalek PB, et al. The natural history of asymptomatic carotid disease in patients undergoing cardiovascular surgery. *Surgery.* 1981;90:1075–1083.
15. Thompson EJ, Patman RD, Talkington CM. Asymptomatic carotid bruit: long-term outcome of patients having endarterectomy compared with unoperated controls. *Ann Surg.* 1978; 188:308–316.
16. O'Donnell TF, Callow AD, Willet C, et al. The impact of coronary artery disease on carotid endarterectomy. *Ann Surg.* 1983;198:705–712.
17. Poldermans D, Boersma E, Bax JJ, et al. The effect of bisoprolol on perioperative mortality and myocardial infarction in high-risk patients undergoing vascular surgery. *N Engl J Med.* 1999; 341:1789–1794.
18. Brenner BJ, Brief DK, Alpert J, et al. The risk of stroke in patients with asymptomatic carotid stenosis undergoing cardiac surgery: a follow-up study. *J Vasc Surg.* 1987;1:269–279.
19. Hertzer NR, Loop FD, Beven EJ, et al. Surgical staging for simultaneous coronary and carotid disease: a study including prospective randomization. *J Vasc Surg.* 1989;9:455–463.
20. Roach GW, Kanchuger M, Mangano CM, et al. Adverse cerebral outcomes after coronary bypass surgery. *N Engl J Med.* 1996;335:1857–1863.
21. Coyle KA, Gray BC, Smith RB, et al. Morbidity and mortality associated with carotid endarterectomy: effect of adjunctive coronary revascularization. *Ann Vasc Surg.* 1995;9:21–27.
22. Mackey WC, Khabbaz K, Bojar R, et al. Simultaneous carotid endarterectomy and coronary bypass: perioperative risk and long-term survival. *J Vasc Surg.* 1996;24:58–64.
23. Darling RC III, Dylewski M, Chang BB, et al. Combined carotid endarterectomy and coronary artery bypass grafting does not increase the risk of perioperative stroke. *Cardiovasc Surg.* 1998;6:448–452.

24. Faggioli GL, Curl GR, Ricotta JJ. The role of carotid screening before coronary artery bypass. *J Vasc Surg*. 1990;12:724–731.
25. Moore WS, Barnett HJM, Beebe HG, et al. Guidelines for carotid endarterectomy: a multidisciplinary consensus statement from the ad hoc committee, American Heart Association. *Stroke*. 1995;26:188–201.
26. Plestis KA, Ke S, Jiang ZD, et al. Combined carotid endarterectomy and coronary artery bypass: immediate and long-term results. *Ann Vasc Surg*. 1999;13:84–92.
27. Curl GR, Pillai L, Raza ST, et al. Staged vs combined carotid endarterectomy in coronary bypass patients. Abstract presented at the Ninth Eastern Vascular Society Meeting, Buffalo NY, May 1995.
28. Hobson RW II. CREST (Carotid Revascularization Endarterectomy versus Stent Trial): background, design and current status. *Semin Vasc Surg*. 2000;13:139–143.
29. Wylie EJ, Effeney DJ. Surgery of the aortic arch branches and vertebral arteries. *Surg Clin North Am*. 1979;59:669–680.
30. Riles TS, Imparato AM, Posner MP, Eikelboom BC. Common carotid occlusion: assessment of the distal vessels. *Ann Surg*. 1984;199:363–366.
31. Kieffer E, Sabatier J, Koskas F, Bahnini A. Atherosclerotic innominate artery occlusive disease: early and long-term results of surgical reconstruction. *J Vasc Surg*. 1995;21:326–337.
32. Berguer R, Morasch MD, Kline RA. Transthoracic repair of innominate and common carotid artery disease: immediate and long-term outcome for 100 consecutive surgical reconstructions. *J Vasc Surg*. 1998;27:34–42.
33. Queral LA, Criado FJ. The treatment of focal aortic branch lesions with Palmaz stents. *J Vasc Surg*. 1996;23:368–375.
34. Queral LA, Criado FJ. Endovascular treatment of aortic arch occlusive disease. *Semin Vasc Surg*. 1996;9:156–163.
35. Levien LJ, Benn CA, Veller MG, Fritz VU. Retrograde balloon angioplasty of brachiocephalic or common carotid artery stenoses at the time of carotid endarterectomy. *Eur J Vasc Endovasc Surg*. 1998;15:521–527.
36. Berguer R, Morasch MD, Kline RA. A review of 100 consecutive reconstructions of the distal vertebral artery for embolic and hemodynamic disease. *J Vasc Surg*. 1998;27:852–859.
37. Sottiurai VS, Lyons R, Omlie W, et al. Combined carotid endarterectomy and vertebral transposition or bypass for cerebral and vertebrobasilar insufficiency. *Vasc Surg*. 2000;34:137–146.
38. Cahan MA, Killewich LA, Kolodner L, et al. The prevalence of carotid artery stenosis in patients undergoing aortic reconstruction. *Am J Surg*. 1999;178:194–196.
39. Deville C, Kerdi S, Madonna F, et al. Infrarenal abdominal aortic aneurysm repair: detection and treatment of associated carotid and coronary lesions. *Ann Vasc Surg*. 1997;11:467–472.
40. Sprung J, Jones FD, Rosen JS, et al. Asymptomatic carotid stenosis and stroke during neck surgery. *Otolaryngol Head Neck Surg*. 1996;115:568–572.
41. Rechtweg J, Wax MK, Shah R, et al. Neck dissection with simultaneous carotid endarterectomy. *Laryngoscope*. 1998;108:1150–1153.

25

Vertebral Artery Disease

Mark D. Morasch, MD

INTRODUCTION

The syndrome of brain stem ischemia, which most often results from diseases involving the extracranial vertebral artery (VA), is well understood by few and is frequently misdiagnosed. In contradistinction to the focal symptoms of carotid/hemispheric ischemia, the symptoms associated with poor brain stem perfusion are multiple, varied, and often vague. Moreover, there is reluctance on the part of many clinicians to pursue aggressively through angiography or to correct surgically accessible lesions that may be responsible for these syndromes. In addition, there are a significant number of medical conditions that mimic vertebrobasilar ischemia and may confound patient selection.

ANATOMY

One reason that the pathophysiology of vertebrobasilar ischemia is less well understood than carotid/hemispheric ischemia is that the peculiar anatomy of the vertebral artery has made it less accessible to surgical reconstruction and to postmortem examination. The surgical anatomy of the paired vertebral arteries has traditionally been divided into four parts. The first portion of the VA begins at its origin from the posteriosuperior aspect of the proximal subclavian artery. This segment ends as it passes into the foramen of the transverse process of the sixth cervical vertebra. The proximal segment is usually <4 cm long. It can be quite tortuous, and usually no branches emanate from this segment. The proximal VA is accessible in the base of the neck in a position medial to the anterior scalene muscle and behind the jugular vein, where it lies between the cervical sympathetics and the longus colli muscle. On the left, the thoracic duct, as it enters the jugulosubclavian confluence, must be divided to access the proximal VA.

The second segment of the VA ascends in the neck, passing through the foramina of the transverse processes of the sixth through second cervical vertebrae. This portion is generally considered inaccessible as it travels through an osteomuscular tunnel composed of vertebral bone and intertransversarium muscle, lies adjacent to the anterior ramus of each respective cervical root, and is intimately surrounded by a dense plexus of veins and cervical sympathetic nerve fibers. Segmental arterial branches emanate from the second portion of the VA and supply blood to the surrounding musculoskeletal structures and to the nerve roots of the spinal cord itself. Collateral circulation from the external carotid and subclavian arteries may serve to maintain patency of a proximally occluded vertebral artery via these segmental branches.

The third portion of the VA begins at the point where it exits the transverse process of the second cervical vertebra and travels over a short distance to where it penetrates the atlanto-occipital membrane. This segment courses superolaterally between the axis and the atlas, and here it is accessible for surgical reconstruction. This portion is relatively redundant, which allows for the exceptional rotational mobility of the atlanto-axial joint. After passing through the transverse process of the atlas, the artery courses medially behind the articular process, passing beneath the posterior occipito-atlantal ligament and entering the skull at the atlanto-occipital membrane to become intradural.

The third portion of the VA is approached surgically between C2 and C1, where it lies deep to the levator scapula muscle and is crossed anteriorly by the anterior ramus of the C2 nerve. A dense plexus of veins intimately surrounds this segment. The artery at this level receives one or more important collateral branches from the occipital or ascending cervical arteries. In cases of proximal vertebral artery occlusion, these anastomotic collaterals allow for continued patency of the more distal VA (Figure 25–1A, B). Above C1, the VA is more difficult to approach as it is covered by short, thick musculature and the surrounding venous plexus is at its most dense.[1]

After passing through the atlanto-occipital membrane, the fourth segment of the VA penetrates the dura mater and enters the cranial vault through the foramen magnum. As it becomes intracranial, the VA ascends in front of the medulla oblongata to end at the lower portion of the pons. Here, it meets the contralateral VA at midline to form the basilar trunk. As this fourth segment penetrates the dura, the adventitial layer and the external elastic lamina both disappear. As a result, the arterial wall thins significantly. Because of this anatomic change, it is usually inadvisable to vigorously instrument the fourth portion of the vertebral artery with embolectomy catheters or dilators during surgical reconstruction, or with angioplasty balloons in the interventional radiology suite as irreparable damage to the vessel may occur.

The paired vertebral arteries are often asymmetric. The left VA is often the larger of the two. It is not uncommon for one VA to be hypoplastic or absent. Rarely, one VA ends in a posterior inferior cerebellar artery (PICA), and has no confluence with the contralateral VA. The vertebral arteries usually arise from their respective subclavian arteries but in 6% of patients the left VA arises directly from the aortic arch. When this anomaly occurs, the left VA often enters the vertebral foramina at a level above C6. Also, in 7% of patients, the VA enters the transverse vertebral process not at C6, but lower in the neck at C7, making the proximal artery harder to expose and more difficult to manipulate surgically. This situation is rarely noted preoperatively.

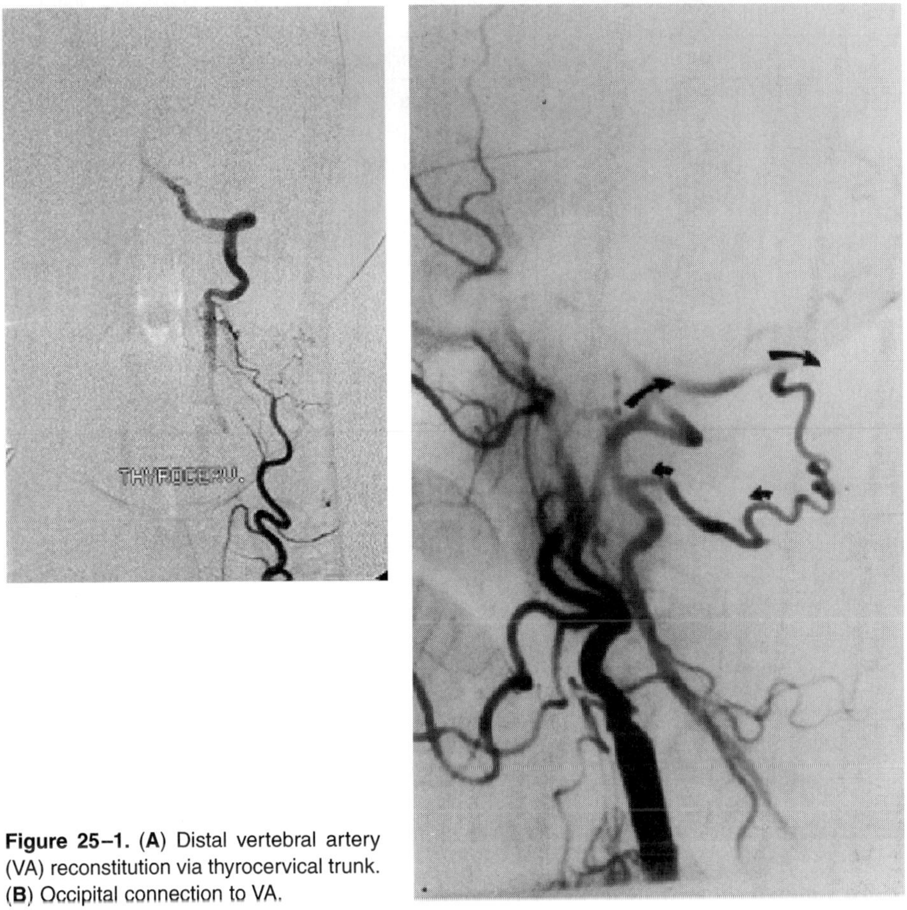

Figure 25–1. (**A**) Distal vertebral artery (VA) reconstitution via thyrocervical trunk. (**B**) Occipital connection to VA.

PATHOPHYSIOLOGY

The mechanisms of vertebrobasilar ischemia are varied. As a result, the clinical manifestations of vertebrobasilar ischemia are also numerous. In addition, patient selection can be confounded by the many medical conditions that mimic vertebrobasilar ischemia (Table 25–1). The symptoms associated with brain stem ischemia are often vague and are certainly not as distinct as those associated with carotid/hemispheric ischemia. Vertebrobasilar ischemia, which effects the temporo-occipital areas of the cerebral hemispheres as well as segments of the brain stem and cerebellum, characteristically produces bilateral symptoms. The classic symptoms of vertebrobasilar ischemia are dizziness, vertigo, diplopia, perioral numbness, alternating parathesiae, tinnitus, dysphasia, dysarthria, and imbalance. Other common symptoms include oscillopsia, blurred vision, ambliopia, drop attacks, and quadriplegia.[2] Lateral medullary syndrome can result when perfusion to a single PICA is compromised.

TABLE 25–1. ALTERNATIVE DIAGNOSES

Medical Conditions that Mimic Vertebrobasilar Ischemia
Cardiac arrhythmia
Pacemaker malfunction
Labyrinthine dysfunction
CPA tumors
Hypoglycemia
Antihypertensive medications
Cerebellar degeneration
Myxedema
Electrolyte imbalance
Others

In general, the ischemic mechanisms can be broken down into those that are hemodynamic and those that are embolic. Hemodynamic symptoms occur as a result of brain stem hypoperfusion and can be precipitated by postural changes or by transient reduction in cardiac output. Proximal subclavian artery occlusive disease may result in hemodynamic ischemic symptoms as a result of subclavian steal. For hemodynamic symptoms to occur as a result of VA disease proper, significant pathology must be present in both of the paired vertebral arteries and compensatory contribution from the carotid circulation, through the circle of Willis, must be incomplete. Alternately, hemodynamic symptoms may follow intermittent extrinsic compression of the vertebral arteries. This can result from arterial impingement from cervical osteophytes or following extreme neck rotation. Ischemia from hemodynamic mechanisms rarely results in tissue infarction; rather, symptoms are short lived, repetitive, and more of a nuisance than a danger. Such hemodynamic symptoms can be hazardous, however, if they happen to occur during critical activities, such as driving.

Traditionally, most neurologists have considered vertebrobasilar symptoms to be purely the result of hemodynamic ischemia. For many years, it was felt that patients suffered from diminished or inadequate blood flow only; hence the term *vertebrobasilar insufficiency,* which is still used, often incorrectly, to describe the syndrome. This was the same interpretation given to carotid ischemia in the early 1970s until the embolic mechanism was widely recognized and became accepted. Since the early 1980s, there has been mounting evidence from detailed pathologic study to indicate that most of the infarctions in the vertebrobasilar territory and up to one-third of vertebrobasilar ischemic syndromes are the result of emboli to the posterior circulation.[3] Emboli result in subclinical or clinical brain stem and posterior hemispheric stroke, and are usually the result of microembolization from proximal sources, including the heart and the aortic arch, or the subclavian, vertebral, and basilar arteries. Plaques found in the subclavian and vertebral arteries have been shown to harbor the same degenerative characteristics as the carotid artery. These include intraplaque hemorrhage, ulceration, and surface thrombus. Emboli can arise from atherosclerotic lesions; intimal defects caused by extrinsic compression or repetitive trauma; and rarely from fibromuscular lesions, Takayasu's or radiation arteritis, aneurysms, or dissections. Compared to hemodynamic mechanisms of ischemia, emboli are more likely to cause fatal infarcts or leave patients with permanent and debilitating strokes.

DIAGNOSIS

The precise diagnosis of a surgically treatable cause for vertebrobasilar ischemia begins with an accurate assessment of the presenting symptom complex. This must be followed by thorough efforts to exclude other causes for patient symptoms. Certain prescription medications can mimic vertebrobasilar ischemia; therefore, patient medications require thorough review. Investigation must be undertaken to exclude inner ear pathology, including rare cerebellar-pontine angle tumors. A cardiac source may be the most common cause of brain stem ischemia, especially in elderly patients. Generally, a complete cardiac work-up, including electrocardiographic (ECG) and Holter monitoring, should be carried out. Because patients often present with a combination of cerebral hemispheric and posterior circulation symptoms, investigation of the carotid circulation is usually warranted.

The ultimate diagnosis and treatment of surgically correctable causes of vertebrobasilar ischemia can remain elusive as a result of difficulties identifying and then defining the offending lesion. Duplex ultrasound is an excellent tool to detect lesions at the carotid bifurcation. In addition, ultrasound imaging can diagnose great vessel pathology, confirm subclavian steal, and sample intracranial velocities. Duplex has become a useful tool for identifying flow velocity changes and stenosis in the vertebral artery as well as reversal of flow down a VA. As such, duplex has become an invaluable screening tool for patients with vertebrobasilar symptomatology. Detection of abnormalities by ultrasound often leads to an accurate diagnosis on follow-up arteriographic evaluation. However, the absence of ultrasonographic defects does not necessarily rule out the possibility of significant vertebral artery pathology.

Small embolic infarctions of the brain stem generally cannot be detected by computed tomography, which is the imaging technique of choice for diagnosing hemispheric pathology. In contrast to traditional computed tomography (CT) scans, transaxial magnetic resonance (MR) images can readily diagnose both acute and chronic posterior fossa infarcts (Figure 25–2). Transaxial MR images should be obtained routinely in all patients suspected to have suffered embolic infarction in the distribution of the posterior circulation.

In addition, we are presently evaluating magnetic resonance angiography (MRA) as a tool for identifying vertebral artery pathology. Recent developments in MR imaging show great promise for safe, noninvasive, detailed evaluation of both the extracranial and intracranial vasculature. New contrast-enhanced MRA techniques provide full-image coverage of the supra-aortic trunks and the carotid and vertebral arteries (Figure 25–3).

Selective subclavian and vertebral angiography remains the gold standard for preoperative evaluation of patients with vertebrobasilar ischemia. Some surgeons still consider angiography to be mandatory prior to surgical reconstruction. The most common site of disease, the VA origin, may not be well imaged with ultrasound or MRA,

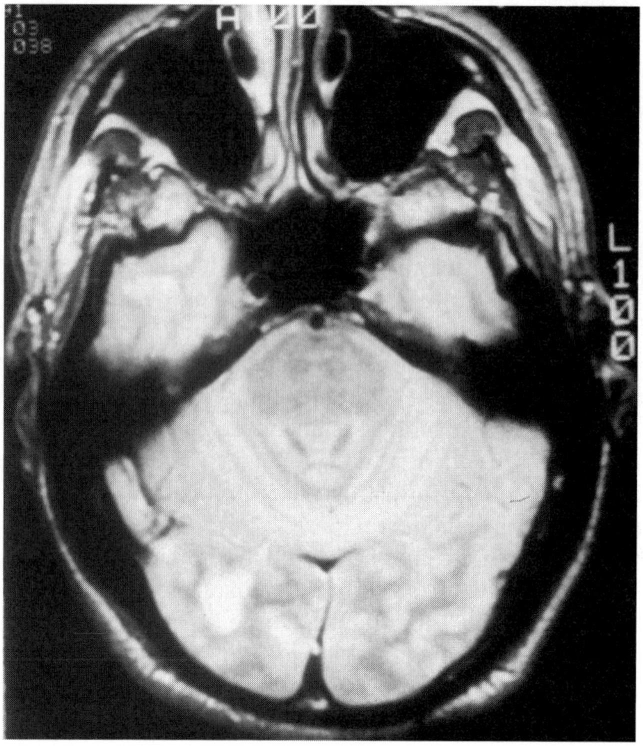

Figure 25–2. Magnetic resonance image (MRI) showing cerebellar infarct.

and in fact often can be displayed only with oblique projections that are not part of standard arch evaluation. Patients with VA compression syndromes who suffer from positional symptoms should undergo dynamic angiography, which incorporates provocative positioning (Figure 25–4). Delayed images may demonstrate reconstitution of an occluded extracranial VA through existing cervical connections.

SURGICAL RECONSTRUCTION

Accumulated experience has shown that, with appropriate surgical intervention, predictable resolution of hemodynamic symptoms and cessation of embolic events can occur. In addition, VA reconstruction is attended by fewer ischemic complications than carotid surgery, and appears to have better long-term results.

Identifiable pathology in the first segment of the VA consists, fundamentally, of atherosclerotic lesions at the origin of the VA. These ostial lesions generally originate in the subclavian artery and are smooth and fibrous in nature. These lesions most commonly produce hemodynamic-type symptoms when found in conjunction with contralateral VA abnormalities or in circumstances in which the vertebrals do not communicate, one forming the basilar artery and one ending in a PICA. These ostial lesions

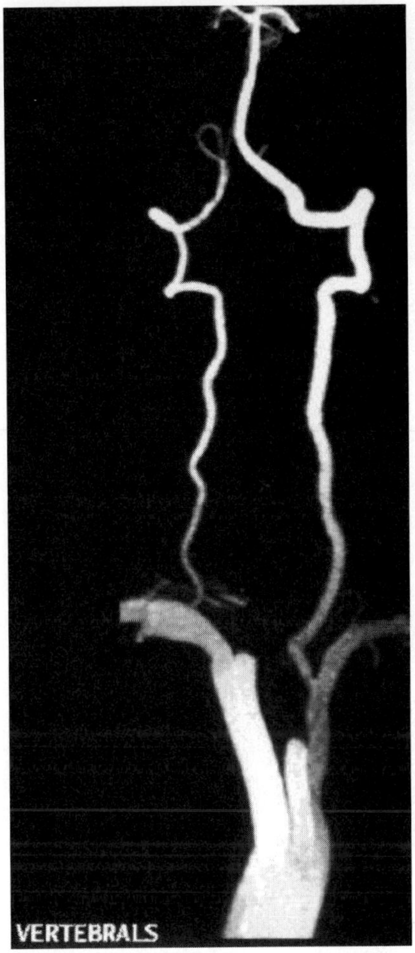

Figure 25–3. Selective vertebral MR angiogram.

also have been known to ulcerate and embolize; however, this occurs infrequently. A number of operations have been described to treat these offending ostial lesions. The original operations to correct proximal VA lesions consisted of direct vertebral or transsubclavian endarterectomies with or without patch angioplasty reconstructions. Vein bypasses taking origin from the more distal subclavian or carotid artery also have been popular forms of reconstruction in the past. Vein bypasses are now usually reserved for situations in which the VA cannot be transposed because of limited length or significant disease in the adjacent donor artery. Transposition of the proximal VA onto the common carotid artery is the most commonly performed reconstruction.

Proximal vertebral transposition is performed following an oblique skin incision over both heads of the sternocleidomastoid muscle at the base of the neck. The two muscle bellies are split, the common carotid artery is retracted medially, and the jugular vein and vagus nerve are moved laterally. On the left side, the thoracic duct is ligated. The vertebral vein is identified in the mediastinum adjacent to the sympathetic

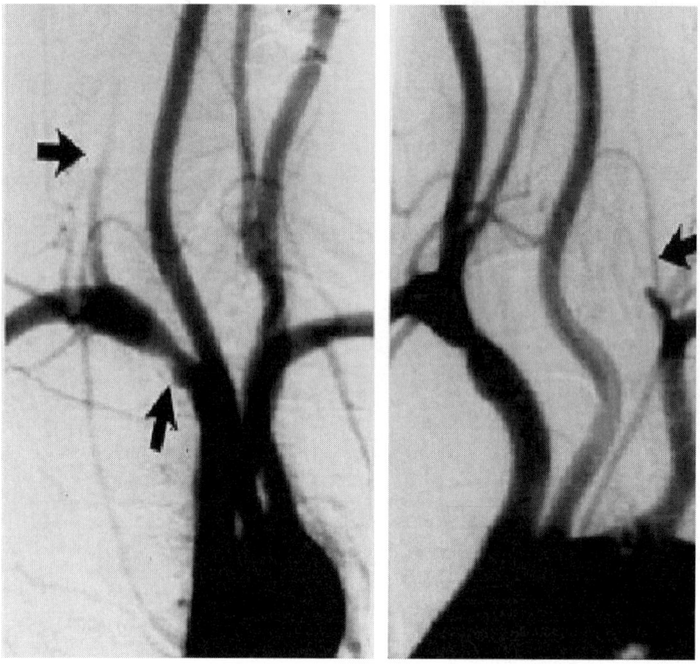

Figure 25–4. Dynamic bilateral VA occlusions.

chain. The vein is ligated and then divided to expose the proximal VA near its origin from the subclavian artery. The first segment of the VA must be mobilized completely from its origin at the subclavian artery to the point where it disappears beneath the tendon to the longus coli muscle. Care must be taken to preserve the sympathetic nerve trunks that ascend with the artery lest a postoperative Horner's syndrome result. Following complete dissection of both the VA and the adjacent segment of carotid artery, the surgeon must judge whether there is adequate length and mobility to swing the VA to a site of implantation on the common carotid. Following systemic anticoagulation with heparin, the VA is divided at its origin and oversewn proximally. The distal VA is then pulled from underneath the sympathetic trunks, spatulated for anastomosis, and transposed to an appropriate site on the posterolateral aspect of the common carotid. The common carotid arteriotomy is created with a cardiac punch and the anastomosis is performed using 7-0 monofilament suture. As with all vertebral reconstructions, completion arteriography is performed prior to closing the incision (Figure 25–5).

The second segment of the VA is the site of origin of a wide variety of disorders. External compression is most likely to occur in a part of the second segment. External compression is an important mechanism for temporary occlusion and, occasionally, for thrombosis or dissection of the VA. Vertebral artery compression syndromes are most frequently caused by osteophytes, the edge of the transverse foramina, and the intervertebral joints. Rotation or extension of the neck usually triggers compression of the VA in its second segment. Vertebral artery compression can be demonstrated radi-

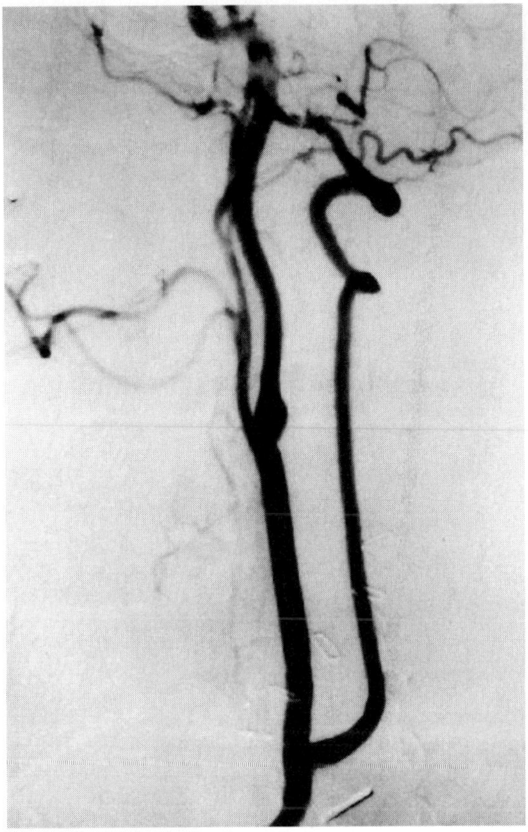

Figure 25–5. Proximal vertebral to common carotid artery transposition.

ographically and linked to specific symptoms through techniques of dynamic arteriography. These studies include radiographic contrast injection with the patient's neck in the symptom-producing position.

The second segment of the VA is also a common site for aneurysmal degeneration of the VA (Figure 25–6 A, B) as well as a frequent site for embolizing atherosclerotic plaques (Figure 25–7) and fibromuscular diseases. Direct surgical reconstruction of the VA in its second segment is very rarely undertaken. However, a number of extrinsic lesions can be corrected to relieve kinking or compression of the artery in this segment. A laminectomy is usually necessary to expose this segment of the VA for purposes of treating a traumatic injury.

Reconstruction of the distal VA is usually performed at the C1–C2 level. For more distal pathology, the VA can also be accessed surgically above the level of the transverse process of C1. The third portion of the VA is vulnerable to direct trauma and stretch injuries that can lead to intimal damage and thrombosis/embolization and dissection. It is also in this segment that the VA is particularly prone to arteriovenous fistula formation and aneurysmal degeneration. Such pathology most likely is the result of an occult traumatic injury.

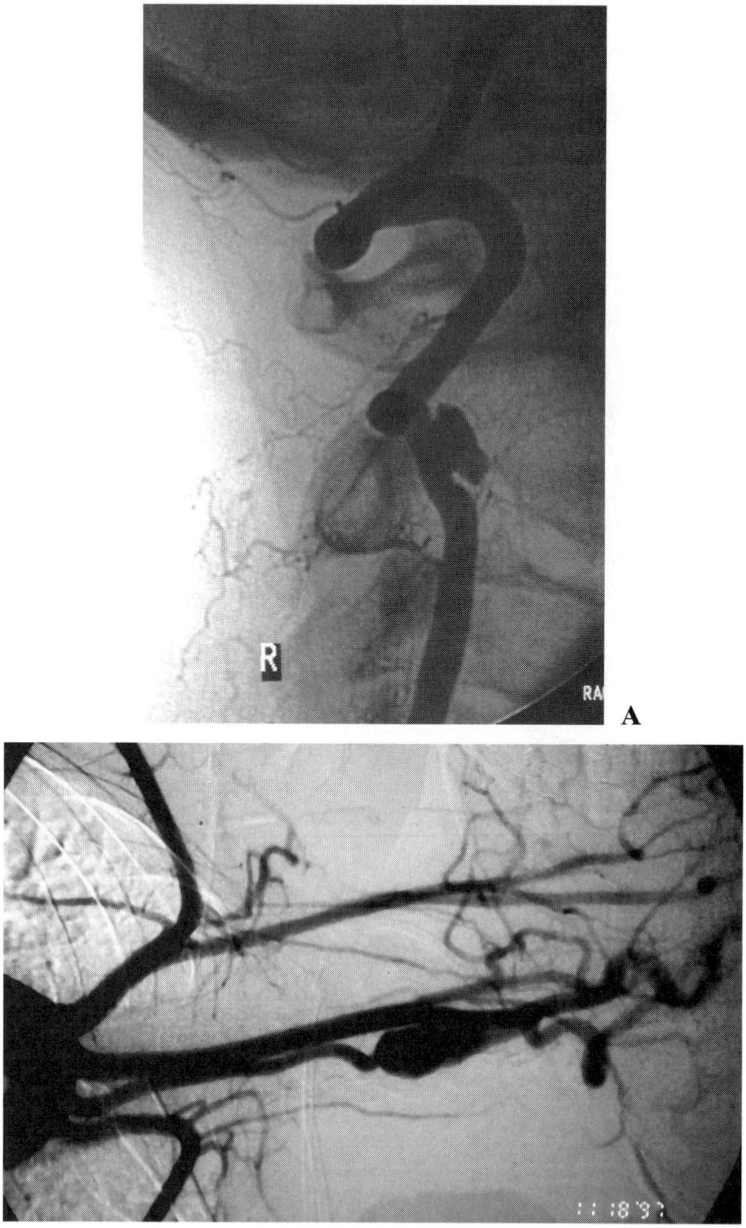

A

B

Figure 25–6. (**A, B**) Vertebral artery aneurysm.

A proximal VA occlusion is the most commonly identified lesion. As mentioned previously, the third segment of the VA can be maintained following a proximal VA occlusion by any of a number of collaterals from the external carotid or subclavian arteries to the more distal VA. This can be exploited in reconstructing the third segment of the VA.

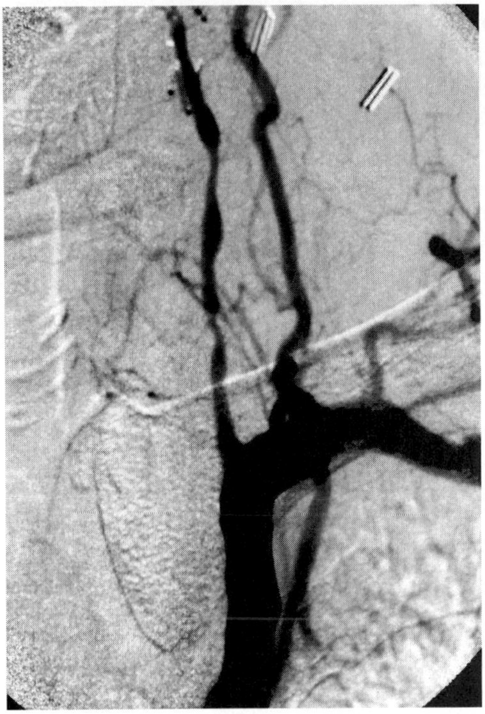

Figure 25–7. Atherosclerotic VA can be a source for emboli.

The techniques most often used to reconstruct the distal VA include saphenous vein bypass from the common carotid, subclavian, or proximal vertebral artery. Transposition of the external carotid or hypertrophied occipital artery to the distal VA and transposition of the distal VA to the side of the distal internal carotid artery have also been described.[4] We took a novel approach to the treatment of symptomatic VA aneurysm that includes carotid to distal vertebral bypass combined with intraoperative transfemoral catheterization of the proximal vertebral artery and coil embolization.

The distal VA at the level of C1–C2 is approached through a standard incision over the anterior border of the sternocleidomastoid muscle. The dissection proceeds between the anterior border of the sternocleidomastoid muscle and the posterolateral wall of the internal jugular vein. The spinal accessory nerve must be identified and isolated as it exits from beneath the digastric muscle and passes over the jugular vein. The transverse process of C1 can be palpated posteriorly at this level, and this bony prominence marks the upper limit of dissection for this approach to the VA. The levator scapula muscle is then divided completely near its insertion. At this level, the anterior ramus of the C2 nerve exits from beneath the anterior border of the levator muscle and divides into two or three branches. This nerve root is carefully divided as well to expose the bulging VA beneath. Bipolar cautery is then used to coagulate the branches of the venous plexus that intimately adhere to the VA at this level. The VA can then be controlled circumferentially with a Silastic loop after passing a small angled clamp behind it. Recall that multiple collateral branches join the distal VA at this level, and care must be taken to avoid their avulsion. With the distal VA exposed at this level, it can easily be controlled inferiorly and superiorly with a small, C-shaped vascular clamp. With the patient anticoagulated and flow through the VA controlled in this manner, a longitudinal arteriotomy is then created on the anterior aspect of the vessel, and a venous bypass conduit or transposed artery can be anastomosed directly to the side of the VA using 7-0 or 8-0 monofilament suture (Figure 25–8). For proximal embolizing lesions the VA is clipped or tied off proximal to the anastomosis. Alternatively, if there is adequate length of VA following complete exposure of the vessel, it can be transected transversely, spatulated, and transposed onto the side of a segment of the distal internal carotid artery.

When using a vein for bypass, we prefer a valveless segment of the greater saphenous vein from the thigh. It is useful to map this segment of vein preoperatively to assure adequate diameter >3.5 mm. When an external carotid or occipital artery transposition is anticipated, it is important that there be no disease narrowing the vessel at its origin from the carotid bifurcation. The external carotid must then be skeletonized to the level of the internal maxillary artery to assure adequate length. The occipital artery, however, often has more than adequate length, but its caliber is adequate only if it has become hypertrophied over time, as in the case of a longstanding occipital–vertebral connection.

Rarely is it necessary to reach the distal VA at a level above C1. If this is anticipated preoperatively, the patient is placed in a park-bench position and the incision is carried posteriorly to allow division of the upper insertion of the sternocleidomastoid and splenius capitis muscles. The transverse process of C1 and part of its posterior arch are resected to expose the VA and the rich venous plexus that surrounds it. Saphenous vein bypass to this segment is generally the only viable option for reconstruction.

Intraoperative completion imaging using digital angiography is necessary for all types of VA reconstruction. A significant number of reparable technical flaws may be identified, and repair can prevent reconstruction failure.

Segment four of the VA is rarely diseased. Infrequent lesions consist of atheroscle-

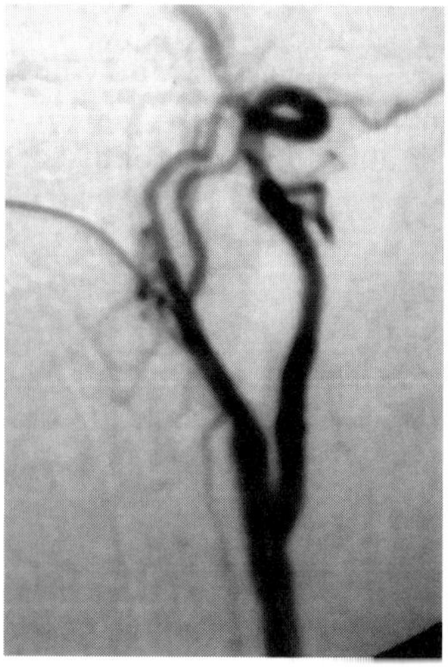

Figure 25–8. Carotid to distal VA bypass.

rotic plaques that appear to localize to the level of the atlanto-occipital membrane. Successful balloon angioplasty has been reported. Also, in rare cases, intracranial revascularization including fourth-segment endarterectomy, occipital to posterior inferior cerebellar artery bypass, and superficial temporal to superior cerebellar artery reconstructions have been described in the neurosurgical literature, but with mixed results.

RESULTS

Results following both proximal and distal VA reconstructions are generally equal to or better than those reported in series reviewing other forms of cerebrovascular revascularization; this includes large series reviewing CEA. In a review of 369 proximal and distal VA reconstructions, Berguer et al.[5] reported 5-yr patency rates of 80%, and in the latter half of the series, the combined stroke and death rates were <2%. Another series that looked closely at distal VA reconstruction alone reported 4 deaths, all from stroke, from a group of 100 patients who underwent the procedure. Secondary reconstruction patency was 80% after 10 yr in this review, and 83% of patients from this series were cured of symptoms or substantially improved.[6] McNamara and Berguer[7] reported a series of 37 patients who underwent combined carotid and vertebral revascularization and noted two deaths and a single stroke.

With experience, surgeons can perform vertebral artery reconstruction with low risk to the patient. The patency rates are excellent, and the vast majority of patients experience long-term benefits such as prevention from brain stem, cerebellar, and posterior hemispheric stroke.

REFERENCES

1. Berguer R. Suboccipital approach to the distal vertebral artery. *J Vasc Surg.* 1999;30:344–349.
2. Rancurel G, Kieffer E, Arzimanoglou A, Vitte E, Freyss G. Hemodynamic vertebrobasilar ischemia: differentiation of hemodynamic and thromboembolic mechanisms. In Berguer R, Caplan LR, eds. *Vertebrobasilar Arterial Disease.* St. Louis: Quality Medical Publishing, Inc.; 1992:40–51.
3. Yates PO. Atheromatous lesions of the vertebral arteries and brain infarction. In Berguer R, Caplan LR, eds. *Vertebrobasilar Arterial Disease.* St. Louis: Quality Medical Publishing, Inc.; 1992:3–10.
4. Berguer R, Kieffer E. *Surgery of the Arteries to the Head.* New York: Springer-Verlag; 1992.
5. Berguer R, Flynn LM, Kline RA, Caplan L. Surgical reconstruction of the extracranial vertebral artery: management and outcome. *J Vasc Surg.* 2000;31:9–18.
6. Berguer R, Morasch MD, Kline RA. A review of 100 consecutive reconstructions of the distal vertebral artery for embolic and hemodynamic disease. *J Vasc Surg.* 1998;27:852–859.
7. McNamara MF, Berguer R. Simultaneous carotid–vertebral reconstruction. *J Cardiovasc Surg.* 1989;30:161–164.

26

Distal Bypasses in the Diabetic Patient

Cameron M. Akbari, MD, and Frank W. LoGerfo, MD

Diabetes mellitus is found in more than 5% of the US population, and the incidence is increasing, with more than 500,000 new cases diagnosed annually.[1] Multiple epidemiologic studies spanning several decades have established a clear link between diabetes and vascular disease. The Framingham Study[2] of more than 5000 subjects demonstrated that diabetes is a powerful risk factor for atherosclerotic coronary and peripheral arterial disease. It is a contributing factor for half of all lower extremity amputations performed in the United States, and it has been estimated that the relative risk for amputation is 40 times greater among people with diabetes.[3] Despite significant advances in the prevention and treatment of peripheral vascular disease, diabetes continues to be the single strongest cardiovascular risk factor for the development of critical leg ischemia and limb loss.[4]

Problems of the diabetic foot are the most common cause for hospitalization in diabetic patients, with an annual health-care cost of more than $1 billion.[5] Diabetic foot ulceration affects 15% of all diabetic individuals during their lifetime, with an annual incidence of 3%, and is clearly a significant risk factor in the pathway to limb loss.[6] Fundamental to diabetic limb salvage is a thorough understanding of the diabetic foot, because all treatment is ultimately directed toward this uniquely complex biologic milieu.

GENERAL CONSIDERATIONS

One of the greatest impediments in understanding vascular disease in patients with diabetes is the misconception that they have an untreatable occlusive lesion in the arteriolar microcirculation, which in turn would suggest that any attempt at correction of ischemia is futile in these patients. This idea of so-called small-vessel disease probably originated from a retrospective study demonstrating the presence of periodic acid–Schiff (PAS)-positive material occluding the arterioles in amputated limb specimens from diabetic patients.[7] However, subsequent prospective anatomic staining and arterial casting studies have demonstrated the absence of an arteriolar occlusive lesion.[8,9] Further evidence comes from physiologic studies of femoropopliteal bypass grafts in diabetic and nondiabetic patients in which direct vasodilator administration into these grafts demonstrates a comparable fall in peripheral resistance between the two groups.[10] These data, coupled with a vast clinical experience of nearly three decades of successful arterial reconstruction in diabetic patients, have thoroughly dispelled the hopeless notion of diabetic small-vessel disease.[11]

Although there is no occlusive lesion in the diabetic microcirculation, other structural changes do exist.[12] Nonocclusive capillary basement thickening may be found in the diabetic microcirculation. Although this does not lead to narrowing of the capillary lumen, consequences include impaired leukocyte migration and increased susceptibility to infection, as well as a diminished maximal hyperemic response following injury. Diabetes also affects the axon reflex. Normally, nociceptive C-fiber stimulation (by injury) causes the secretion of active peptides, such as substance P, that directly and indirectly (through mast cell release of histamine) cause vasodilation and increased permeability. This neurogenic vasodilatory response is impaired in diabetes, further reducing the hyperemic response when it is most needed—that is, under conditions of injury and inflammation. All of these changes contribute to a functional microvascular impairment in the diabetic foot.[13]

Due to these complex microvascular and leukocyte abnormalities, it is not surprising that classic signs of infection, such as erythema and rubor, are often absent in the infected diabetic foot. Fever, chills, and leukocytosis may be absent in up to two-thirds of diabetic patients with extensive foot infections, and hyperglycemia is often the sole presenting sign. Because a benign-appearing superficial ulcer may rapidly progress to a potentially fatal infection, a thorough evaluation for infection in these patients is mandatory. Therefore, prompt control of infection, with incision and drainage of all infected tissue planes and broad-spectrum antibiotics, assumes first priority in diabetic foot management.[14]

The role of neuropathy in the pathogenesis of the diabetic foot is also considerable: it afflicts as many as 50% to 60% of all patients and is present in more than 80% of diabetic patients with foot lesions. Sensory nerve fiber involvement leads to loss of the protective sensation of pain, whereas motor fiber destruction results in small muscle atrophy in the foot. Consequently, the metatarsals are flexed with metatarsal head prominence and "clawing" of the toes. This leads to abnormal pressure points on the bony prominence without sensation, with subsequent erosion and ulceration. Meanwhile, autonomic neuropathy in the foot causes loss of sympathetic tone, which results in increased arteriovenous shunting and inefficient nutrient flow. Autonomic denervation of sweat glands leads to cracking of dry skin, which further predisposes the diabetic foot to skin breakdown and ulceration.[15]

PREOPERATIVE EVALUATION

All limb salvage efforts in the diabetic patient will fail unless ischemia has been appropriately evaluated and treated. Fundamentally, this requires an awareness of the unique biology of the diabetic foot, and knowledge of the nature and pattern of vascular disease in the diabetic patient (Figure 26–1). Microcirculatory and endothelial dysfunction,[16] sensorimotor neuropathy, and loss of the neurogenic inflammatory response predispose the diabetic foot to ulceration even with moderate ischemia. In this milieu, maximal circulation is required to heal an ulcer, and correction of even a moderate degree of ischemia facilitates healing significantly. Therefore, preoperative evaluation should be directed toward the goal of restoring normal arterial pressure to the target area.

A variety of noninvasive arterial tests may be ordered in the evaluation for ischemia. However, in the presence of diabetes, all of these tests have significant limitations. Medial arterial calcinosis occurs frequently in diabetic patients and is characterized by a nonobstructive calcification of the vessel wall at the media layer; its presence can result in noncompressible arteries with artifactually high segmental systolic pressures and ankle–brachial indices. Segmental Doppler wave forms and pulsed volume recordings are unaffected by medial calcification. However, evaluation of these waveforms is primarily qualitative, and not quantitative. In addition, the quality of the waveforms is affected by peripheral edema, cuff size, and motion artifact, and the presence of ulceration may preclude accurate cuff placement.

The limitations of noninvasive testing emphasize the importance of a thorough bedside evaluation. The single most important aspect is the status of the foot pulse. The absence of a palpable foot pulse strongly suggests ischemia, and this finding alone is an indication for contrast arteriography in the clinical setting of tissue loss, poor healing, or gangrene. Concern for contrast-induced renal failure should not mitigate against a high-quality angiogram of the entire lower extremity circulation. The incidence of contrast nephropathy is not higher in the diabetic patient without preexisting renal disease, even with the use of ionic contrast.[17,18] The more costly non-ionic agents should be reserved for the diabetic patient with compromised renal function. Even in this group, the concern for contrast nephropathy should not delay arteriography, as it seldom requires dialysis for treatment. More recently, attention has focused on the roles of magnetic resonance angiography (MRA), carbon dioxide angiography, and duplex scanning as replacements for contrast arteriography. However, each has its own limitations, and although we have selectively used these modalities, we continue to rely heavily on a high-quality contrast arteriogram for most of our patients requiring distal arterial reconstruction.

Whatever preoperative imaging modality is chosen prior to arterial reconstruction, it is mandatory that consideration be given to the pattern of lower extremity vascular disease in patients with diabetes. Although atherosclerosis is the cause of lower extremity ischemia in both diabetic and nondiabetic patients, there is a difference in the pattern and location of the atherosclerotic process.[19] Diabetic patients are more likely to have atherosclerotic disease affecting the infrageniculate arteries, with sparing of the foot arteries. Conversely, the superficial femoral and popliteal arteries are less likely to be affected by the occlusive process, which allows these vessels to serve as an inflow source for distal bypass grafts.

Because the foot vessels are often spared by the atherosclerotic occlusive process, even when the tibial arteries are occluded, it is essential that arteriograms not be termi-

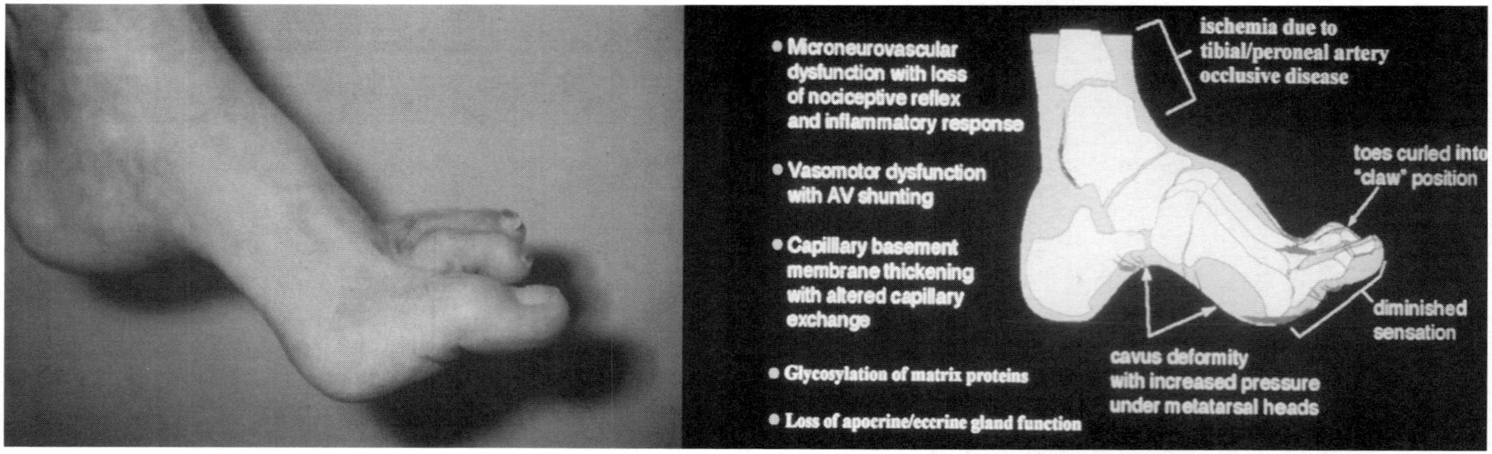

Figure 26–1. Underlying pathophysiology of the diabetic foot predisposing to foot ulceration. The combination of sensorimotor neuropathy, microvascular dysfunction, matrix abnormalities, and atherosclerotic vascular disease ultimately leads to ulceration and poor healing. (*From Akbari CM, LoGerfo FW. Diabetes and peripheral vascular disease. J Vasc Surg 1999;30:373–384, with permission.*)

nated at the midtibial level. The complete infrapopliteal circulation should be incorporated, including the foot vessels (Figure 26–2). Both anteroposterior and lateral foot views should be included to differentiate branch vessels and to visualize all stenoses. Excessive plantar flexion should be avoided, as this can impede visualization of flow in the dorsalis pedis artery.

TECHNICAL CONSIDERATIONS

The primary goal of infrainguinal arterial reconstruction in the ischemic diabetic foot is to bypass to an outflow artery that is in direct continuity with the foot, thereby restoring normal arterial pressure to the target area. Although proximal bypass to the popliteal or proximal tibioperoneal arteries may restore foot pulses, more distal revascularization is often needed to achieve this goal—again, owing to the pattern of occlusive disease in the diabetic patient. Similarly, although excellent results have been reported with peroneal artery bypass, the peroneal artery is not in continuity with the foot vessels and may not achieve the maximal flow required for healing, particularly at the forefoot level. Therefore, we reserve peroneal artery bypass for those rare circumstances in which there is no dorsalis pedis or posterior tibial artery in continuity with the foot, or when limited venous conduit length mitigates against more distal bypass.

Autogenous vein grafting to the dorsalis pedis artery represents a technical advance that provides durable and effective limb salvage for ischemic diabetic foot ulceration.[20] The dorsalis pedis artery is exposed through a longitudinal incision 1 cm distal to an imaginary transverse line between the distal malleoli and 1 cm lateral to the ex-

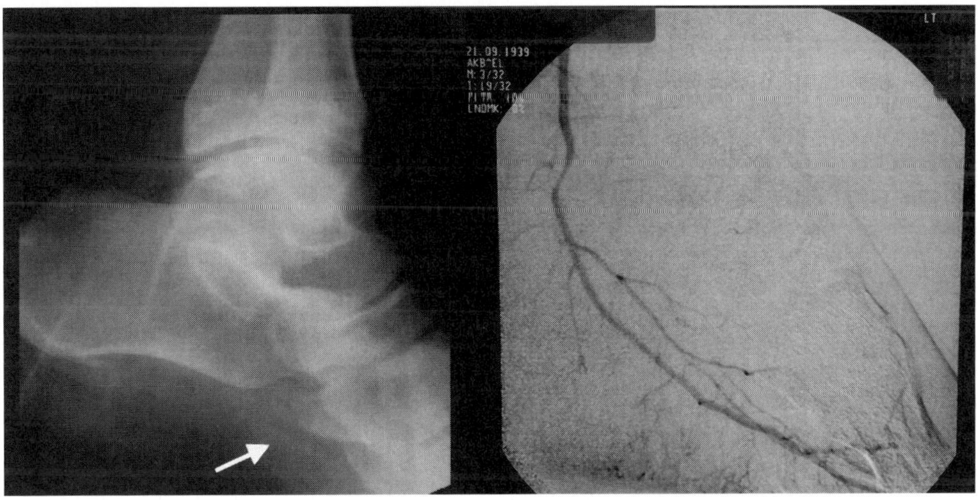

Figure 26–2. Two arteriograms of the foot of the same patient with a heel ulcer. On the left is a conventional angiogram showing only a minimally opacified plantar artery (*white arrow*). Because of no available target outflow artery, amputation was recommended. Repeat arteriogram using digital subtraction techniques is shown on the right, illustrating a patent distal posterior tibial artery. Successful bypass was performed.

tensor hallucis longis tendon. A continuous-wave Doppler probe may be used preoperatively to mark the location of the artery. Experience has shown that the artery is less likely to be calcified at the intermalleolar level. The incision is deepened through the fascia, and the artery is found just beneath the inferior margin of the extensor retinaculum. The dorsalis pedis artery gives off a lateral tarsal branch proximally, then bifurcates into deep plantar and dorsal metatarsal arteries distally. Rarely, the preoperative arteriogram may not demonstrate the dorsalis pedis artery in the presence of an audible Doppler signal over the dorsum of the foot. Under such circumstances, exploration is reasonable as outlined previously. Once the artery is exposed, control is obtained proximally, and distal and longitudinal arteriotomy performed. Careful attempts are made at passage of a 1-mm coronary dilator distally, followed by heparinized saline injection through a 10-cc syringe and a 20-gauge angiocatheter. If injection cannot be performed or if the dilator cannot be passed, the procedure is terminated. With improved arteriographic techniques to visualize the pedal vessels, such as with digital subtraction angiography, blind exploration is now rarely performed.

In the patient with an ischemic heel ulcer, first consideration should be given to the posterior tibial or plantar arteries if they are patent by preoperative imaging. The distal posterior tibial artery is found in the hollow just behind the medial malleolus, halfway between the bone and the Achilles tendon. Again, a Doppler probe may be used to mark its location preoperatively. A longitudinal incision is performed and carried down through the fascia, on which the artery may be visualized. If more distal dissection is required, such as for plantar artery exposure and bypass, the distal dense fascia and flexor retinaculum are divided. This exposes a trifurcation, with a medial calcaneal branch running directly posteriorly toward the heel, followed by the medial and lateral plantar arteries approximately 1 cm beyond the calcaneal branch. If further exposure of the plantar arteries is required, the muscle fibers of the abductor hallucis muscle may be divided.

For control of the distal arterial segment, we prefer Silastic vessel loops instead of vascular clamps. Wide exposure of the artery may unmask a soft segment suitable for vessel loop control. However, in occasional cases, severe calcification of the distal artery may be encountered, precluding conventional attempts at obliteration of flow. In these cases, we use intraluminal vessel occluders (Figure 26–3). Our technique involves careful dissection, taking care not to fracture the calcification, followed by encirclement with loops. Arteriotomy is made, and no attempts are made at endarterectomy or "cracking" the plaque. The luminal diameter is determined by gentle passage of coronary dilators, and an intraluminal bulb-tipped vessel occluder is placed proximally and distally. The correct size of the occluder is typically 0.25 mm larger than the largest coronary dilator that could be passed distally.

The distal location of the dorsalis pedis and posterior tibial arteries theoretically necessitates a long venous conduit, which is often not attainable. However, by using the popliteal or distal superficial femoral artery as an inflow site, a shorter length of vein may be used, with excellent long-term patency. This is particularly true in the diabetic patient—again, due to the pattern of atherosclerotic disease. This avoids dissection in the groin and upper thigh, a common location for wound complications. In addition, the shorter length of saphenous vein obviates the need for foot extension of the vein

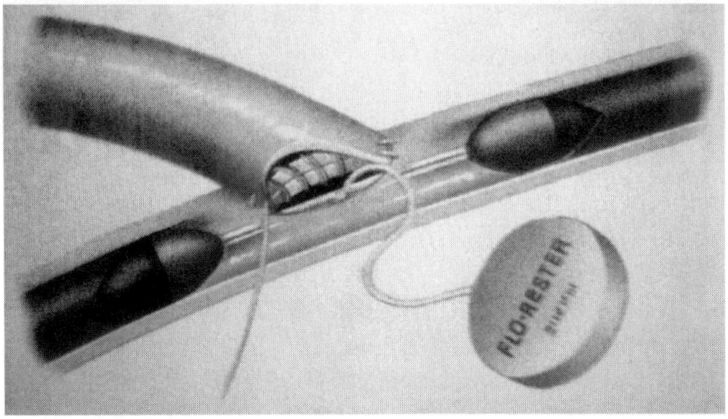

Figure 26–3. Illustration of an intraluminal vessel occluder.

harvest incision, which is parallel to the one required to expose the paramalleolar and inframalleolar arteries; this avoids the resultant skin bridge that may occasionally become ischemic from undue tension. If a skin bridge is created, as with an *in situ* bypass, care must be taken to create the subcutaneous graft tunnel proximal, and not through, the skin bridge (Figure 26–4).

The vein graft can be prepared as an *in situ*, reversed, or nonreversed graft, without any significant difference in outcome.[21] Therefore, we advocate a flexible approach, taking advantage of the technical strategy best suited to the individual vascular anatomy. The *in situ* technique minimizes size mismatch between the graft and native arteries, eliminates the need to completely mobilize the vein, and may prevent inadvertent twisting of the graft. We use the *in situ* technique for most infrageniculate distal bypass grafts originating from the common femoral artery. Although the valves in the vein graft may be lysed blindly, we prefer to cut the valves under direct angioscopic guidance using a flexible valvulotome (Figure 26–5). This also allows for assessment of the saphenous vein to detect intraluminal abnormalities and can help direct endoluminal interventions that upgrade the quality of the conduit and improve patency.

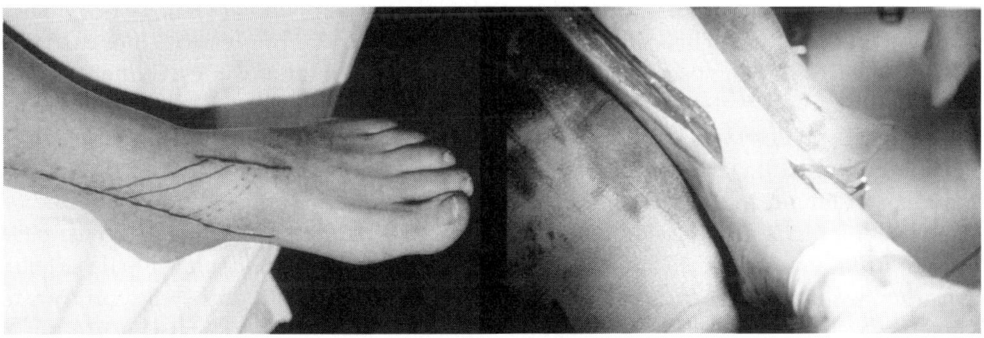

Figure 26–4. The subcutaneous tunnel to the dorsalis pedis artery should be made proximal (*solid line*) and not through (*dotted line*) the skin bridge. The picture on the right illustrates the vein graft brought through the correct configuration.

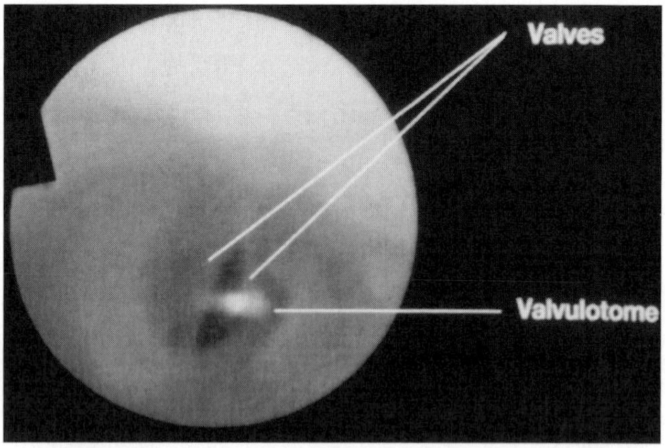

Figure 26–5. Angioscopy-guided valve lysis.

If the distal superficial femoral or popliteal artery is used as an inflow site, the harvested vein graft may be prepared using nonreversed vein with the valves cut either blindly or, preferably, under direct vision with the angioscope. If there is no significant size mismatch or if the saphenous vein is larger at the ankle, the graft may be used in the reversed configuration. In either case, the graft is usually placed back in its native bed in the lower leg, with care taken to avoid kinking or twisting, and then brought through a subcutaneous tunnel to the paramalleolar outflow artery.

We continue to advocate an all-autogenous policy for infrainguinal revascularization, and in our opinion, prosthetic grafts should not be used for distal bypasses. When ipsilateral saphenous vein is not available, several alternatives exist for autogenous conduit. Although the contralateral saphenous vein is an obvious alternative, several considerations limit its use in the diabetic patient. Contralateral leg vein may not always be present in this population of patients, who often require multiple cardiovascular interventions. More importantly, we and others have found that diabetes is a strong risk factor for subsequent contralateral limb bypass, with almost 60% of patients requiring contralateral bypass at 3 yr. Therefore, our approach has been to use arm vein grafts as the first alternative in the absence of ipsilateral saphenous vein. The cephalic, basilic, or upper arm basilic–cephalic loop vein grafts may be harvested. Once the vein has been harvested, angioscopic evaluation is crucial, as many of these patients have undergone multiple venipunctures and cannulations with resultant scarring and weblike synechiae. Angioscopy allows for detection and correction of many of these areas (Figure 26–6) and allows for precise valve lysis within these thin-walled veins. Damaged segments within the graft that cannot be corrected angioscopically should be resected.[22]

Once the distal anastomosis is completed, intraoperative assessment may be performed, usually with a hand-held sterile Doppler probe. Any abnormal signals should be further evaluated with intraoperative arteriography. For *in situ* grafts, the entire graft is interrogated for residual arteriovenous fistulae, which are then ligated. Care must also be taken in closure of the distal incision with either a subcutaneous suture or interrupted fine nonabsorbable closure in place of skin staples. Postoperative edema is common, and can be minimized by elevating the leg and limiting ambulation.

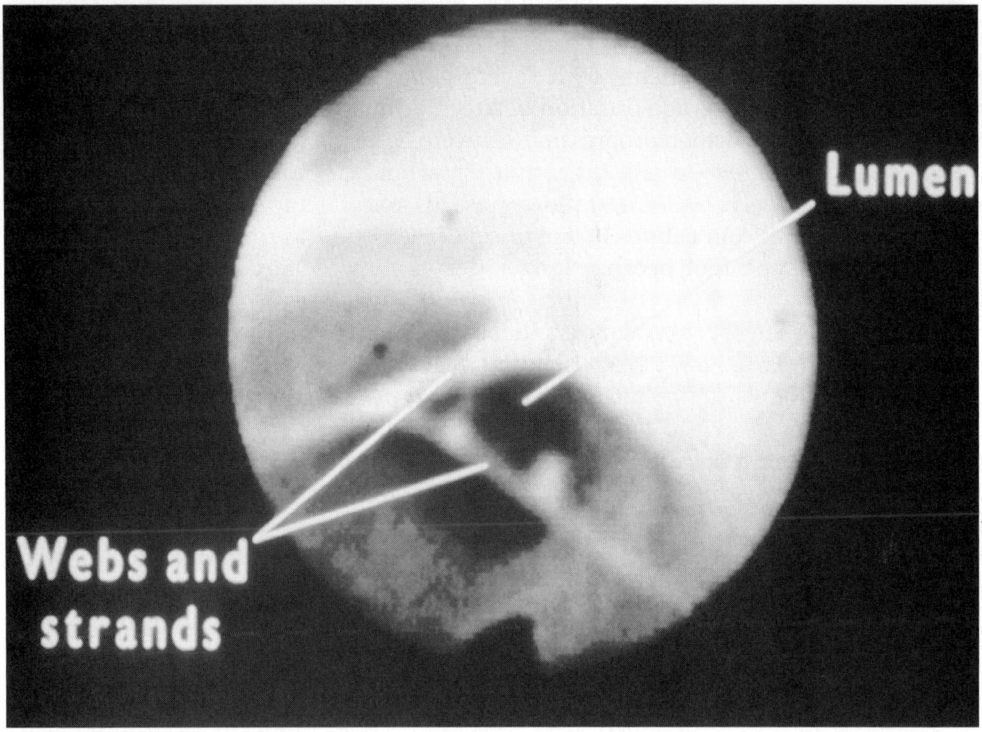

Figure 26–6. Abnormalities detected by angioscopy include webs and strands (seen here), which can often be lysed with a valvulotome. More extensive abnormalities require resection of that segment.

RESULTS

Our initial report of dorsalis pedis arterial bypass demonstrated technical feasibility and short-term durability of the procedure, with patency and limb salvage rates approaching 90% at 3 yr.[23] We subsequently reported on a more extensive 8-yr experience encompassing 384 vein grafts to the dorsalis pedis artery in 367 patients.[24] Ninety-five percent (95%) of the patients had diabetes mellitus, and all procedures were performed for limb-threatening ischemia. The superficial femoral or popliteal artery served as the inflow source in 60% of the patients—again, consistent with the familiar pattern of atherosclerotic disease in the diabetic limb. Twenty-nine grafts (7.5%) failed within the first 30 days, but 19 were successfully revised when a correctable technical problem was found at reoperation. The perioperative in-hospital mortality rate was 1.8%, and the actuarial primary and secondary patency and limb salvage rates were 68%, 82%, and 87%, respectively, at 5-yr follow-up.

Active infection in the foot is not a contraindication to dorsalis pedis bypass, as long as the infectious process is controlled. Adequate control implies resolution of cellulitis, lymphangitis, and edema, especially in areas of proposed incisions required to expose the distal artery or saphenous vein. We reported the results of 56 vein bypasses to the dorsal pedal artery in patients with ischemic foot lesions complicated by infection, including 15 patients with severe gangrene, osteomyelitis, and/or deep space abscess.[25] The average duration between admission and bypass was 10 days, and no patient had further progression of necrosis prior to bypass. Although there was a 12% wound infection rate, the primary graft patency and limb salvage was 92% and 98%, respectively, at 36-mo follow-up. This report emphasizes the need for a timely progression from active control of severe infection to revascularization in the complicated diabetic foot because longer delays may jeopardize chances for limb salvage.

As noted earlier, severe circumferential calcification of the distal artery may be encountered. We reported a 6-yr experience with 101 bypass grafts to severely calcified, unclampable outflow arteries, including 40 grafts to pedal or tarsal/plantar arteries, using the techniques described previously.[26] At 2-yr follow-up, the primary patency, secondary patency, and foot salvage rates were 66%, 69%, and 77%, respectively, rates that were not significantly different from procedures performed on patients without severe arterial calcification.

The diabetic patient with heel ulceration or gangrene poses a formidable problem, especially in the absence of a patent posterior tibial artery. Our large experience with dorsalis pedis artery bypass has allowed us to examine its role and efficacy in the treatment of ischemic heel lesions.[27] Over a 6-yr period at our institution, 96 patients underwent pedal bypass for heel ulceration. When compared to a similar cohort of 336 patients with forefoot lesions undergoing dorsalis pedis bypass, there were no differences at 5 yr with respect to primary patency, secondary patency, or limb salvage. More importantly, dorsalis pedis bypass accomplished complete healing in 87% (84/96) of heel lesions, with healing rates being independent of the presence or absence of an intact pedal arch, and it allowed for a limb salvage rate of almost 90% at 5 yr.

In an effort to dispel concerns regarding long-term graft patency, limb salvage, and survival among diabetic patients, we reviewed our experience with lower extremity revascularization in a largely diabetic population of nearly 1000 patients followed 5 yr or longer.[28] A total of 962 vein grafts were performed on 843 patients, of which 83% (795 grafts) were in patients with diabetes. Minimum follow-up was 5 yr and extended up to 9 yr. The dorsalis pedis or plantar/tarsal arteries served as the outflow artery in 271 (35%) of the diabetic patients. Cumulative 5-yr primary graft patency was 74.7% overall, with no difference among patients with and without diabetes (DM 75.6% vs. NDM 71.9%, p = NS). The secondary graft patency rate was 76.2% for the entire cohort, and was also similar between the diabetic and nondiabetic group (DM 77% vs. NDM 73.6%, p = NS). Most importantly, 5-yr limb salvage and survival rates were virtually identical in diabetic and nondiabetic patients. The overall limb salvage rate was 87.1% (DM 87.3% vs. NDM 85.4%, p = NS). Survival at 5 yr was 58.1% in the entire cohort (DM 58.2% vs. NDM 58.0%, p = NS). These data strongly emphasize that concern for long-term mortality, limb loss, and graft patency in diabetic patients is unwarranted, and should not prevent aggressive attempts at distal bypass required for limb salvage.

CONCLUSION

Our knowledge of the pathophysiology of the diabetic foot has allowed for an orderly treatment plan that incorporates those principles. Specifically, recognition of the pattern of vascular disease in diabetes has made distal infrainguinal arterial bypass grafting an integral element of our treatment plan. At our institution, there has been a significant reduction in every category of lower limb amputation since 1984, and concomitant with this reduction has been an increase in the number of patients undergoing arterial reconstruction with a greater application of the dorsalis pedis bypass graft.[29] Success with distal bypass grafting, especially the dorsalis pedis bypass, has become the single most important technical advance enabling us to take advantage of our understanding of vascular disease and implement our management plan.

REFERENCES

1. American Diabetes Association. Diabetes: 1993 Vital Statistics. 1993.
2. Ruderman NB, Haudenschild C. Diabetes as an atherogenic factor. *Prog Cardiovasc Dis.* 1984;26:373–412.
3. Nathan DM. Long-term complications of diabetes mellitus. *N Engl J Med.* 1993;328:1676–1685.
4. Dormandy J, Heeck L, Vig S. Predicting which patients will develop chronic critical leg ischemia. *Semin Vasc Surg.* 1999;12:138–141.
5. Grunfeld C. Diabetic foot ulcers: etiology, treatment, and prevention. *Adv Intern Med.* 1991; 37:103–132.
6. Reiber GE, Boyko EJ, Smith DG. Lower extremity foot ulcers and amputations in diabetes. In: National Diabetes Data Group, ed. *Diabetes in America,* 2nd ed. Washington: National Institutes of Health, 1995:409–428.
7. Goldenberg SG, Alex M, Joshi RA, Blumenthal HT. Nonatheromatous peripheral vascular disease of the lower extremity in diabetes mellitus. *Diabetes.* 1959;8:261–273.
8. Strandness DE Jr, Priest RE, Gibbons GE. Combined clinical and pathologic study of diabetic and nondiabetic peripheral arterial disease. *Diabetes.* 1964;13:366–372.
9. Conrad MC. Large and small artery occlusion in diabetics and nondiabetics with severe vascular disease. *Circulation.* 1967;36:83–91.
10. Barner HB, Kaiser GC, Willman VL. Blood flow in the diabetic leg. *Circulation.* 1971;43: 391–394.
11. LoGerfo FW, Coffman JD. Vascular and microvascular disease of the foot in diabetes. *N Engl J Med.* 1984;311:1615–1619.
12. LoGerfo FW. Vascular disease, matrix abnormalities, and neuropathy: implications for limb salvage in diabetes mellitus. *J Vasc Surg.* 1987;5:793–796.
13. Akbari CM, LoGerfo FW. Diabetes and peripheral vascular disease. *J Vasc Surg.* 1999;30:373–384.
14. Akbari CM, Pomposelli FB, Jr. The diabetic foot. In: Perler B, Becker G, eds. *A Clinical Approach to Vascular Intervention,* 1st ed. New York: Thieme Medical Publishers. 1998;211–218.
15. Akbari CM, LoGerfo FW. The micro- and macrocirculation in diabetes mellitus. In: Veves A, ed. *A Clinical Approach to Diabetic Neuropathy,* 1st ed. New York: Humana Press. 1998;319–331.
16. Akbari CM, Saouaf R, Barnhill DF, Newman PA, LoGerfo FW, Veves A. Endothelium-dependent vasodilatation is impaired in both micro- and macrocirculation during acute hyperglycemia. *J Vasc Surg.* 1998;28:687–694.

17. Parfrey PS, Griffiths SM, Barrett BJ, et al. Contrast material–induced renal failure in patients with diabetes mellitus, renal insufficiency, or both. A prospective controlled study. *N Engl J Med.* 1989;321:395–397.
18. Schwab SJ, Hlatky MA, Pieper KS, et al. Contrast nephrotoxicity: a randomized controlled trial of a nonionic and ionic contrast agent. *N Engl J Med.* 1989;320:149–153.
19. Menzoian JO, LaMorte WW, Paniszyn CC, et al. Symptomatology and anatomic patterns of peripheral vascular disease: differing impact of smoking and diabetes. *Ann Vasc Surg.* 1989;3:224–228.
20. Akbari CM, LoGerfo FW. Saphenous vein bypass to pedal arteries in diabetic patients. In: Yao JST, Pearce WH, eds. *Techniques in Vascular and Endovascular Surgery.* Norwalk, CT: Appleton and Lange. 1998;227–232.
21. Pomposelli FB Jr, Jepsen SJ, Gibbons GW, et al. A flexible approach to infrapopliteal vein grafts in patients with diabetes mellitus. *Arch Surg.* 1991;126:724–729.
22. LoGerfo FW, Akbari CM. Arm vein grafts for lower extremity arterial reconstruction. In: Ernst CB, Stanley JC, eds. *Current Therapy in Vascular Surgery,* 4th ed. Philadelphia: Mosby. (in press).
23. Pomposelli FB Jr, Jepsen SJ, Gibbons GW, et al. Efficacy of the dorsal pedis bypass for limb salvage in diabetic patients: short-term observations. *J Vasc Surg.* 1990;11:745–752.
24. Pomposelli FB Jr, Marcaccio EJ, Gibbons GW, et al. Dorsalis pedis arterial bypass: durable limb salvage for foot ischemia in patients with diabetes mellitus. *J Vasc Surg.* 1995;21:375–384.
25. Tannenbaum GA, Pomposelli FB Jr, Marcaccio EJ, et al. Safety of vein bypass grafting to the dorsal pedal artery in diabetic patients with foot infections. *J Vasc Surg.* 1992;15:982–990.
26. Misare BD, Pomposelli FB Jr, Gibbons GW, et al. Infrapopliteal bypasses to severely calcified outflow arteries: two year results. *J Vasc Surg.* 1996;24:6–16.
27. Berceli SA, Chan AK, Pomposelli FB Jr, et al. Efficacy of dorsal pedal artery bypass in limb salvage for ischemic heel ulcers. *J Vasc Surg.* 1999;30:499–508.
28. Akbari CM, Pomposelli FB Jr, Gibbons GW, et al. Lower extremity revascularization in diabetes: late observations. *Arch Surg.* 2000;135:452–456.
29. LoGerfo FW, Gibbons GW, Pomposelli FB Jr, et al. Trends in the care of the diabetic foot: expanded role of arterial reconstruction. *Arch Surg.* 1992;127:617–621.

27

Factors Influencing the Long-Term Success of Infrainguinal Bypass

Kellie R. Brown, MD, and Jonathan B. Towne, MD

The success of infrainguinal arterial reconstruction is influenced by changes in the anatomic and hemodynamic characteristics of the inflow artery, the outflow artery, and the bypass conduit. The two disease processes that primarily affect long-term patency are the progression of atherosclerosis and the development of fibrointimal hyperplasia. The progression of atherosclerosis in the inflow and outflow arteries can result in a diameter-reducing stenosis that threatens bypass patency. The development and progression of fibrointimal hyperplasia to diameter-reducing lesions resulting in bypass failures are related to injurious effects of modifying a poor-quality venous conduit, correcting technical errors, handling the vein, and performing the anastomosis. The superior long-term patency rates in recent series of vein bypasses (i.e., *in situ* and reversed) have largely been attributed to improved surgical technique and increase in experience of the vascular surgeon.[1–3] Operative decisions regarding the selection and management of the inflow artery, outflow artery, and venous conduit can have a significant impact on long-term patency. In addition, status of the runoff bed and graft revision after threatened or failed bypass similarly affect long-term outcome. This chapter discusses these factors and the impact they have on infrainguinal bypass patency.

VEIN QUALITY

As the number of technical errors decrease with additional surgical experience, the quality of the vein has emerged as the most important factor determining the need for modification of the bypass conduit. We define a good-quality vein as a thin-walled vein, >2 mm internal diameter, with or without a bifurcated segment, that has a glistening endothelial flow surface.

MODIFIED VEIN

A modified conduit is defined as the need to re-explore the bypass because of residual valve leaflet requiring a venotomy for valve lysis, valvulotome injury, torsion of the vein conduit, anastomotic stricture, formation of platelet aggregates on the endothelial flow surface, or replacement of a sclerotic, varicose, or small-diameter vein with a free vein segment harvested from elsewhere. Modification techniques include vein patch angioplasty, primary repair, resection and venovenostomy, and resection and interposition of a translocated vein graft into the vein bypass. If a technical error occurs, or if a poor-quality segment of vein is identified, the short segment of abnormal vein can be modified and the modified vein used as conduit. The long-term patency of vein bypasses constructed by both *in situ* and reversed techniques is decreased, however, when the ipsilateral saphenous vein is inadequate and requires modification.

In a study from our institution of 361 consecutive *in situ* infrainguinal bypasses, 23% of the 361 saphenous vein conduits required modification at the time of *in situ* bypass grafting to successfully complete the procedure.[1] The secondary procedure was performed to correct an inadequate vein in 10% of the bypasses and technical problems related to vein preparation or vascular construction in 13% (Table 27–1). The primary patency at 4 yr for bypasses requiring modification was 50%, which was significantly less than the rate of 70% for nonmodified bypass conduits. Also, the secondary patency for bypasses requiring modification was 72%, which was significantly less than the patency for nonmodified bypass conduits, which was 84%. Forty percent of the *in situ*

TABLE 27–1. MODIFICATION OF 86 *IN SITU* SAPHENOUS VEIN CONDUITS PERFORMED TO CORRECT INADEQUATE VEINS (37 OF 361, 10%) OR TECHNICAL FAILURE OF ADEQUATE VEINS (49 OF 361, 13%)

	Type of Reconstruction				
Lesion	*Vein Patch*	*Primary Repair*	*Resection Venovenostomy*	Interposition Vein Segment	Totals
Adequate vein					
Vein injury	9	19	1	—	29
Anastomotic stenosis	3	1	—	1	5
Retained valve	4	—	—	—	4
Bypass torsion	2	—	2	—	4
Platelet aggregates	4	—	—	—	4
Low-flow state	—	—	—	3	3
					49
Inadequate vein					
Sclerotic segment	8	—	2	12	22
Previously used	—	—	—	7	7
Small diameter	—	—	1	4	5
Varicosity	1	2	—	—	3
					37

From Bergamini TM, Towne JB, Bandyk DF, et al: *J Vasc Surg.* 1991;13:137–147. Reprinted with permission.

saphenous vein bypasses with modified conduits required revision in the postoperative period compared to 22% of the nonmodified conduits. Therefore, as can be seen with the previously mentioned data, modification of the venous conduit at the time of the initial bypass significantly reduces bypass patency. However, it should be noted that the decline in the secondary patency of the modified bypasses compared to the nonmodified bypasses was due to the poor patency of conduits that were thrombosed at the time of revision. The modified bypasses that were patent at the time of revision had a secondary patency rate equivalent to that of the nonmodified bypasses. The secondary patency rate for modified thrombosed bypasses was 47% at 4 yr, a level comparable to other reports.[4,5] The poor outcome of procedures on thrombosed conduit veins coupled with the excellent patency of patent bypass revisions underscores the importance of monitoring the graft hemodynamics with a surveillance protocol in order to detect the failing bypass prior to thrombosis.

In a series of reversed vein grafts, Taylor et al.[3] reported that the primary patency of grafts with inadequate ipsilateral saphenous vein (68%) was significantly decreased compared to grafts with adequate ipsilateral saphenous vein (80%). The secondary patency of grafts with inadequate vein (77%) was also decreased compared to grafts with adequate vein (84%), but the two were not statistically compared. Similarly, a significant decline was documented in this series with the use of an inadequate vein that underwent modification. The *in situ* technique has the advantage of using the ipsilateral saphenous vein (90%) more frequently in comparison to the reversed vein grafts (55%).[3] The reason for this difference in vein utilization is unclear, but is probably related to the use of smaller diameter veins for the *in situ* bypass. The ability to use the ipsilateral saphenous vein for the length of the bypass can significantly decrease the number of conduits requiring modification and preserves the contralateral saphenous vein for bypass of the opposite extremity (performed in 9% of patients in our series). It is clear, however, that no matter which technique is employed, intraoperative modification of the conduit should result in normal blood flow hemodynamics if early bypass patency is to be expected.[6] Long-term patency is dependent on careful postoperative hemodynamic surveillance to identify and correct new lesions that can develop.

Vein Size

Vein size is a factor that can affect long-term patency of infrainguinal bypasses. We measured the vein diameter from operative angiograms in 187 bypasses.[7] In 10 patients, the vein diameter was 2.0 to 2.9 mm; in 73 grafts, the diameter was 3.0 to 3.9 mm; and 98 grafts were >4 mm in diameter. No vein <2 mm in diameter was used. The 30-day patency of veins <3 mm was 86%, compared to 93% for 3.0 to 3.9 mm grafts and 98% for grafts >4 mm. Long term, there was no difference between the three groups, demonstrating that long-term patency was not affected by vein diameter. Leather et al.[8] also noted no difference in patency for vein grafts <3 mm. Wengerter et al.,[9] however, reported significantly decreased patency rates for reversed veins <3 mm compared with reversed vein grafts with greater diameters. Therefore, it is important to use a conduit of suitable size. Vein grafts <2 mm should not be used, but veins <3 mm have adequate long-term results. If the vein is very small, the *in situ* technique may be beneficial.

Vein Type

In the face of inadequate greater saphenous vein, arm vein or lesser saphenous vein can be used for the conduit. Often, two pieces of vein must be pieced together to obtain adequate length for bypass. Weaver et al.[10] followed 56 lesser saphenous vein (LSV) grafts, 29 of which were LSV alone. Cumulative patency at 3 yr for these grafts was 60%, with a 93% limb salvage rate. There were 14 grafts in this series which were composed of LSV spliced with another piece of autogenous vein. Cumulative patency for these grafts was 38% at 3 yr, with a 72% limb salvage rate. Therefore, although LSV is not as durable as greater saphenous vein, the patency and limb salvage rate are acceptable as an alternative when no greater saphenous vein is available.

Arm vein is another option for autogenous vein material in the absence of greater saphenous vein. Chalmers et al.[11] reported on a series of 42 lower extremity bypass grafts using arm vein. Two-year primary and secondary patency rates in this series were 46% and 85%, respectively. This compares with a series of 520 lower extremity arm vein bypasses reported by Faries et al.[12] Seventy percent (70%) of these bypasses used a single segment of vein, and 30% involved splicing two pieces of arm vein together for bypass. The 3-yr primary and secondary patency rates were 68.9% and 70.3%, respectively. The 5-yr primary and secondary patency rates were 54.5% and 57.5%, respectively, and there was no significant difference between single-segment or spliced-vein bypass grafts. Given these patency rates, it is clear that although greater saphenous vein is preferable when available, arm vein or LSV is a viable option for autogenous lower extremity bypass. In addition, the type of vein used does influence the patency rate of the bypass graft, but splicing two pieces of vein together does not seem to significantly affect the long-term patency of these bypasses.

Aneurysmal Degeneration of the Conduit

An interesting correlation noticed with thrombosed vein grafts is the development of aneurysmal vein conduit degeneration. Aneurysmal degeneration of saphenous vein grafts is an infrequent late finding, with only a few cases described in the literature.[13–19] We found 8 such grafts in a series that evaluated 72 lower extremity grafts functioning for at least 5 yr.[20] Two-thirds (62%) of the grafts had become occluded and undergone either a thrombectomy or thrombolysis many months before the diagnosis of vein graft aneurysm. Three grafts with aneurysms had no history of occlusion, and two of these were reversed saphenous vein grafts. We postulate that a transmural ischemic injury can occur at the time of graft thrombosis or vein retrieval. This alters the integrity of the vein graft wall, which predisposes to subsequent aneurysm formation. Vein graft aneurysms have been described as atherosclerotic in nature, but this may be a result of an ongoing repair of ischemic injury rather than the primary cause of the aneurysm.

INFLOW ARTERY REVISION

Occlusive or aneurysmal disease of the femoral artery may require vascular repair to make this vessel suitable as an inflow source for a femoral distal graft. Femoral artery repairs also adversely affect the long-term patency of distal bypasses. In our series of 361 distal bypasses, severe atherosclerotic disease of the common femoral artery was present in 12% of cases and was treated by endarterectomy, patch angioplasty, or replacement with an interposition prosthesis to complete the proximal anastomosis.[1] The primary patency at 3 yr was significantly lower for bypasses originating from diseased inflow arteries requiring reconstruction (45%) compared to bypasses for inflow arteries not reconstructed (89%). Revision of the vein bypass was not significantly different for those with (34%) and without (25%) a reconstructed inflow artery. However, 53% of the revisions on bypasses with reconstruction of the inflow artery were to correct a problem with the reconstruction or progression of atherosclerotic disease of the outflow artery, compared to 18% of the revisions on bypasses with no reconstruction of the inflow artery. In the follow-up period, *in situ* bypass revision for anastomotic or outflow artery stenosis was significantly more frequent for bypasses with reconstructed inflow arteries (16%) compared to bypasses originating from nonreconstructed inflow arteries (4.5%). Decline in primary patency was not due to failure of the reconstruction in the inflow artery, but was associated with the severity of the preexisting atherosclerotic disease of the patient undergoing bypass. The secondary patency was maintained with bypass surveillance and elective revision. Therefore, inflow artery disease requiring modification prior to bypass seems to be a marker for disease severity. Significantly more of these patients require bypass revision due to disease progression than patients in whom inflow artery revision was unnecessary.

INFLOW AND OUTFLOW VESSEL LOCATION

The site of the inflow artery does not seem to affect secondary patency of infrainguinal bypasses. Both Leather et al.[8] and Wengerter et al.[9] observed this. Our institution also did not find an affect attributable to location of inflow.[1] There may be a difference in patency for grafts with different outflow locations, however. In our study mentioned previously, the primary and secondary patency rates were 63% and 81%, respectively, at 5 yr, with no difference seen for tibial as compared to popliteal outflow. The site of the distal anastamosis was the above-the-knee popliteal artery in 2%, the below-the-knee popliteal artery in 29%, and the tibial artery in 68%. This is at variance with the work of Taylor and his group,[3] who report a significant decrease in primary patency for reversed vein grafts to the tibial arteries (69%) compared to the below-the-knee popliteal artery (80%). The secondary patency for reversed vein grafts to infrapopliteal arteries (77%) was also decreased compared to below-the-knee popliteal artery (80%), but the two were not statistically compared. A significant decrease in cumulative patency for reversed vein grafts compared to the *in situ* bypass to the tibial outflow artery has also been noted by Rutherford et al.[21] and Fogle et al.[22] However, a randomized multicenter trial of 125 patients failed to demonstrate a difference between reversed and *in situ* infrapopliteal bypass patency.[23] It should be noted that in this study, in patients with vein diameter of <3 mm, the *in situ* technique was superior.

The use of the peroneal artery as an outflow vessel has historically been an area of controversy in vascular surgery.[24–28] However, frequently the peroneal artery is the only patent tibial vessel, especially in diabetic patients.[29–30] The 5-yr primary and secondary patency rates in our series of 77 consecutive peroneal bypasses performed between 1981 and 1990 were 61% and 97%, respectively.[33] Shortell et al.[31] reported a series of 62 peroneal bypasses, 17 of which were prosthetic, and observed a primary patency of 56% at 2 yr. There was a 75% patency if the peroneal had no stenosis at the time of bypass. These patency rates are comparable to other tibial bypasses, and illustrate the fact that if the peroneal artery is the only outflow option, it can be used with reasonable success. Therefore, although there is seemingly a difference in patency rates when tibial vessels are used as outflow compared to popliteal outflow, it matters less which tibial vessel is used as the outflow vessel.

Bypasses to vessel below the ankle have also been described. In general, these also have a reasonable success rate. In an analysis of 432 pedal bypasses done for tissue loss, Berceli et al.[32] found a 5-yr primary patency rate of 61.6% and a secondary patency rate of 66.8%. They also found 90% forefoot healing and 86.5% heel healing with bypass in a mean of 139 days. These patency rates are lower than with tibial bypasses in general, but do allow significant wound healing.

STATUS OF RUNOFF

We have been unable to determine any discriminant effect of the status of the pedal arch on the success of distal bypass grafting. Our series of 77 peroneal artery bypasses mentioned previously demonstrated that the presence of a patent dorsalis pedis or posterior tibial artery on the intact pedal arch did not significantly influence primary or secondary patency.[33] The 5-yr secondary patency rates for patients with a patent dorsalis pedis or posterior tibial arch was 88%. In addition, in a study of 432 pedal bypasses, the presence of an intact pedal arch did not significantly improve the bypass patency rate.[32] The inability to develop an outflow assessment score that predicts the success of lower extremity bypass has been confirmed by the results of Synn et al.[34] and Shortell and coworkers.[31] To date there is no preoperative or intraoperative evaluation that reliably predicts which bypass grafts are going to be successful.

SURGEON EXPERIENCE

In order to determine the effect of surgeon experience on graft patency, we compared our experience from 1981 to 1985, which consisted of 179 *in situ* bypasses, to our experience from 1986 to 1989, which consisted of 182 *in situ* bypasses, to identify variables that have improved with increasing surgical experience.[1] This comparison revealed no significant difference in the number of diabetic patients, indications for surgery, total number of conduits undergoing modification, the vein diameter of the conduits, the in-

TABLE 27–2. COMPARISON OF CLINICAL AND ANATOMIC FACTORS BETWEEN THE FIRST 179 CASES (1981–1985) AND THE SUBSEQUENT 182 CASES (1986–1989) OF *IN SITU* SAPHENOUS VEIN BYPASSES

Factor	No. of Bypasses (%)	
	1981–1985	*1986–1990*
Diabetes mellitus	75(42)	81(45)
Tobacco use	149(42)	155(44)
Indication		
Critical limb ischemia	169(94)	166(91)
Popliteal artery aneurysm	8(5)	7(4)
Claudication	2(1)	9(5)
Conduit		
Modified	50(29)	36(20)
No modification	124(71)	145(80)
Vein diameter		
<3.0 mm	6(5)	8(10)
3.0–3.9 mm	48(44)	27(35)
≥4.0 mm	56(51)	42(55)
Inflow artery		
Diseased/reconstructed	16(9)	22(13)
No reconstruction	157(91)	153(87)
Outflow artery		
Popliteal	56(31)	59(32)
Tibial	123(69)	123(68)
Bypass revision	55(31)	40(22)

From Bergamini TM, Towne JB, Bandyk DF, et al. *J Vasc Surg.* 1991;13:137–147. Used by permission.

flow or outflow artery, or the number of bypasses undergoing revision (Table 27–2). A significant decrease in the number of technical errors encountered in preparing the saphenous-vein conduit for *in situ* bypass is documented for the latter half of the experience (Table 27–3). The primary patency improvement for the second half compared to the first half of the experience was not statistically significant. The secondary patency rate was significantly improved in the latter half of the series compared to the first half. The secondary patency rate of the revised bypasses at 3 yr was not significantly different for the latter half (86%) compared with the first half (80%) of experience. The number of bypasses thrombosed at the time of revision decreased for the second-half compared to the first-half experience, but was also not significantly different. The secondary patency at 3 yr of the bypasses not undergoing revision did significantly improve in the latter-half (97%) compared to the first-half (83%) of the experience. Thus, long-term patency of the *in situ* saphenous vein bypass was improved by meticulous technique and increasing surgical experience.

TABLE 27–3. TECHNICAL ERRORS ENCOUNTERED IN PERFORMING THE *IN SITU* SAPHENOUS VEIN BYPASS COMPARING THE FIRST 179 CASES (1981–1985) TO THE SUBSEQUENT 182 CASES (1986–1989)

Technical Error	1981–1985	1986–1989
Valvulotome injury	20	9
Anastomotic stenosis	5	0
Bypass torsion	5	0
Residual valve leaflet	4	0
Total (%)[a]	34(18)	9(5)

[a] Total number of technical errors for the first half compared to the second half is significantly different, $P = 0.0001$ (χ^2 analysis).

From Bergamini TM, Towne JB, Bandyk DF, et al: *J Vasc Surg.* 1991;13:137–147. Reprinted with permission.

GRAFT REVISION

Long-term graft structure is affected by postoperative revisions. Approximately one half (53%) of the grafts in our series, followed at least 5 yr, had undergone at least one revision either to repair the conduit or to maintain inflow or outflow.[1] These revised conduits contained a majority of the significant graft-threatening lesions detected on follow-up, whereas grafts that had never been modified tended to be normal in appearance. During the early postoperative period, all revisions involved the conduit and were necessary to correct technical errors such as retained valves, arteriovenous fistulas, twisted grafts, and the use of an unsuitable vein segment. Between 1 and 24 mo after operation, grafts were usually revised because of stenotic lesions at the anastomosis and valve sites. This tended to portend future problems, and only 17% of these conduits were normal by color duplex ultrasonography at late follow-up. After 2 yr, the grafted extremities were more affected by the ongoing atherosclerotic process. Progression of inflow and outflow disease necessitated two-thirds of the late revisions.

SUMMARY

Vein quality, including vein size, type, and need for modification, is the most important factor in determining long-term bypass patency. Inflow artery revision, inflow and outflow vessel location, and runoff status are less important, but still influential in determining long-term outcome of lower extremity bypass. It is not clear that either the reversed or *in situ* technique is superior in most situations; however, in patients with small vein diameters (<3 mm) *in situ* bypasses have longer patency. Surgeon experience is important, especially with the *in situ* technique, and can confer a better outcome. In addition, close surveillance of these bypasses is critical, because graft revision prior to thrombosis is vastly superior to revision after thrombosis.

REFERENCES

1. Bergamini TM, Towne JB, Bandyk DF, et al. Experience with *in situ* saphenous vein bypasses during 1981 to 1989: Determinant factors of long-term patency. *J Vasc Surg.* 1991;13:137–147.
2. Leather RP, Shah DM, Chang BB, et al. Resurrection of the *in situ* saphenous vein bypass: 1000 cases later. *Ann Surg.* 1988;208:435–442.
3. Taylor LM, Edwards JM, Porter JM. Present status of reversed vein bypass grafting: five-year results of a modern series. *J Vasc Surg.* 1990;11:193–206.
4. Whittemore AD, Clowes AW, Couch NP, et al. Secondary femoropopliteal reconstruction. *Ann Surg.* 1981;193:35–42.
5. Belkin M, Donaldson MC, Whittemore AD, et al. Observations on the use of thrombolytic agents for thrombotic occlusion of infrainguinal vein grafts. *J Vasc Surg.* 1990;11:289–296.
6. Schmitt DD, Seabrook GR, Bankyk DF, et al. Early patency of *in situ* saphenous vein bypasses as determined by intraoperative velocity waveform analysis. *Ann Vasc Surg.* 1990;4:270–275.
7. Towne JB, Schmitt DD, Seabrook GR, et al. The effect of vein diameter on patency of *in situ* grafts. *J Cardiovasc Surg.* 1991;32:192–196.
8. Leather SP, Shah DM, Karmody AM. Intrapopliteal arterial bypass for limb salvage: increased patency and utilization of the saphenous vein use *"in situ." Surgery.* 1981;90:1000–1008.
9. Wengerter KR, Veith FJ, Gupta SK, et al. Influence of vein size (diameter) on infrapopliteal reversed vein graft patency. *J Vasc Surg.* 1990;11:525–531.
10. Weaver FA, Barlow CR, Edwards WH, et al. The lesser saphenous vein: autogenous tissue for lower extremity revascularization. *J Vasc Surg.* 1987;5:687–692.
11. Chalmers RT, Hoballah JJ, Kresowik TF, et al. The impact of color duplex surveillance on the outcome of lower limb bypass with segments of arm veins. *J Vasc Surg.* 1994;19:279–288.
12. Faries PL, Arora S, Pomposelli FB Jr, et al. The use of arm vein in lower-extremity revascularization: results of 520 procedures performed in eight years. *J Vasc Surg.* 2000;31:50–59.
13. Davidson ED, DePalma RG. Atherosclerotic aneurysm occurring in an autogenous vein graft. *Am J Surg.* 1972;124:112–114.
14. DeWeese JA. Aneurysms of venous bypass grafts in the lower extremities. *J Cardiovasc Surg.* 1973;14(suppl):271–273.
15. De La Rocha AG, Peixoto RS, Baird RJ. Atherosclerosis and aneurysm formation in a saphenous vein-graft. *Br J Surg.* 1973;60:72–73.
16. Sassoust G, Moreau J, Courchia G, et al. Deterioration of *in-situ* vein bypasses: anatomic study of 11 cases. *Ann Vasc Surg.* 1988;2:345–348.
17. Kelly PH, Julsrud JM, Dyrud PE, et al. Aneurysmal rupture of a femoropopliteal saphenous vein graft. *Surgery.* 1990;107:468–470.
18. Peer RM, Upson JF. Aneurysmal dilation in saphenous vein bypass grafts. *J Cardiovasc Surg.* 1990;31:668–671.
19. Straton CS, Beckmann CF, Jewell ER. Aneurysm formation in distal saphenous vein bypass grafts as a cause of graft failure. *Cardiovasc Intervent Radiol.* 1991;14:167–269.
20. Reifsnyder T, Towne JB, Seabrook GR, et al. Biologic characteristics of long-term autogenous vein grafts: a dynamic evolution. *J Vasc Surg.* 1993;17:207–217.
21. Rutherford RB, Jones DN, Bergentz SE, et al. Factors affecting the patency of infrainguinal bypass. *J Vasc Surg.* 1988;8:236–246.
22. Fogle MA, Whittemore AD, Corch NR, Mannich JA. A comparison of *in situ* and reversed saphenous vein grafts for infrainquinal reconstruction. *J Vasc Surg.* 1987;5:46–52.
23. Wengerter KR, Vieth FJ, Gupta SK, et al. Prospective randomized multicenter comparison of *in situ* and reversed vein infrapopliteal bypasses. *J Vasc Surg.* 1991;13:189–199.

24. Reichle FA, Tyson RR. Femoroperoneal bypass: evaluation of potential for revascularization of the severely ischemic lower extremity. *Ann Surg.* 1975;181:182–185.
25. Dardik H, Ibrahim IM, Sprayregen S, Dardik I. Revascularization of the peroneal artery. *Surg Gynecol Obstet.* 1976;143:946–948.
26. Dardik H, Ibrahim IM, Dardik II. The role of the peroneal artery for limb salvage. *Ann Surg.* 1979;189:189–198.
27. Graham JW, Hanel KC. Vein grafts to the peroneal artery. *Surgery.* 1981;89:264–267.
28. Szilagyi DE, Hageman JH, Smith RF, Elliott JP, Brown F, Dietz P. Autogenous vein grafting in femoropopliteal atherosclerosis: the limits of its effectiveness. *Surgery.* 1979;86:836–851.
29. Karmody AM, Leather RP, Shah DM, Corson JD, Naraynsingh V. Peroneal artery bypass: a reappraisal of its value in limb salvage. *J Vasc Surg.* 1984;1:809–816.
30. Dible JH. *The Pathology of Limb Ischemia.* Edinburgh: Oliver & Boyd, 1966:37–71.
31. Shortell CK, Ouriel K, DeWeese JA, Green RM. Peroneal artery bypass: a multifactorial analysis. *Ann Vasc Surg.* 1992;6:15–19.
32. Berceli SA, Chan AK, Pomposelli FB, et al. Efficacy of dorsal pedal artery bypass in limb salvage for ischemia heel ulcers. *J Vasc Surg.* 1999;30:499–508.
33. Plecha EJ, Seabrook GR, Bandyk DF, et al. Determinants of successful peroneal artery bypass. *J Vasc Surg.* 1993;17:97–106.
34. Synn AL, Hoballah JJ, Sharp WJ, et al. Vein bypass to the peroneal artery for lower extremity tissue loss: are there angiographic predictors of failure? *Am J Surg.* 1992;164:276–280.

28

Diabetic Foot Infections

David L. Steed, MD

INTRODUCTION

Diabetic foot ulcers continue to be a difficult problem in the United States. It is estimated that there are 16 million patients with diabetes in this country. Between 10% and 15% of patients are at risk for ulceration at some point during the course of their illness. This means that 1 million to 2 million patients have the potential to develop a foot ulcer. These open wounds are a potential portal of entry for bacteria that lead to infection. Complications of foot ulcers are the leading cause for hospitalization in diabetic patients and cost the health-care system billions of dollars each year.[1] One-quarter of all admissions in diabetic patients are for foot wounds. Twenty percent (20%) of diabetic patients are hospitalized at least once in their life for a foot infection.[2] If treatment of an infected diabetic foot ulcer is unsuccessful and amputation is necessary, the cost increases. Not only is there the cost of care, but also the cost of human pain and suffering as well as lost wages if the patient cannot return to work. Between 60% and 70% of amputations in diabetic patients are necessitated by infection.[3] The likelihood of amputation in a patient with diabetes is 15 to 40 times greater than the general population. The surgical morbidity and mortality in these patients is quite high; as many as half of these patients may be dead within 3 to 5 yr.

ETIOLOGY

Diabetic foot ulcers occur most commonly because of neuropathy or peripheral vascular disease. It is estimated that two-thirds of the patients have neuropathy alone. In the other one-third, half of them have vascular disease with ischemia alone and half have both vascular disease and neuropathy. The neuropathy is a motor, sensory, and autonomic neuropathy. Because of the motor neuropathy, there is atrophy of the small intrinsic muscles of the foot, leading to imbalance between the flexor and extensor muscle groups in the foot. Thus, the bones of the foot are not held in proper alignment. The pull of the tendons in an improper direction results in stresses on the foot that change the shape of the foot and lead to pressure in areas where weight is not normally borne. Changes such as claw toe and Charcot deformities develop. The metatarsal heads become prominent and there is forward migration of the plantar fat pad. Limited joint mobility as a result of glycosylation of collagen leads to stiff joints; this in turn reduces the ability to redistribute pressure off the bony prominences. Autonomic neuropathy results in dry skin, which cracks. There is almost always callus formation. There is also a loss of ability to thermoregulate the temperature of the skin. The autonomic neuropathy is associated with arteriovenous shunts and dilitation of arterioles. All these factors increase the risk of ulceration. Pressure on the foot in the face of a sensory neuropathy leads to ulceration, especially in patients who do not wear custom shoes designed to relieve pressure. The open wound then serves as a site for entry of bacteria.

These patients may also have significant peripheral vascular disease. Diabetes is a risk factor for atherosclerosis. There is arteriovenous shunting because of the autonomic neuropathy. Thus, nutrient flow to the skin of the foot is further reduced. This increases the risk of skin breakdown, reduces the chance of healing, and increases the opportunity for infection. Diabetic patients are known to have altered leukocyte function, including phagocytosis, chemotaxis, and bacterial killing function. The function of complement may also be altered. All these factors together result in an increased chance of infection in diabetic patients.

EVALUATION

Assessment of the patient with diabetes and a foot ulcer begins with a complete and thorough history and physical examination. Patients may have a history of coronary artery and cerebrovascular disease, suggestive of generalized atherosclerosis. They may also give a history of claudication or pain, and parasthesias at rest. Risk factors, including smoking, hypertension, hyperlipidemia, and diabetes, especially poor glucose control, are important to note. Muscle wasting of the hand and Charcot deformity of the foot are signs of peripheral neuropathy. The Semmes–Weinstein monofilament wire system is used to evaluate neural sensory threshold and quantify severity of peripheral neuropathy.[10] A foot that is insensate to the finer monofilament wires is at increased risk for ulceration.

The vascular exam includes a detailed evaluation of all the pulses. Noninvasive vascular studies should be performed on patients with foot ulceration unless pulses are clearly palpable. In patients with diabetes, the atherosclerotic process may lead to rigid arteries, causing falsely elevated pressure measurements and improper assessment of blood supply. A more accurate test of blood flow to the foot is the great toe digital artery pressures rather than ankle pressures. The digital arteries are spared from the atherosclerotic process to some degree, and pressure measurements in the digital arteries are less likely to be falsely elevated. Pulse volume recordings or Doppler-derived waveforms may also be useful. Findings of dampened waveforms and a normal ankle pressure are indicative of calcified arteries and falsely elevated ankle pressures.

A valuable test in these patients is the measurement of transcutaneous oxygen tension ($TcPO_2$). Using electrodes placed directly on the skin, $TcPO_2$ measurement reflects the perfusion of the skin. In general, the $TcPO_2$ is approximately 80% of the arterial oxygen tension (PO_2), such as would be measured from an arterial blood gas sample. The accepted normal $TcPO_2$ value in a patient breathing room air is ≥55 mm Hg. A value ≥30 mm Hg suggests the presence of adequate tissue perfusion for wound healing to occur. Most patients with ischemic ulceration have a $TcPO_2$ on the dorsum of the foot of <10 mm Hg.[4]

Infection impedes wound healing. Increased levels of bacteria reduce healing by competing with cells involved in repair for nutrients and oxygen and by increasing metabolic wastes. Infection disrupts the wound healing process by prolonging the inflammatory phase of healing, depleting the components of the complement cascade, disrupting normal clotting mechanisms, altering leukocyte function, and inhibiting granulation tissue formation.

INFECTION

In most cases, diabetic patients who develop an infection in their foot present with the signs of inflammation. The foot is warm, red, swollen, tender, and painful with motion, and there may be abnormal discharge. Even patients with severe neuropathy with limited sensation in their feet may develop pain when infection is present. Diabetic patients may also develop present with a swollen red foot from acute Charcot changes. Differentiating acute Charcot changes from infection and cellulitis may be quite difficult. There are many cases in which acute Charcot changes have been treated with antibiotics. The treatment of acute Charcot changes is casting which will only compound the situation if infection is present. Distinguishing acute Charcot changes from infection becomes critical in deciding how to treat the diabetic patient with a swollen erythematous foot.

All chronic wound are colonized with bacteria without infection. Wounds that are infected and not simply colonized have the signs of inflammation, including erythema, induration, tenderness, warmth, and pain with motion. Infected wounds are often malodorous before cleansing. The diagnosis of infection may be obvious if the patient is febrile, and pus is found exuding from an open wound of the foot. Unfortunately, not many patients present with such unequivocal signs and symptoms. White blood cell counts are often normal. The erythrocyte sedimentation rate may be elevated. Poor glycemic control is quite common when infection is present.

Osteomyelitis

Plain x-rays may be of value in screening for osteomyelitis. Periosteal elevation and bone erosion can be seen in osteomyelitis but at times are difficult to distinguish from acute Charcot changes. If one develops osteomyelitis, the typical change seen on x-ray may not develop for up to 3 weeks, as there is a significant time lag until the bony cortex erodes. Thus, a "normal" foot x-ray suggests that either osteomyelitis is not present or, if it is, it has been present for <3 weeks. Bone scans and radiolabelled white blood cell scans have been used to make the diagnosis of osteomyelitis. Unfortunately, bone scans show inflammation but are not pathognomonic for infection. Triple-phase bone scans have excellent sensitivity but low specificity and may be "positive" in areas of osteoarthropathy. Although white blood cell scans may be somewhat better, they are still not as specific as might be hoped. Indium-III leukocyte scans may be accurate when coupled with triple-phase bone scans, but are quite expensive. Magnetic resonance has been used to make the diagnosis of osteomyelitis and may be quite helpful. Unfortunately, this imaging modality is expensive and is too costly to be used as a screening procedure.

It has been suggested that osteomyelitis should be suspected in any wound in which the bone can be felt when probing with a sterile cotton tipped applicator. If the applicator probes to what seems to be bone, osteomyelitis may be present in as many as 85% of cases. This technique then serves as a good screening tool for osteomyelitis. The ability to probe to bone justifies a debridement of the wound. If osteomyelitis is present, it is best treated surgically with removal of the infected bone. Antibiotics are then needed only as long as there is soft-tissue infection. Prolonged antibiotic therapy for osteomyelitis is unnecessary if the infected bone is removed.

Wound Management

What is an infected wound? All wounds, except those made under sterile conditions such as in the operating room through clean tissue planes, are colonized with bacteria. It may be quite difficult to determine by physical examination whether a wound is infected. Wounds can only be assessed accurately by quantitative bacteriology. If there are $>10^5$ bacteria per gram of tissue as determined by quantitative bacteriology counts, then the wound is infected and must be treated with antimicrobial therapy. Wounds with fewer bacteria need not be treated. The one exception to this rule is *Streptococcus.* If any streptococci are found in the wound, then they must be treated, even if the number of bacteria is not $>10^5$. Topical antibiotics are quite effective in reducing colony counts in granulation tissue. Even saline-moistened gauze, changed frequently, reduces the number of bacteria in a wound.

What bacteria are commonly present in a diabetic wound? In wounds that have been present for <1 mo, the most common organisms found are *Staphylococcus* and *Streptococcus*[5–7] (Table 28–1). These gram-positive organisms are commonly isolated from the skin. If the wound has been open for >1 mo or so, enteric organisms are likely to be present. These include *Proteus* and *Pseudomonas.* Diabetic patients commonly develop polymicrobial infections, including both gram-positive and gram-negative microorganisms. In addition, 25% of diabetic patients have anaerobic bacteria in their wounds. These factors should be considered when choosing an antibiotic before any culture results are known.

How should diabetic foot wounds be cultured? Many diabetic wounds are covered with a black eschar and have no drainage. If patients present with cellulitis and a dry black eschar, there is no benefit to swabbing the dry eschar as the culture yields only skin contaminants that have no bearing on the bacteria responsible for cellulitis. Similarly, some patients present with an open wound that is not draining. Again, a surface swab in this setting is unlikely to find the bacteria responsible for cellulitis. The samples

TABLE 28–1. BACTERIOLOGY OF DIABETIC FOOT INFECTION

Infection	Cases (%)
Staphylococcus	61
Polymicrobial	58
Streptococcus	50
Anaerobic	19
Enterococcus	16
Diphtheroides	14
Proteus mirabilis	13
Peptostreptococcus	11
Bacteroides	8
Pseudomonas	8
Escherichia coli	6
Klebsiella	6

From: McCauley R, Linares H, Herndon D, Robson M, Heggers J. *In vitro* toxicity of topical antimicrobial agents to human fibroblasts. *J Surg Res.* 1989;46:267–274.

that are most accurate in determining the bacteria causing infection are cultures of pus or tissue taken from the deepest part of the wound at the time of debridement. Without cultures of pus or debrided tissue, it is probably better to "play the odds" when choosing an antibiotic than to choose one based on a culture from a surface swab.

Antibiotic Therapy

Antibiotic therapy should be started before the results of cultures are available. In general, mild infections can be treated with oral antibiotic agents.[8,9] If there is no improvement within 48 hr, the patient should be hospitalized and parenteral therapy begun. Diabetic wounds are best treated initially with cephalosporins or penicillin derivatives as they are active against gram-positive organisms.[10] This can be coupled with an antibiotic effective against anaerobes. In wounds present for longer periods of time or in more complicated wounds, a quinolone antibiotic may be better.

Antibiotics given systemically are critically important in managing infected wounds; however, systemic antibiotics alone are of little value in reestablishing bacterial balance in wounds heavily laden with bacteria.[11] They offer the greatest potential for reducing wound infection when tissue levels are bacterocidal within the first 4 hr of wounding. Systemic antibiotics, whether given orally or intravenously, do not achieve adequate concentrations in granulation tissue to be effective. Lowering bacterial counts in granulation tissue can be achieved to a much greater degree by using water-based topical antibiotic creams, including gentamicin sulfate, silver sulfadiazine, or mafenide acetate.[12] Unfortunately, these agents may have a deleterious effect on the principal cells of wound healing, including fibroblasts and keratinocytes.[13] It is important to keep this concept in mind when treating an infected wound. It may make more sense to use a topical antibiotic cream until the colony count is reduced, then change treatment to a less noxious agent, such as saline-moistened gauze, until healing has been accomplished.

Dressings

The proper care of the diabetic foot ulcer involves wound cleansing and dressing changes. In general, harsh soaps should not be used in the cleansing of wounds. Agents such as iodine, peroxide, and alcohol kill viable cells, including fibroblasts and epithelial cells as well as bacteria. If they are to be used, they should be diluted. Gentle soap, such as common bath soap, is less toxic to the wound and is an effective cleanser.

The purpose of dressings and dressing changes is to provide an element of protection for viable tissues, avoid desiccation, and remove necrotic tissue along with microorganisms. The current trend is toward keeping the wound moist in order to provide an optimal environment for wound healing. The saline-dampened gauze provides a moistened wound environment as well as gentle debridement. Newly developed hydrocolloid dressings retain moisture and allow for autolytic debridement by allowing autologous serum enzymes to lyse tissues.

Debridement

Debridement is particularly useful in managing a patient with an infected diabetic foot ulcer. Debridement serves several functions. It removes devitalized tissue that supports bacterial growth and thereby allows topical antibiotic therapy to penetrate into the tissues where needed. Removing devitalized tissue rids the wound of a culture medium for bacteria. The tissue on the surface of a wound is often heavily laden with bacteria. Removing this tissue likely reduces bacterial colony counts. Debridement is also a good method to find undrained pockets of pus. Widely debrided wounds with a good blood supply quickly begin to granulate. Patients with inadequate circulation should not be debrided because the deeper tissue desiccates if not kept moist; these wounds must be revascularized. Debridement should also be avoided in patients with medical conditions that impair wound healing or if there is a risk of exposing deeper structures such as joint space. In this setting, debridement must be coupled with a plan for tissue coverage.

Debridement can be accomplished in a variety of ways. The quickest and most efficient method of debridement is surgical debridement with a knife or scissors. The procedure can usually be performed under local or regional anesthesia with minimal risk. In fact, some patients with severe sensory neuropathy require no analgesia or anesthesia. Many of these patients have a good blood supply, and bleeding must be controlled. For these reasons, these procedures are best performed in an operating room by a surgeon.

Mechanical debridement can be accomplished by applying saline-moistened gauze to a wound and allowing it to dry before being removed. This technique is effective in removing dead tissue and fibrin from a wound; however, it may be associated with significant pain when removing the gauze. There may also be bleeding. Some newly formed epithelium may stick to the gauze as well, and be damaged as the gauze is removed.

Autolytic debridement occurs when the wound is covered by an occlusive dressing, allowing enzymes active in the wound to liquify necrotic material. It is selective, noninvasive, and painless. The necrotic material is a good culture medium for bacteria, and the dressing must be changed frequently enough so as not to allow bacterial counts to become too high. This treatment is not favored for an infected wound.

Enzymatic debridement is useful in patients who cannot tolerate surgery or in patients in long-term care facilities. There are several enzymatic debriding agents available that break down necrotic material and allow it to be washed away. As the necrotic material can be a culture medium for bacteria, these agents are often used with an antibiotic powder to keep bacterial counts low. This method of debridement is less efficient than surgical debridement, and thus most appropriate for patients without access to surgical debridement, such as patients in extended care facilities in which moving the patient may be difficult.

Biologic agents can be used for debridement, although there is some reluctance to do so. Maggots have been used to debride wounds. In fact, sterile maggots have been bred and raised for the specific purpose of debriding wounds; however, many patients and their health-care providers find this form of therapy unappealing.

Debridement serves other purposes as well. In addition to removing dead tissue and bacteria, debridement causes some bleeding, thereby attracting platelets into the wound. The platelets control hemorrhage locally, but also begin the healing process by releasing growth factors. These growth factors are found in large quantities in the alpha granules of platelets and contain multiple growth factors involved in healing. In fact, preparations of growth factors isolated from platelets are commercially available for the treatment of wounds and are known as *platelet releasates*. The platelets control the wound environment for the first 48 hr after wounding until monocytes invade the wound, become tissue macrophages, and assume the role of modulating wound repair still through growth factors.

Debridement also removes senescent cells from the wound bed. The primary cell of wound healing is the fibroblast. It has been shown that fibroblasts harvested from chronic wounds are less efficient at replicating and making protein than fibroblasts taken from the same patient at a different site. Debridement of the chronic wound bed allows these inefficient fibroblasts to be replaced by younger fibroblasts, which can better participate in the wound healing process.

Irrigation may be coupled with debridement to cleanse a wound. Water or saline are usually adequate to remove unwanted material from the wound. Commercial cleansers may have an antimicrobial component, but when used routinely may be toxic to the cells involved in wound repair. Irrigation with pulsed lavage should use pressure adequate to remove debris but not so forceful so as to cause tissue damage. Use of whirlpool therapy is controversial, but probably of limited benefit.

Duration of Therapy

Once antibiotic therapy has been initiated, it may be difficult to be certain when this therapy should be stopped. Traditionally, antibiotic therapy has been continued for 7, 10, or 14 days without good evidence to support such a decision. Severe infections, especially those involving bone, may be continued for 6 weeks. The clinical picture is often more complicated in patients who have been treated with several antibiotics, perhaps for varying lengths of time. It has been suggested that antibiotic therapy can be stopped if a patient has been afebrile for 48 hr, has no sign of inflammation, and meets the following criteria: (1) absolute white blood cell count <8000 lmm^3; (2) polymorphonuclear count <60%; (3) band count <3%. If the patient has none of these and antibiotics are stopped, the recurrent infection rate will be 2% or less, irrespective of how long the patient has been on antibiotics.

SUMMARY

Thus, in summary, infections in diabetic foot ulcer are a major problem and lead to limb loss. Infections must be sought diligently and thoroughly, and treated aggressively and properly. Patients with limited arterial circulation lose their limbs when an infection develops from minor trauma, and antibiotics cannot be delivered in adequate concentrations to the wound. To reduce amputations in diabetic patients, prevention of foot wounds is critical.

REFERENCES

1. Public Health Service. *Health People 2000: National Health Promotion and Disease Prevention Objectives: Full Report with Commentary.* Washington, DC: US Department of Health and Human Services; Publication PHS 91-50212, 1991.
2. Reiber G, Boyko E, Smith D. Lower extremity foot ulcers and amputations in diabetes. In *Diabetes in America,* NIH publication 95-1468, National Institutes of Health, Bethesda, MD; 1995.
3. Reiber G, Pecoraro R, Koepsell T. Risk factors for amputation in patients with diabetes mellitus. *Ann Intern Med.* 1992;117:97–101.
4. Steed D. Foundations of good ulcer care. *Am J Surg.* 1998;176 (Suppl 2A):20S–25S.
5. Frykberg R, Veves A. Diabetic foot infections. *Diabet Metab Rev.* 1996;12:255–270.
6. Eckman M, Greenfield S, Mackey W, et al. Foot infections in diabetic patients. *JAMA.* 1995;273:712–720.
7. Criado E, DeStefano A, Keagy B, Upchurch G, Johnson G. The course of severe foot infections in patients with diabetes. *Surg Gyn Obstet.* 1992;175:135–140.
8. Caputo G, Cavanaugh P, Ulbrecht J, Gibbons G, Karchmer A. Assessment and management of foot disease in patients with diabetes. *N Engl J Med.* 1994;331:854–860.
9. Lipsky B, Pecoraro R, Larson S, Hanley M, Abroni J. Oupatient management of uncomplicated lower extremity infections in diabetic patients. *Arch Int Med.* 1990;150:790–797.
10. Robson M. Wound infection: a failure of wound healing caused by an imbalance of bacteria. *Surg Clin North Am.* 1997;77:637–650.
11. American Diabetes Association Consensus Conference. The diabetic foot. *Diab Care.* 1999;21: 598–604.
12. Kulan J, Robson M, Heggers J, Ko F. Comparison of silver sulfadiazine, providine iodine, and physiologic saline in the treatment of chronic pressure ulcers. *J Am Geri Soc.* 1981;29:232–235.
13. McCauley R, Linares H, Herndon D, Robson M, Heggers J. *In vitro* toxicity of topical antimicrobial agents to human fibroblasts. *J Surg Res.* 1989;46:267–274.

29

Prosthetic and Surgical Considerations in the Rehabilitation of Amputees

Todd Kuiken, MD, PhD

The quality and type of amputation performed greatly affect the rehabilitation outcome of the patient. It is important for surgeons performing amputations to appreciate all the factors affecting the patient's function, including amputation level, gait dynamics, and the eventual use of a prosthesis. In this chapter, we discuss orthotic, prosthetic, and surgical issues as they relate to the various amputation levels.

TOE AND RAY AMPUTATION

Toe amputations are probably the most common amputations performed. This is a very successful amputation level, as there is minimal impairment and the patient can be expected to have a normal gait without the use of a prosthesis. If multiple toes are amputated, a full-length shoe insert with toe filler should be considered to minimize anterior movement of the foot in the shoe, decrease pressure on the end of the remaining toes, and protect the toes. If there is a tender distal metatarsal head associated with the amputation, a shoe insert with a carbon-fiber, full-length footplate can be used to minimize pressure on the distal head of the metatarsal during the rollover and toe-off phases of gait.

With ray amputations, the length of the foot is still preserved and normal gait mechanics can be expected. Once again, a shoe insert with toe filler can be very useful to keep the now narrowed forefoot from moving excessively from side-to-side in the shoe. Excessive movement of the foot in the shoe can lead to friction and skin breakdown. Pressure is concentrated on the remaining distal metatarsal heads during the rollover and toe-off phases of walking. A total-contact shoe insert also helps to distribute pressure throughout the remaining foot, preventing plantar surface callus formation and pressure sores. If there is pain during rollover or toe-off, or if there are problems with skin breakdown, a carbon-fiber footplate glued on the bottom of a foot orthosis effectively stiffens the shoe and minimizes pressure on the distal metatarsal heads during rollover and toe-off.

With forefoot surgery, including amputations, it is frequently desirable to minimize weight bearing to allow wound healing. Unfortunately, many elderly dysvascular patients cannot ambulate with a "nonweightbearing" restriction to a leg. This confines the patient to a wheelchair, decreases their independence and can even necessitate a stay in a nursing home. Other options worth considering are the use of a wedge shoe or a patellar-tendon bearing (PTB) orthosis. A wedge shoe is an inexpensive device that looks like a cast shoe with a large heel and minimal sole under the forefoot (Figure 29–1). The wedge shoe forces the patient to place the weight on the heel; the forefoot of the shoe does not touch the floor, thus there is minimal pressure and movement in the forefoot. It is important to ensure that the patient learns to use the shoe correctly with a physical therapist. If used incorrectly, the patient walks as if wearing high-heeled shoes, increasing pressure of the forefoot and having the opposite of the desired effect. A PTB orthosis is a custom-made bypass weightbearing device (Figure 29–2). It is designed to take much of the weight off of the patient's foot and transfer the weight to their patellar tendon and calf—it is intended to work much like a transtibial prosthesis. Although the PTB orthosis can reduce the pressure on the plantar surface of the foot, it is a modest reduction (probably <50%). The PTB orthosis does not work well in patients with significant volume changes in their leg. When using either the wedge shoe

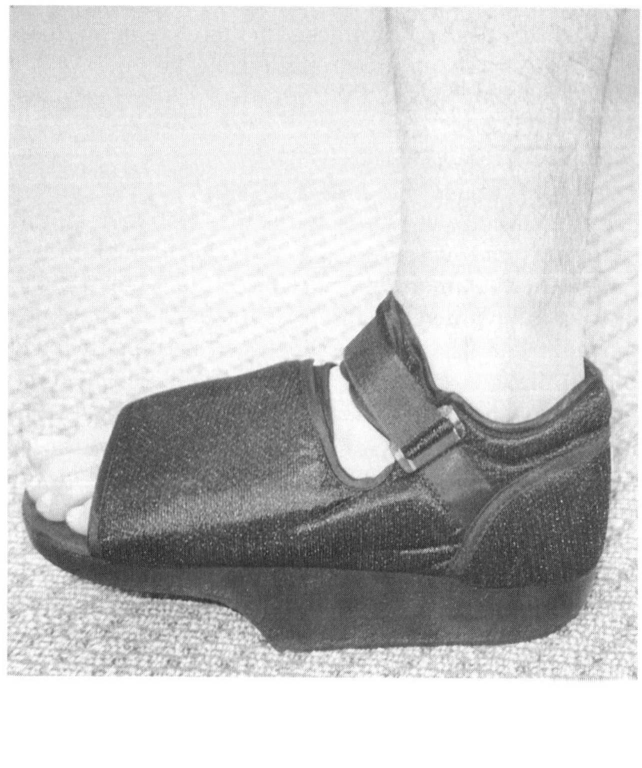

Figure 29–1. Wedge shoe used to minimize forefoot weightbearing.

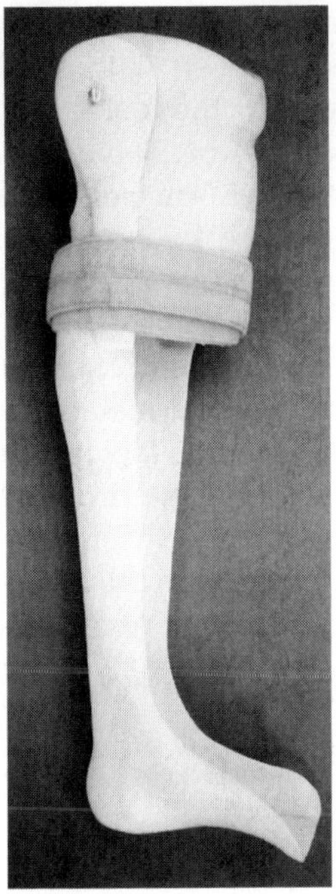

Figure 29–2. Patellar-tendon bearing orthosis. Weightbearing occurs through the patellar-tendon and the calf, thereby decreasing weightbearing through the foot.

or PTB orthosis, it may be necessary to provide the patient with a shoe build-up for the contralateral limb so that they have even functional leg lengths.

Although the single toe amputation generally does not require foot orthosis, the patient with the dysvascular foot also frequently has significant degenerative joint disease. Therefore, many of these patients require special footwear to prevent skin breakdown in the fragile dysvascular foot or to heal wounds of the foot. There are three main goals for the footwear. The foot should be supported in the best biomechanical position possible. Pressure should be evenly distributed throughout the entire plantar surface of the foot. This frequently means that reliefs must be made to minimize pressure on prominent boney deformities (i.e., a depression is made in the foot orthosis to accommodate the bony prominence). Finally, there should be adequate room in the shoe to accommodate foot deformities and prevent excessive pressure. At the same time, the shoe should not be so big that the foot is loose in the shoe. A shoe that is too big can lead to problematic friction and shear forces.

If hammertoe or claw toe deformities are present in the remaining foot, a high toe box or extra-depth shoe is necessary to give the toes room and prevent breakdown on the dorsal surface of the toes. Bunions and hallux valgus are common foot deformities. As the protruding first metatarsal head rubs on the side of the shoe, excessive callus formation and skin breakdown are frequent problems. A leather shoe can be stretched a bit to accommodate a mild deformity. With larger deformities, an extra-wide shoe is needed to provide more room in the forefoot and minimize rubbing. A foot orthosis with a high medial wall and a relief for the metatarsal head can also minimize pressure and friction over this bony prominence.

The dysvascular foot is frequently associated with excessive pronation of the foot and flattening of the arch. For this condition, a total-contact foot orthosis with good medial support (or a medial wedge) should be considered to support the foot better, help align the ankle, and protect the foot from spots of excessive pressure. Sometimes an extra-wide shoe is also necessary. In severe cases, the first cuneiform bone can protrude, causing excessive pressure on the underlying skin and skin breakdown. Here, good shoes and a foot orthosis with an appropriate relief are essential for wound healing.

When a distal metatarsal head protrudes down in the plantar surface of the foot farther than its neighbors, it is said to have *dropped*. Because the dropped metatarsal head protrudes down, there is greater pressure on the plantar surface of the foot in this area with standing and walking. This leads to callus formation under the dropped metatarsal head, and can lead to pressure ulcerations. A total-contact foot orthosis with a relief under this metatarsal head helps redistribute the pressure, minimizes callus formation, and allows healing of such wounds. A metatarsal bar or metatarsal pad is frequently placed under the shaft of the metatarsal to relieve some of the pressure under the distal metatarsal head (Figure 29–3).

PARTIAL FOOT AMPUTATION

The transmetatarsal amputation is a very common and successful amputation level. Although the patient can walk without the use of a prosthesis, gait mechanics are abnormal. The foot is shortened; therefore, toe-off is reduced, the stride is shortened, and we see drop-off in the gait. A total-contact foot orthosis with soft toe filler and a three-quarter

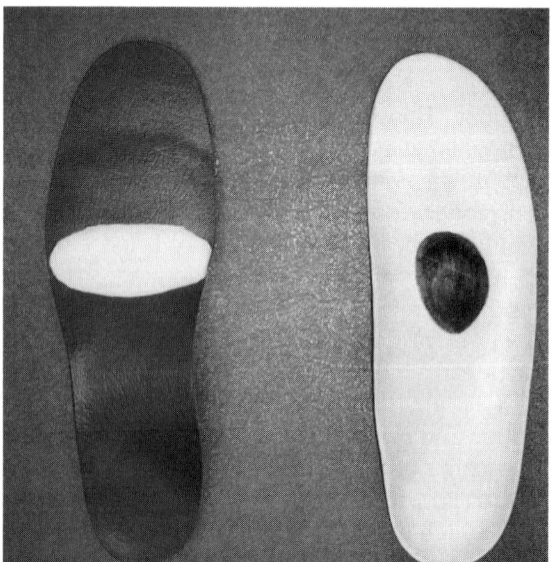

Figure 29–3. Metatarsal bar and metatarsal pad on a foot orthosis.

length carbon-fiber footplate is required to protect the foot and normalize gait mechanics. The total-contact foot orthosis redistributes pressure throughout the remaining foot and gives good medial support. Soft toe filler is required. A stiff toe filler gets pushed onto the anterior–superior part of the foot (usually right on the suture line), and this can cause wound breakdown (Figure 29–4). The three-quarter length carbon-fiber footplate is essential to restore the functional length of the foot and protect the distal transect metatarsal bones. Without this foot plate, the orthosis and shoe "break" (bend) at the end of the foot on the amputation, pushing the toe-filler into the top of the wound and keeping the foot length too short.

The tarsometatarsal (Lisfranc) amputation and the transtarsal (Chopart) amputation are problematic for several reasons. The remaining foot is so short that there is no effective lever arm. The remaining ankle is essentially useless. Balance is also lost between flexion and extension with these midfoot amputations. The very large and strong plantar flexors are still intact, whereas the primary dorsiflexor (the anterior tibialis) is compromised. More importantly, the foot is so short that the ground reaction force cannot counterbalance the strong plantar flexors. Therefore, the overpowering plantar flexion leads to equinovarus deformities and anterior bony prominences that are painful and prone to skin breakdown. Another problem with midfoot amputation is that they are very difficult to fit with a good prosthesis. A simple foot orthosis is inadequate and an ankle foot orthosis (AFO)-type of device is necessary. The AFO adds bulk around the hindfoot and makes it difficult for the patient to wear matching shoes. Furthermore, the AFO-type devices cannot be made with significant energy storage properties. This means that higher level activities such as running and jumping are very difficult. Due to these difficulties, we recommend that midfoot amputations <u>not</u> be performed.

ANKLE DISARTICULATION

The ankle disarticulation, or Syme's amputation, has a number of advantages and disadvantages. The primary advantages are that there is a long residual limb and it is an

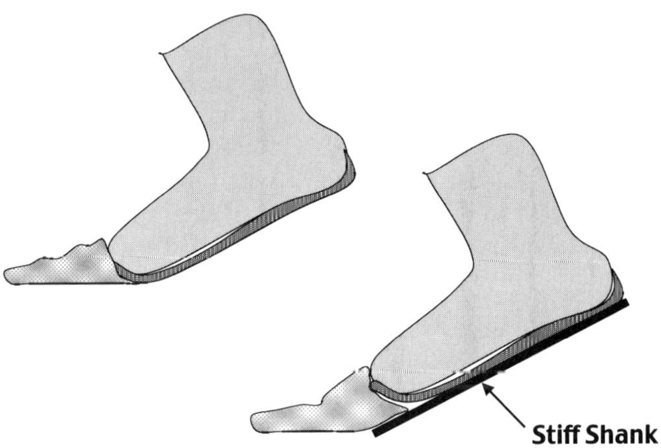

Figure 29–4. Transmetatarsal amputation foot orthosis. Without a stiff footplate, the shoe and orthosis bend at the end of the residual foot. With the three-quarter length carbon-fiber footplate, the functional foot length is restored and the end of the foot is protected.

end weight–bearing amputation. This may allow the amputee to ambulate without a prosthesis. However, when doing so, there is a significant limb length discrepancy (1½–3 in.) and no foot for rollover. This makes for an awkward and inefficient gait pattern. In our experience, most Syme's amputees do not ambulate without a prosthesis. Those who do only walk around their homes for short periods of time.

The main disadvantages are the bulkiness of the prosthesis and the lack of room for a prosthetic foot. The distal residual limb is quite bulbous because the malleoli are still in place. The socket must accommodate this bulbous end, and the resulting prosthesis is bulky, fairly heavy, and has poor cosmesis. There is also little room left for a prosthetic foot with the Syme's amputation. Although dynamic response feet are made for Syme's amputations, the lever arms are fairly short and they do not store as much energy as other prosthetic feet. Also, there is no room for multi-axle feet or ankle units with the Syme's amputation. These shortcomings should be discussed with the patient prior to surgery so that they have appropriate expectations.

The Syme's amputation is worth consideration in a well-perfused limb. However, if there are concerns about wound healing or progression of peripheral vascular disease, these risks may outweigh its advantages. Revision rates as high as 50% have been reported necessary in diabetic and dysvascular patients.[1]

TRANSTIBIAL AMPUTATION

The transtibial or below-the-knee amputation is the most common major amputation of the lower extremity.[2] A standard transtibial amputation (as advocated by Burgess[3]) is performed one-third of the way down the tibia. At this length the bulk of the posterior compartment muscles are available for a flap, and they provide good soft-tissue coverage over the distal tibia. The goal of surgery should be a cylindrically shaped residual limb; bulbous residual limbs delay fitting with a prosthesis.

Long transtibial amputations are sometimes performed to save as much residual limb length as possible.[4] The argument made for such amputations is to give patients the longest lever arm possible for improved prosthetic function and to decrease energy expenditure.[5] However, no functional muscle attachments are saved with a long transtibial amputation, and there is no mechanical advantage if there is an efficient socket limb interface. Modern total-contact sockets and suspensions systems clearly provide adequate and efficient interface systems. A standard-length transtibial residual limb is long enough to provide excellent control and energy transfer into the prosthesis. Furthermore, the long transtibial amputation is associated with multiple complications.[6,7] With a longer transtibial amputation the posterior compartment muscles have tapered so that there is less soft tissue available to cover the tibia and pad the end of the residual limb. Long transtibial residual limbs usually become bony. As the gastrocnemius muscles atrophy, the distal tibia and fibula become prominent. Bony prominences make it more difficult to provide a comfortable prosthetic fit. Frequently, the lack of soft tissue leads to a focus of excessive pressure on the skin and skin breakdown.[8] These pressure sores can be painful; they reduce or eliminate the use of the prosthesis and sometimes necessitate surgical revision. For patients with peripheral vascular disease, tissue perfusion is also an issue. The longer residual limb often has relatively decreased perfusion distally and is slower to heal or even fails to close, necessitating a surgical revision. Finally, the long transtibial amputation does not leave as much room for modern prosthetic componentry. Many more prosthetic components are available today that greatly enhance the function and comfort of the prosthesis. These include energy storage feet, multi-axle feet and ankle, vertical shock pylons, tibial rotators, torsion absorbers, and suction sock suspension systems (Figure 29–5). All of these components require some vertical space in the prosthesis. With a long transtibial amputation, there is frequently not enough room to include all of the components that may benefit an active amputee. The standard length transtibial amputation allows more room for a greater number and variety of prosthetic components. Therefore, we recommend only standard length transtibial amputations be performed; from one-third to at most, one-half of the tibial length.

KNEE DISARTICULATION

The knee disarticulation is an uncommon amputation that is performed on <1% of patients. It is an unpopular amputation level because the long bulbous residual limb creates many problems. The prosthetic socket and knee unit lengthens the thigh component of the knee disarticulation prosthesis. Therefore, when the patient sits down, the prosthesis sticks out 1½–2½ inches beyond the other leg. This is cosmetically undesirable, and can make it difficult for the patient to sit in tight spaces such as cars, church pews, and public transportation. This problem can be minimized with an outside hinge knee unit, but then the patient's clothes tend to get caught in these hinges. Furthermore, the femoral condyles make the residual limbs quite bulbous distally. When the socket is added over the condyles, the prosthesis looks much larger than the intact limb.

However, the knee disarticulation does have some significant advantages over a transfemoral amputation. It is an end weight–bearing amputation; therefore, the socket

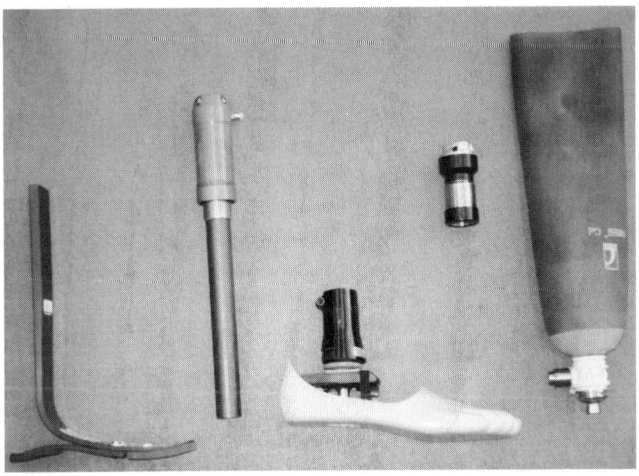

Figure 29–5. Transtibial prosthetic components that require vertical space. From left to right: High-profile energy storage foot, vertical shock pylon, low-profile energy storage foot with multiaxial ankle, tibial rotator, and silicone suction suspension system.

on the knee disarticulation need not come all the way up to the ischium, as with a transfemoral amputation. The adductor magnus and the tensor fascia lata (TFL) remain attached to the medial and lateral condyles, respectively, so it is generally a stronger residual limb. Finally, supracondylar suspension can be used, which is very convenient.

Zimmerman and Houben[9] performed a shortening osteotomy of the femur after through-the-knee amputation in attempt to preserve the advantages of the knee disarticulation while minimizing its disadvantages. With this procedure the femoral condyles are saved, which allows for end weight–bearing and supracondylar suspension. The knee hinge of the prosthesis can resume a more natural height, normalizing the appearance of the gait and making it easier to sit in confined spaces. The attachments of the TFL and adductor magnus are preserved. Finally, soft-tissue mobilization over the shortened bone can allow better coverage of the residual limb with traumatic amputation. This technique is worthy of consideration for selected traumatic and dysvascular amputees.

TRANSFEMORAL AMPUTATION

For transfemoral amputation, maximizing the length of the residual limb is the primary surgical goal. Another important surgical goal is to stabilize the femur within the residual limb. Myodesis of the adductor magnus and the quadriceps to the femur followed by myoplasty of the hamstrings to the posterior of the adductor magnus is recommended.[10] Myoplasty alone is inadequate; this does not restore normal muscle length, nor does it allow for adequate control of the femur. The femur is too mobile within the residual limb, the distal femur can be a focus of excessive pressure causing pain, and the transfer of energy into the prosthesis is probably compromised.

It is often challenging to fit obese patients with a transfemoral prosthesis. Excessive soft tissue is difficult to pull into the prosthetic socket; it can cause "pistoning" of the femur within the residual limb and can decrease the transfer of energy into the prosthesis, thereby decreasing the efficiency of the gait. One of the most common problematic spots is the "adductor roll." This is an accumulation of fat at the proximal anteromedial thigh. When the patient dons their transfemoral socket, it is often difficult if not impossible to pull this fatty area down into the socket. It then rolls up at the top of the socket and becomes pinched between the socket and the pubic bone. If a patient has an obvious adductor roll, consider surgical removal or reduction of this roll at the time of amputation. Another occasionally problematic area is the end of the residual limb. Although adequate distal soft tissue is necessary to pad the distal femur, excessive distal soft tissue should be avoided.

HIP DISARTICULATION AND TRANSPELVIC AMPUTATION

With the hip disarticulation and hemipelvectomy amputation, there is obviously no residual limb. The patient is fit with a "bucket" as opposed to a socket. The bucket fits around the pelvis and has a hole in the bottom for the remaining limb to fit through.

During stance phase on the side of the amputation, the patient's weight is born through the remaining ischium and ilium. Therefore, one of the major goals of surgery is to provide adequate soft-tissue padding of the remaining pelvis. With adequate soft-tissue coverage of the bony structures, the patient can wear the prosthesis comfortably and walk quite well.

SUMMARY

The rehabilitation of the amputee starts before the surgery is performed. It is important to inform the patient as fully as possible not only about their surgical options and prognosis, but also about their functional or prosthetic options and prognosis. Patient acceptance of the amputation is better if the patient feels he or she has participated in the decision-making process. The rehabilitation process proceeds more smoothly and successfully if the patient understands the consequences of the choices made.

Information about the rehabilitation process and encouragement about their prognosis greatly helps calm the patient's fears and adjust to their new disability. In general, we can be very optimistic and encouraging to patients who are facing limb loss. More than 80% of patients with lower limb amputation ambulate to within one level of the preamputation function out of a 7-level scale.[11] When possible, it is worthwhile to have a rehabilitation specialist (a physiatrist) assess and counsel the patient prior to surgery.

Clearly, the type and quality of the amputation are both critically important for the rehabilitation of the patient. It is important for the surgeon to understand all of the issues at play when performing the amputation. There should be no hesitation to discuss surgical options and decisions with the entire rehabilitation team. The varied input can only lead to better outcomes. Finally, the amputation should not be viewed as a failure to save the limb. It is a reconstructive surgery that is essential to maximize the patient's function and quality of life.

REFERENCES

1. Sarmiento A, Warren WB. The evaluation of lower extremity amputations. *Surg Gynecol Obstet.* 1969;129:799.
2. Kay HW, Newman JD. Relative incidence of new amputations. *Orthoc Prosthet.* 1975;29:8.
3. Burgess EM, The below-knee amputation. *Bull Prosthet Res.* 1968;10:9–25.
4. Yamanaka M, Kwong P. The side-to-side flap technique in below-the-knee amputation with long stump. *Clin Ortho Rel Res.* 1985:201;75–79.
5. Waters R, Perry J, Antonelli D, Hislop H. Energy cost of walking of amputees: the influence of level of amputation. *J Bone Joint Surg.* 1976;1:42–46.
6. Scully SP, Harrelson JM. Amputation and limb substitution. In: Sabiston DC, ed. *Textbook of Surgery: The Biological Basis of Modern Surgical Practice,* 15th ed. WB Saunders Co. 1997:1452–1458.
7. Ouriel K, Green RM. Arterial disease. In: Shires et al., eds. *Principles of Surgery,* 7th ed. New York: McGraw-Hill. 1999:931–1003.
8. Silver-Thorn MB, Childress DS. Parametric analysis using the finite element method to in-

vestigate prosthetic interface stresses for persons with trans-tibial amputation. *J Rehab Res Dev.* 1996;33:227–238.

9. Zimmerman KW, Houben PFJ. Shortening osteotomy of the femur after through knee amputation. IXth World Congress of the International Society of Prosthetics and Orthotics. p. 348.
10. Gottschalk, F. Transfemoral amputation. In: Bowker JH, Michael JW, eds. *The Atlas of Limb Prosthetics: Surgical, Prosthetic, and Rehabilitation Principle,* 2nd ed. St. Louis: Mosby. 1992:509–533.
11. Pinzur MS, Littooy F, Daniels J, et al. Multidisciplinary preoperative assessment and late function in dysvascular amputees. *Clin Ortho Rel Res.* 1992:281;239–243.

30

Thoracic Outlet Syndrome and Cumulative Trauma

Herbert I. Machleder, MD

INTRODUCTION

Ergonomic characteristics of the workplace have changed dramatically through the course of the 20th century. Workers compensation claims, previously dealing predominantly with back and lung complaints, are now largely a consequence of cumulative trauma injuries to the upper extremity. With this evolution has come an increasing awareness of the neurovascular compressive abnormalities. Disorders, particularly at the thoracic outlet, often originate in a congenital anomaly or variation of normal, followed by musculotendonous and bony hypertrophy as a consequence of repetitive movements. It is these effort-related developments that commonly elevate often silent anatomic variations to levels of symptomatic clinical relevance (Figure 30–1).

THE CLINICAL SYNDROMES

Arterial Compression

From the extensive literature discussing symptomatic cervical ribs, came the recognition that ischemic symptoms of the hand could follow as a consequence of thoracic outlet compression. The subclavian artery can be compressed, either against a cervical rib by the anterior scalene muscle or between the normal first thoracic rib and overlying clavicle. At the site of compression, a spectrum of changes can be observed ranging from mild intimal injury and irregularity, which can give rise to mural thrombus and subsequent embolization, to poststenotic dilatation and small aneurysm formation. Repetitive episodes of embolization with progressive obliteration of the distal vessels account for the attacks of Raynaud's symptoms that in some cases are followed by ischemia and digital gangrene.

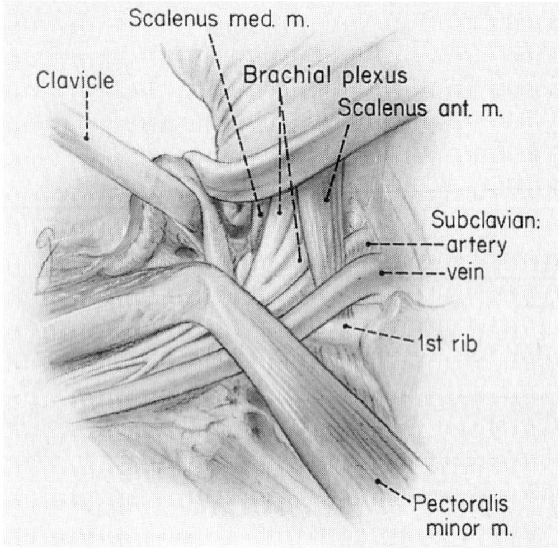

Figure 30–1. Anterior view of thoracic outlet, with clavical reflected laterally. (*From Machleder HI, ed. Vascular Disorders of the Upper Extremity, 3rd ed., Futura Press, Armonk, NY, 1999.*)

The angiographic appearance may underestimate the pathologic changes by disclosing only very subtle luminal abnormalities, particularly when the patient is supine. This disparity between the angiographic appearance and operative findings reflects the similar underestimation of the magnitude of mural thrombus, propagating clot and poststenotic dilatation. On occasion, minor areas of irregularity with associated thrombus may be more demonstrable on computed tomographic (CT) or magnetic resonance imaging (MRI) scan. Often, no bony abnormality is encountered, and posttraumatic changes in the anterior scalene muscle may account for the compression.

Presenting History and Physical Signs

Patients with arterial compression may in the early stages have symptoms suggestive of autonomic dysfunction, such as unilateral cold hypersensitivity, Raynaud's phenomenon, episodes of rubor, and recurrent mild edema. The disorder may often be attributed erroneously to a collagen vascular disease. The unilaterality of the symptoms should suggest strongly that this is more likely an embolic or neurovascular compressive process.

As the disorder progresses there are episodes of cold-induced ischemia, fingertip pain, and frank punctate ischemic ulcers at the paranichial area. Examination occasionally shows splinter hemorrhages in the nail beds. Digital plethysmography often shows dampened waveform shapes in the affected fingers with evidence of digital artery occlusion. Once again, the unilaterality must suggest to the examiner the possibility of an axillosubclavian artery lesion or central embolizing source.

Alternatively, in the face of complete occlusion, patients complain of aching of the hand and arm with exercise. This is usually associated with cold hypersensitivity or cold intolerance in the hand and fingers. Although a misnomer, this symptom is often referred to as *arm claudication* because of its similarity to the exercise-induced lower extremity symptoms of arterial insufficiency. At this stage, Doppler-derived segmental arterial pressures of the upper extremities is clearly abnormal.

Arteriography is almost invariably required, recognizing the problems of interpretation discussed previously. The studies should be performed with the arm in the neutral position and then with the arm place in abduction, at a right angle to the thorax. Failure to use stress positions results in many false-negative or incomplete studies.

Treatment

Treatment of these patients should be prompt surgical repair, to avoid progressive loss of the outflow vessels from repetitive embolization. Our standard approach has been removal of the first thoracic rib to decompress the thoracic outlet and facilitate a normal anatomic reconstruction. When there is poststenotic dilatation of the axillosubclavian artery, aneurysmal formation, or complete obstruction, resection and direct repair or interposition graft provides a durable correction of the abnormality. In patients who have developed severe autonomic changes or reflex sympathetic dystrophy, cervicothoracic sympathectomy provides additional relief of symptoms when coupled with vascular reconstruction. Two recent surgical series outline the full spectrum of vascular abnormalites, emphasizing the evaluation and treatment[1,2] (Figure 30–2).

Brachial Plexus Compression

Physical Examination

Patients with neurogenic thoracic outlet syndrome (TOS) often incur symptoms in the overhead position (abduction and external rotation, AER) typically developing numbness of the fourth and fifth fingers and ulnar aspect of the forearm. They rapidly note

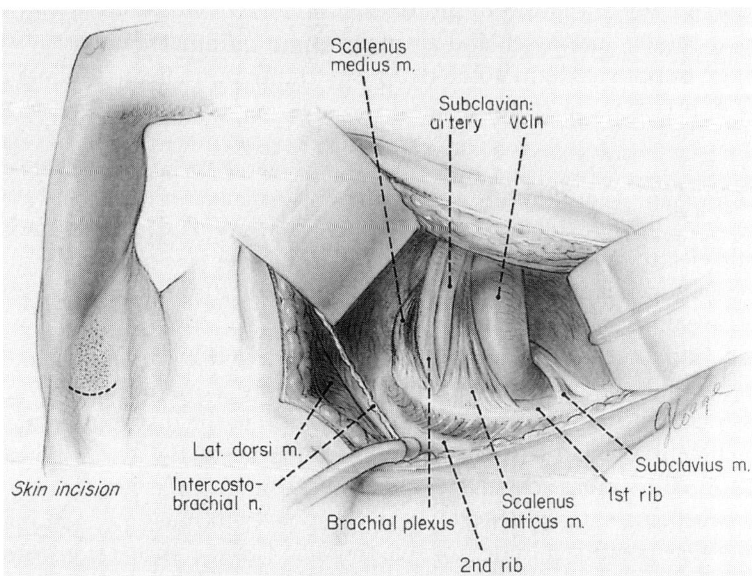

Figure 30–2. View of thoracic outlet from the transaxillary surgical approach. (*From Machleder HI, ed. Vascular Disorders of the Upper Extremity, 3rd ed., Futura Press, Armonk, NY, 1999.*)

impairment in strength and endurance with exercise in AER. When fatigue occurs in this position, a bruit can often be auscultated inferior to the lateral third of the clavicle over the axillary artery. This positional neurovascular compression affects mechanics, painters, stone masons, electricians, and others who work with arms in abduction. The symptom characteristics can be replicated on physical examination by having the patient clench and unclench the fingers with arms elevated, the so-called elevated arm stress test (EAST). The EAST or AER maneuver has been studied in industrial workers in Sweden and found to correlate both with symptoms at work and with the presence of nocturnal dysesthesias.[3] During elevated arm exercise, the hand often becomes pale and shows reactive hyperemia on resuming the neutral position.

Characteristically, there is tenderness over the anterior scalene muscle and hypersensitivity to clavicular percussion on the affected side. This hypersensitivity is very often associated with a positive Tinnel's sign at the brachial plexus. In addition, fine finger movement and grip strength become progressively impaired as patients develop difficulty performing tasks in both the AER position and with their arms in neutral positions. This accounts for the disabilities seen in many patients from industrial and white-collar repetitive motion occupations.

The loss of tactile ability and fine motor coordination is a consequence of impairment in the C8–T1 nerve root contribution to both median and ulnar nerves. Median nerve–innervated muscles such as the opponens pollicis and lumbricalis–interossei on the radial side are supplied completely by the C8–T1 roots. The flexor pollicis longus and brevis as well as the abductor pollicis brevis derive substantial innervation from C8–T1, as does flexor digitorum profundus and sublimis.

Most of the ulnar innervated muscles derive their entire innervation from C8–T1. These include the flexor digitorum profundus (fingers 3 and 4), adductor pollicis, dorsal interossei, palmar interossei, and abductor digiti quinti. The motor innervation of the fifth finger; opponens digiti quinti and flexor digiti quinti is predominantly from inferior trunk of brachial plexus (C8–T1).

Electrophysiologic Examination

When advanced, the neurogenic symptom complexes of TOS can be associated with characteristic electrophysiologic changes. Similar to other peripheral compression syndromes, one would not expect to see evidence of denervation and reinervation unless atrophy and weakness are evident clinically.

Nerve conduction, electromyography, and F-wave determinations are often normal in patients with neurogenic thoracic outlet compression. In more advanced stages of compression there may be evidence of denervation in the distribution of the inferior trunk of the brachial plexus. In these cases, the ulnar nerve F-wave response may likewise be abnormal. A more sensitive evaluation of the brachial plexus may be accomplished by measuring somatosensory evoked responses for median and ulnar nerves in neutral and stress positions. In neurogenic thoracic outlet compression there may be a characteristic loss of amplitude at the brachial plexus (or Erb's point) potential. Occasionally, there is an increase in latency. These changes have been documented in the literature with pre- and postoperative studies.[4]

We have found the EMG-guided scalene muscle block to be the most useful test in the diagnosis of neurogenic thoracic outlet compression syndrome. Jordan and Machleder[5] published initial results using this modality.

Radiologic Studies

Chest and cervical spine x-rays are obtained regularly, particularly in patients in the third decade of life and older. Neither the CT nor MRI scan has demonstrated any particular usefulness in evaluating the thoracic outlet compression syndromes. Their current application is confined to research protocols. Arteriography and venography are used in the particular settings in which arterial insufficiency or venous obstruction is a prominent component of the clinical picture. These tests should be performed with the arms in neutral position (at the sides) and again with the arm abducted (humerus at right angles to the chest).

Conservative Management

From the initial physiotherapy management program described by Peet at the Mayo Clinic, there have been additions and modifications. In France, Aligne and Barral[6] reviewed the general principles of physical therapy as improving and strengthening the muscle groups that they consider *openers* of the thoracic outlet area. These are the middle and superior segments of the trapezius, the levator scapulae, and the sternocleidomastoid muscles. This is performed concomitantly with relaxation of the muscle group called *closers:* anterior and middle scalene, subclavius, pectoralis minor, and pectoralis major. They recognized that moderate to severe cases should be referred for surgical treatment, but reported a 70% success rate with physical therapy when the following criteria were met:

1. early entrance into the physical therapy program
2. absence of bony abnormalities
3. symptoms are neurologic only, without vascular compromise
4. physical therapy is combined with exercises done at home

They recognized poor outcomes in cases where there was antecedent cervical trauma, and with what they termed "moderate-to-average severity, combining vascular and neurological involvement."[6]

Venous Compression

The Paget–Schroetter variant of thoracic outlet compression, spontaneous or effort-related thrombosis of the axillosubclavian vein, is a disabling thoracic outlet disorder affecting young, otherwise healthy individuals. At the time of Hughes' original report, the primary therapy was surgical thrombectomy in an attempt to restore normal upper extremity venous hemodynamics. In fact, despite increasing recognition of early rethrombosis, primary surgical therapy remained the standard approach until the early 1980s when techniques for local catheter directed thrombolytic therapy were popularized.

A number of authors studied and reported on the natural history of the disorder, providing a yardstick against which therapeutic advances could be measured. Untreated patients with Paget–Schroetter's syndrome can be expected to have varying degrees of disability as a consequence of chronic venous hypertension and/or recurrent episodes of venous thrombosis. This disability incidence ranges from a low of 25% reported by Linblad from Sweden, 40% reported by Gloviczki from the Mayo Clinic, to 47% reported by Donayre and 74% by Tilney. In addition, there is a small incidence of pulmonary embolism.

The underlying cause of Paget–Schroetter's syndrome is now recognized to be a mechanical abnormality at the costoclavicular portion of the axillosubclavian vein, with superimposed thrombosis resulting in the complexity of the clinical manifestations. The acute thrombosis is almost invariably in an area of chronic compression and stricture of the axillosubclavian vein at the thoracic outlet. The vein is compressed between a hypertrophied scalene or subclavius tendon and the first rib. A large exostosis is often found at the costoclavicular junction.

Presenting History and Physical Signs

Patients, who are very often tradesmen or competitive athletes, suddenly notice severe and uniform swelling of one upper extremity. This usually occurs in the absence of any recognizable trauma. In addition to edema, the arm has a slight rubor or cyanosis, often erroneously suggesting a cellulitis but without fever or any other systemic signs or symptoms. The patient may notice prominence of the upper extremity veins or be aware of collateral veins appearing around the shoulder or lateral pectoral region. Ordinarily there is minimal pain, except in the axilla, where pain and tenderness may occur over the course of the axillary vein. If untreated, the swelling often resolves in a few days to several weeks and the patient is remarkably asymptomatic at rest. Symptoms of swelling, tightness, heaviness, and easy fatigue, occasionally associated with vasomotor changes of pallor and sweating, occur with various levels of upper extremity activity. These symptoms are particularly exacerbated in warm weather or other situations stimulating vasodilation in the upper trunk and arms.

Demographic Characteristics

A group of 76 consecutive patients studied at UCLA gives an accurate description of the contemporary demographic characteristics in this disorder.[7,8] In the initial study of 50 patients, there were 31 men with a mean age of 24 yr and a range of 14 to 50 yr, and 19 women with a mean age of 38 yr and a range of 23 to 51 yr. The women as a group are significantly older ($p < 0.0001$). Forty-seven (94%) of these patients were right-hand dominant, and in 33 patients (66%) the dominant hand was the symptomatic side.

All but 1 of the men had been engaged in vigorous physical activity at the time of the episode of swelling and cyanosis, including 10 who were student athletes. Eleven women were engaged in relatively sedentary occupations, whereas eight were working in activities involving upper extremity effort, including three who were student athletes. (The student athletes included five weight lifters, three baseball players, two swimmers, and one each tennis, volleyball, and rowing crew competitors.) As a group then, 38 (76%) of the patients had the episode associated with effort and 12 (24%) were sedentary. As a good characterization of their customary activities, 15 patients were engaged in competitive sports, 18 were laborers and 17 were white-collar workers.

Physical Examination

The physical examination varies depending on the interval between occurrence and examination. In patients who have had an acute episode of thrombosis, the characteristics outlined previously are readily evident to the examiner. In patients who have an established thrombus with collateral venous development there may be surprisingly few physical findings during the interval periods, and the examiner may need to examine the patient after exercise. A series of push-ups, particularly in a warm room, often discloses the underlying difference between the two arms. The edema may be quite minimal under these circumstances, although a general duskiness is evident, as well as increased prominence of the collateral veins. With further exercise the patient often complains of pain in the collateral veins, particularly in the supraclavicular, pectoral, or axillary regions. In addition, these veins may be tender. However, the rapid resolution after rest discounts the impression of phlebitis.

It should be recognized that a tradesperson normally has a 1 to 1.5 cm increase in circumference at the biceps in the dominant compared to the nondominant arm, and a 0.5 to 1 cm asymmetry at the forearm. Measurements, if made, should be done before and after exercise.

Because of extensive and progressive collateral development, the disparity between symptoms and signs increases with time. However, in most patients the resistance in the collaterals is such that symptoms almost invariably increase with increasing work of the arm. In a remarkably similar characteristic to patients with other forms of thoracic outlet compression syndrome, these individuals complain of severe exacerbation when the arm is used in the outstretched or overhead position. This position leads to rapid fatigue and typical dysesthesias in the C8–T1 dermatomal distribution. Signs of sympathetic hyperreactivity are also present to a variable degree, although true causalgia is very uncommon in this disorder.

Diagnosis

Patients presenting with a swollen arm without an obvious etiology such as cellulitis, insect bite, trauma, or other possible cause should undergo axillosubclavian venography. Venography is preferentially performed in two supine positions: with the arm at the patient's side and with the humerus at right angles to the chest wall. Unfortunately, duplex ultrasound scanning and magnetic resonance angiography are reported to be inaccurate for venous assessment in the area of the retroclavicular space.[9]

Thrombolytic and Anticoagulant Therapy

Immediately after verification of the diagnosis, patients should be treated by catheter-directed fibrinolytic therapy into the thrombus, when this is available. Heparin is administered concomitantly and continued until therapeutic anticoagulation with coumadin (warfarin sodium) can be accomplished. Although streptokinase has been used successfully in axillosubclavian vein thrombosis, much of the reported experience suggests the superiority of urokinase for this disorder; consequently, urokinase was generally considered to be the preferred agent, until withdrawn from availability by the FDA in 1999. In 1999 and 2000, rTPA has successfully replaced urokinase, although adequate reports have not yet appeared in the literature.

The staged approach is based on the effectiveness of thrombolytic therapy, as reported by Zimmerman in 1981. The case reports of Taylor and Porter (1985) and then Perler and Mitchel (1986) added surgical treatment of the underlying anatomic abnormality and the use of selective transluminal angioplasty to this new therapeutic design. In 1989, Kunkel and Machleder[10] reported the results of a definitive, staged, multidisciplinary approach to the problem that had been initiated at UCLA. The results of this approach in a series of 50 consecutive patients was published in 1993.[11]

Surgical Treatment

To avoid rethrombosis, surgical therapy has been delayed following successful thrombolysis and anticoagulation. Drawing from experience with lower extremity venous thrombosis and studies of upper extremity venous endothelium, a 4-week period of anticoagulation with coumadin is preferable prior to definitive treatment of the underlying structural abnormality. With increasing skill in thrombolytic techniques and earlier diagnosis, the consequences of endothelial injury has been reduced. This has enabled the elimination of the "delay" stage in selected patients. In these cases, the treatment protocol is completed on the initial hospital admission (i.e., thrombolysis and decompressive surgery). Evaluation of success with this modified protocol must await publication of the results of current studies.

If the underlying anatomic abnormality is not corrected surgically, recurrent episodes of thrombosis can be expected to occur in many of this group of patients. Prior to definitive therapy, 34% of the patients in our series had multiple venographically verified recurrent episodes of thrombosis. The contralateral vein was studied venographically in 34 patients (68%). Five of these patients (15%) had an episode of thrombosis of the contralateral axillosubclavian vein, and 18 (53%) had evidence of ≥50% compression. The vein was normal in 11 patients and not studied in 16 patients. One patient had a clinically diagnosed and angiographically proved pulmonary embolus associated with the initial thrombotic event (Figure 30–3).

Surgical treatment is recommended if one or the other of the following conditions are met:

1. An underlying compressive abnormality is demonstrated venographically, following restoration of vein patency
2. If symptomatic patients with an occluded vein demonstrated obstruction of the venous collaterals with abduction of the arm

Transaxillary first-rib resection is considered the procedure of choice in this situation, based on the extensive literature documenting long-term results, effectiveness of decompression, and the excellent anatomic visualization of the area.

Transluminal Balloon Venoplasty

Postoperative transluminal angioplasty can be used when the subclavian vein does not return to a normal configuration (if a residual stricture is demonstrated on postoperative venogram). The continued presence of collateral venous channels following operation generally signifies that the residual stricture may be hemodynamically significant.

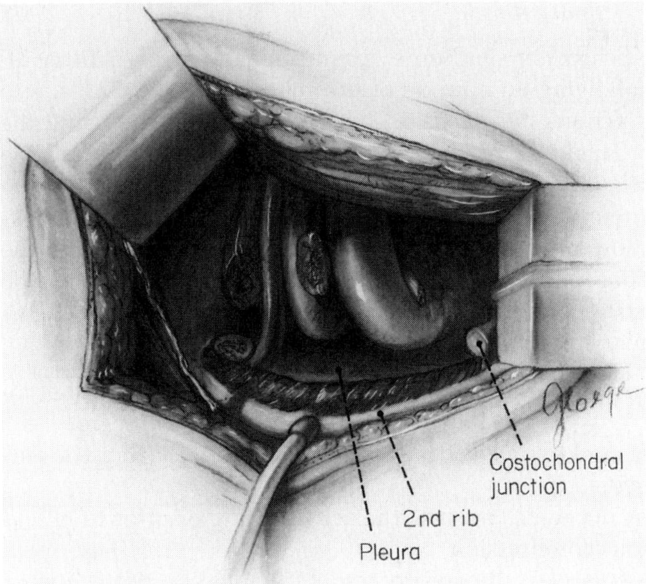

Figure 30–3. View of decompression of the thoracic outlet structures after removal of the first rib. Note the detachment of the subclavius tendon behind the axillo-subclavian vein. (*From Machleder HI, ed. Vascular Disorders of the Upper Extremity, 3rd ed., Futura Press, Armonk, NY, 1999.*)

Results of Treatment

The objectives for correcting the underlying disorder are as follows:

1. Relief of the venous hypertension
2. Correction of compression of both the axillary–subclavian and the collateral veins
3. Prevention of further episodes of thrombosis

These objectives have been achieved with first-rib and subclavius tendon resection. After surgical decompression of the costoclavicular space, no patient experienced a recurrent episode of thrombosis. Viewed from another perspective, 29 of 35 patients (83%) who underwent transaxillary first-rib resection were asymptomatic at the conclusion of the study. Twenty-two of these had a patent and normal appearing vein with 13 patients having residual occlusion. The three patients who remained symptomatic postoperatively all had residual venous occlusion.

The most significant determinant of ultimate vein patency was establishment of patency at the outset with medical therapy ($p = 0.0003$). Nevertheless, recanalization has been observed, even in chronically occluded veins, when the external compression is relieved. In the group of patients who remained symptomatic or disabled, there was a significantly higher incidence of contralateral vein occlusion ($p = 0.05$), or inability to open the ipsilateral vein by initial medical therapy ($p = 0.03$). Of 35 patients who underwent first-rib resection, 30 (86%) were essentially symptom-free (25 completely, 5 with minimal symptoms) and engaged in unrestricted normal activity. Five patients had residual symptoms, and two of these patients remained disabled for their usual occupations.

Summary

In the natural history of Paget–Schroetter syndrome, resumption of normal activity after a period of recuperation (following an episode of thrombosis) frequently leads to symptoms of upper extremity venous hypertension that is exacerbated by using the arms in the overhead position. This position can be demonstrated venographically to further occlude collateral vessels in the thoracic outlet. A number of patients develop more extensive symptoms of neurogenic TOS accompanied by positional numbness and dysesthesias. Anticoagulation may protect the collateral vessels and interrupt the period of active clot propagation, producing a better functional result than would be expected from the natural history of the thrombotic event. Our experience at UCLA with this disorder can be summarized as follows:

1. Local thrombolytic agents were the most effective means for reestablishing venous patency.
2. With clot dissolution, the underlying compression of the vein at the thoracic outlet could be demonstrated.
3. Balloon angioplasty was not undertaken in the acute setting or prior to relieving the musculotendonous compression.
4. The acute phlebitic process was allowed to resolve, under the protection of coumadin, for 4 to 12 weeks. At that time, it could be determined more effectively which patients would require additional therapy.
5. Removal of the first rib decompresses the axillosubclavian vein and the thoracic outlet collaterals, permitting the vein to regain its normal configuration (particularly in younger patients with more acute onset of compression).
6. Postoperative transluminal balloon venoplasty was used in patients with more chronic compression in whom the vein had become stenotic. Improvement of the luminal configuration was accomplished without the necessity for venous reconstructive procedures.

Patients with Paget–Schroetter syndrome have a symptom complex that often reflects more extensive neurovascular compression at the thoracic outlet than that which might result from venous hypertension alone. Although thrombolytic therapy can restore patency of the axillosubclavian vein, first-rib resection is necessary to relieve the external compression. This procedure was very effective in patients who had restoration of subclavian vein patency, and to a lesser degree in patients with residual occlusion.

OPERATIVE MANAGEMENT OF TOS

Surgical Approaches

There are three main surgical approaches to relief of thoracic outlet compression: transcervical, posterior, and transaxillary. In the hands of skilled surgeons who recognize the underlying bony or soft-tissue abnormalities that cause compression of the neurovascular structures, the particular surgical approach is of lesser significance. Each approach is capable of accomplishing the same ends and tends to vary by surgical training and skill, concepts about the underlying pathophysiology, and inclination.

The anterior approach has the historical advantage of being the primary exposure and the vantage point from which the anatomy has always been exposed and studied. There have been many variations of operative technique, from simple excision of a cervical rib to division of the anterior scalene muscle and/or middle scalene muscle to excision of the scalene muscle and resection of the first rib.

This last approach suffered from a high incidence of failures during the "scalenous anticus syndrome" era, when the operation was applied to patients who had radicular symptoms predominantly in the upper plexus or median nerve distribution. This era antedated the understanding of cervical disc and neuroforaminal disease as well as an understanding of carpal ligament compression of the median nerve. The failures were attributed to faulty diagnosis as well as inadequacies of the procedure. The primary technical failure was reattachment of the severed end of the scalene muscle to the deep cervical fascia with subsequent reappearance of neurocompressive symptoms. This procedural deficiency has been corrected by scalenectomy, wherein the entire portion of the anterior scalene muscle that overlies the brachial plexus is removed.

The importance of soft-tissue abnormalities has been emphasized by many authors and has encouraged some to reconsider the anterior supraclavicular approach.[12] In an attempt to incorporate the advantages of both the supraclavicular and transaxillary approaches, Qvarfordt and colleagues[13] reported on the combined surgical approach. Sanders and Pearce[14] emphasized very similar results with three different operative approaches that were performed in a setting of considerable expertise and operative experience: transaxillary rib resection, scalenectomy, and supraclavicular rib resection. In this study, there were 80% good results at 1 to 2 yr and 70% good results at 5 to 10 yr of follow-up evaluations.

Summary

It has become evident that operative effectiveness depends more on recognition of anomalies and the compressing elements than on the particular route chosen for surgical exposure of the thoracic outlet. Despite diagnostic and therapeutic concerns, excellent success rates in the 90% range are reported from many countries with the transaxillary approach.[15,16] The safe performance of first-rib resection by this route has been emphasized by Roos[17] and Machleder.[18] The posterior approach, proposed by Clagget and furthered by others, has largely been abandoned, except for complex recurrent problems.

Follow-up Care

Follow-up evaluations by the surgical team have been a reliable indicator of the response to operation. Lindgren and coworkers[19] from Sweden had the following to say: "The outcome of surgery as evaluated by the surgeon correlated well with the record of sick-leave from the regional social insurance offices." They further stated, "a long preoperative period of sick-leave due to symptoms of TOS did not exclude the possibility of a successful operation."[19]

Although excellent relief of neurovascular compressive symptoms can be expected from surgical correction, there are some patients who are troubled by residual regional muscle pains referred to as *fibrositis* or the more generalized condition of *fibromyalgia*. It is perhaps most important that these patients be returned to some regular activity despite continued symptoms. There are growing proponents of progressive activity rather than rest to treat this condition. As with carpal tunnel syndrome and neuroforaminal or disc disease, a good therapeutic result depends on careful rehabilitative measures.

CONCLUSION

In their most obvious manifestations, the congenital and acquired abnormalities recognized in association with the thoracic outlet compression syndrome are considered discreet anomalies. However, they should more properly be viewed as part of a continuum of developmental variation. The particular spectrum of developmental variations seen may be significant as predisposing elements when complicated by either increased functional requirements or a change in muscle fiber type (or isoforms of myosin) consequent to trauma.

Greater resilience of the arterial and venous system seems to result in relatively innocuous symptoms until compression reaches levels of hemodynamic significance or structural damage. It is evident that the threshold for neurogenic symptoms from the brachial plexus is lower than that of the vascular system.

Coincident with the range and continuum of developmental abnormalities, there is a range and continuum of compression of the normal structures which traverse the thoracic outlet area. Symptoms associated with the extremes of the compressive abnormalities are easy to distinguish because they represent the "classical" cases:

1. Paget–Schroetter axillosubclavian vein occlusion
2. Hand ischemia from thrombosis or embolization from the compressed or aneurysmal subclavian artery
3. The "wasted hand" of cervical band compression of the brachial plexus

In addition to these end-stage conditions, it is important to recognize the full spectrum of symptoms that can arise from neurovascular compression at the thoracic outlet. The lessor degrees of compression are often disabling in settings of specific physical or occupational requirements.

REFERENCES

1. Gelabert HA, Machleder HI: Diagnosis and management of arterial compression at the thoracic outlet. *Ann Vasc Surg*. 1997;11:359–366.
2. Durham JR, Yao JST, Pearce WH, Nuber GM, McCarthy III WJ. Arterial injuries in the thoracic outlet syndrome. *J Vasc Surg*. 1995;21:57–70.
3. Toomingas A, Hagberg M, Jorulf L, Nilsson T, Burstrom L, Kihlberg S. Outcome of the Abduction External Rotation test among manual and office workers. *Am J Indust Med*. 1991;19:215–227.
4. Siivola J, Sulg I, Pokela R. Somatosensory evoked responses as diagnostic aid in thoracic outlet syndrome. *Acta Chir Scand*. 1982;148:647–652.

5. Jordan SE, Machleder HI. Diagnosis of thoracic outlet syndrome using electrophysiologically guided anterior scalene blocks. *Ann Vasc Surg.* 1998;12:260–264.
6. Aligne C, Barral X. Rehabilitation of patients with thoracic outlet syndrome. *Ann Vasc Surg.* 1992;6:381–389.
7. Machleder HI. Evaluation of a new treatment strategy for Paget–Schroetter's syndrome. *J Vasc Surg.* 1993;17:305–317.
8. Machleder HI. Thrombolytic therapy and surgery for primary axillosubclavian vein thrombosis: current approach. *Sem Vasc Surg.* 1996;9:46–49.
9. Haire WD, Lynch TG, Lund GB, Lieberman RP, Edney JA. Limitations of magnetic resonance imaging and ultrasound-directed (duplex) scanning in the diagnosis of subclavian vein thrombosis. *J Vasc Surg.* 1991;13:391–397.
10. Kunkel JM, Machleder HI. Treatment of Paget–Schroetter syndrome: a staged, multidisciplinary approach. *Arch Surg.* 1989;124:1153–1158.
11. Machleder HI. Evaluation of a new therapeutic strategy for treatment of Paget–Schroetter syndrome: axillary–subclavian vein thrombosis. *J Vasc Surg.* 1993;17:305–317.
12. Sanders RJ, Raymer S. The supraclavicular approach to scalenectomy and first rib resection: description of technique. *J Vasc Surg.* 1985;2:751–763.
13. Qvarfordt PG, Ehrenfeld WK, Stoney RJ. Supraclavicular radical scalenectomy and transaxillary first rib resection for the thoracic outlet syndrome. A combined approach. *Am J Surg.* 1984;148:111–116.
14. Sanders RJ, Pearce WH. The treatment of thoracic outlet syndrome: a comparison of different operations. *J Vasc Surg.* 1989;10:626–634.
15. Carty NJ, Carpenter R, Webster JHH. Continuing experience with transaxillary excision of the first rib for thoracic outlet syndrome. *Br J Surg.* 1992;79:761–762.
16. Leffert RD, Perlmutter GS. Thoracic outlet syndrome. Results of 282 transaxillary first rib resections. *Clin Orthop.* 1999;368:66–79.
17. Roos DB. Essentials and safeguards of surgery for thoracic outlet syndrome. *Angiology.* 1981;32:187–193.
18. Machleder HI. Transaxillary operative management of thoracic outlet syndrome. In: Ernst CB, Stanley JC, eds. *Current therapy in vascular surgery,* 2nd ed. Philadelphia: BC Decker, Inc. 1991:227–230.
19. Lindgren SHS, Ribbe EB, Norgren EH. Two-year follow-up of patients operated on for thoracic outlet syndrome. Effects on sick-leave incidence. *Eur J Vasc Surg.* 1989;3:411–415.

31

Management of Vascular Access Complications

S. Ram Kumar, MD, Vincent L. Rowe, MD, and Fred A. Weaver, MD

During the 1990s, the capability and ease of vascular access has resulted in a marked increase in the number of vascular access procedures. Temporary or permanent central access of the venous system is now used routinely for the administration of medication, chemotherapy, parenteral nutrition, and acute or chronic hemodialysis. This allows many chronic therapeutic interventions—for instance, chemotherapy—to move from the in-patient to the ambulatory setting. In addition, with about 40,000 new patients developing end-stage renal disease in the United States every year, consistently larger numbers of patients now require permanent arteriovenous (AV) vascular access for hemodialysis.[1] The average lifespan of patients on dialysis has also been on the rise, and is currently estimated at around 5.5 yr. Taken together, these developments have put enormous pressure on the need for and maintenance of permanent vascular access, which continues to be the "Achilles' heel" of the hemodialysis population. With the increase in vascular access procedures comes a wide spectrum of complications. Appropriate management of complications is critical to minimizing morbidity and extending the use of the access in a medically compromised patient population.

PERCUTANEOUS VENOUS ACCESS

Short-term central venous access is usually established percutaneously via the subclavian, jugular, or femoral veins. Complications that follow percutaneous procedures can be categorized as acute, which generally result from technical misadventures, and late, which are consequences of long-term intravascular devices.

Acute Complications

Technical errors when placing a venous access catheter lead to a variety of immediate complications, some of which may have lethal consequences. Operator experience minimizes the incidence of errors in percutaneous access procedures.[2] In a prospective study of 1303 central venous cannulations done in the intensive care unit or operating room,[3] a 6.9% acute complication rate was reported. The most common complication varies depending on the vein chosen for access. When the internal jugular is used, arterial injury is the most frequent (5.2%)[3]; and when the subclavian is chosen, pneumothorax is the most common complication (2.5%).[4]

Pneumothorax

Inappropriate direction or depth of the needle during subclavian or internal jugular venous access can puncture the pleura, particularly in thin, cachectic, or emphysematous patients, resulting in a pneumothorax. Aspiration of air during implantation implies violation of the parietal pleura. An immediate indication of a pneumothorax such as severe respiratory distress is rare. Because clinical findings alone do not reliably identify complications following percutaneous subclavian or internal jugular catheterization, a routine postplacement chest radiograph is necessary.[5]

For most pneumothoraces, commercially available small chest tubes with a self-contained drainage system are adequate. A formal tube thoracostomy is only rarely required. Small pneumothoraces (<15% lung volume) may be observed with serial evaluation by chest x-ray. If the pneumothorax increases in size or symptoms develop, a chest tube is needed.

If a subclavian or internal jugular catheterization is unsuccessful, attempts on the contralateral side should be avoided until a pneumothorax is ruled out. Ultrasound-guided cannulation of the internal jugular[6] and femoral veins[7] has been performed with improved technical success and reductions in access time and complications.

On occasion, simultaneous perforation of a great vessel and pleura may occur, resulting in a hemothorax or hemomediastinum. This requires formal tube thoracostomy and careful observation. It is important to remove the catheter, as it may actually "stent" the vessel open and accentuate the bleeding diathesis. Persistent bleeding into the pleural cavity may necessitate a thoracotomy. Rarely, the brachial plexus or thoracic duct may be injured during percutaneous catheterization. Immediate catheter removal is usually all that is necessary, and long-term sequelae are rare.

Arterial Injury

Clinically significant hemorrhage from a punctured or lacerated common carotid or subclavian artery most frequently follows a cervical approach to the internal jugular vein. Difficulty in passing the guidewire or resistance to the introduction of the catheter into the vessel is a sign of potential arterial cannulation. If the catheter is indeed placed in the artery, the sheath should be removed and local compression applied for 10 to 15 min. If the patient is anesthetized, general anesthesia should be aborted, the patient awakened, and a neurologic exam performed. If the exam is normal and no cervical hematoma is present, the patient can be observed. Patients with an expanding hematoma with or without airway compromise require neck exploration and arterial repair. The presence of a cervical thrill or bruit indicates an AV fistula or intimal flap, whereas a pulsatile mass suggests an underlying pseudoaneurysm. An abnormal neurologic exam may be indicative of an underlying common or internal carotid occlusion or flap. Color-flow duplex scan can provide a rapid assessment of vascular structures and direct further surgical therapy. An abnormal duplex exam should be followed by diagnostic arteriography and carotid exploration and repair, if indicated.

Long-Term Complications

The type of the indwelling catheter (temporary or cuffed), the patient's underlying condition, and the extent of catheter care dictate the onset of late complications. Most late complications relate to either venous thrombosis or sepsis. Other complications include malfunction or fracture of the catheter and embolization into the heart or pulmonary vascular tree.

Thrombosis

The reported rates of catheter-related venous thrombosis vary widely between 3% and 70%,[8] in part because several factors contribute to the risk of catheter-induced venous thrombosis.[9] These include the number of attempts at catheter placement, the duration of catheterization, the composition and stiffness of the catheter, catheter diameter and length, position of the distal tip of the catheter, the composition of the infusate, and the indication for placement of the catheter. Proximal and distal propagation of the thrombus determines whether clinical symptoms are produced. Most focal short-segment occlusions remain asymptomatic, as venous collaterals decompress the extremity, whereas thrombosis that extends centrally is more likely to cause symptoms. Inability to withdraw blood from the catheter, pain, limb edema, and dilated superficial veins suggest catheter-induced venous thrombosis. Color-flow duplex scan can be used to screen for venous thrombosis; however, thrombi proximal to the clavicle and first rib may be missed by a duplex exam. Pulmonary embolism complicates about 15% of upper extremity catheter-related central venous thrombotic events, and can be life-threatening.[10]

Management of catheter-induced venous thrombosis in an asymptomatic patient without complications is controversial. Routine use of low-dose, unfractionated, or low-molecular-weight heparin or low-dose warfarin has been recommended.[11] When symptoms develop, extremity elevation and systemic anticoagulation is required. Depending on the need for catheter salvage, functioning catheters may be removed.

Thrombosis of the catheter is the most common cause of cuffed-catheter dysfunction. Instillation of 1 mg tPA into the catheter with a 30- to 60-min dwell time may restore patency. If unsuccessful, the catheter can be exchanged over a guidewire.

Catheter-Related Sepsis

A potentially life-threatening complication of percutaneous catheter placement is sepsis, with a reported incidence of 0.08 to 0.14 episodes per 100 catheter days.[8] Organisms commonly implicated in catheter-related sepsis are *Staphylococcus aureus* and *Streptococcus* spp. Fungal infections like *Candida* are usually superinfections in a patient on long-term antibiotic therapy. When catheter-related sepsis is suspected, the catheter should be removed and cultured to identify the causative organism. Culture of blood drawn through the catheter may also be helpful in the diagnosis.

Occasionally, a catheter infection can result in septic thrombophlebitis. Initially, this is best treated by removal of the catheter and systemic antibiotics directed at the causative organism plus anticoagulation. A vast majority of cases resolve with this therapy. Rarely, surgical exploration and thrombectomy of the infected thrombus or resection of the infected venous segment may be required. There is evidence to suggest that dissolution of the infected thrombus with thrombolytic agent may provide a more rapid resolution and fewer treatment failures.[12] The lytic agent is best administered via catheters placed directly into the thrombus to optimize drug delivery, limit the necessary dose, and minimize hemorrhagic complications.

Catheter exit-site or tunnel infections with cuffed catheters can be managed by topical and systemic antibiotics. Catheter-mediated bacteremia requires hospitalization and parenteral antibiotics based on culture. If the patient remains symptomatic despite antibiotic therapy for >36 hr, the catheter should be removed.[13] Systemic antibiotics must be continued for 3 weeks and new permanent access should not be placed until cultures have been negative for ≥48 hr after cessation of antibiotics.[13]

The most significant factor in minimizing catheter-related infection is careful, aseptic technique during placement and care of the catheter. Routine antibiotic prophylaxis or changing catheters at prescribed time-intervals have not shown uniformly to be of benefit.

ARTERIOVENOUS ACCESS FOR HEMODIALYSIS

Vascular access complications are a major cause of morbidity in patients with end-stage renal disease on maintenance hemodialysis. Complications related to AV access account for almost 20% of hospitalizations in these patients. The interval between access placement and the need for remedial procedures has been decreasing throughout the 1990s, whereas the expenditure for reestablishing patency has become substantially higher.[1]

Primary patency of AV accesses at 1 yr varies between 40% and 60% and is largely dependent on the type of access (Table 31–1). In a retrospective review of 483 procedures, Ascher et al.[14] reported a 72% 1-yr primary patency rate: 84% for native AV fistulas and 54% for AV grafts. The NKF/DOQI recommends a cumulative patency rate of at least 70% at 1 yr, 60% at 2 yr, and 50% at 3 yr for all AV accesses.[13]

Complications that lead to vascular access failure are multiple, with graft thrombosis accounting for the vast majority. Infections and hemodynamic complications, which include steal syndrome, extremity venous hypertension, and neurologic dysfunction, make up the remainder. The management of AV access complications relies on a multidisciplinary approach involving nephrologists, vascular surgeons, interventional radiologists, and dialysis personnel. The ultimate goal is preservation of vascular access.

The Failing or Thrombosed Graft

Thrombosis of AV access accounts for more than 80% of all complications,[15] with a reported rate of 0.81 episodes per patient per year.[16] The likelihood of thrombosis de-

TABLE 31–1. SELECTED REPORTS OF PATENCY RATES OF NATIVE AV FISTULAS AND PROSTHETIC AV GRAFTS AT ONE YEAR

	One-Year Patency Rates			
	AV Fistulas		*AV Grafts*	
Reference	Primary (%)	Secondary (%)	Primary (%)	Secondary (%)
Ascher et al.[14]	84		54	
Kherlakian et al.[36]		71		75
Palder et al.[15]		60		80
Tellis et al.[37]		33		62
Kinnaert et al.[38]		88		
Rohr et al.[17]		62		
Silcott et al.[39]		75		
Munda et al.[40]				67
Puckett and Lindsay[41]				95
Rizzuti et al.[42]				76
Tordoir et al.[43]				74

pends on multiple factors, including the type of access, anatomy of the graft or fistula, site of anastomosis, and selection of graft material (autogenous versus prosthetic).

Immediate thrombosis in the operating room results from an inadequate vein, compromised arterial inflow or venous outflow, hypercoagulability states, or a technical error. Ensuring >3 mm venous diameter for autogenous fistulas[17] or >4 mm outflow venous diameter for prosthetic grafts maximizes technical success, assuming arterial inflow is adequate (i.e., a palpable pulse). Technical errors, such as narrowing the inflow artery or kinks or sharp turns in the graft, must be avoided. Anastomotic venous stenosis resulting from intimal hyperplasia accounts for the majority of late access thrombosis.[18] Arterial stenosis and central venous stenosis are less common causes.

It has been demonstrated that a failing hemodialysis access can be detected prior to thrombosis by adopting a routine monitoring protocol at intervals of <1 mo.[13] A decrease in the Kt/V values, indicating inefficient dialysis, loss of thrill over the fistula or graft, and increased venous pressure on dialysis, are signs of a failing AV access. By establishing a baseline at the first use of the access site, dynamic or static venous dialysis pressures can be used to prospectively evaluate outflow stenoses.[19] Trends in pressure measurements are more predictive of access stenosis than any single pressure measurement. Flow measurements performed by ultrasound velocity in blood dilution can also be done on-line during dialysis and provide a reliable, valid, and inexpensive monitoring tool for stenosis.[20] Patients suspected of a failing access should be referred for color-flow duplex scanning. Focal increases in velocity either within the access or at either anastomosis should be followed up with angiography.

A venous stenosis, angiographically demonstrated to be >50%, causing hemodynamic, functional, or clinical deterioration, should be corrected. In a prospective study of 265 patient-years of monitored dialysis, Schwab et al.[19] showed that prompt intervention by a combination of angioplasty and surgical revision in AV accesses with elevated venous dialysis pressures reduced the occurrence of thrombosis to 0.15 episodes per patient-year of dialysis in contrast to 1.4 episodes in untreated patients.

Both surgical revision and percutaneous transluminal angioplasty (PTA) may be used. Early reocclusions are more frequent following surgery.[21] Elastic recoil of the AV access following PTA may require stent placement. This, however, should be reserved for upper-arm access, as stents placed in the forearm, particularly across the elbow, are less effective and uncomfortable for the patient. In-graft stenoses in prosthetic grafts can be managed by removal of debris using percutaneous thrombectomy devices. In patients with restenosis following angioplasty, repeat PTA is of little benefit. In this situation, surgical correction is recommended.[13] Reported experience on the relative benefits of the surgical revision versus PTA in the management of AV access stenosis is mixed (Table 31–2).[21,22] Prospective randomized studies comparing outcomes of the two procedures are required to establish the preferred treatment option.

Thrombosis of AV grafts has traditionally been managed by surgical thrombectomy. Graft thrombectomy and plastic repair of the causative venous anastomotic stenosis, either by widening the lumen with a patch or by constructing the venous anastomosis on a different vein or at a more proximal site on the same vein, is usually necessary. In some institutions, thrombectomy is followed by intraoperative balloon angioplasty rather than surgical revision. Grafts that thrombose in the absence of a mechanical obstruction usually fail early. About 15% of surgically managed grafts fail immediately, and another 15% reocclude in 3 mo—the most common cause for reocclusion being a residual untreated vascular stenosis. Postoperative swelling at the operative site does not usually restrict immediate use of the access site. Wound-related complications, however, are not uncommon. Thrombectomy is rarely successful in AV fistulas, and usually necessitates creation of a new access.

Alternatives to surgical thrombectomy are thrombolysis and percutaneous mechanical thrombectomy. Neither of these approaches has any role to play in the treatment of early thrombosis (<30 days postimplantation), as most early thromboses result from technical failures and hence mandate surgical correction or a new access. Throm-

TABLE 31–2. COMPARISON OF PATENCY FOLLOWING PTA VERSUS SURGICAL INTERVENTION FOR THE MANAGEMENT OF AV ACCESS STENOSIS

	One-Year Patency After Intervention	
Reference	*PTA (%)*	*Surgery (%)*
Brooks et al.[22]	25	50
Dapunt et al.[21]	31	19
Beathard[44]	38[a]	
Glanz et al.[45]	45	
Gmelin et al.[46]	91	
Kanterman et al.[47]	41[a]	
Lumsden et al.[48]	10[a]	
Mori et al.[49]	25	
Turmel-Rodrigues et al.[23]	82	

[a] Primary patency rate. All others are secondary patency rates.

bolysis has been reported with widely varying success rates, using differing techniques and a variety of lytic agents. At our institution, we use a "criss-cross" catheter technique, with the catheter ends directed toward the arterial and venous ends of the graft; 1 mg tPA is injected into each catheter.

Following thrombolysis, balloon angioplasty is used to treat residual stenoses. The addition of stent deployment following angioplasty of elastic stenoses has further extended the utility of an endovascular approach.[23] The highest rate of rethrombosis occurs in the first month after PTA, and repeat intervention is required at some point in more than half the patients.[24] A nondilating stenosis or aneurysmal disease in the access or efferent vessel is not amenable to angioplasty and requires surgical revision.

Retrospective studies show that angioplasty has about an 80% initial success rate, with unassisted patency rates comparable to, or even better than, surgical revision (Table 31–3). In a recent, prospective, randomized trial that compared the efficacy of surgical or endovascular techniques in restoring dialysis access functions, Marston et al.[25] reported comparable immediate patency rates in both groups (83% in the surgical and 72% in the endovascular group), but surgical management resulted in significantly longer primary patency compared to endovascular management (25% and 9% patency at 12 mo, respectively). Currently, recommendations for the management of thrombotic occlusions of AV access vary with institution. In our center, thromboses that occur beyond 30 days of access placement are preferentially managed by endovascular therapy and thrombolysis; for other institutions, surgical thrombectomy remains the initial treatment of choice.

Mechanical thrombectomy can be achieved using a number of commercially available devices, including the balloon embolectomy catheter, or oscillation maceration probes with or without suction capabilities. PTA and stent implantation can be used to complement thrombectomy. Although, anecdotal reports suggest that mechan-

TABLE 31–3. COMPARISON OF PATENCY AFTER INTERVENTION FOR AV ACCESS OCCLUSION

	One-Year Patency after Intervention		
Reference	Thrombolysis with PTA (%)	Surgical Thrombectomy and Revision (%)	Surgical Thrombectomy with PTA (%)
Marston et al.[25]	9[a]	25[a]	
Polak et al.[50]	12 (6 mo)[a]	11 (6 mo)[a]	
Summers et al.[51]	20[a]	20[a]	
Brotman et al.[52]		2.5	
Palder et al.[15]		60	
Puckett et al.[41]		36[a]	
Beathard[16]	46		
Cohen et al.[24]	69 (16)[a]		
Gmelin et al.[46]	50		
Valji et al.[53]	51 (26)[a]		
Bitar et al.[54]		17 (at 6 mo)[a]	28 (at 6 mo)[a]
Smith et al.[55]			58 (at 5 mo)[a]

[a] Primary patency rate. All others are secondary patency rates.

ical thrombectomy is at least as effective as thrombolysis, we have not found this to be so.

Infection

Uremia is a strong immunosuppressant, impairing several aspects of neutrophic function and cell-mediated immunity. Vascular-access infection is the second major cause of mortality and morbidity in patients requiring chronic hemodialysis. The overall infection rate of AV access is 21%.[26] Single organisms are responsible for more than 80% of the infections, and *Staphylococcus aureus* has been reported as the causative organism in from 70% to 90% of cases.

Infections occurring in the immediate postoperative period result from contamination during construction of the access, whereas those occurring later are related to repeated needle puncture for hemodialysis. In the early stages of infection, local erythema and tenderness predominate, and systemic bacteremic effects are uncommon. Neglected infections lead to the formation of abscesses, skin dehiscence and drainage, false aneurysms or anastomotic disruption. Severe complications, including loss of limb, metastatic abscesses, and endocarditis with fatal outcomes, have been reported.[27]

Poor personal hygiene and dialysis access technique are common causes of infection, and hence patient and staff education on infection control measures is critical. Proper techniques of cannulation and skin and catheter care significantly decrease the incidence of infection. Meticulous adherence to aseptic techniques during and after establishment of the access is mandatory. The value of perioperative antibiotics for native AV fistula placement is limited; however, prophylactic antibiotic therapy during the placement of AV graft using prosthetic material has been shown to minimize infectious complications.[28,29]

In a vast majority of cases, an established infection of an AV graft requires both antibiotic and surgical therapy. The choice of antibiotic depends on the bacteriology of the infection, but whereas sensitivities are pending, staphylococcal, streptococcal, and gram-negative coverage must be achieved. Incision and drainage of infected material is usually required to control infections adequately.

Management of sepsis in an established AV graft depends on the severity and spread of infection (Figure 31–1). Regardless of the extent, infection in a graft placed within 1 mo warrants graft excision.[13] For older grafts with a focal infection in the body, distant from the anastomoses, drainage, wound care, and frequent dressing changes may be adequate. Segmental replacement of the infected portion of the graft can be performed by dividing the graft proximal and distal to the site of infection and interposing a new graft segment routed through clean tissue planes. In the absence of tissue necrosis, abscess formation, or bacteremia, segmental bypass can be performed as a single-stage procedure. Segmental bypass yields graft salvage rates of about 50%; positive blood cultures, especially gram-negative sepsis, are associated with lower salvage rates.

Extensive graft infection, anastomotic involvement with or without a false aneurysm, systemic sepsis, or the presence of metastatic abscesses necessitates total graft excision. Several approaches are available to deal with the arteriotomy site following complete graft excision. Simple arteriotomy closure is usually not possible without narrowing the lumen of the artery. Arterial continuity can be maintained by vein

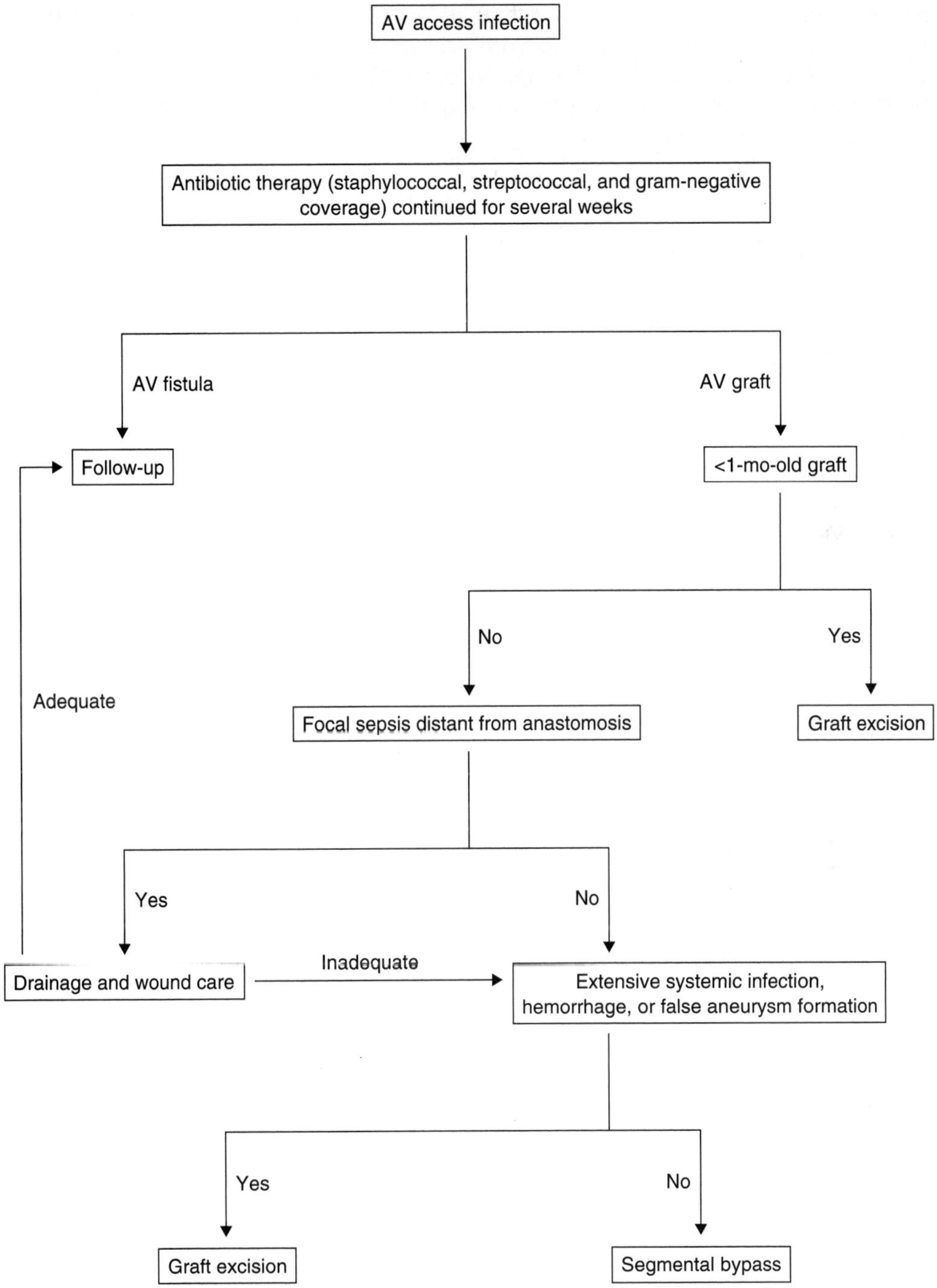

Figure 31–1. Algorithm for the management of established infection in an AV access.

patch repair if the arterial wall is not infected. If the arterial wall is infected, arterial ligation is the only option. In patients with proximal brachial artery or dominant radial artery involvement, distal tissue loss may occur. In these instances, bypass or arterial reconstruction with autogenous conduits is required. If the brachial artery is ligated distal to the profunda brachii, critical limb ischemia is uncommon, although limited midarm or calf claudication could ensue. Management of skin loss due to underlying infection may on occasion warrant subsequent skin grafting or rotation of muscle flaps for coverage.

Infections in AV fistulas are uncommon and respond well to antibiotic therapy alone. Infected perifistula hematomas require incision and drainage. Rarely, septic emboli may necessitate ligation of the fistula.[13]

Pseudoaneurysms

Aneurysms develop frequently in AV fistulas and usually have a benign course.[13] Unless the aneurysm involves and compromises the arterial anastomosis, excision is not mandatory. Although the incidence of aneurysmal dilatation is far lower with the use of newer PTFE grafts, they do develop false aneurysms secondary to repetitive needle trauma and graft degeneration. Expanding large pseudoaneurysms that threaten the viability of overlying skin, aneurysms more than twice the diameter of the native graft, and infected aneurysms must be corrected surgically. In the absence of infection, interposition replacement with a new graft is sufficient.

Hemodynamic Complications

The establishment of an AV access leads to an increase in cardiac output, reduced systemic vascular resistance, and increased venous pressure. Depending on the diameter of the AV communication, these changes could be significant enough to cause extremity hemodynamic complications.

Neurologic Dysfunction

Symptomatic arterial insufficiency, or *steal syndrome,* is rare, with a reported incidence between 1% and 2%. It is particularly common in diabetics with preexisting neuropathy and diffuse occlusive vascular disease. Uremia can also potentiate the development of neuropathic symptoms. Symptomatic steal rarely results from autogenous fistulas because some accommodation to the fistula flow occurs with time. AV grafts, particularly those with inflow at the brachial artery, are most prone to steal phenomena. Steal is manifested by paresthesias involving the palm and fingers. Minimal symptoms usually resolve spontaneously. If symptoms progress, especially with motor involvement, surgical repair is necessary.

Surgical approaches to limit arterial steal have in the past included banding the graft, to restrict arterial inflow and reduce steal, or ligation. Both procedures were unsatisfactory because they inevitably resulted in graft thrombosis and the need for creation of a new AV access, which may also cause symptomatic steal. In 1988, Schanzer et al.[30] described a new procedure in which the inflow artery is ligated just distal to the arterial anastomosis and a bypass constructed from the artery proximal to the arterial anastomosis to the artery distal to the ligation. In their experience, all patients who underwent the arterial ligation-bypass procedure for the management of symptomatic steal[31] showed immediate neurologic improvement. The cumulative patency of the access was 73% at 1 yr and 45.5% at 2 yr. The patency for the bypass itself was 95.6% at 2 yr. Currently, this technique is the procedure of choice for patients with progressive symptoms due to steal phenomena.

The construction of an AV access may also lead to compression of the median nerve within the carpel tunnel, due to either venous hypertension at the wrist or limb edema. Symptomatic carpal tunnel syndrome is characterized by nocturnal pain and/or paresthesia in the distribution of the median nerve in the hand. Thenar wasting occurs late in the course of the disease. When diagnosed early, compression on the median nerve can be released by division of the transverse carpal ligament and neurilemmal sheath, which provides symptomatic relief and minimizes permanent neurologic dysfunction.[32]

Venous Hypertension

Arterialization of the venous system by the construction of an AV fistula can lead to increased venous pressures, which in the presence of venous outflow obstruction results in limb swelling, cyanosis, and pain. Venous obstruction is usually caused by a previously unrecognized central venous thrombosis or stenosis. In many cases this obstruction is a consequence of prior percutaneous access of the subclavian veins.[33] Because duplex scanning is limited in detecting the location of axillosubclavian vein stenoses or subclavian/innominate occlusions, symptomatic patients should undergo venography for diagnosis.

Management of venous hypertension caused by a central venous stenosis can be challenging. Endovascular methods of dilatation are ideally suited to treat these lesions and balloon angioplasty alone is initially successful in most cases (Figure 31–2). Most initial failures are because of the fibrotic nature and elastic recoil properties of these lesions. Primary use of self-expanding wall-stents across lesions with elastic recoil and a significant residual stenosis after dilatation improves initial success rates, but several studies have questioned their long-term efficacy.[34,35] Vesely and colleagues[34] reported primary patency rates of 90% at 1 mo following stenting of central venous stenoses; however, patency rates declined to 25% at 1 yr. When stenosis recurs, the lesions are usually located at the ends of the stent and are amenable to repeat dilatation. Using such an approach, Haage et al.[35] reported secondary patency rates of 97% after 6 and 12 mo, 89% after 24 mo, and 81% after 36 and 48 mo. Surgical repair of central venous stenosis is now rarely performed. Venovenous bypass or internal jugular turndown procedures are now reserved for occlusive lesions of the axillosubclavian veins.

Effective use of vascular access has revolutionized medical care, especially the management of end-stage renal disease. A variety of vascular access procedures are now available to the vascular surgeon. Although the benefits of vascular access far outweigh the associated risks, a large spectrum of complications has been reported. Appropriate management of these complications extends the life of the access, and in many instances, the life of the patient as well.

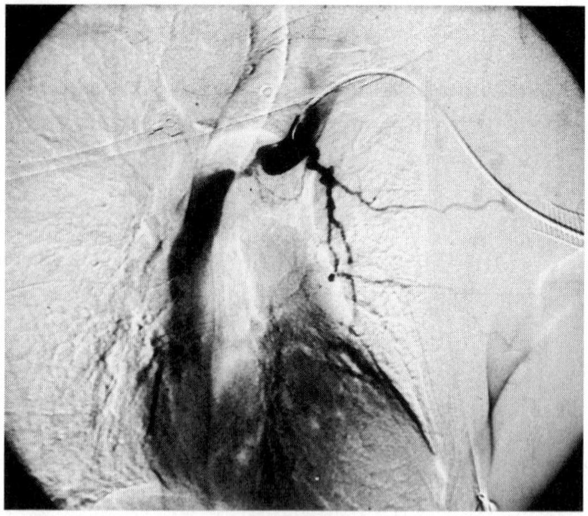

A

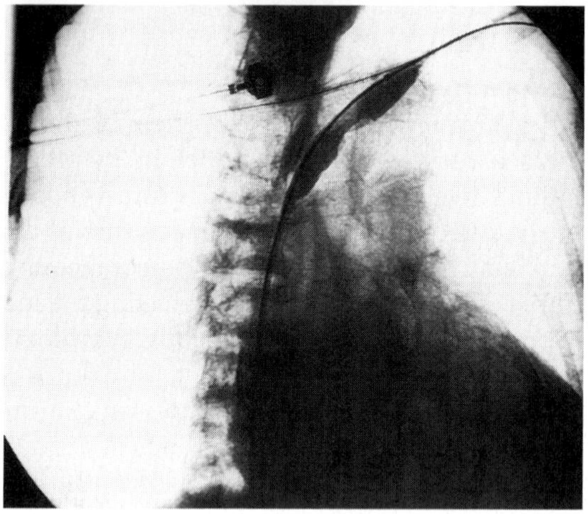

B

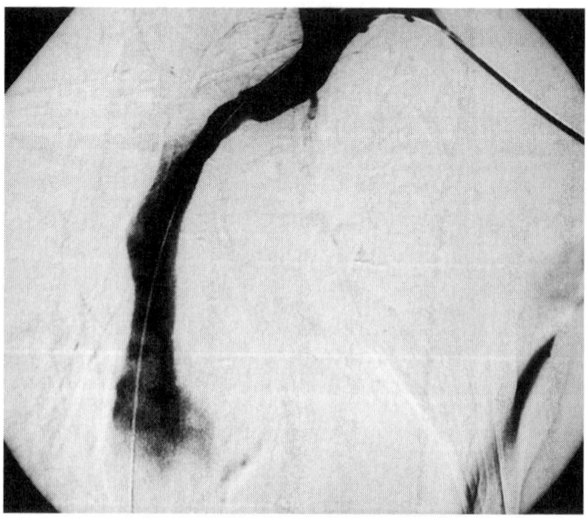

C

Figure 31–2. (**A**) High-grade right innominate vein stenosis following long-term venous access is managed by percutaneous transluminal balloon angioplasty (**B**). Follow-up venogram shows minimal residual stenosis (**C**).

REFERENCES

1. US Renal Data System: VI. Causes of death. *Am J Kid Dis.* 1995(suppl);26:S93–S102.
2. Parsa MH, Tabora F. Central venous access in critically ill patients in the emergency department. *Emerg Med Clin North Am.* 1986;4:709–744.
3. Yilmazlar A, Bilgin H, Korfali G, Eren A, Özkan U. Complications of 1303 central venous cannulations. *J Roy Soc Med.* 1997;90:319–321.
4. Hye RJ, Stabile BE. Complications of percutaneous vascular access procedures and their management. In: Wilson SE, ed. *Vascular Access: Principles and Practice,* 3rd ed. St. Louis; Mosby-Year Book, Inc. 1995.
5. Gladwin MT, Slonim A, Landucci DL, Gutierrez DC, Cunnion RE. Cannulation of the internal jugular vein: is post-procedural chest radiography always necessary? *Crit Care Med.* 1999;27:1819–1823.
6. Denys BG, Uretsky BF, Reddy PS. Ultrasound-assisted cannulation of the internal jugular vein: a prospective comparison to the external landmark-guided technique. *Circulation.* 1993;87:1557–1562.
7. Kwon TH, Kim YL, Cho DK. Ultrasound-guided cannulation of the femoral vein for acute hemodialysis access. *Nephrol Dial Transplant.* 1997;12:1009–1012.
8. Lowell JA, Bothe A Jr. Venous access: preoperative, operative, and postoperative dilemmas. *Surg Clin North Am.* 1991;71:1231–1246.
9. Clagett GP, Eberhart RL. Artificial devices in clinical practice. In: Colman RW et al, eds. *Hemostasis and Thrombosis: Basic Principles and Clinical Practice,* 3rd ed. Philadelphia, PA: Lippincott, 1994:1348–1365.
10. Monreal M, Raventos A, Lerma R, et al. Pulmonary embolism in patients with upper extremity DVT associated to venous central lines—a prospective study. *Thromb Haemost.* 1994;72:548–550.
11. Prandoni P, Bernardi E. Upper extremity deep vein thrombosis. *Curr Opin Pulm Med.* 1999;5:222–226.
12. Seigel EL, Jew AC, Delcore R, Iliopoulos JI, Thomas JH. Thrombolytic therapy for catheter-related thrombosis. *Am J Surg.* 1993;166:716–718.
13. NKF-DOQI clinical practice guidelines for vascular access. National Kidney Foundation–Dialysis Outcomes Quality Initiative. *Am J Kid Dis.* 1997;30(4 Suppl 3):S150–S191.
14. Ascher E, Gade P, Hingorani A, et al. Changes in the practice of angioaccess surgery: impact of dialysis outcome and quality initiative recommendations. *J Vasc Surg.* 2000;31:84–92.
15. Palder SB, Kirkman RL, Whittemore AD, Hakim RM, Lazarus JM, Tilney NL. Vascular access for hemodialysis: patency rates and results of revision. *Ann Surg.* 1985;202:235–239.
16. Beathard GA. Thrombolysis versus surgery for the treatment of thrombosed dialysis access grafts. *J Am Soc Nephrol.* 1995;6:1619–1624.
17. Rohr MS, Browder W, Frentz GD, McDonald JC. Arteriovenous fistulas for long-term dialysis: factors that influence fistula survival. *Arch Surg.* 1978;113:153–155.
18. Kumpe DA, Cohen MA. Angioplasty/thrombolytic treatment of failing and failed hemodialysis access sites: comparison with surgical treatment. *Prog Cardiovasc Dis.* 1992;34:263–278.
19. Schwab SJ, Raymond JR, Saeed M, Newman GE, Dennis PA, Bollinger RR. Prevention of hemodialysis fistula thrombosis: early detection of venous stenoses. *Kid Int.* 1989;36:707–711.
20. Krivitski NM. Theory and validation of access flow measurement by dilution technique during hemodialysis. *Kid Int.* 1995;48:244–250.
21. Dapunt O, Feurstein M, Rendl KH, Prenner K. Transluminal angioplasty versus conventional operation in the treatment of hemodialysis fistula stenosis: results from a 5-year study. *Br J Surg.* 1987;74:1004–1005.

22. Brooks JL, Sigley RD, May KJ Jr, Mack RM. Transluminal angioplasty versus surgical repair for stenosis of hemodialysis grafts. A randomized study. *Am J Surg.* 1987;153:530–531.
23. Turmel-Rodrigues LA, Blanchard D, Pengloan J, et al. Wallstents and Craggstents in hemodialysis grafts and fistulas: results for selective indications. *J Vasc Interv Radiol.* 1997;8:975–982.
24. Cohen MA, Kumpe DA, Durham JD, Zwerdlinger SC. Improved treatment of thrombosed hemodialysis access sites with thrombolysis and angioplasty. *Kid Int.* 1994;46:1375–1380.
25. Marston WA, Criado E, Jaques PF, Mauro MA, Burnham SJ, Keagy BA. Prospective randomized comparison of surgical versus endovascular management of thrombosed dialysis access grafts. *J Vasc Surg.* 1997;26:373–380; discussion, 380–381.
26. Adams WJ, Thompson JF, Liounis B, Ekberg H, Rotenko I. The Allen Brown shunt: a useful option for vascular access. *Am J Surg.* 1991;162:24–30.
27. Francioli P, Masur H. Complications of *Staphylococcus aureus* bacteremia. Occurrence in patients undergoing long-term hemodialysis. *Arch Intern Med.* 1982;142:1655–1658.
28. Bennion RS, Hiatt JR, Williams RA, Wilson SE. A randomized, prospective study of perioperative antimicrobial prophylaxis for vascular access surgery. *J Cardiovasc Surg (Torino)* 1985;26:270–274.
29. Zibari GB, Gadallah MF, Landreneau M, et al. Preoperative vancomycin prophylaxis decreases incidence of postoperative hemodialysis vascular access infections. *Am J Kid Dis.* 1997;30:343–348.
30. Schanzer H, Schwartz M, Harrington E, Haimov M. Treatment of ischemia due to "steal" by arteriovenous fistula with distal artery ligation and revascularization. *J Vasc Surg.* 1988;7:770–773.
31. Haimov M, Schanzer H, Skladani M. Pathogenesis and management of upper-extremity ischemia following angioaccess surgery. *Blood Purif.* 1996;14:350–354.
32. Bosanac PR, Bilder B, Grunberg RW, Banach SF, Kintzel JE, Stephens HW. Post-permanent access neuropathy. *Trans Am Soc Artif Intern Organs.* 1977;23:162–167.
33. Surratt RS, Picus D, Hicks ME, Darcy MD, Kleinhoffer M, Jendrisak M. The importance of preoperative evaluation of the subclavian vein in dialysis access planning. *Am J Roentgen.* 1991;156:623–625.
34. Vesely TM, Hovsepian DM, Pilgram TK, Coyne DW, Shenoy S. Upper extremity central venous obstruction in hemodialysis patients: treatment with Wallstents. *Radiology.* 1997;204: 343–348.
35. Haage P, Vorwerk D, Piroth W, Schuermann K, Guenther RW. Treatment of hemodialysis-related central venous stenosis or occlusion: results of primary Wallstent placement and follow-up in 50 patients. *Radiology.* 1999;212:175–180.
36. Kherlakian GM, Roedersheimer LR, Arbaugh JJ, Newmark KJ, King LR. Comparison of autogenous fistula versus expanded polytetrafluoroethylene graft fistula for angioaccess in hemodialysis. *Am J Surg.* 1986;152:238–243.
37. Tellis VA, Kohlberg WI, Bhat DJ, Driscoll B, Veith FJ. Expanded polytetrafluoroethylene graft fistula for chronic hemodialysis. *Ann Surg.* 1979;189:101–105.
38. Kinnaert P, Vereerstraeten P, Toussaint C, Van Geertruyden J. Nine years' experience with internal arteriovenous fistulas for hemodialysis: a study of some factors influencing the results. *Br J Surg.* 1977;64:242–246.
39. Silcott GR, Vannix RS, DePalma JR. Repair versus new arteriovenous fistulae. *Trans Am Soc Artif Intern Organs.* 1980;26:99–104.
40. Munda R, First MR, Alexander JW, Linnemann CC Jr, Fidler JP, Kittur D. Polytetrafluoroethylene graft survival in hemodialysis. *JAMA.* 1983;14;249:219–222.
41. Puckett JW, Lindsay SF. Midgraft curettage as a routine adjunct to salvage operations for thrombosed polytetrafluoroethylene hemodialysis access grafts. *Am J Surg.* 1988;156:139–143.

42. Rizzuti RP, Hale JC, Burkart TE. Extended patency of expanded polytetrafluoroethylene grafts for vascular access using optimal configuration and revisions. *Surg Gynecol Obstet.* 1988;166:23–27.
43. Tordoir JH, de Bruin HG, Hoeneveld H, Eikelboom BC, Kitslaar PJ. Duplex ultrasound scanning in the assessment of arteriovenous fistulas created for hemodialysis access: comparison with digital subtraction angiography. *J Vasc Surg.* 1989;10:122–128.
44. Beathard GA. Percutaneous transvenous angioplasty in the treatment of vascular access stenosis. *Kid Int.* 1992;42(6):1390–1397.
45. Glanz S, Gordon DH, Butt KM, Hong J, Lipkowitz GS. The role of percutaneous angioplasty in the management of chronic hemodialysis fistulas. *Ann Surg.* 1987;206:777–781.
46. Gmelin E, Winterhoff R, Rinast E. Insufficient hemodialysis access fistulas: late results of treatment with percutaneous balloon angioplasty. *Radiology.* 1989;171:657–660.
47. Kanterman RY, Vesely TM, Pilgram TK, Guy BW, Windus DW, Picus D. Dialysis access grafts: anatomic location of venous stenosis and results of angioplasty. *Radiology.* 1995;195:135–139.
48. Lumsden AB, MacDonald MJ, Kikeri DK, Harker LA, Allen RC. Hemodialysis access graft stenosis: percutaneous transluminal angioplasty. *J Surg Res.* 1997;68:181–185.
49. Mori Y, Horikawa K, Sato K, Mimuro N, Toriyama T, Kawahara H. Stenotic lesions in vascular access: treatment with transluminal angioplasty using high-pressure balloons. *Intern Med.* 1994;33:284–287.
50. Polak JF, Berger MF, Pagan-Marin H, Aruny JE, Meyerovitz MF. Comparative efficacy of pulse-spray thrombolysis and angioplasty versus surgical salvage procedures for treatment of recurrent occlusion of PTFE dialysis access grafts. *Cardiovasc Intervent Radiol.* 1998;21: 314–318.
51. Summers S, Drazan K, Gomes A, Freischlag J. Urokinase therapy for thrombosed hemodialysis access grafts. *Surg Gynecol Obstet.* 1993;176:534–538.
52. Brotman DN, Fandos L, Faust GR, Doscher W, Cohen JR. Hemodialysis graft salvage. *J Am Coll Surg.* 1994;178:431–434.
53. Valji K, Bookstein JJ, Roberts AC, Davis GB. Pharmacomechanical thrombolysis and angioplasty in the management of clotted hemodialysis grafts: early and late clinical results. *Radiology.* 1991;178:243–247.
54. Bitar G, Yang S, Badosa F. Balloon versus patch angioplasty as an adjuvant treatment to surgical thrombectomy of hemodialysis grafts. *Am J Surg.* 1997;174:140–142.
55. Smith TP, Cragg AH, Castaneda F, Hunter DW. Thrombosed polytetrafluoroethylene hemodialysis fistulas: salvage with combined thrombectomy and angioplasty. *Radiology.* 1989;171:507–508.

32

Finger Gangrene

Lloyd M. Taylor, Jr., MD, Gregory L. Landry, MD, Gregory L. Moneta, MD, James M. Edwards, MD, and John M. Porter, MD

Vascular surgeons see many patients with gangrenous lesions of the toes. Nearly all such patients have severe atherosclerosis. Diagnosis rarely presents a challenge. Without effective revascularization, inevitable disease progression eventually results in limb loss in the majority of patients affected. Appropriate diagnostic evaluation and standard approaches to treatment of these lesions form a large portion of everyday vascular practice.

In contrast, finger gangrene is infrequently encountered in most vascular practices. Atherosclerosis is an unusual cause of finger gangrene, with most cases resulting from a large variety of primary diseases, many of which are only rarely treated by vascular surgeons. Not surprisingly, diagnosis is paramount and may be difficult, and both treatment and prognosis differ considerably from the routine approach to atherosclerotic lower extremity ischemia.

Since the early 1970s, the Division of Vascular Surgery at Oregon Health Sciences University has maintained a long-term clinical research project devoted to the diagnosis, treatment, and long-term follow-up of patients with hand and finger ischemia. More than 1500 patients have been enrolled, including more than 300 patients with finger gangrene. This chapter briefly describes the pathophysiology, diagnosis, and treatment of finger gangrene based on our experience with this large number of patients.

PATHOPHYSIOLOGY

Two features distinguish upper extremity ischemia: (1) vasospasm plays a prominent role in the nature of the symptoms which occur, and (2) the available collateral circulation in the upper extremities vastly exceeds that of the lower extremities. Knowledge of normal and abnormal vasospasm leads to understanding of upper-extremity ischemic symptoms. Knowledge of the role of collaterals leads to understanding of the natural history and prognosis of finger gangrene.

Normal Upper-Extremity Vasospasm

The hands, like the head and neck, are involved in regulating heat loss/conservation for the whole body. This means that resting blood flow exceeds nutritional requirements, there are many functional arteriovenous shunts, and flow to the hands and fingers varies greatly in response to ambient and body temperature and somewhat in response to emotional states. Cooling of the entire body or of only the hands normally results in marked reduction of hand and finger blood flow caused by spasm of palmar and digital arteries. A similar response occurs with strong emotions.

Abnormal Upper-Extremity Vasospasm (Raynaud's Syndrome)

It is normal for hand and finger blood flow to decrease in response to cold or emotions. Complete spastic closure of digital arteries resulting in cessation of flow is abnormal. When this occurs, the stereotypical symptoms that occur are known as *Raynaud's syndrome*. When digital artery flow ceases, pallor occurs. As vasospasm relaxes, the initial arterial blood is rapidly desaturated, producing cyanosis. Postischemic hyperemia ensues, producing rubor. Many Raynaud's episodes do not include all three classic color changes. Raynaud's episodes last from a few minutes to, at most, 1 to 2 hr.

Digital artery closure resulting in Raynaud's syndrome can occur through two distinctly different mechanisms (Figure 32–1).[1] In *vasospastic Raynaud's syndrome*, normally patent digital arteries have intermittent complete closure due to an abnormally forceful spastic response to cold. In *obstructive Raynaud's syndrome*, digital arteries with reduced intraluminal pressure caused by fixed arterial obstructive disease have intermittent complete closure as a result of the normal vasospastic response to cold.

Nearly all patients with upper extremity ischemia, regardless of cause, complain of Raynaud's syndrome. Because of this, physicians may be tempted to attribute symptoms of severe ischemia, including fixed cyanosis or pallor, constant ischemic pain, and ischemic ulceration/gangrene to abnormal vasospasm. Central to understanding the pathophysiology of finger gangrene is the knowledge that, with a single rare exception, this is never the case.

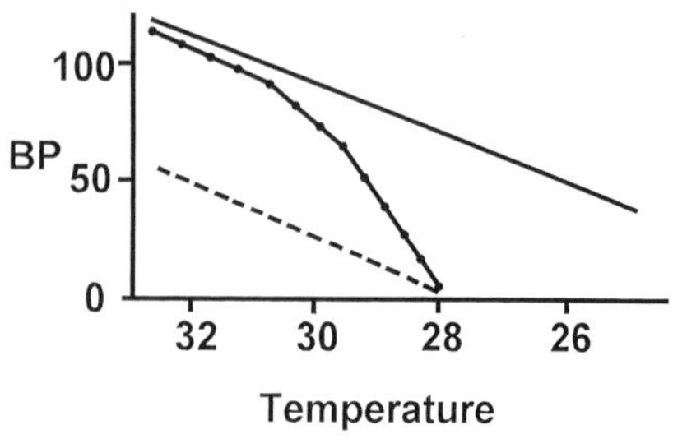

Figure 32–1. Pathophysiology of Raynaud's syndrome: Normal vasospastic response to cold results in reduced finger blood pressure but maintenance of flow (*solid line*). In vasospastic Raynaud's syndrome, normally patent arteries have an abnormally strong vasospastic response to cold, resulting in digital artery closure and cessation of flow (*solid line with dots*). In obstructive Raynaud's syndrome, abnormal arteries with preexisting obstruction become completely closed with cessation of flow as a result of normal cold-induced vasospasm (*dashed line*).

> Symptoms caused by abnormal vasospasm are intermittent, and the involved extremity is asymptomatic and normal in appearance and to examination between attacks. Consequently, all symptoms of severe upper extremity ischemia, including ischemic rest pain, fixed cyanosis, ischemic ulceration, and gangrene, are caused by fixed arterial obstruction, not by vasospasm.

The single exception to this rule occurs when abnormal vasospasm is caused by toxins or medication as is the case with ergotism.[2]

Collateral Vessels in the Pathophysiology of Finger Gangrene

Collaterals in the upper extremity are more plentiful than in the lower extremity. In contrast to the lower extremities, progression of ischemia to extensive gangrene requiring major limb amputation is extremely rare in the upper extremities, regardless of etiology or treatment. The extensive collateral network also means that considerable progression of occlusive disease including occlusion of major limb arteries is well tolerated and indeed may be asymptomatic. This is particularly true of diffuse small artery disease. Symptoms occur only after extensive disease exists. When disease progression finally results in occlusion of additional arteries/collaterals, the symptoms that occur may be erroneously interpreted as an indication of an acute disease process when in fact the opposite is true. The abundance of collateral supply in the upper extremity is the most important reason why classification of finger gangrene cases into acute and chronic causes based on symptoms is misleading and not clinically relevant.

DIAGNOSIS

Symptoms of severe finger ischemia, including constant ischemic pain, ischemic ulceration, and finger gangrene, establish the presence of permanent arterial obstruction with reduced finger blood pressure. The task of the clinician is to determine the underlying cause of arterial obstruction. Our experience indicates that it is useful and clinically relevant to classify the various disorders producing ischemia according to whether the affected vessels are large arteries (proximal to the wrist) or small arteries (distal to the wrist). In a few cases, finger ischemia results from digital artery obstruction by embolic material that originates in proximal large artery lesions. Although these patients are rare, they are the group most amenable to surgical correction, thus the diagnostic approach must include methods to detect this pattern. The large number of diverse disorders that may produce finger gangrene are listed in Table 32–1 according to this classification.

History

Large artery obstructive disease is suggested when symptoms of exercise-induced muscle pain accompany finger ischemia. Symptoms confined to the hands and fingers may result from large or small artery disease or from embolization. *Embolization of distal small arteries from proximal large artery sources should be suspected whenever symptoms are unilat-*

TABLE 32–1. CAUSES OF FINGER GANGRENE

- **Vasospasm**
  - Ergotism
- **Arterial obstruction**
  - **Large artery causes**
    - Atherosclerosis
    - Thoracic outlet compression by bony abnormalities
    - Arteritis
      - Takaysu's
      - Giant cell
    - Fibromuscular disease
  - **Small artery causes**
    - Connective tissue disease
      - Scleroderma
      - Rheumatoid arthritis
      - Mixed connective tissue disease
      - Systemic lupus erythematosus
    - Myeloproliferative disease
      - Thrombocytosis
      - Leukemia
      - Polycythemia
    - Buerger's disease
    - Hypersensitivity angiitis
    - Cold injury
    - Henoch–Schonlein purpura
    - Cytotoxic drugs
    - Hypercoaguable states
      - Heparin antibodies
      - Malignancy
      - Deficiencies
        - Antithrombin III
        - Protein S
        - Protein C
      - Factor V Leiden
      - Prothrombin gene mutation
      - Hyperviscosity syndromes
        - Macroglobulinemia
        - Cryoglobulinemia
        - Myeloma
  - **Proximal large artery sources of embolism to distal small arteries**
    - Ulcerated or stenotic atherosclerotic plaques
      - Aortic arch
      - Innominate artery
      - Subclavian artery
    - Aneurysms
      - Innominate artery
      - Subclavian artery
      - Axillary or brachial artery
      - Ulnar artery

eral. Although further testing may reveal that the involvement is in fact bilateral, unilateral symptoms from diffuse small artery disease are rare.

The history should include specific questions to elicit causes of environmental or occupational exposure known to be related to finger ischemia, such as ergot exposure, vibrating tool use, vinyl chloride exposure, and use of the hands as a hammer (carpenters, mechanics, etc.). Diabetes or symptoms of atherosclerotic disease at other sites, smoking history, and any history of connective tissue or hematologic disorders should also be specifically considered.

Physical Examination

Palpation of normal axillary, brachial, radial, and ulnar pulses establishes that finger ischemic lesions are the result of small artery obstruction. A proximal large artery embolic source should be suspected if the findings are unilateral. Cervical ribs and aneurysmal dilation of the subclavian/axillary arteries should be sought by palpation (Figure 32–2).

Typically diffuse small artery occlusive disease involves multiple fingers, although there may be a range of ischemic symptoms from Raynaud's syndrome only in those least affected, through cyanosis to ischemic ulceration and gangrene in the worst. Is-

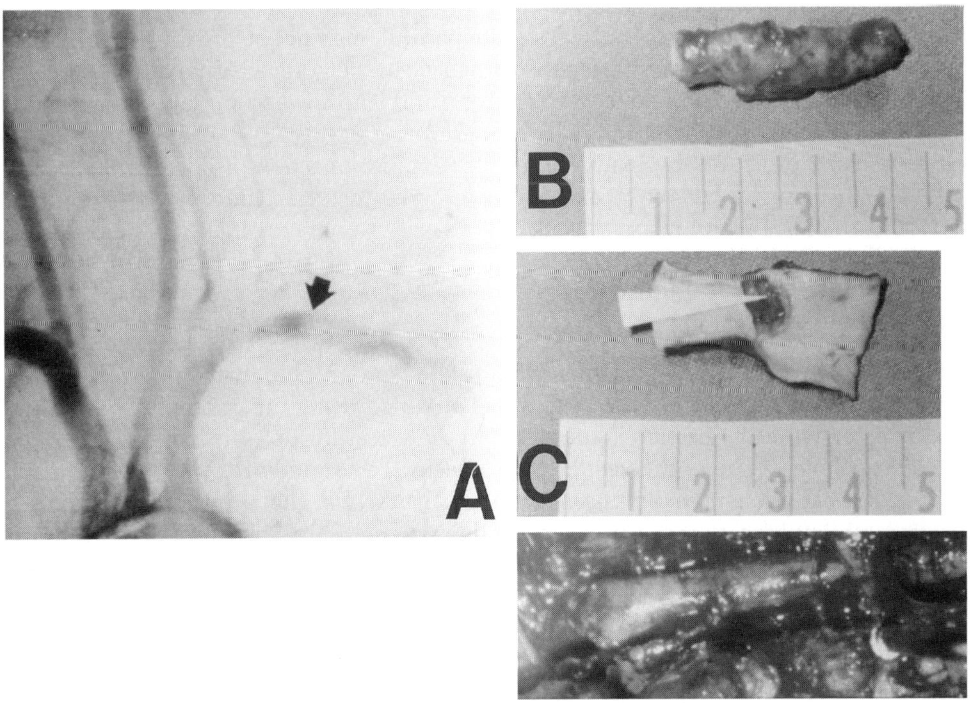

Figure 32–2. Proximal large artery source of emboli which occluded distal small arteries. (**A**) Arteriogram showing subclavian artery aneurysm in a patient with a cervical rib. (**B**) The excised aneurysm. (**C**) Aneurysm opened showing adherent intraluminal thrombus, the source of the emboli.

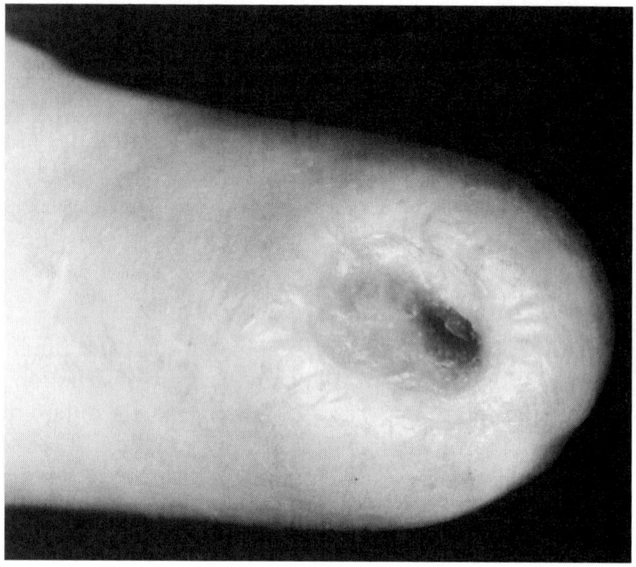

Figure 32–3. Typical small painful ischemic fingertip ulcer in a patient with scleroderma.

chemic fingers, although nearly always quite painful, may not be obviously ischemic in appearance, especially to inexperienced primary care personnel. Any painful finger ulcers should be suspected of an ischemic origin, and lead to vascular laboratory evaluation (Figure 32–3). Drainage of calcific material is diagnostic of scleroderma. The ischemic lesions produced by inadvertent intra-arterial injection of illicit drugs may be especially difficult to diagnose due to the evasive historical information frequently given by addicts. Careful inspection usually reveals an obvious injection site.

Vascular Laboratory Evaluation

Bilateral arm segmental pressures and Doppler analog waveforms are used to detect and confirm large artery obstruction. Photoplethysmographic fingertip arterial waveforms combined with finger blood pressures obtained using the photoplethysmograph as a detector with finger cuffs is the most accurate test for detecting digital artery obstruction. When positive, this test is quite specific for digital artery obstruction.[3] The test is not ideally sensitive. Because each finger has two digital arteries, one can be obstructed while patency of the other maintains normal finger blood pressure. Because finger cuffs are applied at the base of the fingers, it is possible for the finger blood pressure obtained to be normal despite the presence of considerable distal digital arterial occlusive disease.

Digital arterial embolization from a proximal large artery source is suggested when finger blood pressures and waveforms are abnormal in the affected hand and normal in the contralateral asymptomatic hand. The suggestion is even stronger when positive vascular laboratory findings are confined to the symptomatic digits. In contrast, if only one hand is symptomatic but the vascular laboratory testing shows bilateral involvement, intrinsic small artery obstructive disease is the most likely explanation.

Radiographic Examination

Chest radiographs should be performed to detect bony abnormalities of the thoracic outlet (cervical rib, abnormal first rib or clavicle). Hand radiographs may detect calcinosis cutis, as is seen in scleroderma and mixed connective tissue disease.

Arteriography

Detailed arteriograms of upper-extremity vessels from the aortic arch to the fingers should be performed in patients with symptomatic large artery obstruction and in all patients with suspected embolic occlusion of distal small arteries. Arteriograms are not required in patients with noninvasive findings showing diffuse bilateral small artery obstructive disease when laboratory studies clearly diagnose connective tissue disease, a defined hematologic disorder, or other known cause of small artery obstruction as listed in Table 32–1.

In our practice, arteriograms are obtained in patients with finger gangrene and probable small artery disease in whom a definite diagnosis cannot be made based on laboratory testing (see section entitled "Laboratory Evaluation"). This is both because the arteriographic appearance may be diagnostic (example: fibromuscular disease) and because proximal large artery sources of distal emboli may be impossible to detect without arteriography.

Upper-extremity arteriography, including adequate views of palmar and digital arteries, is challenging.[4] Normal vasospasm, especially in response to catheters, may mimic fixed obstruction of large and small arteries (Figure 32–4). Magnification views, external warming of the hands, and intra-arterial vasodilators may be necessary to produce images of diagnostic quality. Digital subtraction images, particularly from older machines, may not have sufficiently high resolution to delineate digital artery disease.

Most upper-extremity arteriograms should be bilateral, even if only one extremity is symptomatic. This is because the bilateral nature of diffuse small artery occlusive disease allows differentiation from embolic obstruction of digital arteries that should nearly always be unilateral. This is especially important when proximal atherosclerotic lesions are suspected as the source of digital emboli. Bilateral small artery disease may prove that the atherosclerosis is simply coexsistant with the independent small artery disease, instead of causative as would be the case if the small artery lesions were unilateral.

Echocardiography

A few patients with finger gangrene caused by embolic digital artery occlusion may not be found to have a proximal embolic source by routine arteriography. This occurs when the proximal source consists of friable thrombus (frequently mobile) adherent to the wall of the ascending aorta/aortic arch, adjacent to the origins of the brachiocephalic vessels. Because of the very high flow rates in the proximal aorta, high contrast density is necessary for arteriography in this region, but the high density contrast used may obscure thrombus from view. Transesophageal echocardiography is particularly suitable for visualizing such lesions and should be performed in patients suspected of proximal embolic sources in whom arteriography fails to reveal a source.

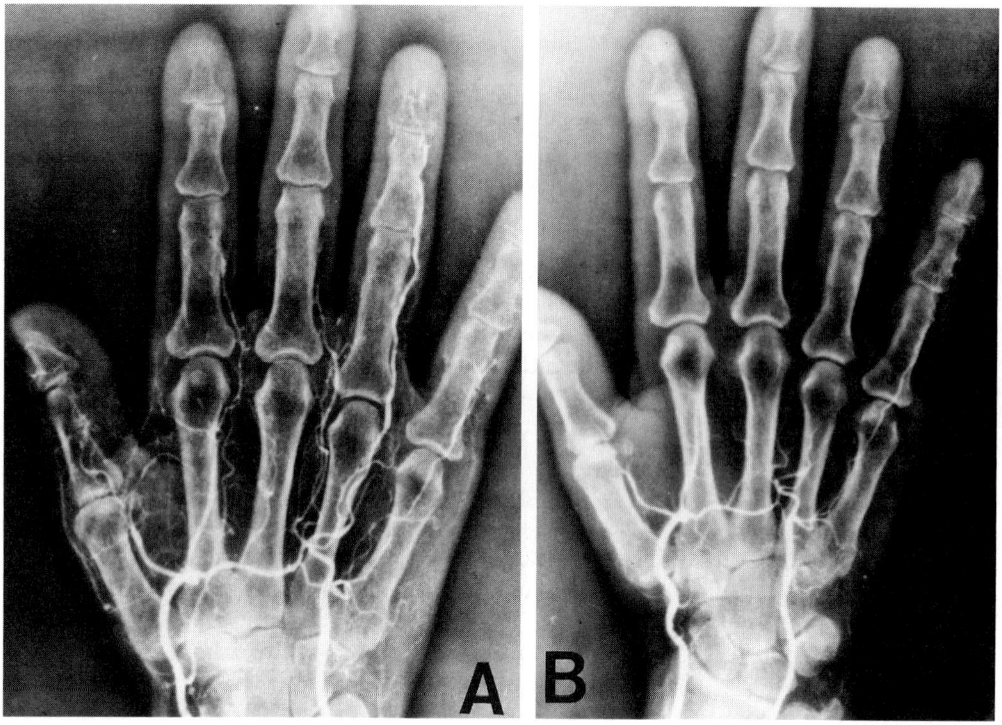

Figure 32–4. Hand arteriogram showing persistence of normal cold-induced vasospasm despite extensive small artery obstruction. (**A**) Arteriogram shows extensive occlusions of palmar and digital arteries. (**B**) After the hand is immersed in icewater, vasospasm occurs.

Laboratory Evaluation

The presence of finger gangrene establishes that fixed arterial obstructive disease is present. Some of the disorders producing these symptoms are obvious from the history (e.g., ergot intoxication; trauma; previous dialysis access procedures; occupational exposure, such as carpenter or mechanic) and others from physical exam (e.g., cervical rib, subclavian aneurysm). Others are clearly diagnosed by arteriography (e.g., aneurysms, ulcerated atherosclerotic plaques, ulnar artery fibrodysplasia). For a significant number of patients, however, particularly patients with diffuse small artery disease, laboratory evaluation is essential for diagnosis. A list of the laboratory tests obtained routinely and in special circumstances is shown in Table 32–2. Most patients with finger gangrene from named connective tissue diseases have typical positive laboratory evaluations that allow positive diagnosis. For patients with no positive laboratory tests and vascular laboratory or arteriographic evidence of diffuse multiextremity small artery occlusions, two possibilities exist: Buerger's disease and what we have chosen to call hypersensitivity angiitis. Diagnostic criteria for Buerger's disease have been established.[5] Extensive bilateral small artery obstruction in the absence of any laboratory features of connective tissue disease, hypercoaguable states, hematologic abnormality, or other

TABLE 32–2. LABORATORY TESTING FOR PATIENTS WITH FINGER GANGRENE

All patients
Complete blood count with platelet count
Urinalysis
Multichemistry screen
Erythrocyte sedimentation rate
Antinuclear antibody
Rheumatoid factor
Large artery vasospasm
No tests; caused only by ergotism
Small artery obstruction
Serum protein electrophoresis
Hep-2 antinuclear antibody
Extractable antinuclear antibody
Anti-native DNA antibody
Cold agglutinins
Protein C
Protein S
Antithrombin III
Anticardiolipin antibody
Heparin-associated antibodies
Factor V Leiden
Prothrombin gene mutation
Large Artery Obstruction
Lipid panel
Glucose

identified cause has been called *hypersensitivity angiitis* based on the presumption that it has an immune origin and the fact that such patients almost always suffer a discrete symptomatic episode followed by gradual improvement through collateral vessel formation without recurrence.

Diagnosis of Finger Gangrene in Patients with End-Stage Renal Disease

Finger gangrene is especially frequent in end-stage renal disease (ESRD) patients. Many such patients have severe diabetes, atherosclerosis, or connective tissue disease. Severe calcific small artery disease is common in ESRD patients, partly as a result of the calciphylaxis that complicates hyperparathyroidism. In addition, many patients have had multiple arterial surgical procedures performed on the upper extremities for dialysis access, further complicating the picture. For all these reasons, arteriography should be used liberally in ESRD patients. Arterial occlusions resulting from surgical complications respond well to standard vascular reconstruction. Hemodynamic steal from arteriovenous shunts is common and responds well to vascular reconstruction, the so-called DRIL (distal revascularization, interval ligation) procedure.[6] Some ESRD patients have distal arterial occlusions that may be treated with vein bypass distal to the wrist,[7] a procedure we perform infrequently with mixed results. Although the hemodynamic improvement invariably produced some symptomatic improvement, most patients died within 6 mo, emphasizing that finger gangrene in ESRD patients in the absence of large artery causes is a manifestation of end-stage disease.

NATURAL HISTORY OF FINGER GANGRENE

Regardless of cause, the natural history of finger gangrene is markedly different from that associated with the more familiar lower extremity gangrene. This is largely because of the abundant collateral supply available in the upper extremities, particularly in the hands and fingers. Extensive experience indicates two general facts:

1. For the vast majority of patients with finger gangrene, the disease is worst at the time of initial presentation; progressive gangrenous changes and need for limb amputation are rare.[8]
2. Regardless of cause, the factor most closely associated with prognosis is cigarette smoking. Patients who cease smoking almost never loose tissue; patients who cannot stop, not infrequently do.

There are a few exceptions. Failure to recognize or treat ergot intoxication and proximal sources of emboli may result in marked progression of ischemia. Digital gangrene from malignancy and other untreated (or untreatable) hypercoaguable states is much more likely to progress than that from other causes. The relationship of prognosis to smoking is most important in Buerger's disease, but is also strong in many other conditions. In a review of finger gangrene from all causes, excepting patients with malignancy, extensive tissue loss occurred only in persistent smokers, regardless of the underlying cause of ischemia.[9]

For the vast majority of patients with finger gangrene, appropriate treatment results in disease stabilization. Recovery is the rule following treatment for large artery obstruction and proximal sources of emboli. For those with chronic small artery diseases, recurrent symptomatic episodes are common, but progression to major tissue loss is extremely rare (Figure 32–5).

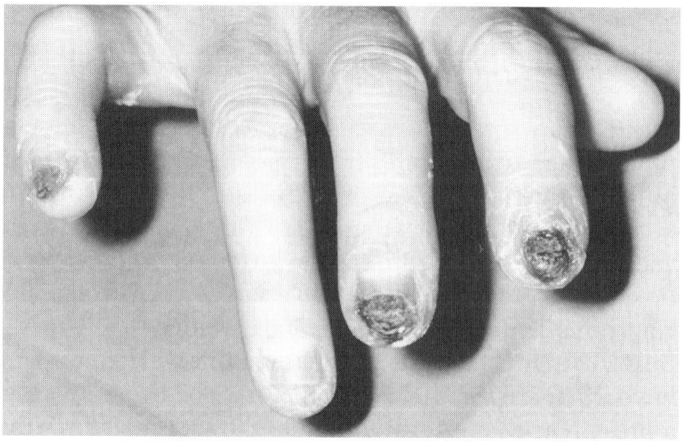

Figure 32–5. Fingertip gangrene in a patient with diffuse small artery disease. With dressing changes and cleansing, the lesions healed over a period of several months. Surgery was not required.

TREATMENT OF FINGER GANGRENE

Arterial Reconstruction

Obviously, large artery obstructions should be relieved and proximal sources of emboli should be eliminated using standard techniques of arterial reconstruction in patients with finger gangrene. Our preference is to use autogenous vein grafting for all arteries distal to the subclavian. We prefer subclavian to carotid transposition operations, if possible, to treat proximal subclavian lesions. If not possible, prosthetic carotid subclavian bypass is satisfactory. Our preference is to use aneurysm excision and autogenous saphenous vein interposition grafting for subclavian artery aneurysms, accompanied by excision of the causative bony abnormalities.[10]

For inflammatory large artery arteriopathies (Takayasu's arteritis, giant cell arteritis), surgery is best delayed until appropriate anti-inflammatory medication has reduced the level of disease activity (as judged by sedimentation rate, reduction of systemic symptoms, etc.). Operations performed in the face of active disease have a high recurrence rate.

The natural history of upper extremity ischemia is relevant to the timing of arterial reconstruction. Most patients with acute symptoms of finger ischemia or gangrene have chronic arterial disease that has been gradually producing increasing arterial obstruction that has finally become sufficiently severe to produce symptoms. This is particularly true of proximal embolic sources. Most patients with subclavian aneurysm, for example, have had multiple embolic episodes, only the most recent of which have produced symptoms. Because most of the arterial occlusions are in fact chronic, catheter thromboembolectomy is rarely successful, nor is intra-arterial lytic therapy. Emergency operations are rarely indicated. Careful patient evaluation, including detailed arteriography when appropriate, is essential to first establish a clear diagnosis. Elective surgery, when appropriate, should be planned to revascularize patent distal vessels rather than to restore patency to occluded segments, which is rarely possible.

Vasodilator Therapy

The fact that Raynaud's symptoms accompany almost all episodes of finger gangrene has led to the frequent assumption that vasospasm is somehow involved in the pathophysiology of finger gangrene. This is simply not true. Finger gangrene is caused only by fixed arterial obstruction. It is obviously axiomatic that vasodilator therapy will not result in improvement in fixed arterial obstructions. The fact that finger gangrene has a natural history characterized by stabilization/improvement in the vast majority of cases has misled many observers to attribute benefit to the use of vasodilator medications or sympathetic blocks/sympathectomy. In fact, no controlled study has ever shown benefit for use of vasodilators in finger gangrene, regardless of the therapeutic agent or cause of disease. The same can be said for sympathetic blocks/sympathectomy. We do not use vasodilator medications or sympathetic blocks/sympathectomy for treatment of finger gangrene.

Anticoagulant Treatment

We use heparin anticoagulation to treat patients with acute symptoms of finger gangrene while diagnostic studies are underway. Patients with cardiac or central aortic sources of emboli require long-term warfarin anticoagulation. This medication is also used for patients with documented hypercoaguable states and patients with finger gangrene as a complication of malignancy.

Smoking Cessation

Regardless of cause, the prognosis for finger ischemia is improved markedly by smoking cessation. This fact must be communicated clearly to patients at the initial and all subsequent encounters. Use of prescription aids to smoking cessation, such as nicotine patches and gum and/or wellbutrin, is appropriate. Patients are helped by understanding that smoking cessation is a process, not an event. Most persons who stop smoking successfully do so over a period of 1 to 3 yr and have an average of six abstinence/relapse cycles. Positive reinforcement of this pattern assists patients; condemnation of the relapses may well interrupt it. Many patients identify repeated positive encouragement to stop smoking from health professionals, family, and friends as the most important influence leading to tobacco abstinence.

Treatment of Ischemic Lesions

Given the overall natural history of finger gangrene, treatment of the ischemic lesions must be conservative. Ischemic ulcers are treated with soap-and-water scrubs, antibiotics when cellulitis is present, and protective bandaging. Healing is the rule, especially if smoking cessation is achieved, but the time required for healing is typically prolonged and is measured in months. Debridement of clearly necrotic tissue or exposed bone is appropriate.

Amputations in gangrenous fingers should be limited to excision of clearly necrotic segments only. Formal ray amputations, including metacarpal excisions, are almost never necessary (Figure 32–6).

Pain Management

As anyone who has mistakenly struck his/her finger with a hammer knows (and who has not?), the fingers are extraordinarily sensitive to pain. Treatment of finger gangrene requires special attention to pain management. Conservative treatment of ischemic finger ulcers requires adequate pain relief during the period of waiting for healing to occur. Narcotics are required, frequently at rather high doses and for unusually prolonged periods given the relative size of the lesions. Adequate pain relief is necessary if patients are to continue normal activities, especially occupational activities. No patient can make progress toward smoking cessation in the absence of adequate pain relief. We have found consultation with pain management specialists useful in finger ischemia patients.

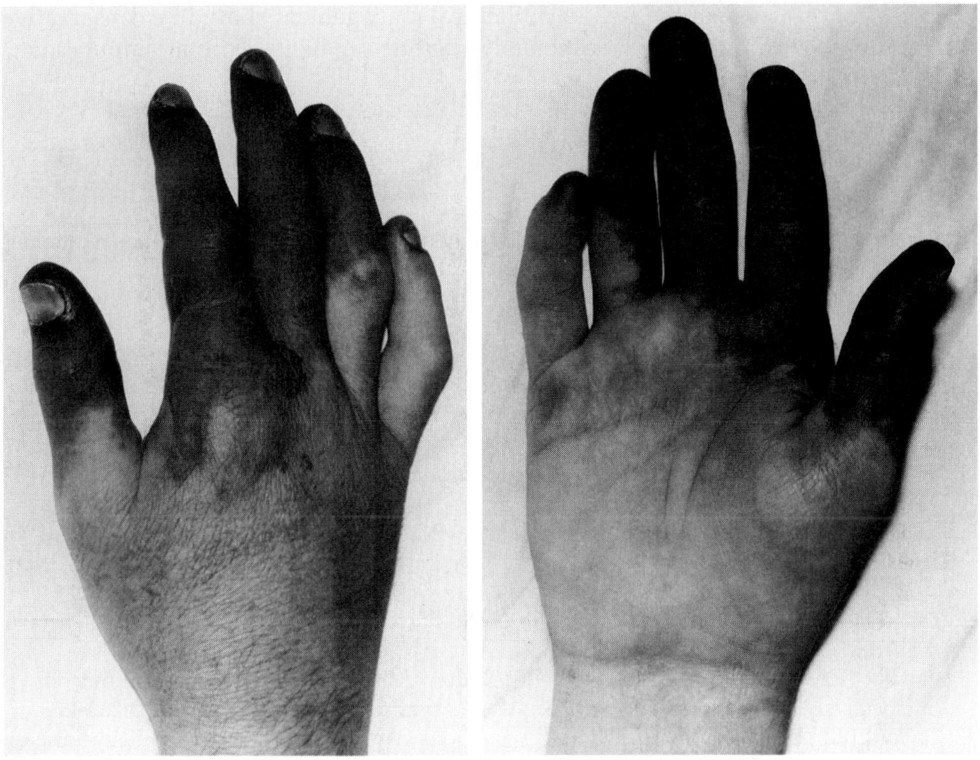

A B

Figure 32–6. (**A**) Volar and (**B**) palmar views of extensive finger ischemia following intra-arterial injection of illicit drugs. There was an obvious injection site in the radial artery. Despite the extent of the lesions, healing occurred after prolonged observation. Only the tips of the thumb, index, and middle fingers required amputation.

SUMMARY

Central to understanding the pathophysiology of finger gangrene is the knowledge that it results only from fixed permanent arterial occlusions. Although normal vasospasm may persist in the presence of extensive occlusive disease, it is never the cause of finger gangrene. Thus, the task of the physician is first to diagnose the cause of the arterial occlusions then to treat it appropriately. Given the diverse causes of hand and finger artery obstruction, extensive diagnostic testing may be necessary. Reconstruction of obstructed large arteries or of proximal large artery sources of emboli to distal small arteries is indicated.

The natural history of finger gangrene is one of stabilization and improvement in the vast majority of cases. Progression to extensive tissue loss is rare. This is because of the extensive collaterals that exist in the upper extremity. Smoking cessation is critical, regardless of the cause of the ischemia. Surgical management should be conservative, with amputation limited to unquestionably necrotic segments. Formal amputation of entire fingers is rarely necessary.

REFERENCES

1. Porter JM, Snider RL, Bardana EJ, et al. The diagnosis and treatment of Raynaud's phenomenon. *Surgery.* 1976;80:756.
2. Merhoff CG, Porter JM. Ergot intoxication: historical review and description of unusual clinical manifestations. *Ann Surg.* 1974;180:773–779.
3. Holmgren K, Baur GM, Porter JM. The role of digital photoplethysmography in the evaluation of Raynaud's syndrome. *Bruit.* 1981;5:19.
4. Rosch J, Porter JM, Gralino B. Cryodynamic hand angiography in the diagnosis and management of Raynaud's syndrome. *Circulation.* 1977;55:807–810.
5. Mills JE, Taylor LM Jr, Porter JM. Buerger's disease in the modern era. *Am J Surg.* 1987; 154:129–132.
6. Schanzer H, Schwartz M, Harrington E, Haimov M. Treatment of ischemia due to "steal" by arteriovenous fistula with distal artery ligation and revascularization. *J Vasc Surg.* 1988;7:770–773.
7. Dalman RL, Nehler MR, Harris EJ, Taylor LM Jr, Porter JM. Upper extremity bypass distal to the wrist. *J Vasc Surg.* 1992;16:633–642.
8. Landry GL, Edwards JM, McLafferty RB, Taylor LM Jr, Porter JM. Long-term outcome of prospectively analyzed patients with Raynaud's syndrome. *J Vasc Surg.* 1996;23:263–271.
9. Taylor LM Jr, Baur GM, Porter JM. Finger gangrene caused by small artery occlusive disease. *Ann Surg.* 1981;193:453–461.
10. Nehler MR, Taylor LM Jr, Moneta GL, Porter JM. Surgical treatment of upper extremity ischemia from subclavian artery aneurysm. *Arch Surg.* 1997;132:527–532.

33

Upper-Extremity Injuries in Athletes

William H. Pearce, MD, and James S.T. Yao, MD, PhD

INTRODUCTION

Upper extremity arterial injuries in athletes are probably more common than recognized. Professional athletes of all sports who engage in repetitive activities are at risk. There are two mechanisms by which upper-extremity arteries are injured (Table 33–1): overuse and direct trauma. Muscle hypertrophy and abnormal positioning (i.e., hyperabduction) damage arteries by stretch or repeated compression. Stretch injuries injure the intima, which leads to intimal hyperplasia or endofibrosis. Arterial injuries resulting from repetitive compression are similar to the arterial lesions seen with popliteal artery entrapment. The arterial pathology includes intimal hyperplasia with occlusion and aneurysm formation. Distal emboli are frequent, either from irregular intima or aneurysms. Direct blunt external trauma is the second mechanism of arterial injury. Palmar and digital arteries are the arteries most susceptible to injury (sports-related hypothenar and palmar artery syndromes). These patients present with digital ischemia and seasonal Raynaud's phenomenon.

The nature of athletic arterial injury in the upper extremity is unique to the sport played. Arterial injuries of the subclavian, axillary, and branch arteries occur in baseball pitchers and volleyball players.[1–3] Interestingly, similar injuries have not been reported in tennis players or swimmers who overuse the upper extremity in a similar fashion. This difference is related to the mechanics of shoulder motion in these different sports. Small differences in the location of the humeral head in relationship to the axillary artery is key. We have had several baseball players who, with the change of their pitching motion, develop effort vein thrombosis. Obviously, the change precipitates a more proximal injury. Unlike these venous injuries, the arterial injuries are more insidious and may take years to manifest.

As patients, professional and college athletes are difficult to manage because their

TABLE 33–1. SPORT

Overuse		Direct Trauma	
Pitching Volleyball Kayaking	Subclavian axillary artery	Catching Frisbee Handball	Palmar arch
		Volleyball (forearm)	

livelihood and scholarships are dependent on their performance. Tremendous pressure is exerted by parents and the athletes themselves to return as soon as possible to their sport. Thus, there is a temptation to overlook what appears to be relatively minor arm or hand complaint, which can result in a disastrous outcome.[4] This chapter reviews the mechanisms and patterns of injury, diagnosis, and treatment of upper-extremity arterial injuries in athletes.

MECHANISMS OF INJURY

The anatomy of the thoracic outlet is complex and compact. The subclavian–axillary arteries transverse several well-defined anatomic spaces (retroscalene, costoclavicular, and subpectoral spaces). Muscular hypertrophy of the anterior scalene or pectoralis muscle may produce dynamic compression of either the subclavian or axillary arteries. Hypertrophy of the subclavian muscle does not affect the arterial structures, but does affect the subclavian vein (effort thrombosis).[5]

The shoulder is a dynamic joint, suspended from the thorax by the clavicle and opposing pulls of the pectoralis major and minor anteriorly, rhomboids, latissimus posteriorly, superiorly by the trapezius, and inferiorly by the latissimus dorsi and serratus longus.

Imbalance by hypertrophy of any muscle alters the relationship of the anatomic structure of the thoracic outlet. For example, an enlarged subclavius muscle is associated with venous thrombosis. Hypertrophy of the anterior scalene muscle produces arterial compression of the subclavian artery in athletes.[6] Similarly, axillary artery impingement is produced by an enlarged pectoralis minor muscle. McCarthy et al.[6] reported on five patients who had branch occlusions either of the suprascapular artery or the posterior circumflex humeral arteries. These occlusions of secondary branch arteries were thought to be related to the hypertrophy of the muscle associated with the artery. In 1995, the most recent Northwestern experience was reported.[7] In this study, patients were found to have axillary artery occlusion produced by hyperextension and hyperabduction. One patient was found to have an aneurysm of the posterior circumflex humeral artery. Axillary artery injury is produced by stretching the artery over the humeral head as the arm is hyperabducted (Figure 33–1). The axillary artery is fixed to the chest wall by the thoracodorsal artery and to the arm by the anterior and posterior humeral circumflex arteries. Repetitive stretch injuries produced intimal damage and endofibrosis.

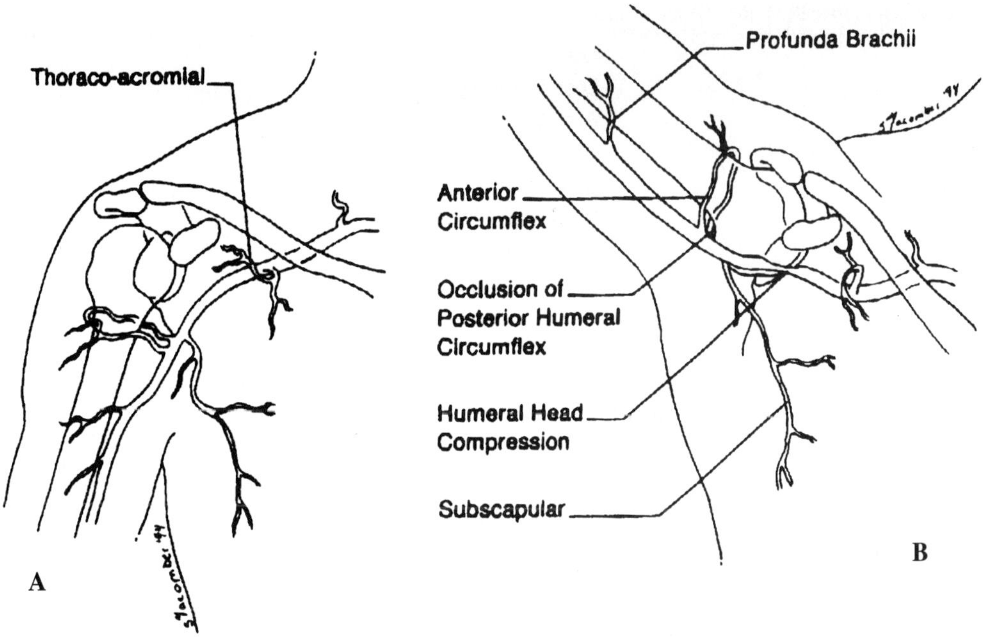

Figure 33–1. The arterial blood supply to the upper extremity is the subclavian axillary artery. The axillary artery is tethered on both sides of the shoulder joint by the **(A)** thoracoacromial arteries and **(B)** the anterior and posterior humeral circumflex arteries. Because of this tethering, the axillary artery is stretched and occluded with abduction and external rotation. (*With permission from J. Vasc. Surg.* 1995;21:65, *Mosby Inc.*)

CLINICAL MANIFESTATION

The clinical manifestations of arterial injury in athletes are variable and difficult to recognize. Table 33–2 lists the most common presenting symptoms. In pitchers, lack of control rather than loss of velocity is the most common symptom. Interestingly, the majority of these patients present each spring following training camp. At the start of the season in cold climates, numbness and coldness of the fingertips develops from an obstructive Raynaud's phenomenon. It is rare for these patients to present late in summer as the ambient temperature has warmed. Arm fatigue and arm pain is a late symptom, suggesting subclavian stenosis or occlusion. Rarely, proximal propagation of a subclavian clot produces cerebral embolization. Arm fatigue is more common in tennis players, kayakers, and weight lifters, similar to a neurogenic thoracic outlet.

EVALUATION

Patients with suspected arterial injuries and distal embolization are first evaluated with noninvasive tests followed by complete upper-extremity arteriography. Upper-extremity

TABLE 33–2. PRESENTING SYMPTOMS

Loss of control
Loss of velocity
Arm fatigue
Stroke
Digital gangrene
Raynaud's phenomenon
White fingers

segmental limb pressures with digital pressures is necessary to document the presence of digital artery occlusion.[8,9] Cold immersion testing is not necessary. Duplex scanning is used to evaluate the axillary and subclavian arteries. For patients with suspected humeral head compression, the patient's arm is placed in the abducted and externally rotated position, with transaxillary ultrasonic evaluation of the axillary arteries. Arteriography is performed with the patient's arm in the neutral position and with maximal abduction and external rotation. It is very important that the patient duplicate the pitching motion, or the motion that is most commonly used in the athlete's sport (Figures 33–2 and 33–3).

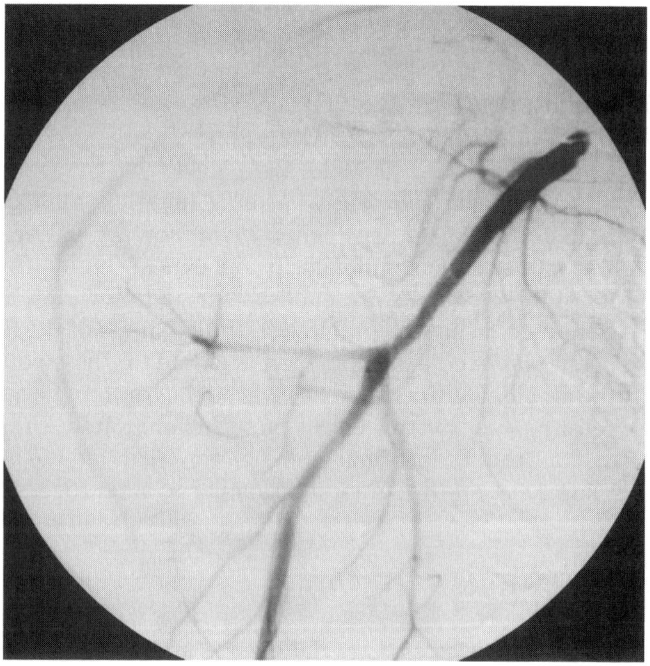

Figure 33–2. Right upper-extremity arteriogram in a professional baseball pitcher demonstrating abnormality of the axillary artery just proximal to the circumflex humeral vessels.

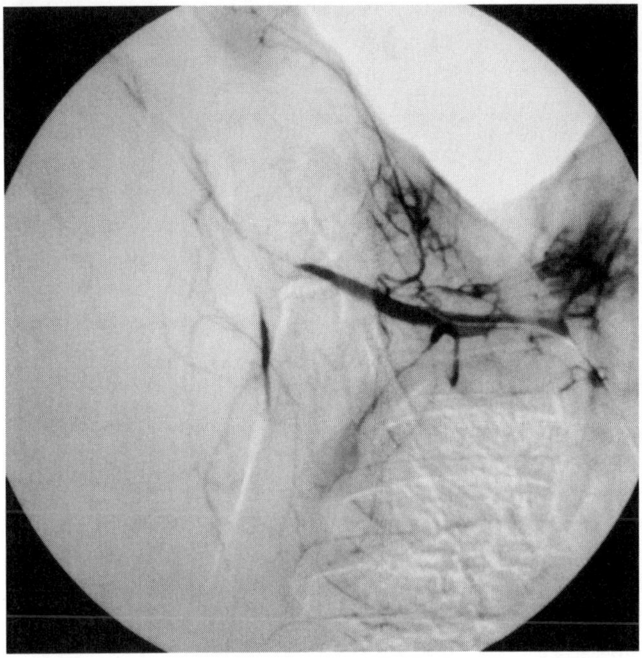

Figure 33–3. With the arm abducted and externally rotated, the impingement and abnormality becomes much more apparent.

TREATMENT

Once diagnosed, the treatment options focus on removing the source of distal embolization and treatment of hand and digital ischemia. In our series, thrombolytic therapy was used in five patients to dissolve or remove distal clots from the brachial, forearm, and palmar vessels (Figure 33–4). With the distal circulation cleared of emboli, attention can then be focused in the treatment of the proximal arterial lesion. The surgical treatments from the two series reported from Northwestern are listed in Table 33–3. In the majority of instances, hypertrophied muscles were resected. All arterial injury reconstructions were performed with saphenous vein. The most difficult patients to treat, however, are those with humeral head compression of the axillary artery, producing endofibrosis. There are two surgical options: One may chose to lengthen the artery with an interposition graft using the greater saphenous vein, or simply place a vein patch over the narrower artery to enlarge the vessel. This procedure allows flow with maximal compression. The surgical exposure of these patients is transaxillary, as seen in Figure 33–5. The operative procedure is complicated by fibrosis of the neurovascular bundle in this location. The repetitive trauma to the neurovascular bundle trauma has resulted in scarring of the adjacent structure and fixes the artery in one position. Care is taken to avoid injury to the adjacent brachial plexus. Once the artery has been dissected along with the neurovascular structures, the artery gains additional mobility and relocates with arm movement.

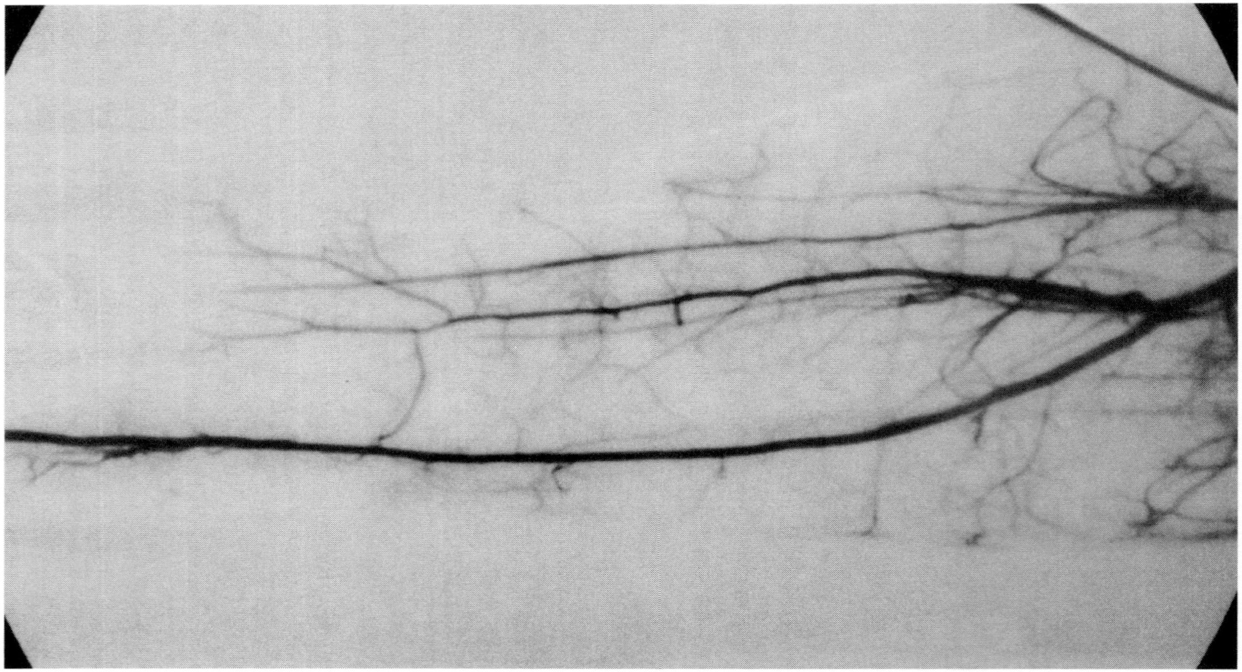

Figure 33–4. Distal arteriogram of the previous patient demonstrating distal embolization at the ulnar artery.

TABLE 33–3. OPERATION

- Muscle resection
  - Anterior scalene
  - Pectoralis minor
- First rib resection
- Vein patch angioplasty
- Interposition graft
- Ligation of side branch
- Distal bypass

QUADRILATERAL SPACE SYNDROME

The quadrilateral space is another important location for arterial trauma in the athlete. The quadrilateral space syndrome was described in 1983 by Cahill and Palmer.[10] The quadrilateral space is located in the back of the shoulder between the torso and humerus (Figure 33–6), and is bounded by the teres minor superiorly, the long head of the triceps medially, the teres major inferiorly, and the surgical neck of the humerus. The axillary nerve and posterior humeral circumflex artery (PHCA) passes through the space. The neurologic symptoms manifest by intermittent paresthesia in the upper extremity and pain that is poorly localized to the posterior aspect of the shoulder. The diagnosis can be made with arteriography and electromyography (EMG). In professional athletes, this space acts as a double nutcracker that crushes the PHCA, producing either occlusion or aneurysm formation. Aneurysms of the PHCA have been reported in professional pitchers as well as college volleyball players. In each instance, the aneurysm had thrombosis of the PHCA produced distal embolization. With each contraction of the quadrilateral space, clot is forced into the axillary artery, producing the distal embolization.

The diagnosis of patients with quadrilateral space syndrome is made by arteriography with the arm fully abducted and externally rotated. The aneurysm of the PHCA is not seen, but a flush occlusion or slight dimpling of the axillary artery in the region of the posterior circumflex humeral artery is seen (Figure 33–7). The aneurysm can only

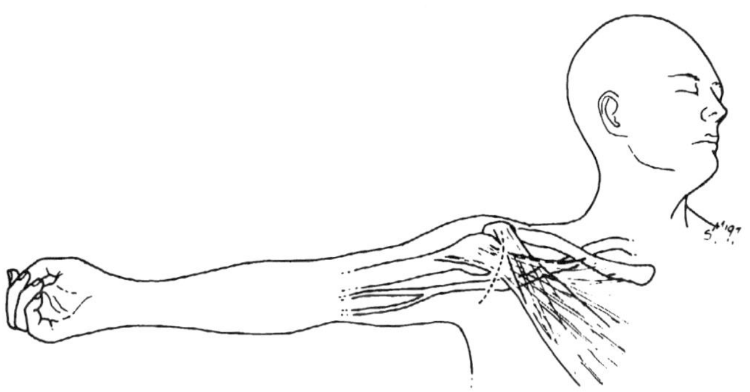

Figure 33–5. Surgical approach to the third portion of the axillary artery through an axillary incision. The pectoralis minor and major are retracted. No incision of the muscle is required.

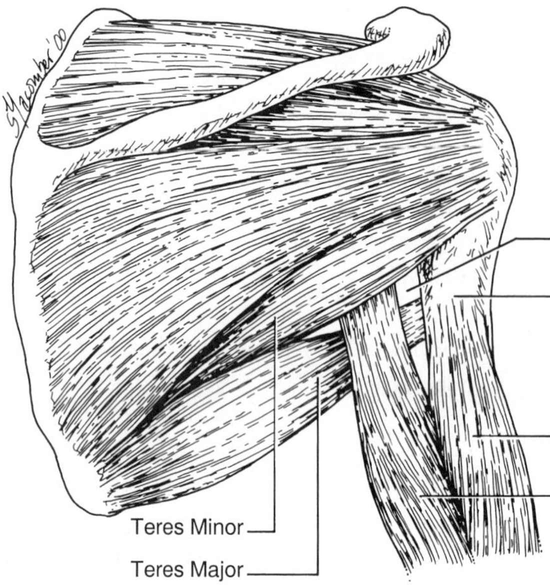

Figure 33–6. The posterior aspect of the right shoulder. The quadrilateral space is formed by the terres minor superiorly, terres minor inferiorly, the long head of the triceps medially, and the humerus laterally. With the arm abducted and externally rotated, the space is occluded.

be found at surgery. In one of our patients, computed tomography (CT) of the shoulder did not reveal the aneurysm. The treatment of patients with PHCA has been varied because of the rarity of this lesion. We treated two patients with ligation and patching of the axillary artery. This procedure removes the embolic source and avoids narrowing of the axillary artery. The distal emboli were treated with thrombolytic therapy.

HAND ISCHEMIA FROM DIRECT INJURY

The Palmar artery and the digital arteries are prone to direct trauma in baseball catchers and Frisbee, volleyball, and handball players.[6,9,11–13] The repetitive trauma to the Palmar arch is similar to patients presenting with hypothenar hammer syndrome. The common digital arteries as well as the superficial Palmar arch are compressed between the external trauma and the bony structures of the hand. Repeated trauma produces digital artery occlusion (Figures 33–8 and 33–9). Recently, Ferris and coworkers[14] from Portland found that many of the arteries removed in patients with the hypothenar hammer syndrome were, in fact, patients with fibromuscular dysplasia. It is unclear whether this observation is related to the trauma or is a preexisting condition. In this study, Ferris found that the opposite extremity contained arterial lesions similar to the hand that was subjected to the repeated trauma.

Nonetheless, Bartel et al.[9] studied professional athletes who found that digital artery

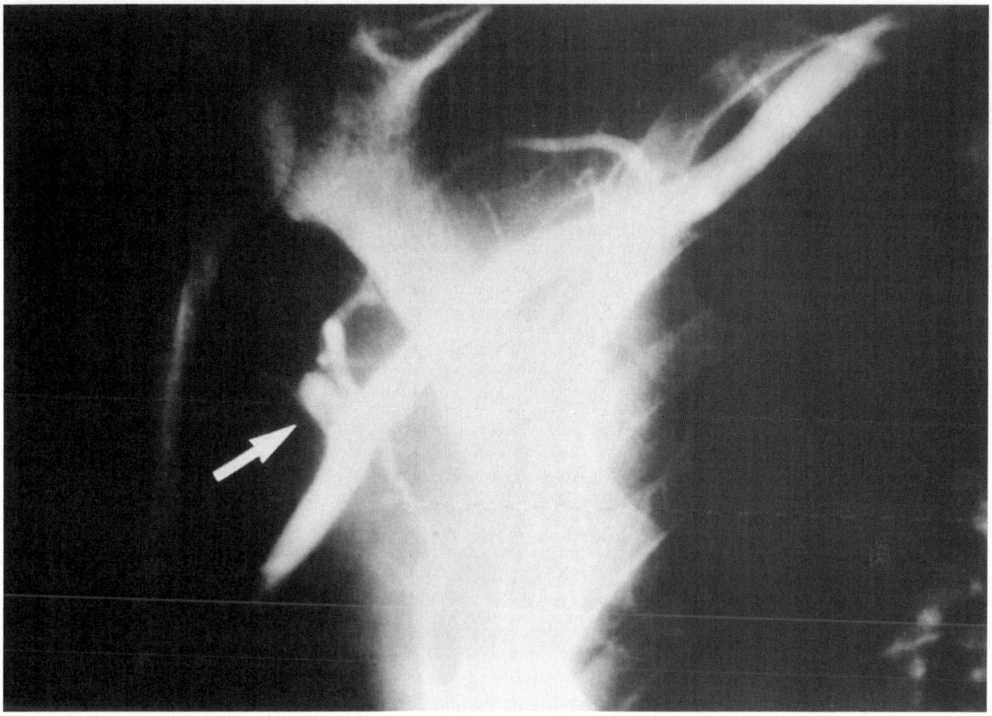

Figure 33–7. A 32-year-old pitcher with distal embolization who is found to have this abnormality on arteriography. Surgical exploration demonstrated aneurysm of the posterior humeral circumflex artery with intramural thrombus.

occlusions were almost as common as patients using vibratory tools (Figure 33–10). Attempts to pad gloves were unsuccessful because the sound of the impact of the ball striking the catcher's mitt was intimidating to batters. This study has not been repeated. Unfortunately, patients with digital artery trauma do not respond to thrombolytic therapy. Aspirin is used to maintain arterial patency. Vasoconstrictive agents such as caffeine, nicotine, and chewing tobacco should be avoided. Patients with hand ischemia either from proximal embolization or from direct arterial trauma present with obstructive Raynaud's phenomenon in the cold. As a result of this, the patients lose the feel of the ball, and as a result, loss of control.

CONCLUSIONS

Arterial injuries in professional and college athletes are not uncommon. All patients with hand symptoms who have exposed their upper extremities to repetitive extreme motions should be suspected of having arterial injuries. If left untreated, these lesions progress either to digital gangrene with tissue loss or with proximal propagation and

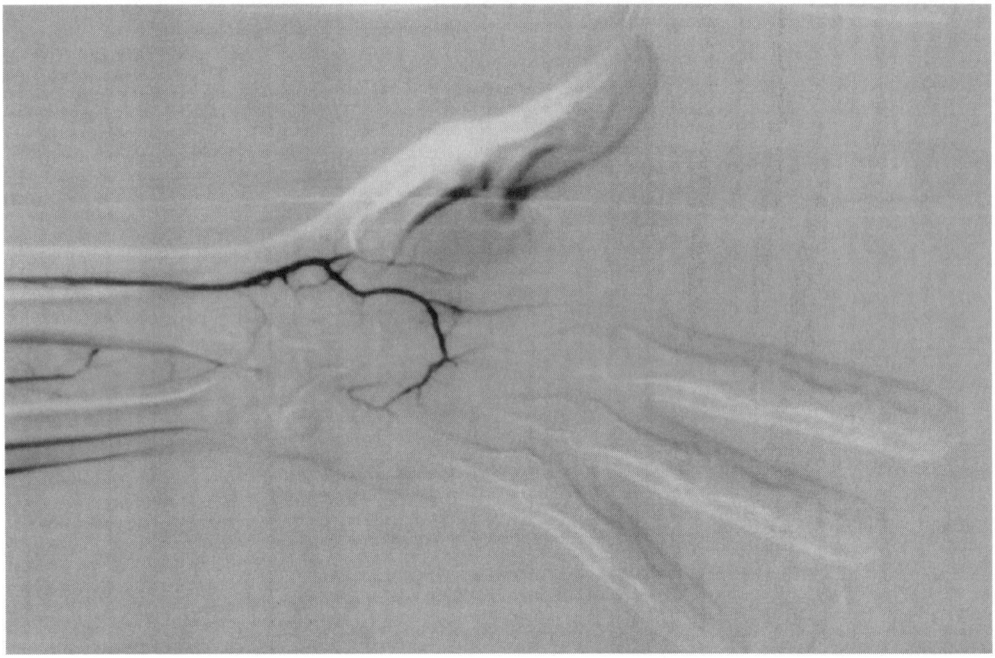

Figure 33–8. Distal hand arteriography demonstrating an occlusion of the distal radial artery. This injury occurred in a baseball catcher with what appears to be hypothenar hammer syndrome.

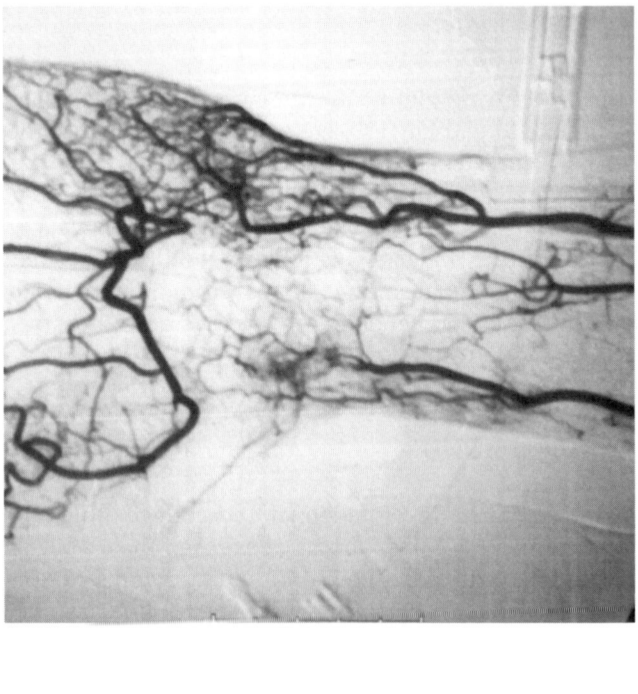

Figure 33–9. Diffuse palmar arch injury. This is a result of direct trauma to the palmar arch.

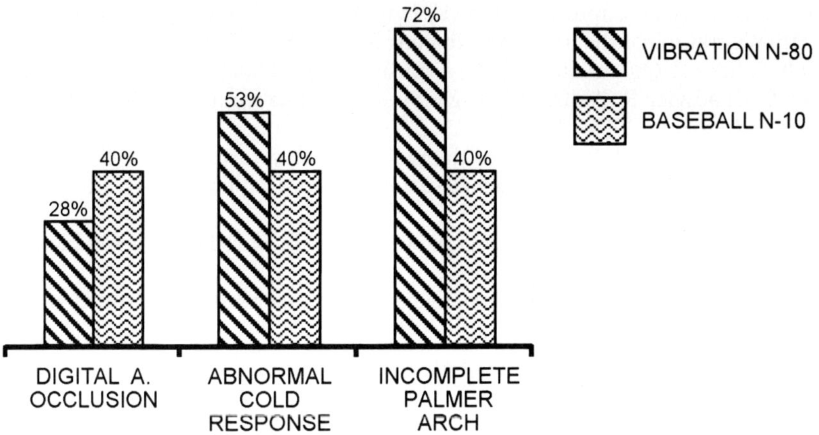

Figure 33–10. The incidence of digital artery occlusion and incomplete palmar arches of workers using vibratory tools and baseball players. Allen Press, Inc. *Bruit.* 1984;8:17.

cerebral vascular embolization. The diagnosis is made with contrast arteriography with the arm in the position of maximum stress on the shoulder. Treatment is varied, including surgical reconstructions and thrombolysis. Mobilization of the axillary artery and patching are important in patients presenting with humeral head compression. Aneurysms of branch vessels and occlusions are treated best with ligation. Rarely, it may be necessary to perform reconstructions in the palm secondary to the hypothenar hammer syndrome. In many instances, these patients return to their athletic endeavors, despite these significant arterial lesions.

REFERENCES

1. Tullos H, Erwin W, Woods G, et al. Unusual lesions of the pitching arm. *Clin Orth.* 1972; 88:169–182.
2. Itoh Y, Wakano K, Takeda T, et al. Circulatory disturbances in the throwing hand of baseball pitchers. *Am J Sports Med.* 1987;15:264–269.
3. Rohrer M, Cardullo P, Pappas A, Wheeler H. Axillary artery compression and thrombosis in throwing athletes. *J Vasc Surg.* 1990;11:761–769.
4. Fields W, Lemak N, Ben-Menachem Y. Thoracic outlet syndrome: review and reference to stroke in a major league pitcher. *Am J Neuorad.* 1986;7:73–78.
5. Molina J. A new surgical approach to the innominate and subclavian vein. *J Vasc Surg.* 1998; 27:576–581.
6. McCarthy W, Yao J, Schafer M, et al. Upper extremity arterial injury in athletes. *J Vasc Surg.* 1989;9:317–327.
7. Durham J, Yao J, Pearce W, Nuber G, McCarthy W. Arterial injuries in the thoracic outlet syndrome. *J Vasc Surg.* 1995;21:57–70.
8. Rosi G, Pichot O, Bosson J, Calabrese G, Carpentier P. Echographic and Doppler screening of the forearm arteries in professional volleyball players. *Am J Sports Med.* 1992;20:604–606.

9. Bartel P, Blackburn D, Capron L, Payne K, Flinn W, Yao J. The value of non-invasive tests in occupational trauma of the hands and fingers. *Bruit*. 1984;8:15–18.
10. Cahill B, Palmer R. Quadrilateral space syndrome. *J Hand Surg*. 1983;8:65–69.
11. Lowrey C, Chadwick R, Waltman E. Digital vessel trauma from repetitive impact in baseball catchers. *J Hand Surg*. 1976;3:236–238.
12. Kostianen S, Orava S. Blunt injury of the radial and ulnar arteries in volley ball players. A report of three cases of the antebrachial–palmar hammer syndrome. *Br J Sports Med*. 1983; 17:172–176.
13. Vayssairat M, Priollet P, Capron L, Hagege A, Housset E. Does karate injure blood vessels of the hand? *Lancet*. 1984;2:529.
14. Ferris B, Taylor L, Oyama K, et al. Hypothenar hammer syndrome: proposed etiology. *J Vasc Surg*. 2000;31:104–113.

34

Complications Related to Percutaneous Arterial Access and Arterial Closure Devices

Michael R. Lepore Jr., MD,
and Samuel R. Money, MD, FACS

INTRODUCTION

Complications related to cardiac catheterization and percutaneous arterial access have been well recognized and treated by surgeons dating back to when the first cardiac catheterizations were performed. Endovascular procedures, which require vascular access, are becoming more frequent within the field of vascular surgery. The 1990s contributed major technological advances to the treatment of peripheral vascular and cardiac disease in the form of these endovascular surgical techniques. In turn, the introducer-sheath diameters have increased, along with their concurrent use leading to more complex interventions. Superimpose the increasing use of anticoagulants and platelet inhibitors and the potential for vascular complications from percutaneous access seems likely to increase as well.

The industry has answered with improvements in ultrasound technology to aid in the identification and treatment of complications from percutaneous arterial access. In addition, various vascular closure devices have been developed in an attempt to improve hemostasis and reduce the complications related to arterial access. A new set of complications has been born out of the use of these devices. We present some of the different vascular complications, new closure devices, and discuss their respective methods of treatment.

PERCUTANEOUS VASCULAR COMPLICATIONS

Although some newer techniques of radial artery access for coronary procedures are being used, the most common site for access to the arterial circulation continues to be the femoral artery. The current trend toward endovascular therapies for peripheral vascular and cardiac disease has led to percutaneous access that necessitates sheath diameters that are 8 Fr to 9 Fr. The larger diameter sheaths are necessary to accommodate the larger stents and balloons that are being used for treatment. The complications, however, have not changed: pseudoaneurysm, arteriovenous fistula, uncontrolled hemorrhage (possibly retroperitoneal), and vascular occlusion.[1]

Fortunately, for the increasing number of patients undergoing these procedures, vascular occlusion and uncontrolled hemorrhage are typically the least common complications. Most surgeons would agree that these complications require immediate surgical exploration, with treatment dictated by the respective etiology of occlusion. Treatment of the other complications has changed somewhat since the early 1990s.

PSEUDOANEURYSMS

Pseudoaneurysm formation has been recognized as one of the most common complications following arterial access. In the past, the treatment has been open surgical repair of the involved artery, evacuation of hematoma, and possible drain placement. This not only necessitated further hospitalization, but also led to the accompanying potential problems of open surgical repair for the patient. The same form of treatment is sometimes required today for more complicated vascular injuries secondary to percutaneous arterial access. However, newer and less invasive techniques have evolved.

In the early 1990s the technique of ultrasound-guided pseudoaneurysm compression was introduced. This requires a dedicated sonographer to apply between 10 and 120 min of compression to the "neck" of the pseudoaneurysm. The technique has the obvious labor-intensive drawback of occupying a significant amount of time for the sonographer. The procedure has a reported initial success rate of 60% to 90%, obviating the need for surgical repair in these cases. However, recurrence rates have been reported to be as high as 25% to 30%.[2–4] Ultrasound-guided compression typically requires sedation and has even lower success rates, not only in larger (>3–4 cm) pseudoaneurysms but also for patients receiving anticoagulation or antiplatelet therapy. This represents a significant number of today's patients who undergo percutaneous procedures.

More recently, the use of ultrasound has been combined with thrombin injection for much improved results. An overall success rate of 96% has been reported in the largest series in which approximately 25% of the patients were on some form of anticoagulation. The technique still requires a dedicated sonographer who aids in localization of the respective pseudoaneurysm, but for a significantly shorter period of time. Under ultrasound guidance, a needle is introduced directly into the pseudoaneurysm, taking care not to cross into the supplying artery (Figure 34–1). Thrombin is then injected into the pseudoaneurysm, and near-immediate thrombosis is observed on the ultrasound

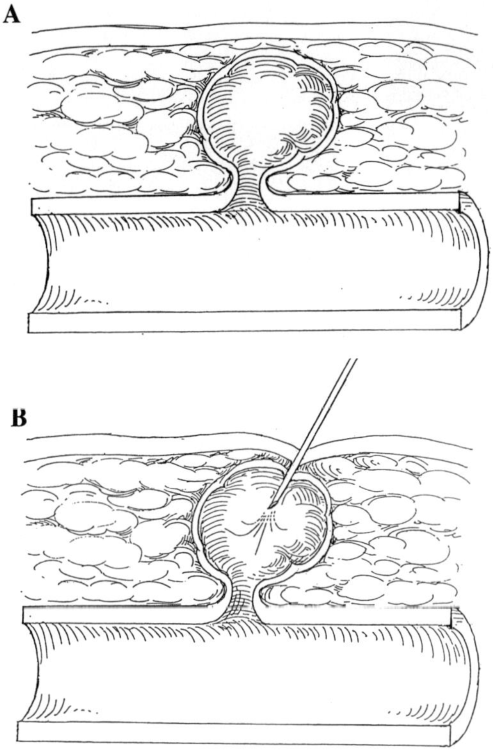

Figure 34–1. (**A**) Illustration depicting a common femoral artery pseudoaneurysm in a sagittal view. (**B**) A needle is introduced into the pseudoaneurysm and thrombin injected.

image (Figure 34–2). The patients require only local anesthetic and can walk 1 hr after the procedure, eliminating the need for hospitalization.[5,6] There is the risk of direct injection of thrombin into the supplying artery; however, only 1 patient in the 83 cases reported experienced this complication, which resolved with heparinization. Newer echogenic needles are now available, making this an even less likely complication.

Although thrombin injection has shown good results, other methods of treatment for pseudoaneurysms are being investigated. One of the newest techniques reported involves the implantation of endovascular covered stents to exclude a pseudoaneurysm or arteriovenous fistula. Early success rates were promising at 88%, but initial follow-up detected an almost 20% failure rate.[7] This, combined with the uncertainty of covered stent–graft implantation in the femoropopliteal region, should make it an investigational treatment at best.

HEMORRHAGE

Fortunately, uncontrolled hemorrhage following percutaneous access is not a common occurrence. The patient may present with obvious bleeding from the access site or growing hematoma formation that cannot be controlled with direct pressure. These pa-

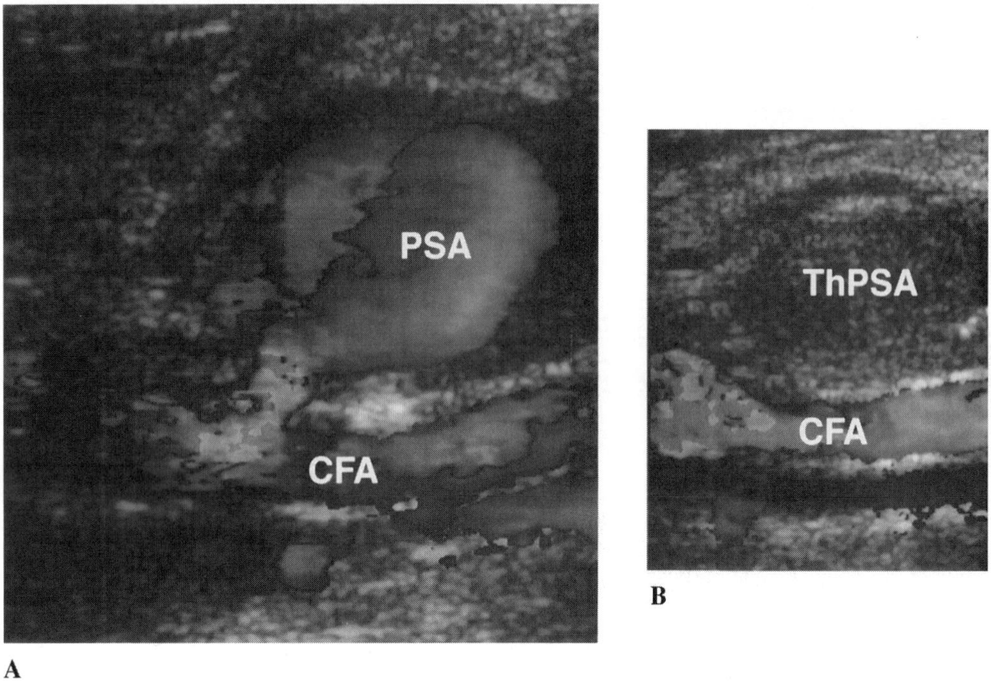

Figure 34–2. (**A**) Color-duplex ultrasonography of a pseudoaneurysm emanating from the common femoral artery. PSA: pseudosaneurysm; CFA: common femoral artery. (**B**) Color-duplex ultrasonography of the same pseudoaneurysm after thrombin injection. Note there is no color flow in the preexisting pseudoaneurysm. ThPSA: thrombosed pseudoaneurysm.

tients require immediate surgical intervention and are likely to have a larger injury to the respective blood vessel than is suspected, such as a laceration or avulsion. This is not a common scenario, but should be treated with the standard vascular principles of adequate exposure with proximal and distal vascular control prior to repair.

It is typically uncontrolled and unrecognized hemorrhage that presents the greatest threat to the patient's life. Patients do not exhibit overt signs of ongoing hemorrhage, but instead may initially present with more subtle clinical signs of bleeding. This may manifest itself as mild blood pressure (hypotension) changes with a concommitant increase in heart rate that improves transiently with fluid administration. When ultimately recognized, a decreasing hemoglobin level verifies the likelihood of a retroperitoneal hematoma. The location of the percutaneous approach (i.e., above the inguinal ligament) also provides clues to this complication. In addition, a computed tomographic (CT) scan not only verifies the suspected complication, but delineates the location and size of the hematoma. The majority of these patients do not require surgical exploration, as the retroperitoneum serves to tamponade the bleeding. The mainstay of treatment revolves around aggressive resuscitation and correction of any underlying coagulopathy prior to consideration of surgical intervention.

CLOSURE DEVICES

As discussed previously, the growing field of endovascular techniques has led to more frequent percutaneous arterial access. Devices have been developed in an attempt to help achieve near-immediate hemostasis and theoretically decrease related complications. There are currently four devices that have recently been introduced and are available on the market today. The design of these devices involves different philosophies of closure. Some of them use collagen-based materials to "plug" the access site; others use procoagulant materials to achieve thrombotic closure of the access site, while another device uses permanent suture to mechanically close the defect in the vessel. We discuss each of these devices and their inherent complications.

The first device, AngioSeal (Sherwood Davis and Geck, St. Louis, MO), involves the use of a collagen plug that is fixed by an absorbable suture to a small, flat, rectangular anchor located intraluminally (Figure 34–3). The initial success rate has been reported in the range of 88% to 92%. The manufacturers state that the learning curve of the operator has an impact on success and improves over time. The deployment of any intraluminal material in this patient population is distressing to many vascular surgeons. In addition, complications related to infection, vessel stenosis, and vascular occlusion/acute ischemia have been reported to be about 2.4%.[8–12] The risk of infection with this device seems excessive when compared to manual compression alone, and may limit its ultimate use.

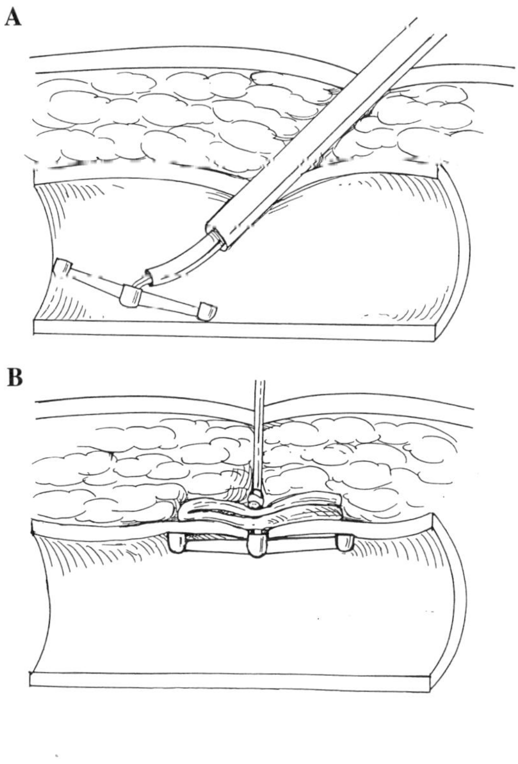

Figure 34–3. (**A**) Angio-Seal device being delivered intraluminally into the common femoral artery. (**B**) Hemostasis is achieved when the intraluminal anchor is tightened to an extraluminal collagen plug by a biodegradable suture.

The second device, VasoSeal (Datascope Corp., NJ), places a collagen plug in the subcutaneous access tract on the extraluminal side of the artery (Figure 34–4). At the time of access, the distance between the skin and the artery is measured for possible use of the device. Once the procedure is completed, the wire is placed back into the vessel and an introducer tissue dilator placed down the tract. The collagen plug is then deployed just above the artery and pressure applied for 2 to 3 min. Immediate hemostasis has been reported to range between 87% and 95%. There has been as high as a 21% hematoma rate seen, but only 1% required surgical exploration.[13] It is likely that the hematoma rate is high because of inadequate compression of the vessel by the collagen plug. The tract is plugged, but the artery continues to bleed into the surrounding subcutaneous tissue. Success rates for patients on either anticoagulation or antiplatelet therapy declined to 79%. Furthermore, the success rate was found to be lower (58.8%) in obese patients (>90 kg).[14] Complications related to embolization of the collagen plug, late bleeding, and infection have been reported to lead to vascular surgical intervention in 5% of patients.[15] Other studies have reported some lower complication rates without the use of heparin, but results have not been duplicated in the more recent literature.[16,17]

The third device, Duett sealing device (Vascular Solutions, Inc., Minneapolis, MN), inflates a small balloon to seal the arterial puncture on the luminal side while a procoagulant is injected (Figure 34–5). The balloon is then deflated and the device removed

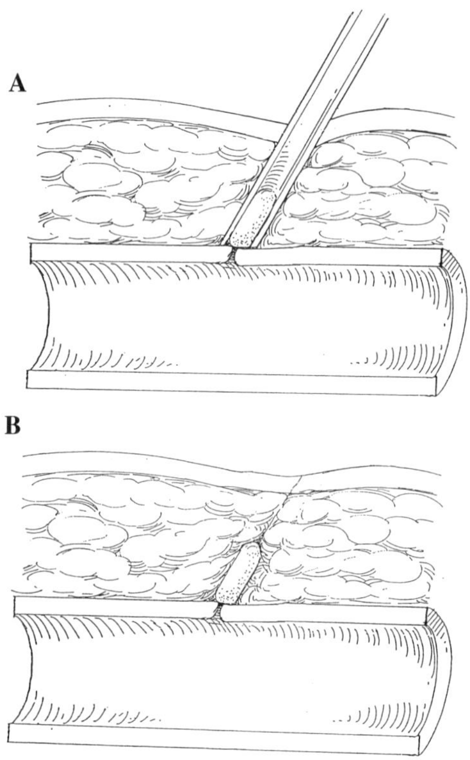

Figure 34–4. (**A**) VasoSeal delivery sheath with collagen plug loaded for placement. (**B**) The collagen plug has been deployed within the subcutaneous tract for direct apposition to the arteriotomy site.

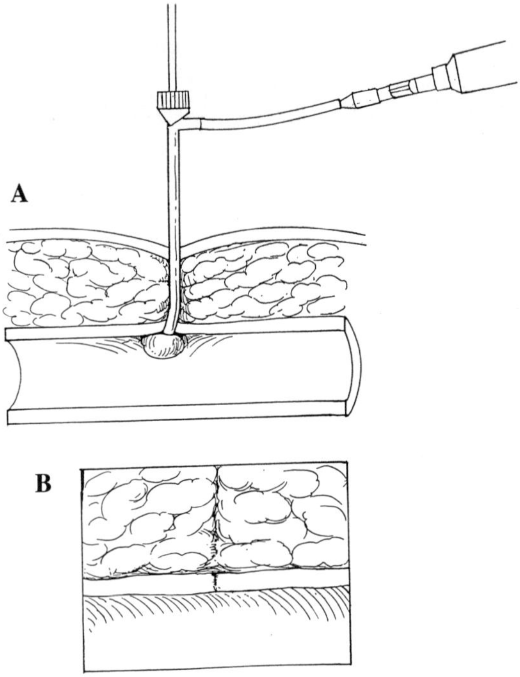

Figure 34–5. (**A**) The Duett-device is in position with the intraluminal balloon inflated to protect the arterial lumen. Procoagulant is injected while the balloon is inflated. (**B**) The device is completely removed with the procoagulant in place to seal the arteriotomy.

followed by 2 min of manual compression. The Duett device was studied in a european multicenter registry consisting of 1587 patients and had a reported 96% deployment rate with successful hemostasis achieved within 2 to 5 min in 95% of the patients. Overall complication rate was 2.6%, including pseudoaneurysms and complete arterial occlusions. Less than 1% of all patients required surgical intervention.[18] Patients on IIb/IIIa platelet receptor antagonists were not excluded from this study.

The fourth device, Perclose (Perclose Inc., Menlo Park, CA) is now FDA approved and will be used with increasing frequency. The device is also placed over a guidewire through the arterial puncture site. Two needles puncture the vessel in a cephalad to caudad orientation and capture a preloaded suture (Figure 34–6). The ends of the suture are brought out through the device, tied extracorporally, and placed against the vessel wall using a knot pusher while the device is removed. In fact, many clinicians are now preclosing a vessel prior to upsizing a sheath. The device is fired and the sutures are placed to the side while the respective procedure is performed. Once the sheath is removed, the sutures are tied and placed against the vessel with the knot pusher for immediate hemostasis. Success with this device is reported to be from 85% to 90%.[14] Complications related to improper deployment or pseudoaneurysm formation postdeployment have been reported in 1.8% of patients. One of the advantages to this device is that the majority of failures are immediately recognized by absence of both sutures or inadequate hemostasis. However, because the needles are small, they are not always successful in penetrating the thickened calcified vessels that may be encountered. If the device is unsuccessful, simple manual pressure is usually sufficient.

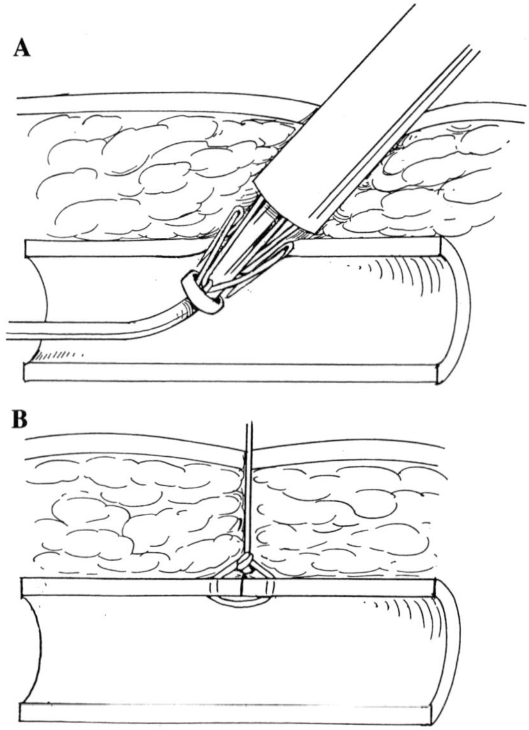

Figure 34–6. (**A**) The Perclose device is inserted into the arteriotomy over a wire. The device needles fire in a cephalad to caudad orientation and capture the suture. (**B**) The suture is tied extracorporally and slid down to the arteriotomy site for closure and near immediate hemostasis.

Although there is no randomized clinical trial that examines the tissue changes postdeployment of the closure devices mentioned, we have experiences with all of them at our institution. Anecdotal observations from our vascular surgeons operating on patients in whom these closure devices have been used indicate a significant inflammatory response in the surrounding tissue. The scarring and inflammation encountered on exploration has been likened to a "reoperative groin." It is important that surgeons who care for patients in whom these devices are used become familiar with them. Knowledge of the specific device can facilitate treatment of the respective complications.

CONCLUSION

Complications related to percutaneous access have been treated by vascular surgeons since the early 1970s. As the technology of percutaneous devices continues to improve, so does both the frequency and complexity of the procedures that are currently being performed using percutaneous arterial access. One of the most important factors that may figure into treatment of these complications is recognition of the respective problem. This may not always happen immediately, and sometimes leads to further related complications from vascular occlusion, blood loss, and infection.

The various closure devices discussed have both positives and negatives associated with their use. During the phase III clinical trial development of the different devices, the reported complication rates were lower than what is being reported in the more current literature. This is likely due to more routine use of these devices. Patients who were enrolled in the original trials were screened and considered "ideal" candidates. It is for that reason that we feel these devices should be used in selected patients and not routinely. Patients who have recently completed thrombolysis, are actively anticoagulated, unable to maintain a supine position for 4 hr, and with relatively normal-caliber vessels are good candidates. However, those patients who are not on any anticoagulants or platelet inhibitors and have heavily calcified smaller caliber arteries should not have a closure device used on their vessels. In addition, for the cost of one device per day, a full-time nurse can be hired to assist in the angio suite and also "hold groins."

These guidelines will not always be followed by all clinicians performing percutaneous arterial access for interventional/endovascular procedures. Vascular surgeons should be familiar with these devices and their appropriate application for their endovascular practice. In addition, familiarity with the related complications may be helpful when considering surgical intervention on consultation.

REFERENCES

1. Kresowik TF, Khoury MD, Miller BV, et al. A prospective study of the incidence and natural history of femoral vascular complications after percutaneous transluminal coronary angioplasty. *J Vasc Surg*. 1991;13:328–336.
2. Field R, Patton CM, Carabasi A, et al. Treatment of iatrogenic femoral artery injuries with ultrasound-guided compression. *J Vasc Surg*. 1992;16:832–840.
3. Cox GS, Young JR, Bruce GR, et al. Ultrasound-guided compression repair of postcatheterization pseudoaneurysms: results of treatment in one hundred cases. *J Vasc Surg*. 1994;19:683–686.
4. Sorrell KA, Feinberg RL, Wheeler JR, et al. Color-flow duplex-directed manual occlusion of femoral false aneurysms. *J Vasc Surg*. 1993;17:571–577.
5. Kang SS, Labropoulos N, Mansour MA, et al. Percutaneous ultrasound guided thrombin injection: a new method for treating postcatheterization femoral pseudoaneurysms. *J Vasc Surg*. 1998;27:1032–1038.
6. Kang SS, Labropoulos N, Mansour MA, et al. Expanded indications for ultrasound-guided thrombin injection of pseudoaneurysms. *J Vasc Surg*. 2000;31:289–298.
7. Thalhammer C, Kirchherr AS, Uhlich F, et al. Postcatheterization pseudoaneurysms and arteriovenous fistulas: repair with percutaneous implantation of endovascular covered stents. *Radiology*. 2000;214(1):127–131.
8. Gonze MD, Sternbergh, III, WC, Salartash K, et al. Complications associated with percutaneous closure devices. *Am J Surg*. 1999;178:209–211.
9. Eidt JF, Habibipour S, Saucedo F, et al. Surgical complications from hemostatic puncture closure devices. *Am J Surg*. 1999;178:511–516.
10. Ward SR, Casale P, Raymond R, et al. Efficacy and safety of a hemostatic puncture closure device with early ambulation after coronary angiography. *Am J Cardiol*. 1998;81:569–572.
11. Goyen M, Manz S, Kroger K, et al. Interventional therapy of vascular complications caused by the hemostatic puncture closure device Angio-Seal. *Cathet Cardiovasc Intervent*. 2000; 49:142–147.

12. O'Sullivan GJ, Buckenham TM, Belli AM. The use of the Angio-Seal haemostatic puncture closure device in high risk patients. *Clin Radiol.* 1999;54(1).
13. Ernst SM, Tjonjoegin RM, Schrader R, et al. Immediate sealing of arterial puncture sites after cardiac catheterization and coronary angioplasty using a biodegradable collagen plug: results of an international registry. *J Am Coll Cardiol.* 1993;21:851–855.
14. Chamberlin JR, Lardi AB, McKeever LS, et al. Use of vascular sealing devices (VasoSeal and Perclose) versus assisted manual compression (Femostop) in transcatheter coronary interventions requiring abciximab (Reopro). *Cathet Cardiovasc Intervent.* 1999;47:143–147.
15. Carere RG, Webb JG, Miyagishima, et al. Groin complications associated with collagen plug closure of femoral arterial punture sites in anticoagulated patients. *Cathet Cardiovasc Intervent.* 1998;43:124–129.
16. Sanborn TA, Gibbs HH, Brinker JA, et al. A multicenter randomized trial comparing a percutaneous collagen hemostasis device with conventional manual compression after diagnostic angiography and angioplasty. *J Am Coll Cardiol.* 1993;22:1273–1279.
17. Gwechenberger M, Katzenschlager R, Heinz G, et al. Use of collagen plug versus manual compression for sealing arterial puncture site after cardiac catheterization. *Angiology.* 1997;48 (2):121–126.
18. Silber S, Tofte AJ, Kjellevand TO, et al. Final report of the european multi-center registry using the Duett vascular sealing device. *Herz.* 1999;24(8):620–623.

35

Blunt Carotid Trauma

Jon M. Burch, MD, and Walter L. Biffl, MD

Historically, blunt carotid injuries (BCI) have been considered rare but potentially devastating. Given the lack of experience with BCI, there is essentially no class I literature to guide their management. This chapter summarizes our experience and the available literature regarding BCI and attempts to clarify some of the major issues surrounding these complex injuries.

ANATOMIC CONSIDERATIONS

The common carotid artery divides into the internal carotid artery (ICA) and external carotid artery at the level of the C3–4 disc space, corresponding to the superior border of the thyroid cartilage. The ICA can be separated anatomically into four segments: cervical, petrous, cavernous, and cerebral (supraclinoid). The cervical portion has no named branches because it ascends ventral to the transverse processes of the C1–C3 vertebral bodies. The petrous segment traverses the carotid canal in the petrous portion of the temporal bone; here, it is at risk of laceration in the setting of a basilar skull fracture. The cavernous portion (also called the *carotid siphon* because of its gentle S shape) is the first part of the ICA within the cranial vault. It is suspended between the layers of the dura mater that form the cavernous sinus. At the anterior clinoid process, the ICA perforates the dura and becomes the supraclinoid, or cerebral, segment.

MECHANISMS OF INJURY

Four fundamental mechanisms of BCI have been identified. Type I injuries result from a direct blow to the neck and account for a minority of BCI. Type II injuries, the most common, result from hyperextension and contralateral rotation of the head and neck. Because the lateral articular processes and pedicles of the upper three cervical vertebrae project more anteriorly than do those of the lower four cervical vertebrae, the distal ICA is prone to stretch injury during cervical hyperextension. This phenomenon may be exacerbated by rotation at the atlantoaxial joint, which may further displace the contralateral C1 lateral mass anteriorly, further exacerbating a stretch injury. Type III injuries result from intraoral trauma, and may be seen in children who have fallen with a hard object in their mouth. Type IV injuries are associated with basilar skull fractures that involve the sphenoid or petrous bones and result in laceration of the artery.

There are numerous case reports in the literature that document BCI following trivial mechanisms that would not ordinarily raise suspicion of such injury. These include virtually any athletic activity, chiropractic manipulation, visiting the hairdresser, head-banging to music, bottoms-up drinking, rapid head turning, and everyday activities such as coughing, shaving, vomiting, nose-blowing, and scolding a child.[1] In view of such reports, there has been some debate over whether spontaneous carotid dissections are a real entity. Spontaneous dissection allegedly accounts for 2.5% of primary strokes. Reported risk factors include hypertension, Marfan syndrome, fibromuscular dysplasia, syphilis, arteriopathies, and Erdheim's cystic medial necrosis. However, it is the contention of some clinicians that it is highly unlikely that dissections are truly spontaneous. Rather, it is believed that these risk factors simply predispose patients to BCI following trivial trauma.

PATHOPHYSIOLOGY

Regardless of the underlying mechanism of injury, the final common pathway of BCI in most patients is intimal disruption. This exposes the thrombogenic subendothelial collagen surface, which promotes platelet aggregation with subsequent embolization or thrombosis. In addition, the intimal tear offers a portal for a dissecting column of blood. Dissection may result in progressive luminal narrowing and subsequent occlusion. Less commonly, partial or complete transection of the artery occurs, resulting in pseudoaneurysm formation or free rupture. Rupture may result in intra- or extracranial hemorrhage or arteriovenous fistula formation.

CLINICAL PRESENTATION

Signs and symptoms associated with the vessel injury itself may suggest the presence of BCI prior to manifestations of cerebral ischemia. Pain (neck, ear, face, or periorbital) is present in up to 60% of patients and is believed to reflect either mural hemorrhage or dissection of the vessel wall. Complaints of such pain are often difficult to elicit in the multiply injured and may be attributed to other injuries. Horner syndrome or oculosympathetic paresis (paratial Horner syndrome) may result from disruption of the periarterial sympathetic plexus. Pupillary asymmetry can have several etiologies in the injured patient. However, if the larger of the pupils is reactive and the smaller pupil is not, BCI should be suspected on the side of the smaller pupil.

Signs or symptoms of cerebral ischemia are absent in many patients with BCI. A latent period between the time of injury and the appearance of clinical manifestations is characteristic of BCI and relates to its pathophysiology. Unless the vessel is immediately occluded, time is required for a platelet plug to form and either limit flow or embolize. In various series, 23% to 50% of patients first developed signs or symptoms of BCI more than 12 hr after the traumatic event. In our experience, 42% of symptomatic patients manifested ≥18 hr postinjury and 2 exhibited symptoms 7 days later.[2] Delayed recognition may occur in the face of multisystem trauma, with critical injuries demanding immediate attention; or head injury, which may preclude a meaningful neurologic examination. In order to make the early diagnosis of BCI it is imperative that the surgeon recognize the signs and symptoms in a trauma patient. These include: (1) hemorrhage of arterial origin from mouth, nose, ears, or wounds; (2) expanding cervical hematoma; (3) cervical bruit in a patient <50 yr old; (4) evidence of cerebral infarction on CT scan; (5) unexplained or incongruous neurologic deficit, transient ischemic attack, amaurosis fugax, or Horner syndrome.

INCIDENCE

The true incidence of BCI is difficult to quantify because many patients remain asymptomatic or a patient's symptoms may be attributed to associated brain injury. It appears, however, that the incidence of BCI is increasing. Recent series have reported incidences of 0.24% to 0.33%.[3–5] The argument that the incidence actually is increasing is supported by the fact that nearly all the patients in the series published through 1997 were symptomatic at the time of diagnosis. By screening asymptomatic individuals, we have further uncovered an epidemic of BCI.[6] Between 1990 and June 1996, prior to screening, our incidence of BCI was 0.1% of blunt trauma admissions. During the $2^1/_2$ yrs following the initiation of a screening protocol, the incidence of BCI was an astounding 1.1% of all blunt trauma admissions to our center![2]

Our experience suggests that there are specific injury patterns and mechanisms that define high risk for BCI. They include: (1) an injury mechanism compatible with cervical hyperextension/rotation or hyperflexion, particularly if associated with displaced or complex midface or mandibular fracture, or closed head injury consistent with diffuse axonal injury of the brain; (2) near-hanging, resulting in cerebral anoxia; (3) seatbelt abrasion or other soft-tissue injury of the anterior neck resulting in significant cervical swelling or altered mental status; (4) basilar skull fracture involving the carotid canal; and (5) cervical vertebral body fracture or distraction injury, excluding isolated spinous process fracture. Based on this screening protocol, 27% of asymptomatic patients undergoing arteriography have been diagnosed with BCI. Further refinement using multivariate analysis revisited Glasgow Coma Score (GCS) ≤6, petrous bone fracture, diffuse axonal brain injury, and LeFort II or III fracture were risk factors for BCI. The only independent predictor of BVI was cervical spine fracture.[7] Furthermore, there is a direct correlation between the number of these predictors and the risk of BCI (Table 35–1).

TABLE 35–1. BLUNT CAROTID ARTERIAL INJURIES—MULTIPLE LOGISTIC REGRESSION ANALYSIS

Carotid Arterial Injury	
Risk Factors = GCS ≤6, Petrous fracture, DAI, LeFort II or III fracture	
No risk factors	20%
Any one risk factor	33–48%
Any two risk factors	56–74%
Any three risk factors	80–88%
All four risk factors	93%

GCS, Glascow Coma Score; DAI, diffuse axonal brain injury.

DIAGNOSTIC EVALUATION

The gold standard for diagnosis of BCI is biplanar cerebral arteriography, and its risks are well known. There are noninvasive diagnostic alternatives for screening asymptomatic patients for BCI; however, diagnostic sensitivity is compromised. Duplex ultrasonography (DUS) is considered the modality of choice for noninvasive imaging of the carotid arteries, although experience in diagnosing BCI is limited. In a recent multicenter review,[3] DUS had an 86% sensitivity for BCI. It was also noted that the lesions missed were located at the base of the skull. Because the large majority of BCI occur near the base of the skull, the unreliability of DUS to detect injuries in this area is a major weakness. Furthermore, although duplex can provide indirect evidence of injuries by detecting turbulence and other flow disturbances, these findings are not reliable in the presence of stenoses <60%. Unfortunately, luminal irregularities that appear innocuous can cause devastating cerebrovascular accidents. Therefore, we do not believe DUS is adequate for BCI screening. Computed tomographic angiography (CTA) is attractive because most multisystem trauma patients have indications for CT scanning. However, our experience has shown that the sensitivity of CTA is no better than DUS. Of all the noninvasive screening modalities, magnetic resonance angiography (MRA) holds the greatest promise to supplant cerebral arteriography. Advantages of MRA include the capability to image the remainder of the head and neck simultaneously and detect cerebral infarction earlier than CT scanning while avoiding contrast. Major impediments are a lack of rapid availability at many institutions and incompatibility of ventilatory and orthopedic fixation equipment with the magnet. Until MRA has been rigorously evaluated, cerebral arteriography remains the predominant screening modality. Recently, transcranial Doppler (TCD) has been used to detect microemboli downstream from ICA dissections that correlate clinical manifestations of stroke. Given this capability, TCD has the potential to guide noninvasively the decision of whether, and how long, to treat BCI.

INJURY GRADING

Carotid arterial injuries are a heterogeneous mix of lesions. It has been suggested that different types of injuries might be managed differently. However, the absence of a for-

TABLE 35–2. BLUNT CAROTID ARTERIAL INJURY GRADING SCALE

Injury Grade	Description
I	Luminal irregularity or dissection with <25% luminal narrowing
II	Dissection or intramural hematoma with ≥25% luminal narrowing, intraluminal thrombus, or raised intimal flap
III	Pseudoaneurysm
IV	Occlusion
V	Transection with free extravasation

mal BCI grading scale has been a major impediment to formulating practice guidelines. We believe that different injury types have distinct implications in terms of response to therapy and ultimate neurologic outcome. Our group developed a grading scale based on the literature and our collective experience with 109 BCI (Table 35–2) and recently reported that stroke incidence increased with BCI injury grade (Table 35–3).[2] However, given the frequent coexistence of severe brain injury with BCI and its even distribution across injury grades, there is no difference in mortality among grades I–IV (Table 35–3).[2] Analysis of treatment related outcomes stratified by injury has led to specific treatment recommendations.

TREATMENT AND OUTCOME

The optimal management of BCI remains controversial. The choices for management include observation alone, nonsurgical therapy, endovascular techniques, and direct surgery. In determining the treatment for an individual, the location and grade of the injury, symptomatology, and associated injuries must be considered.

Observation cannot be considered optimal therapy for symptomatic BCI because reports have established a morbidity of 58% and a mortality of 28%. Because most BCI occur at or above the base of the skull, direct operative intervention is difficult. At least two direct approaches have been described that expose the ICA within the petrous portion of the temporal bone. However, the small series of patients so treated had exces-

TABLE 35–3. STROKE RATE AND MORTALITY OF BLUNT CAROTID ARTERIAL INJURIES STRATIFIED BY INJURY GRADE

	BCI	
Worst Injury Grade	***Stroke (%)***	***Mortality (%)***
I	3	11
II	11	11
III	33	11
IV	44	22
V	100	100

BCI, blunt carotid arterial injury.

sive morbidity and mortality. Extracranial–intracranial bypasses have occasionally been performed, but this approach also remains controversial. As a result, most BCI are not amenable to a surgical solution and nonoperative treatment has become standard therapy.

Recent series have supported anticoagulant therapy for BCI. In 1996, Fabian et al.[4] reported a large experience with BCI, the majority of whom were treated with heparin. Anticoagulation improved neurologic outcome of patients presenting with minor as well as major neurologic deficits.

Based on the findings of a multicenter trial[3] and the report by Fabian et al.,[4] systematic anticoagulation has been considered the treatment of choice for surgically inaccessible lesions in patients without contraindications to heparin. We found that symptomatic patients who were anticoagulated showed a trend toward greater neurologic improvement at the time of discharge than did patients who were not anticoagulated.[6] Table 35–4 shows the combined results from Memphis and Denver and the potential benefit of systemic anticoagulation.[2,4] Another important finding of our series is that identification and treatment of BCI prior to the onset of symptoms appears critical in improving neurologic outcome. In the group as a whole and in those suffering stroke, neurologic outcomes were better. In addition, favorable trends were seen with regard to progression of lesions to higher injury grades, deterioration in neurologic status from diagnosis to discharge, and the occurrence of stroke.

Although our retrospective data support the continued use of anticoagulation, the use of systemic heparin creates some potential problems in patients with multisystem trauma. In an earlier review of 37 patients with BCI, 54% of those treated with systemic heparin had hemorrhagic complications.[6] Sources of hemorrhage included the nasopharynx, gastrointestinal tract, head, fracture sites, liver, and retroperitoneum. Analysis of the partial thromboplastin time (PTT) measurements on all anticoagulated patients did not reveal a direct relationship between the highest measured PTT and the occurrence of hemorrhagic complications. Nevertheless, we modified our protocol as follows. Consideration is given to administering some degree of antithrombotic therapy in symptomatic patients with cerebral intraparenchymal hemorrhage, or fractures in regions with the potential to develop an underlying epidural hematoma; however, anticoagulation is not initiated until follow-up CT scan 24 hr following initial consult excludes a significant change of the lesion. If there has been progression of the injury, anticoagulation is held until CT scans are stable for a 24-hr interval. Anticoagulation is

TABLE 35–4. NEUROLOGIC OUTCOME OF BLUNT CAROTID ARTERIAL INJURIES STRATIFIED BY TREATMENT[a]

Outcome	Systemic Heparin (%)	No Systemic Heparin (%)	*p* Value
Neurologic improvement, diagnosis to discharge	49	19	<0.05
Neurologic deterioration, diagnosis to discharge	5	24	<0.05
Good neurologic outcome	50	30	<0.05
Poor neurologic outcome	30	60	<0.05

[a] Combined experience from Denver[2] and Memphis.[4]

not withheld for punctate intraparenchymal, small subarachnoid, or intraventricular hemorrhages. Our anticoagulation protocol is to begin a heparin infusion at 15 U/kg/hr, without an initial bolus dose. The PTT is measured 6 hr after therapy is started, and the infusion rate is adjusted to maintain the PTT at 40–50 s. With this change in protocol we have witnessed fewer hemorrhagic complications (10% vs. 54%).[6] Fortunately, this change has not been associated with an increase in adverse neurologic events.

Angiographic ICA embolization has not been supported because of concern of brain infarction. Our experience with attempted embolization of the ICA has been confined to grade-V injuries; in each instance, embolization has proved futile.

Deployment of endovascular stents is gaining increasing favor in the treatment of vascular lesions. Our experience consists of 14 patients in whom 18 stents were placed.[8,9] Typically, we deployed stents to treat persistent pseudoaneurysms in an attempt to track down the intima and exclude the pseudoaneurysm from the circulation. In addition, we treated grade-II dissections with luminal stenoses that threaten to occlude the vessel as well as patients with new deficits on adequate medical therapy. Given the risk of stroke during manipulation of devices in an acutely injured artery, we recommend waiting 7 days, if possible, before attempting stent placement. On follow-up arteriography, 16 of the 18 carotid endovascular stents were patent. Of the 14 patients, 3 suffered complications related to endovascular stents, 2 patients had stent thrombosis (1 with cerebral infarction) and 1 had TIA. In all 3 patients there was a period of time preceding the event during which systemic anticoagulation lapsed. This is an important point, because experience with stenting for atherosclerotic carotid disease suggests that antiplatelet agents may be sufficient to prevent thrombosis or embolization. Until more data are available, we cannot recommend anything less than full anticoagulation to cover stents for traumatic pseudoaneurysms. It must be recognized that these devices are not approved for these indications, and their use should be restricted to research protocols.

TREATMENT RECOMMENDATIONS

The accumulation of a relatively large series of BCI (109 BCI in 76 patients) and the development of a grading system allowed the formulation of treatment recommendations for carotid injuries. These recommendations are based in part on data regarding arteriographic progression of lesions in patients treated with and without systemic anticoagulation.[2]

The progression of grade-I lesions is unpredictable. In our series, 7% had progressed to higher-grade lesions on follow-up arteriography. Furthermore, there was a 3% stroke risk associated with grade-I lesions. We could not identify a difference in arteriographic outcome of grade-I BCI as related to treatment, but again, this was not a randomized study. Given the pathogenesis of these lesions, it makes intuitive sense that antithrombotic therapy would be advantageous to prevent ongoing platelet aggregation at sites of intimal disruption. Whether systemic heparin is necessary to achieve this protection is unknown. We are presently enrolling patients in a prospective study in which heparin is being compared with antiplatelet therapy in the treatment of grade-I BCI.

Grade-II lesions are by definition potentially hemodynamically significant; we believe they put the patient at greater risk for adverse events, and thus we have had a lower threshold to anticoagulate patients in the face of multisystem trauma. Despite this aggressive stance, 70% of grade-II injuries progressed to pseudoaneurysm formation or vessel occlusion on heparin therapy, and only 10% healed. Fortunately, just one patient with a grade-II BCI suffered stroke, implying a benefit of anticoagulation. We advise aggressive treatment (including surgical repair of accessible lesions) and follow-up of these injuries. However, the optimal type, dose, and duration of anticoagulation in nonoperative lesions remains to be established.

Grade-III injuries deserve special consideration. These lesions not only put the patient at risk for thromboembolism or continued enlargement with vessel obliteration, but also for rupture with intra- or extracranial hemorrhage. Surgical repair should be considered first-line therapy. However, the arteriogram must be examined carefully to exclude distal injury. Attempts at surgical repair may be met with a friable artery poorly suited for repair, with a distal extent that obviates secure control. Unfortunately, in our experience, grade-III lesions are typically not accessible. Anticoagulation is the second line of therapy; however, it is the collective experience of our group that a few percent resolve with anticoagulation alone. Presumably, heparin reduces the stroke risk, but it is conceivable that it perpetuates the lesion. In terms of progression, we have not found a difference between heparin and no heparin that would suggest such an adverse effect, but we have not randomized treatment groups. Until more data become available, we recommend heparin for inaccessible pseudoaneurysms; if they persist for 7 days, we support the use of endovascular stents under controlled protocols.

Grade-IV BCI, in our experience, has been associated with a high stroke rate (44%), and it appears that heparin therapy is protective against stroke. All of the patients with grade-IV injuries who suffered strokes in our series did so prior to the initiation of anticoagulation. In contrast, none of the patients who had acutely occluded carotid arteries and who were anticoagulated suffered stroke. Thus, we recommend heparin for these injuries.

None of the patients with arterial transection (grade-V injuries) in our series have survived to undergo follow-up arteriography. If surgical control is not possible, we recommend attempts at endovascular embolization or balloon occlusion.

REFERENCES

1. Biffl WL, Moore EE, Elliott JP, Brega KE, Burch JM. Blunt cerebrovscular injuries. *Curr Prob Surg*. 1999;36:507–599.
2. Biffl WL, Moore EE, Offner PJ, Brega, KE, Franciose RJ, Burch JM. Blunt carotid arterial injuries: implications of a new grading scale. J Trauma. 1999;47:845–853.
3. Cogbill TH, Moore EE, Meissner M, et al. The spectrum of blunt injury to the carotid artery: a multicenter perspective. J Trauma. 1994;37:473–479.
4. Fabian TC, Patton JH Jr, Croce MA, Minard G, Kudsk KA, Pritchard FE. Blunt carotid injury: importance of early diagnosis and anticoagulant therapy. *Ann Surg*. 1996;223:513–525.
5. Parikh AA, Luchette FA, Valente JF et al. Blunt carotid artery injuries. *J Am Coll Surg*. 1997;185:80–86.

6. Biffl WL, Moore EE, Ryu RK, et al. The unrecognized epidemic of blunt carotid arterial injuries: early diagnosis improves neurologic outcome. *Ann Surg*. 1998;228:462–470.
7. Biffl WL, Moore EE, Offner, PJ, et al. Optimizing screening for blunt cerebrovascular injuries. *Am J Surg*. 1999;178:517–522.
8. Bernstein SM, Coldwell DM, Prall JA, Brega KE. Treatment of traumatic carotid pseudoaneurysm with endovascular stent placement. *JVIR*. 1997;8:1065–1068.
9. Duke BJ, Ryu RK, Coldwell DM, Brega KE. Treatment of blunt injury to the carotid artery by using endovascular stents: an early experience. *J Neurosurg*. 1997;87:825–829.

36

Injuries of Visceral Vessels

Martin A. Schreiber, MD, and Kenneth L. Mattox, MD

INTRODUCTION

A gunshot wound injury to the splenic artery caused the delayed death of President Garfield in 1881.[1] A fatal stab wound to the portal vein of French President Carnot in 1894 prompted an observing medical student, Alexis Carrel, to develop the triangulation method of vascular anastomosis.[2] In 1963, the world watched on television as a gunshot wound to the aorta and superior mesenteric artery of alleged assassin Lee Harvey Oswald resulted in his death.[3]

Injury to the visceral vessels is infrequently the focus of a single chapter. Such injury, especially to the proximal superior mesenteric artery (SMA) or portal vein, carries a mortality that is comparable to that of the aorta. Due to associated injuries, the degree of hemorrhage and complexities involved in repair of these injuries, a successful outcome frequently involves the use of damage-control techniques.

This chapter addresses injuries to the visceral vasculature, including the celiac axis, SMA, and inferior mesenteric arteries (IMA), their corresponding veins, renal vessels, portal vein, hepatic arteries, and the splenic vessels. The largest single review of wartime vascular injuries was performed by DeBakey and Simeone[4] during World War II and contained 2471 arterial injuries.[4] There were only two (0.08%) reported visceral artery injuries, and both involved the renal arteries. Similar reviews performed during the Korean War and the Vietnam War reveal no visceral artery injuries.[5,6] It is likely that soldiers sustaining these injuries did not survive long enough for diagnosis and treatment. Visceral vein injuries were not included in these reports.

Civilian literature contains significantly different results from military reports. A 30-yr review of 5760 vascular injuries treated at Ben Taub General Hospital between 1958 and 1987 revealed 216 (3.8%) injuries to the mesenteric arteries.[7] In addition, 189 (3.3%) injuries to the portal venous system and 163 (2.8%) injuries to the renal vessels were seen. No injuries of the celiac axis or mesenteric veins were reported. More than

90% of all reported military vascular injuries are in the extremity, whereas more than 65% of civilian vascular injuries are in the trunk.[7]

The majority of visceral vessel injuries are caused by penetrating trauma. If the six published series concerning mesenteric vessel injury since 1978 are combined, a total of 133 of 171 (78%) patients suffered penetrating injury.[8–13] Approximately 75% of penetrating injuries were attributed to firearms whereas 25% were stab wounds. Similarly, approximately 70% to 75% of portal triad injuries are secondary to penetrating trauma.[14,15] Series of renal vessel injuries are generally small in number and contain a mix of blunt and penetrating trauma. The incidence of penetrating renal vessel trauma ranges from 0% to 82%.[16–18]

ANATOMIC CONSIDERATIONS

In reference to visceral vascular injury, the abdomen can be divided into three zones. Zone 1 includes the midline retroperitoneum, and can be divided into the supramesocolic area and the inframesocolic area. The supramesocolic area contains the suprarenal abdominal aorta, celiac axis, proximal SMA, proximal renal artery, and superior mesenteric vein (SMV). The inframesocolic area contains the infrarenal abdominal aorta, IMA and inferior mesenteric vein (IMV), and infrahepatic inferior vena cava. Zone 2 is the upper lateral retroperitoneum and contains the distal renal artery and renal vein. Zone 3 represents the portal–retrohepatic area, and contains the portal vein and hepatic artery.

The celiac axis, SMA, and the left renal artery originate from the aorta and are in close proximity (Figure 36–1). The celiac axis is the largest branch off of the abdominal

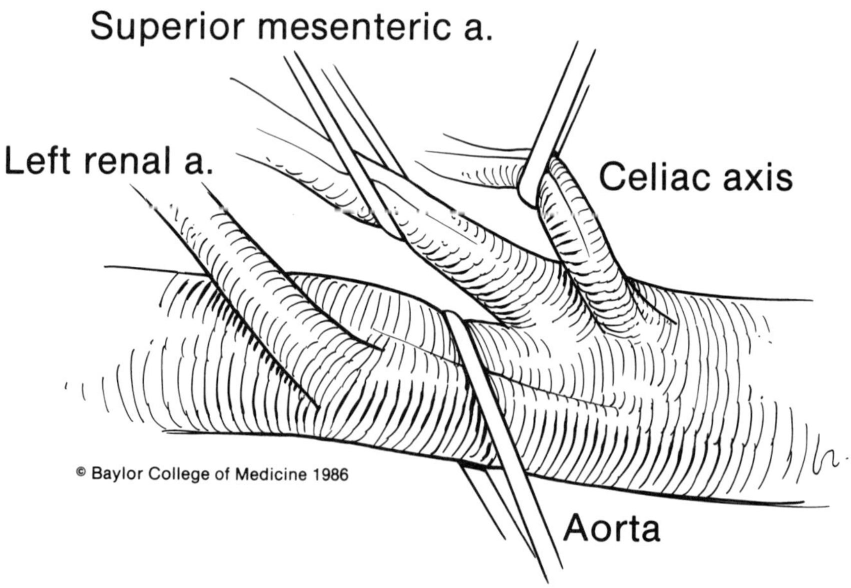

Figure 36–1. The relationship of the celiac axis, superior mesenteric artery (SMA), and renal arteries. These vessels all originate from the aorta in close proximity.

aorta, and it originates between the medial crura of the diaphragm and passes anteriorly above the pancreas where its major branches occur. The artery itself is an average of 1 cm long and is surrounded by dense aponeurotic periaortic nervous tissue, which makes dissection difficult, especially when approached from an anterior position. In nearly 90% of patients, there are three proximal main branches: the left gastric, splenic, and common hepatic arteries. Extensive collateral circulation exists. Numerous variations occur in the remaining 10% of patients.

The first branch of the common hepatic artery is the gastroduodenal artery. Following this branch point, the hepatic artery is known as the *proper hepatic artery,* and it divides into a left and right hepatic artery.

The portal vein is formed at the confluence of the superior mesentric and splenic veins behind the neck of the pancreas. It continues for approximately 7 cm before bifurcating into left and right branches. The portal vein is located posteriorly to the hepatic artery and hepatic duct in the porta hepatis. The IMV drains directly into the splenic vein in most patients.

The SMA arises from the anterior surface of the aorta beneath the pancreas. The middle colic artery is the first major branch. Tributaries of the middle colic artery connect with tributaries of the inferior mesenteric artery via the marginal artery of Drummond and the arc of Riolan. The IMA originates from the anterior aorta at the level of the 3rd lumbar vertebrae.

The American Association for the Surgery of Trauma has developed an abdominal organ injury scoring system, based on the vessel injured and the site of the injury.[19] The organ injury scoring system is shown for visceral vessels (Table 36–1).

DIAGNOSIS

In contrast to extremity vessels, injuries to the visceral vessels have no hard signs suggestive of injury. Intra-abdominal vessels are concealed and are not accessible to external compression. Hemorrhage from these vessels can be massive, even prior to detection. Diagnosis and control are frequently performed simultaneously at the time of celiotomy.

The presentation of the patient is dependent on mechanism of injury, vessel injured, and whether there is a contained hematoma, thrombosis, or active hemorrhage. Patients with contained hematomas can initially be remarkably stable with minimal abnormal findings on abdominal exam.

Hematuria is the most common sign of renal injury in all series and may be present in 80% to 100% of cases.[20–23] However, in patients with major renal vessel injuries, hematuria is frequently absent, or, if present may be only transient.[24] The absence of hematuria does not rule out a renovascular injury.

The evaluation of blunt trauma patients with potential visceral vascular injuries is dependent on the stability of the patient. Unstable patients with obvious abdominal findings are rapidly triaged to the operating room with minimal prior evaluation. Emergency center chest and pelvic radiographs may reveal other potential sources of shock. Focused abdominal sonography for trauma (FAST) can also be a useful test for rapidly ruling out an associated pericardial tamponade as well as for confirming the presence of free abdominal fluid.[25–27]

TABLE 36–1. AMERICAN ASSOCIATION FOR THE SURGERY OF TRAUMA ABDOMINAL VASCULAR ORGAN INJURY SCORE MODIFIED FOR VISCERAL VASCULAR INJURIES

	OIS Grade	AIS-90
Grade I		
Nonnamed superior mesenteric artery or superior mesenteric vein branches		NS
Nonnamed inferior mesenteric artery or inferior mesenteric vein branches	I	NS
Other non-named small arterial or venous structures	I	NS
Grade II		
Right, left, or common hepatic artery	II	3
Splenic artery/vein	II	3
Right or left gastric arteries	II	3
Gastroduodenal artery	II	3
Inferior mesenteric artery, trunk; or inferior mesenteric vein, trunk	II	3
Primary named branches of mesenteric artery (e.g., ileocolic artery) or mesenteric vein	II	3
Grade III		
Superior mesenteric vein, trunk	III	3
Renal artery/vein	III	3
Grade IV		
Superior mesenteric artery, trunk	IV	3
Celiac axis proper	IV	3
Grade V		
Portal vein	V	3

Stable patients with equivocal abdominal findings require additional evaluation. The FAST exam is also useful in these patients to determine the presence or absence of blood in the abdomen. However, the FAST exam is not designed to diagnose visceral vessel injury. Helical computed tomography (CT) with oral and intravenous contrast is frequently used and may reveal either indirect or direct evidence of visceral vessel injury. Indirect evidence includes the presence of free fluid in the abdomen without solid organ injury or the presence of a hematoma in proximity to a vessel. Free fluid without organ injury may be indicative of a visceral vessel injury.

Direct evidence includes the presence of a splenic artery or hepatic artery blush. Absence of a parenchymal nephrogram on one side indicates traumatic renal artery occlusion. Contrast-enhanced helical CT may also visualize dissections and thromboses of the visceral vessels. Helical CT is also a useful tool for identifying those stable blunt trauma patients who might benefit from aortography. The presence of a contrast blush associated with a solid organ injury has been shown to predict failure of nonoperative management.[28] The success rate of nonoperative management in patients with arterial blushes by CT has been shown to increase from 6% to 61% with the use of arteriographic embolization.[29]

Unstable patients with penetrating abdominal injuries or patients with abnormal abdominal examinations also are rapidly triaged to the operating room for control of hemorrhage. Stable patients and patients with modest to moderate hypotension have traditionally undergone one-shot intravenous pyelogram (IVP) preoperatively, with the logic that if a nephrectomy is contemplated intraoperatively, the one-shot IVP ensures that the other kidney is present and functioning. This practice guideline is now in question because three recent reviews of penetrating trauma patients undergoing celiotomy demonstrated that the single-shot preoperative IVP affected management in only 6 out of 519 patients, and these 6 patients all had flank wounds or gross hematuria.[30–32]

INITIAL MANAGEMENT

As is true with all trauma patients, adherence to the principles of the Advanced Trauma Life Support course is indicated. Patients with visceral vascular injuries are at risk for massive hemorrhage. Although intravenous access is recommended, aggressive fluid resuscitation prior to control of bleeding is contraindicated. In a prospective randomized trial of hypotensive patients with penetrating truncal injuries, when resuscitation was delayed until hemostasis, survival was greater than for those who received immediate aggressive resuscitation.[33] The negative effects of immediate aggressive resuscitation include elevation of blood pressure resulting in increased bleeding, hypothermia, and dilution of coagulation factors resulting in coagulopathy.

Emergency center thoracotomy is rarely successful for patients presenting in extremis after isolated abdominal trauma. In a review of 24 studies, only 4.7% of patients with isolated abdominal trauma undergoing emergency center thoracotomy survived.[34]

Once in the operating room, the patient is prepped from chin to knees. Measures are taken to avoid hypothermia, such as the use of warmed fluids, the Bair hugger on exposed areas, and warming of the room. A midline laparotomy incision extending from xyphoid to pubis is made, clot is manually removed from the abdomen, and all four quadrants are packed with laparotomy sponges. Rapid inspection is performed, seeking sites of active bleeding or contained hematoma. Rapid visual assessment of the retroperitoneum, base of the mesentery, and portal triad is performed. Active bleeding can initially be controlled manually. Obvious "black bowel" combined with a mesenteric injury and hypotension are signs of SMA injury.

The decision to use damage control tactics should be made early in the procedure. Patients who have developed hypothermia, acidosis, and coagulopathy intraoperatively rarely survive prolonged definitive procedures.

MANAGEMENT OF SPECIFIC INJURIES

Zone 1 Injuries

When there is active bleeding or hematoma located in the midline supramesocolic area, injuries to the suprarenal aorta, celiac axis, origin of the SMA or renal arteries should be suspected. Proximal control of these injuries can be obtained using at least three techniques. A total left visceral rotation, as popularized by Mattox et al.,[35] may be performed. This maneuver involves reflecting the colon, kidney, spleen, tail of pancreas, and fundus of the stomach to the midline (Figures 36–2 and 36–3). Using this maneuver, the entire abdominal aorta from the hiatus to the bifurcation is exposed. Alternatively, control of the descending aorta in the chest may be obtained by dividing the left crus of the diaphragm and exposing the aorta to the level of the inferior pulmonary vein. In extreme situations, a left anterolateral chest incision allows for further resuscitation. Extension of the abdominal incision into a thoracoabdominal incision creates significant morbidity and rarely provides additional exposure.

Celiac Axis

Options for treating injuries to the celiac axis include ligation, lateral arteriography, and placement of an interposition graft. The choice of treatment should be based on the patient's condition and nature of injury. In the report from Graham et al.[9] from Ben Taub General Hospital, 13 injuries to the celiac axis were described with an overall survival of 62%. The majority of injuries in this series were treated with lateral arteriorraphy. However, 4 patients were treated with ligation, 2 of whom survived with no apparent long-term morbidity or mortality. Complex repairs of the celiac axis are probably not in-

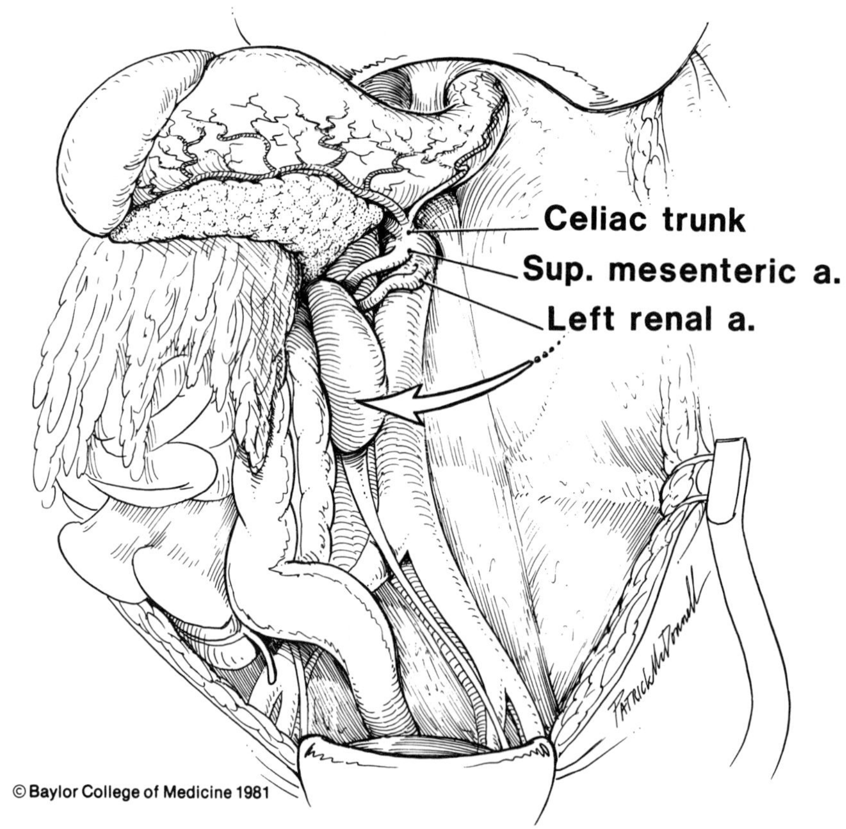

Figure 36–2. Anterior view of the Mattox maneuver.

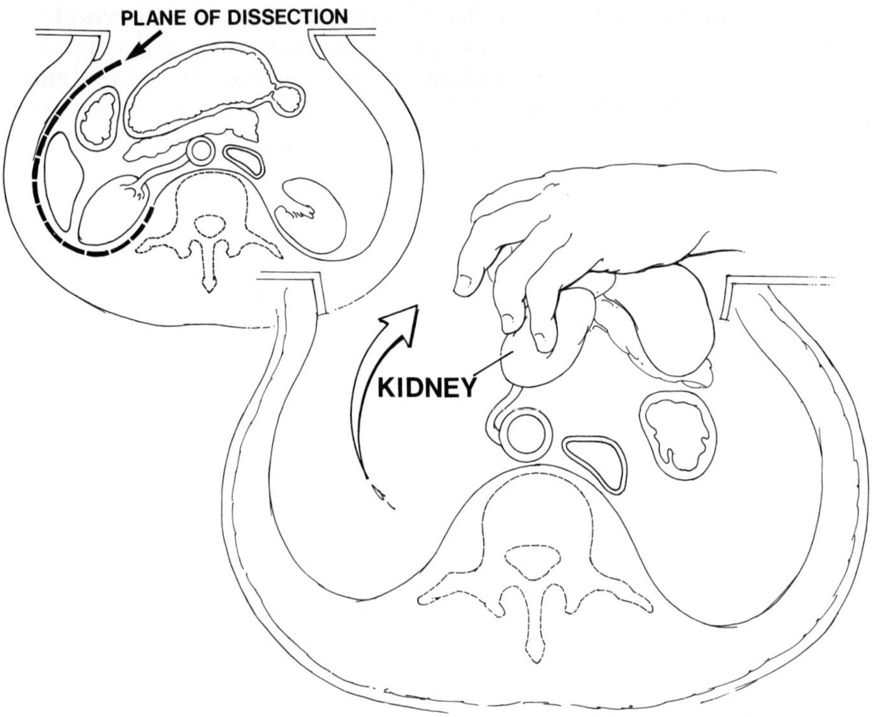

Figure 36–3. Sagittal view of the Mattox maneuver demonstrating the plane of dissection and mobilization.

dicated. In this series of 13 injuries, there was a mean of 5 associated injuries per patient The most commonly injured organs were the liver, pancreas, and lung.

Celiac Artery Branches

Injuries to the left gastric and splenic arteries are difficult to repair, as these vessels are relatively small and surrounded at their origin by dense lymphatic and neurologic tissue. The stomach has a rich collateral blood supply, and there are few if any reasons to repair the left gastric artery, especially in a patient with shock. Injuries to the left gastric and splenic arteries generally should be ligated. The common hepatic artery is a larger artery and may be amenable to lateral arteriography or placement of interposition graft. However, the artery may be ligated for injuries proximal to the gastroduodenal artery due to collateral flow from the mesenteric circulation. Injuries to the hepatic artery distal to the gastroduodenal artery are discussed with other zone 3 injuries.

Superior Mesenteric Artery and Vein

Management of SMA injuries is determined by the site of injury and condition of the patient. Fullen et al.[34] developed an anatomic classification scheme for SMA injuries

(Table 36–2). Proximal lesions have a greater propensity for ischemic bowel complications and mandate an effort at maintaining flow. The anatomic location of the proximal SMA at the base of the mesocolon, posterior to the pancreas, affords a technical challenge to the surgeon. In addition to the left visceral rotation already described, this area can be approached either through the lesser sac or through the base of the mesocolon or small bowel mesentery. The pancreas can also be divided to provide access. However, a postoperative pancreatic fistula has been reported resulting in disruption of an end-to-end anastamosis repair.[9] Proximal control using these approaches is technically difficult due to the proximity of the pancreas, celiac axis, celiac plexus, and the renal arteries.

A review of the 6 largest series published on the management of SMA injuries since 1978 (Table 36–3) reveals that the majority of patients treated underwent primary repair. The majority of these consisted of lateral arteriography, although some included primary reanastomosis. The recent series from LA County reported by Asensio et al.[8] shows a high incidence of ligation as definitive treatment. This article points out that the majority of ligations were performed as a last resort in patients with distal injuries. Extensive efforts were made to restore flow in patients with more proximal injuries.

Another option for patients who are developing the lethal triad of hypothermia, acidosis, and coagulopathy is placement of a temporary intraluminal shunt between the divided ends of the SMA to maintain flow. This is a damage control technique that allows early termination of the surgical procedure, permitting restoration of physiology prior to definitive management.

Superior mesenteric vein injuries are managed by either lateral venorrhaphy or ligation. In their literature review, Donahue and Strauch[37] reported on 110 SMV injuries, of which 70% were treated with lateral venorrhaphy and the remainder were treated with ligation. Overall mortality was 15% in the ligation group and 36% in the primary repair group. Bowel necrosis was uncommon in both groups. Ligation is well tolerated due to collateral flow within the portal system via the IMV and portosystemic collaterals largely from retroperitoneal perforators of Retzius.[38,39]

Venorrhaphy is recommended for easily repaired linear lacerations located in accessible locations, especially in stable patients without concomitant life-threatening injuries. Unstable patients with multiple injuries and difficult to repair SMV injuries should be managed with ligation.

TABLE 36–2. SEGMENTS OF THE SUPERIOR MESENTERIC ARTERY (FULLER CLASSIFICATION)

Zone	Segment of Superior Mesenteric Artery	Grade	Ischemic Category	Bowel Segments Affected
I	Trunk proximal to first major branch (inferior pancreaticoduodenal)	I	Maximal	Jejunum, ileum, right colon
II	Trunk between inferior pancreatico-duodenal and middle colic	II	Moderate	Major segment, small bowel, and/or right colon
III	Trunk distal to middle colic	III	Minimal	Minor segment or segments, small bowel, or right colon
IV	Segmental branches, jejunal, ileal, or colic	IV	None	No ischemic bowel

TABLE 36–3. DISTRIBUTION OF PORTAL TRIAD INJURIES

Reference	Year	1° Repair	IP Graft	Reimplant	Ligation
Graham et al.[9]	1978	38	4	2	1
Lucas et al.[13]	1981	14	1	0	0
Courcy et al.[12]	1984	9	0	0	1
Sirinek and Levine[11]	1985	10	1	0	1
Accola et al.[10]	1986	10	7	2	3
Asensio et al.[8]	1999	14	2	0	18
Total		**95**	**15**	**4**	**24**

Superior mesenteric vessel injuries are commonly associated with multiple injuries that have an impact on management and outcome. The number of associated injuries reported varies from 1.9 to 3.9 injuries per patient. Associated injury to the small intestine is most common, but injuries to other abdominal vessels, the pancreas, stomach, and liver also occur frequently.

Following management of superior mesenteric vessel injuries, intestinal viability is assessed. Second-look operations are not necessarily mandatory. They should be considered in patients who do not have a reliable physical exam postoperatively, patients with combined arterial and venous injury, patients with complex repairs, and patients with questionable intestinal viability at the conclusion of the first operation.[8]

Inferior Mesenteric Artery and Vein

Injuries to the midline inframesocolic area of zone 1 are exposed by reflecting the transverse colon cranially and eviscerating the small bowel to the right. The ligament of Treitz is divided, opening the retroperitoneum and exposing the infrarenal aorta up to the level of the left renal vein and down to the aortic bifurcation.

In the vast majority of patients, injuries to the IMA and IMV can be managed by ligation without negative sequelae. Prior to ligation of the IMA, the surgeon should ensure adequate collateral flow. An extensive collateral circulation exists through anastomoses with branches of the middle colic artery and the lower hemorrhoidal arteries. Patients with advanced atherosclerotic disease of the SMA and the internal iliac artery may not have adequate collateral flow. In addition, previous left colectomy with interruption of the marginal artery also predisposes to colon ischemia. If collateral flow is absent, primary repair should be considered. Patients with inadequate collateral flow and life-threatening injuries or patients who are unstable, should be treated with ligation followed by resection of the resulting ischemic colon.

Zone 2 Injuries

Hematoma or free bleeding from the upper lateral retroperitoneum may be indicative of either a renal parenchymal injury or an injury to the renal vasculature. Lateral hematomas that are not expanding following blunt trauma do not require exploration, especially when renal function has been documented preoperatively by either computed tomography (CT) or intravenous pyelogram. Lateral hematomas resulting from penetrating trauma and found intraoperatively are explored to determine the tract of the injury and rule out a vascular injury.

There are two proposed methods for approaching lateral hematomas in patients with potential renovascular injuries. The classic approach, initially popularized by Scott and Selzman in 1966[41] and later reported by other groups, involves obtaining central vascular control of the renal artery and vein prior to opening the hematoma.[40–43] These studies reported decreased nephrectomy rates, blood loss, and transfusion requirements when vascular control was obtained prior to opening Gerota's fascia. However, the studies were either retrospective or used historical controls.

The second approach to lateral hematomas with potential renovascular injury involves opening Gerota's fascia and assesssing the injury without first obtaining vascular control. If active bleeding is found, the kidney is elevated into the wound and the artery is clamped at either the midline on the left or just lateral to the vena cava on the right. A prospective randomized trial comparing these two methods performed at the University of South Alabama revealed no difference in nephrectomy rate, transfusion requirements, or blood loss.[44] Attempts at obtaining vascular control prior to opening Gerota's fascia in patients with active bleeding may result in prolonged operative times and increased blood loss.[45]

Renal Artery and Renal Vein Injuries

The management of renal vascular injuries is determined by the hemodynamic status of the patient, associated injuries, and the warm ischemia time. Complex vascular repairs should be avoided in unstable patients with multiple injuries. Rapid nephrectomy is the preferred procedure in patients who are developing the lethal triad of hypothermia, coagulopathy, and acidosis.

For patients in whom revascularization is being considered, proximal control of the renal vessels can be obtained by reflecting the transverse colon cranially and retracting the small bowel out of the abdomen to the right side, exposing the base of the small bowel mesentery and retroperitoneum. The retroperitoneum is incised medial to the IMV over the aorta. The incision is carried superiorly to the level of the left renal vein. Superior retraction of the left renal vein exposes the left renal artery. The right renal artery is located slightly superiorly. The right renal vein is isolated by dissection over the vena cava laterally (Figure 36–4).

Combined renal artery and vein injuries are common. In their review of 20 renovascular injuries, Sagalowsky et al.[16] noted four patients with isolated renal artery injury, eight with combined artery and vein injuries, and eight with renal vein injuries. Fifteen injuries were treated with nephrectomy, and five injuries were repaired. One patient undergoing arterial repair subsequently required nephrectomy due to a missed renal vein injury.

Vascular repair should be considered in stable patients without life-threatening associated injuries. Treatment options include lateral repair, resection and reanastomosis, and interposition grafting with either saphenous vein or PTFE. Aortorenal bypass procedures have also been performed. The most critical factors in achieving successful renal function are the time from injury to reestablishment of flow and ongoing patency of repairs.[46]

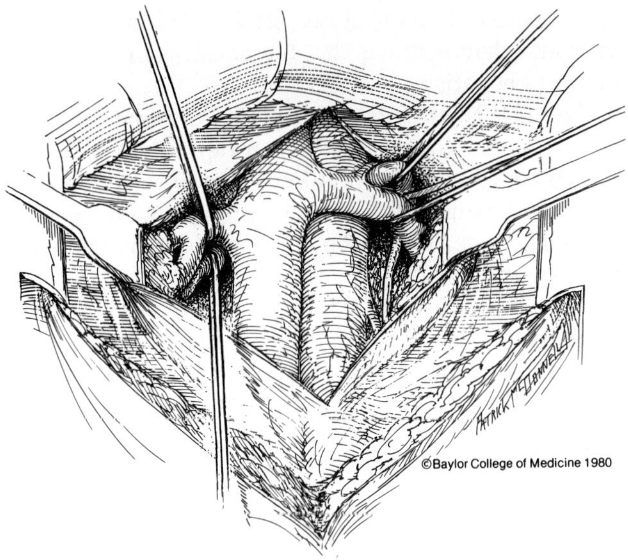

Figure 36–4. The relationship of the renal vessels.

Thrombosis of attempted renal arterial revascularizations is common. In the review by Carroll et al.[46] from UCSF, only two of nine attempted repairs resulted in complete renal preservation. One of these two patients was treated with end-to-end reanastomosis and the other with primary repair of the laceration. The review made by Brown et al.[47] from the Ben Taub General Hospital revealed slightly better results, with 16 of 27 (59.3%) revascularization attempts being successful.

Blunt injury of the renal artery frequently results in traumatic occlusion secondary to arterial stretching and intimal injury. There is a great deal of debate concerning management of these injuries. In a single institution review from Case Western Reserve University, 12 patients with blunt traumatic renal artery occlusion were described and 5 patients underwent attempted revascularization.[48] One patient underwent nephrectomy due to inability to establish flow, 3 had no postoperative renal function, and 1 patient had 9% return of differential function. Of 7 patients with no attempt at revascularization, 3 developed hypertension necessitating nephrectomy at a mean follow-up of 11 mo, and 4 patients were asymptomatic and normotensive in follow-up. In another review, revascularization was successful in restoring some renal function in 80% of patients treated within 12 hr of occlusion and 57% at 18 hr.[49]

Spontaneous recovery of renal function after traumatic occlusion has been reported.[50] Interventional techniques have also been used to manage blunt renal artery injuries. Villas et al.[51] from Temple University has reported the successful use of a Wallstent in managing a right renal artery dissection.

Zone 3 Injuries

The presence of hematoma or active hemorrhage from the area of the porta hepatis may indicate an injury to the hepatic artery or portal vein, possibly in combination with a bile duct injury. Table 36–4 shows the distribution of injured structures in four studies reviewing trauma of the portal triad and demonstrates that the portal vein is the most commonly injured structure in the porta hepatis.

Injuries to the portal triad are rare. The 21 patients reported by Dawson et al.[53] represented only 0.21% of all trauma patients admitted to Harborview Medical Center during the reporting period. Proximal control of the porta hepatis is obtained initially by digital pressure, followed by a Pringle maneuver using a clamp to obtain more definitive control. Placement of an umbilical tape around the hepatoduodenal ligament is dangerous and may cause secondary injury. The Pringle maneuver also helps differentiate bleeding from the porta hepatis versus bleeding from the hepatic veins or retrohepatic vena cava. Cessation of bleeding after applying the Pringle maneuver indicates bleeding from the hepatic artery or portal vein. If bleeding does not cease, it most likely involves the hepatic veins or inferior vena cava.

Portal Vein

The vast majority of patients with portal vein injuries present in shock.[54] Rapid control of hemorrhage in the operating room is critical to survival. Portal vein injuries are difficult to treat due to the posterior location of the structure within the portal triad, the friability of the vessel wall, and high blood flow. The majority of portal vein injuries occur within the body of the portal vein located in the hepatoduodenal ligament, and this area is best exposed by performing a Kocher maneuver. The porta hepatis is dissected and the common bile duct is mobilized to the left. Injuries to the retropancreatic portion of the portal vein require deliberate division of the pancreatic neck to provide exposure.

Similar to other visceral vessels, management of the injury is dependent on the nature of the injury, the presence of other lethal injuries and the patient's physiology. Options for management include ligation, lateral repair, end-to-end repair, and complex repairs. Reported complex repairs include splenic vein to SMV bypass, interposition grafting, and ligation of the distal portal vein followed by end-to-side portacaval shunt. A temporary intravascular shunt has also been used with success in the portal vein at the Ben Taub General Hospital. In this damage control tactic, a carotid shunt was left in the portal vein for 5 days prior to its removal and successful venorrhaphy.

Primary lateral repair is preferred in stable patients with accessible injuries. In a review of portal vein injuries, Stone et al.[54] showed an 80% survival for patients undergoing ligation of the portal vein when lateral repair could not be performed. In this review, survival after ligation was significantly improved when performed early in the

TABLE 36–4. MANAGEMENT OF PORTAL TRIAD VESSEL INJURIES

Reference	Year	Patients	Portal Vein	Hepatic Artery	Bile Duct
Jurkovich et al.[14]	1995	99	55	28	35
Busuttil et al.[15]	1979	21	10	4	14
Sheldon et al.[52]	1985	31	29	3	4
Dawson et al.[53]	1991	21	14	7	4
Total		**172**	**108**	**42**	**57**

operation. Table 36–5 shows the method of treatment used and subsequent survival in three series of portal vein injuries.

Hepatic Artery

Injuries to the hepatic artery are generally well distributed among the right, left, proper, and common hepatic arteries.[14] The hepatic artery is a much smaller vessel than the portal vein, and management of hepatic artery injuries is generally limited to ligation and lateral repair. The normal liver tolerates hepatic artery ligation in the majority of cases because of extensive collateral flow and the fact that approximately 50% of oxygen delivered to the hepatocytes derives from the portal vein.[56–59] Hepatic artery ligation is poorly tolerated in cirrhotic patients and in patients with associated portal vein ligation.

Jurkovich et al.[14] reported 7 patients who underwent primary repair of hepatic artery injuries and 19 patients who underwent ligation out of a total of 28 patients with hepatic artery injury. Mortality was 86% in the patients undergoing repair and 58% in the patients undergoing ligation. Two patients died before any repair could be performed. Ligation resulted in hepatic necrosis in one case.

Associated injuries are extremely common in patients with injuries to the porta hepatis, with one report citing 3.6 associated injuries per patient.[52] The most common associated injuries in order were liver, major vascular, pancreas, and duodenum. The aorta and inferior vena cava were the most commonly associated injured vessels.

Complications of Visceral Vessel Injuries

Complications related to the management of visceral vessel injuries are much more difficult to detect than those related to peripheral vascular injuries. Potential complications include thrombosis, infection, suture line dehiscence and vascular–enteric fistulas. Thrombosis is not uncommon after repairs of vessels like the renal artery, SMA, and hepatic artery, as these are relatively small vessels that are prone to vasoconstriction. In addition, hypotension is common in these patients adding to the potential for thrombosis.

Other complications are associated with the vessel injured and include hepatic and bowel necrosis as well as renal failure. Second-look operations may be indicated after correction of physiologic abnormalities to investigate bowel viability and correct graft thromboses.[60] Infection also occurs as visceral vascular repairs are frequently associated with enteric injuries and therefore contamination.

TABLE 36–5. OUTCOME AFTER VISCERAL VESSEL INJURY

Reference	Patients	Ligation	1° Repair	End-to-End	PCS	Complex
Jurkovich et al.[14]	55	10 (1)	33 (19)	0	0	1 (0)
Stone et al.[54]	46	18 (9)	17 (12)	3 (1)	1 (0)	0
Graham et al.[55]	37	4 (0)	26 (16)	1 (1)	1 (1)	0
Total[a]	**138**	**32 (10)**	**76 (47)**	**4 (2)**	**2 (1)**	**1 (0)**

[a]Numbers in parentheses indicate survival.

TABLE 36–6. SUMMARY LISTING OF INJURY AND OUTCOME OF VISCERAL VASCULAR INJURY[a]

Reference	Year	Celiac	SMA	SMV	RA	RV	IMA	IMV	HA	PV
Asensio et al.[61]	2000	10 (5)	28 (13)	33 (14)	14 (7)	34 (15)	3 (3)	8 (6)	6 (4)	14 (4)
Graham et al.[9]	1978	13 (8)	45 (26)				8 (8)			
Accola et al.[10]	1986		22 (7)							
Courcy et al.[12]	1984		6 (2)	12 (6)						
Lucas et al.[13]	1981		15 (10)							
Jurkovich et al.[14]	1993								28 (9)	55 (20)
Busuttil et al.[15]	1980								4 (3)	10 (5)
Goff and Collin[17]	1998				9 (9)					
Sturm et al.[24]	1975				10 (5)	5 (2)				
Donahue and Strauch[37]	1988			110 (77)						
Haas et al.[48]	1998				12 (11)					
Sirinek and Levine[11]	1985		20 (14)	12 (9)						
Graham et al.[55]	1978			45 (31)				9 (9)		37 (18)
Stone et al.[54]	1982			42 (27)						46 (22)
Petersen et al.[62]	1979									28 (17)
Ivatury et al.[63]	1985									14 (7)
Dawson et al.[53]	1991								6 (3)	13 (4)
Wiencek and Wilson[64]	1986			5 (1)		19 (8)		2 (2)		17 (6)
Carroll et al.[46]	1990				15 (12)	18 (12)				
Cohen et al.[65]	1980			3 (1)		5 (1)				8 (5)
Total		**23 (13)**	**136 (72)**	**252 (166)**	**60 (44)**	**81 (38)**	**11 (11)**	**19 (17)**	**44 (19)**	**242 (108)**
Survival%		56	53	66	73	47	100	89	43	45

[a] Numbers in parentheses indicate survival.

Visceral vascular injuries are commonly associated with massive blood loss and the need for transfusion in patients who survive. This frequently results in the development of the lethal triad consisting of hypothermia, coagulopathy, and acidosis. It is critical for the surgeon to recognize this triad early and terminate the procedure as quickly as possible, allowing restoration of normal physiology in the intensive care unit. Asensio et al.[61] notes that 20% of patients with abdominal vascular injuries required damage control procedures consisting of vessel ligation, bowel stapling, and packing of the abdomen. Prosthetic abdominal wall closure was performed in 12% of patients to deal with the sequelae of ischemia–reperfusion injury, massive resuscitation, and the abdominal compartment syndrome.

OUTCOME

The vast majority of patients who die following visceral vessel injury exsanguinate either prior to arrival, in the operating room, or within 24 hr of admission.[9–11,14,61] Timely control of hemorrhage is the single most important measure that improves survival. Other causes of death include multiple system organ failure with or without adult respiratory distress syndrome, cardiopulmonary arrest, brain death, sepsis, and bowel necrosis (Table 36–6).

SUMMARY

Visceral vascular injuries are most commonly caused by penetrating trauma. They are associated with a high mortality, most commonly secondary to exsanguination. Rapid transportation and control of hemorrhage is critical to survival, and damage control techniques should be used early when the patient is at risk for developing the lethal triad of hypothermia, coagulopathy, and acidosis. Attempts at restoration of blood flow should be used only in stable patients when technically feasible.

REFERENCES

1. Brooks SM. Our assassinated presidents. Bell Publishing Co., New York, 1985:47–72.
2. Edwards WS, Edwards PD. Alexis Carrel, visionary surgeon. Charles C. Thomas Publisher, Springfield, IL. 1974:8–16.
3. The Warren Report. Associated Press Publishers. 1964:224–225.
4. DeBakey ME, Simeone FA. Battle injuries of the arteries in World War II. *Ann Surg*. 1946; 123:534–578.
5. Hughes, CW. Arterial repair during the Korean War. *Ann Surg*. 1958;147:555–561.
6. Rich NM, Baugh JH, Hughes CW. Acute arterial injuries in Vietnam: 1000 cases. *J Trauma*. 1970;10:359–369.
7. Mattox KL, Feliciano DV, Burch J, Beall AC, Jordan GL, DeBakey ME. Five thousand seven hundred sixty cardiovascular injuries in 4459 patients. *Ann Surg*. 1989;209:698–705.
8. Asensio, JA, Berne JD, Chahwan S, et al. Traumatic injury to the superior mesenteric artery. *Am J Surg*. 1999;178(3):235–239.

9. Graham JM, Mattox KL, Beall AC Jr, DeBakey ME. Injuries to the visceral arteries. *Surgery.* 1978;84:835–839.
10. Accola KD, Feliciano DV, Mattox KL, Burch JM, Beall AC Jr, Jordan GL Jr. Management of injuries to the superior mesenteric artery. *J Trauma.* 1986;26:313–317.
11. Sirinek, KR, Levine BA. Traumatic injury to the proximal superior mesenteric vessels. *Surgery.* 1985;98:831–835.
12. Courcy PA, Brotman S, Oster-Granite ML, Soderstrom CA, Siegel JH, Cowley RA. Superior mesentric artery and vein injuries from blunt abdominal trauma. *J Trauma.* 1984;24:843–845.
13. Lucas AE, Richardson JD, Flint LM, Polk HC. Traumatic injury of the proximal superior mesenteric artery. *Ann Surg.* 1981;193:30–34.
14. Jurkovich GJ, Hoyt DB, Moore FA, et al. Portal triad injuries. *J Trauma Inj Infect Crit Care.* 1993; 39:426–434.
15. Busuttil OW, Kitahama A, Cerise E, McFadden M, Lo R, Longmire WP. Management of blunt and penetrating injuries to the porta hepatis. *Ann Surg.* 1980;191:641–647.
16. Sagalowsky AI, McConnell JD, Peters PC. Renal trauma requiring surgery: an analysis of 185 cases. *J Trauma.* 1983;23:128–131.
17. Goff CD, Collin GR. Management of renal trauma at a rural, level I trauma center. *Am Surg.* 1998;64:226–230.
18. Pontius GV, Kilbourne BC, Paul EG. Injuries of miscellaneous intra-abdominal arteries. Rich NM, Cooper FC, eds. WB Saunders Co., Philadelphia, 1978:457–474.
19. Moore EE, Cogbill TH, Jurkovich GJ, et al. Organ injury scaling III: chest wall, abdominal vascular, ureter, bladder, and urethra. *J Trauma.* 1992;33:337.
20. Glenn JF, Harvard BM. The injured kidney. *JAMA.* 1960;173:1189.
21. Banowsky LH, Wolfel DA, Lackner LH. Considerations in diagnosis and management of renal trauma. *J Trauma.* 1970;10:587.
22. DeWeerd JH. Management of renal injuries. *J Internat Coll Surg.* 1958;29:567.
23. Scholl AJ, Ferrier PA. Injuries of the kidney. In *Urology.* Campbell M, ed. Philadelphia: WB Saunders Co., Vol. 2. 1954:863.
24. Sturm JT, Perry JF, Cass AS. Renal artery and vein injury following blunt trauma. *Ann Surg.* 1975;182:696–698.
25. Rozycki GS, Ochsner MG, Schmidt JA, et al. A prospective study of surgeon-performed ultrasound as the primary adjuvant modality for injured patient assessment. *J Trauma.* 1995; 39:492.
26. Rozycki GS, Feliciano DV, Schmidt JA, et al. The role of surgeon-performed ultrasound in patients with possible cardiac wounds. *Ann Surg.* 1996;223:737.
27. Rozycki GS, Ballard RB, Feliciano DV, et al. Surgeon-performed ultrasound for the assessment of truncal injuries, lessons learned from 1540 patients. *Ann Surg.* 1998;228:557.
28. Schurr MJ, Fabian TC, Gavant M, et al. Management of blunt splenic trauma: computed tomographic contrast blush predicts failure of nonoperative management. *J Trauma.* 1995;39:507–513.
29. Davis KA, Fabian TC, Croce MA, et al. Improved success in nonoperative management of blunt splenic injuries: embolization of splenic artery pseudoaneurysms. *J Trauma: Inj Infect Crit Care.* 1998;44:1008–1015.
30. Patel VG, Walker ML. The role of "one-shot" intravenous pyelogram in evaluation of penetrating abdominal trauma. *Am J.* 1997;63:350–353.
31. Stevenson J, Battistella FD. The "one-shot" intravenous pyelogram: is it indicated in unstable trauma patients before celiotomy? *J Trauma.* 1994;36:828–833.
32. Nagy KK, Brenneman FD, Krosner SM, et al. Routine preoperative "one-shot" intravenous pyelography is not indicated in all patients with penetrating abdominal trauma. *J Am Coll Surg.* 1997;185:530–533.

33. Bickell WH, Wall MJ Jr, Pepe PE, et al. Immediate versus delayed fluid resuscitation for hypotensive patients with penetrating torso injuries. *N Engl J Med.* 1994;331:1105–1109.
34. Rhee PM, Acosta J, Bridgemen A, Wang D, Jordan M, Rich N. Survival after emergency department thoracotomy: review of published data from the past 25 years. *J Am Coll Surg.* 2000;190:288–298.
35. Mattox KL, McCollum WB, Beall AC Jr. , Jordan GL, DeBakey ME. Management of penetrating injuries of the suprarenal aorta. *J Trauma.* 1995;15:808–815.
36. Fullen WD, Hunt J, Altemeier WA. The clinical spectrum of penetrating injury to the superior mesenteric arterial circulation. *J Trauma.* 1972;12:656–664.
37. Donahue TK, Strauch GO. Ligation as definitive management of injury to the superior mesenteric vein. *J Trauma.* 1988;28:541–543.
38. Child CG. Portal hypertension. In *Major Problems in Clinical Surgery,* Vol. XIV. Philadelphia: WB Saunders, 1974:1–283.
39. Schwartz SI. Surgical diseases of the liver. New York: McGraw-Hill, 1964.
40. McAninch JW, Carroll PR. Renal trauma: kidney preservation through improved vascular control—a refined approach. *J Trauma.* 1982;22:285–290.
41. Scott RF, Selzman HM. Complications of nephrectomy: a review of 450 and a description of a modification of the transperitoneal approach. *J Urol.* 1966;95:307–312.
42. Carlton CE, Scott R, Goldman M. The management of penetrating injuries of the kidney. *J Trauma.* 1968;8:1071–1083.
43. Cass AS, Ireland GW. Comparison of the conservative and surgical management of the severe degrees of renal trauma in multiple injured patients. *J Urol.* 1973;109:8–10.
44. Gonzalez RP, Falimirski M, Holevar MR, Evankovich C. Surgical management of renal trauma: is vascular control necessary? *J Trauma.* 1999;47:1039–1044.
45. Atala A, Miller FB, Richardson JD, et al. Preliminary vascular control for renal trauma. *Surg Gyn Obstet.* 1991;172:386–390.
46. Carroll PR, McAninch JW, Klosterman P, Greenblatt M. Renovascular trauma: risk assessment, surgical management, and outcome. *J Trauma.* 1990;30:547–552.
47. Brown MR, Graham JM, Mattox KL, Feliciano DV, DeBakey ME. Reovascular trauma. *Am J Surg.* 1980;140:802–805.
48. Haas CA, Dinchman KH, Nasrallah PF, Spirnak JP. Traumatic renal artery occlusion: a 15-year review. *J Trauma.* 1998;45:557–561.
49. Maggio AJ, Brosman S. Renal artery trauma. *Urology.* 1978;11:125.
50. Greenholz SK, Moore EE, Peterson NE, Moore GE. Traumatic bilateral renal artery occlusion: successful outcome without surgical intervention. *J Trauma.* 1986;26:941–944.
51. Villas PA, Cohen G, Putnam SG, Goldberg A, Ball D. Wallstent placement in a renal artery after blunt abdominal trauma. *J Trauma.* 1999;6:1137–1139.
52. Sheldon GF, Lim RC, Yee ES, Petersen SR. Management of injuries to the porta hepatis. *Ann Surg.* 1985;202:539–545.
53. Dawson DL, Johansen KH, Jurkovich GJ. Injuries to the portal triad. *Am J Surg.* 1991; 161:545–551.
54. Stone JJ, Fabian TC, Turkleson ML. Wounds of the portal venous system. *World J Surg.* 1982; 6:335–341.
55. Graham JM, Mattox KL, Beall AC Jr. Portal venous system injuries. *J Trauma.* 1978;18:419–422.
56. Feliciano DV. Surgery for liver trauma. *Surg Clin N Am.* 1989;69:273–284.
57. Ochsner MG, Jaffin JH, Golocovsky M, et al. Major hepatic trauma. *Surg Clin N Am.* 1993; 73:337–352.
58. Mays ET. Hepatic trauma. *Curr Prob Surg.* 1976;13:11.
59. Flint LM, Mays ET, Aaron SW, et al. Selectivity in the management of hepatic trauma. *Ann Surg.* 1977;185:613–618.

60. Carrillo EH, Bergamini TM, Miller FB, Richardson JD. Abdominal vascular injuries. *J Trauma.* 1997;43:164–171.
61. Asensio JA, Chahwan S, Hanpeter D, et al. Operative management and outcome of 302 abdominal vascular injuries. AAST-OIS correlates well with mortality. Trauma Surgery, 52nd Annual Meeting of the Southwestern Surgical Congress, April 11, 2000.
62. Petersen SR, Sheldon GF, Lim RC Jr. Management of portal vein injuries. *J Trauma.* 1979; 19:616–620.
63. Ivatury RR, Rohman M, Nallathambi M, Rao, PM, Gunduz Y, Stahl WM. The morbidity of injuries of the extra-hepatic biliary system. *J Trauma.* 1985;25:967–973.
64. Wiencek RG, Wilson RF. Abdominal venous injuries. *J Trauma.* 1986;26:771–778.
65. Cohen D, Johansen K, Cottingham K, Clayson K, Simonowitz D. Trauma to major visceral veins: an underemphasized cause of accident mortality. *J Trauma.* 1980;20:928–932.

37

The Role of Gut Hypoperfusion in Multiple Organ Failure

Heitham T. Hassoun, MD,
and Frederick A. Moore, MD, FACS

INTRODUCTION

In the mid-1970s, multiple organ failure (MOF) emerged as a new syndrome in intensive care units (ICU) as a result of the ability to keep patients alive with advanced ICU technology. Despite intensive investigation, the pathogenesis of MOF remains elusive. Laboratory and clinical research strongly suggest that the gastrointestinal tract (i.e, the gut) plays a pivotal pathogenic role. Based on our observations and the observations of others, we believe that shock with resulting gut hypoperfusion is an important inciting event. The purpose of this chapter is to provide a brief overview of the role of gut hypoperfusion in the development of time-dependent intermediate outcomes that contribute to the pathogenesis of MOF, including (1) refractory shock, (2) early systemic inflammatory response syndrome (SIRS), and (3) late infections.

HISTORICAL PERSPECTIVE

Although there were early reports in the 1960s of critically ill patients who had developed simultaneous organ failure, in 1973, Tilney et al.[1] were given credit for first describing sequential failure of multiple organs in 18 consecutive patients with ruptured abdominal aortic aneurysms (AAAs) who required postoperative hemodialysis. These authors concluded that this phenomenon occurred as a result of a combination of preexisting disease and hemorrhagic shock. In 1977, Eiseman et al.[2] introduced the term *multiple organ failure* to describe the clinical course of 42 ICU patients with progressive organ failure; half of these patients had an intra-abdominal infection implicated as the inciting event. Thus, sepsis was added to the list of risk factors for MOF. Soon thereafter, Polk and Fry[3] confirmed a consistent association between infection and MOF, and concluded that MOF was the "fatal expression of uncontrolled infection." As a result, research efforts in the early 1980s were focused on determining how the initial traumatic insult promotes infections and how infections caused MOF. In the mid-1980s, observations from Europe by Faist[4] and Goris[5] changed this research focus. They observed that a significant proportion of blunt trauma patients who developed MOF did not have an identifiable infection. They concluded that MOF can occur as a result of an "autodestructive inflammatory response," and research efforts refocused on explaining how a variety of noninfectious insults could cause SIRS that would result in MOF independent of a bacterial infection. Although the early trauma studies observed correctly that infection can cause MOF, later studies demonstrated that early MOF frequently occurs in the absence of infection. *Sepsis syndrome* became a popular term, and bacterial translocation was the proposed mechanism to explain how these noninfected patients could appear to be septic. Widespread interest in this provocative hypothesis focused attention persuasively on the role of the gut in MOF pathogenesis.

UNIFYING CONCEPT

In the late 1980s, the National Institutes of Health (NIH) funded Trauma Research Centers (TRCs) to study MOF. Based on new knowledge, the concepts of MOF pathogenesis continue to evolve.[6] Our most recent rendition is depicted in Figure 37–1. The global

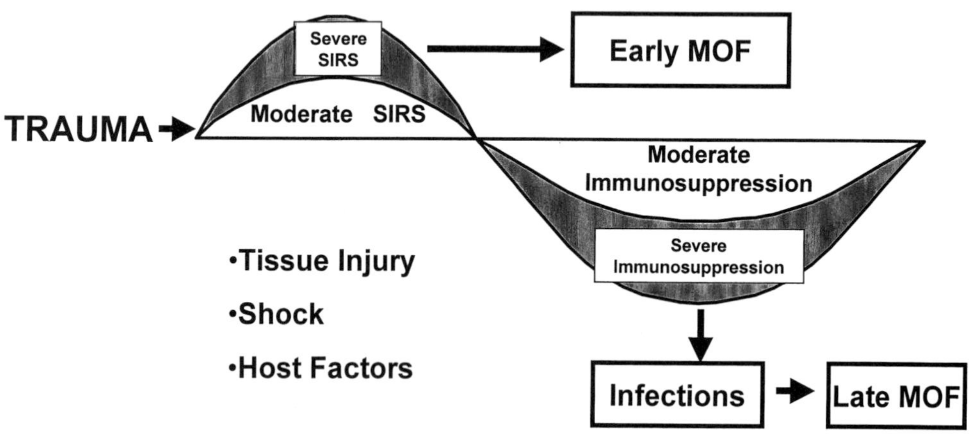

Figure 37–1. Postinjury MOF occurs as a result of a dysfunctional inflammatory response. Conceptual framework for the pathogenesis of postinjury MOF. SIRS: systemic inflammatory response syndrome.

hypothesis is that postinjury MOF occurs as a result of a dysfunctional inflammatory response. Following trauma, patients are resuscitated into a state of systemic hyperinflammation (i.e., SIRS). Mild to moderate SIRS is most likely beneficial (i.e., it is the normal injury stress response), but severe SIRS can precipitate early MOF. The intensity of early SIRS is dependent on (1) the amount of tissue injury, (2) the severity of shock, and (3) a variety of host factors. As time proceeds, negative feedback mechanisms downregulate certain aspects of SIRS to restore homeostasis and potential autodestructive inflammation. This compensatory anti-inflammatory response results in delayed immunosuppression. Again, mild-to-moderate immunosuppression is presumed to be beneficial, but when severe, it is associated with late infections (principally pneumonia) that can worsen early MOF or precipitate late MOF.

GUT HYPOPERFUSION AS AN INCITING EVENT FOR MOF

One focus of clinical research efforts has been the ability to make early predictions concerning those patients who ultimately develop MOF.[7] Readily available clinical parameters associated with MOF were collected prospectively and then analyzed by logistic regression to develop acute prediction models. Indices of shock emerged as strong predictors of MOF. This is consistent with other observations. A strong and consistent temporal association between early shock and the later development of MOF indicates that shock is an important etiologic factor. Laboratory observations confirm that shock induces disproportionate splanchnic hypoperfusion, and with reperfusion, an ischemic gut can cause remote organ injury. In the clinical setting of traumatic shock resuscitation, a number of investigative groups[8–11] (e.g., Chang, Civetta, Ivatury, McKinley, and Rouman) have demonstrated that persistent gut hypoperfusion (documented by gastric tonometry), despite maximal resuscitative efforts, is predictive for MOF and death. Thus, gut hypoperfusion has been implicated as an important inciting event in MOF pathogenesis.

ROLE OF GUT HYPOPERFUSION IN THE PATHOGENESIS OF REFRACTORY SHOCK

In a 1965 review article, Jacob Fine[12] concluded that refractory traumatic shock was caused by the absorption of bacteria and endotoxin (LPS) from the gut in conjunction with shock-induced impairment of the ability of the hepatic reticuloendothelial system to detoxify the portal venous effluent, potentiating the systemic spread of bacteria and LPS. This theory faded from the literature because of a lack of collaborating experimental and clinical data. Experimental work in the mid-1980s, however, revived interest in this phenomenon. Deitch and Berg[13] popularized the term *bacterial translocation,* which they initially defined as "the passage of viable indigenous bacteria from the GI tract through the intact epithelial mucosa to the mesenteric lymph nodes (MLN's) and other organs." In 1990, Alexander et al.[14] expanded this definition to "the passage of both viable and non-viable microbes and microbial products such as endotoxin across an anatomically intact intestinal barrier." Throughout the 1980s these investigators and others performed innovative experiments that elucidated the mechanisms that regulate bacterial translocation (BT). A number of these studies were done in rodent hemorrhagic shock models. In Deitch and Berg's[13] experiments, rats were bled to a mean arterial pressure (MAP) of 30 mmHg for 30, 60, and 90 min. The rats were then sacrificed 24 hr after shock and ileocolic MLNs, spleens, and livers were harvested and then cultured quantitatively. Shock at 30 and 60 min had roughly equivalent effects: half of the MLN cultures were positive, spread to the liver and spleen was <20%, and mortality was 15% and 20%, respectively. In contrast, after 90 min of shock, all MLNs had positive cultures and a significantly greater amount of enteric bacteria (60%) disseminated to systemic organs. Also, mortality increased to 40%. Of note, 35% of these rats had positive blood cultures. In a subsequent study, these authors performed histologic analysis of the ileum and cecum in rats subject to 30 min of shock (again, bled to 30 mmHg). The mucosa was relatively intact 2 hr after shock, but by 24 hr there was frank mucosal damage in both the ileum and cecum. In a similar model (rats bled to MAP of 30 to 35 mmHg for 90 min), Schlag, Redl and associates[15] noted that endotoxin levels in the portal vein increased significantly at the end of 90 min of shock and became evident in the systemic circulation during the first 60 min of resuscitation. Morphologic examination of the gut after shock revealed that both the jejunum and ileum often had areas of mucosal necrosis, but the colon had relatively normal histology. Rush et al.[16] also conducted a series of hemorrhagic shock studies (MAP 30 mmHg until 80% of shed blood returned) in rats. On average, this represents a shock period >4 hr and therefore is a much more severe model than the aforementioned two models. Blood cultures became positive 30 min into the shock period, and bacteremia continued throughout the ensuing 48 hr of observation. In another study, rats were fed *Escherichia coli* labeled with carbon-14 oleic acid. After the same severe hemorrhagic shock insult, half were noted to have increased plasma carbon-14 activity; all animals whose blood cultures were also positive were dead within 80 hr. In contrast, 83% of the animals without plasma carbon-14 activity survived. Moreover, Rush et al.[16] demonstrated that germ-free rats subjected to their shock model had significantly better survival at 24, 48, and 72 hr (62%, 30%, and 25% vs. 24%, 11%, and 5%, respectively).

Although these animal models are logical and consistent, clinical studies indicate that BT (as documented in laboratory models) after shock is an infrequent event in humans. In the Korean conflict, Lindberg et al.[17] found that among 30 soldiers who died, only 3 (10%) had positive blood cultures, and only 3 cultures (8%) were positive in 38 other soldiers who were in shock for an average of 7.3 hr. When their data were corrected for contamination, they estimated the incidence of early bacteremia would be <5% in combat casualties. As a clinical correlate to their rodent experiments, Rush et al.[5] sampled blood within 3 hr of admission in 50 acutely injured patients. Cultures were positive in 10 (56%) of the 18 patients who arrived in shock, compared to 3 (9%) of the 32 patients without shock. Eight (8) of the 10 patients who presented in shock and had positive blood cultures died within 24 hr. Of note, 70% of the bacteria recovered from the blood were gram-positive organisms, but the specific species were not reported. In addition, LPS was assayed in the blood of 10 patients. LPS was not detected in the 6 patients without shock, but was detected in 2 of the 4 patients with shock. Subsequently, our group performed a similar blood culture study in 132 acutely injured patients requiring emergency laparotomy.[6] Cultures were positive in 12 (32%) of 38 patients who arrived in shock, compared to 10 (12%) of 94 patients who were not in shock on arrival. Like Rush et al., we found an exceptionally high incidence of gram-positive organisms. Most notably, coagulase-negative *Staphylococcus* (staph) was isolated in 5 (13%) of the patients with shock and in 6 (7%) of the patients without shock. The exact source of these staph bacteremias is not clear, but they appeared to be of minimal clinical significance; none of the patients developed occult staphylococcal infection, nor did any of them die of refractory shock. In contrast, of the 7 patients with shock who had more typical enteric bacteremias, 6 died within 24 hr of refractory shock, and 4 of the 7 patients had hollow viscous injuries. Therefore, it appears that at least 3 patients had BT. This low incidence of BT early after traumatic shock is consistent with a more recent study by Roumen et al.,[19] who measured serial LPS in 11 patients (5 with ruptured AAA and 6 trauma patients with an ISS ≥25). Six patients (5 with AAAs and 1 with trauma) had endotoxemia at baseline or at 6 hr, but in the patients who survived acute resuscitation, endotoxemia was not demonstrated at 24 or 48 hr. More recently, Endo et al.[20] obtained serial blood samples (0.5, 1, 2, 3, 6, 12, 24, 48, 72, 106, 120, 144, and 168 hr after arrival) in 29 severely injured patients who arrived in shock. Elevated LPS levels were found in only 7 (2%) of 342 specimens.

From these data, we conclude that laboratory studies support the notion that BT is responsible for irreversible shock, but note that they use severe shock insults. In addition, clinical studies document BT in a small number of patients who are moribund on arrival. Whether BT contributes to early patient death or is just an epiphenomena of severe shock is not clear. This is exceedingly difficult to determine because animal and human responses are so different.

THE ROLE OF GUT HYPOPERFUSION IN SIRS AND EARLY MOF

In the late 1980s and early 1990s, the experimental work at a number of TRCs persuasively focused attention on BT. Shock-induced BT was proposed to explain the "sepsis syndrome" (i.e., SIRS without an infection) that characterized early postinjury MOF. In an attempt to recreate the clinical scenario, a nonlethal model of gut ischemia/reperfusion (I/R) induced acute lung injury (ALI) was developed.[21] A relatively short period of gut ischemia (45 min superior mesenteric artery occlusion) followed by 6 hr of reperfusion resulted in the following sequence: (1) gut phospholipase A_2 activation; (2) neutrophils (PMN) sequestration in the gut; (3) circulating PMN priming; (4) circulating PMN adhesion receptor expression; (5) PMN sequestration in the lung; and (6) ALI. Interestingly, when the potential role of BT was investigated in this model, it was surprising to find that plasma LPS levels were elevated to the same level in both the gut I/R and sham laparotomy animals, but the sham laparotomy animals had no evidence of ALI.[22] In addition, the elimination of LPS by pretreatment with monoclonal antibodies did not alter gut I/R–induced ALI. Thus, the reperfused gut appears to be an early source of proinflammatory mediators that cause ALI independent of BT.

Simultaneously with these basic laboratory studies, a parallel study was performed in the trauma ICU.[23] The specific purpose was to determine whether early BT via the portal vein occurred in patients who survive resuscitation but are at high risk for MOF. Twenty (20) patients [30% (6) of whom later developed MOF] requiring emergency trauma laparotomy, had a portal vein catheter placed. Portal venous blood was obtained at laparotomy and again at 6, 12, 24, and 48 hr and at 5 days postinjury. Simultaneous systemic blood samples were also obtained. The blood samples were cultured for bacterial growth, and surprisingly, they were virtually sterile. Only 9 (2%) of 212 cultures were positive. In the portal blood, 5 grew coagulase-negative *Staphylococcus,* two grew *Proprionibacterium acnes,* and one grew an *Acinobacter* spp. The only positive systemic blood culture grew *Staphylococcus aureus* in a patient who had simultaneous *S. aureus* pneumonia. In addition, the blood samples in the first 48 hr were assayed for LPS, complement fragment C_{3a}, tumor necrosis factor (TNF), and interleukin 6 (IL-6). As expected, C_{3a} and IL-6 levels were elevated, but LPS was not detected and TNF levels were not different from normal controls. Hoch et al.[24] confirmed these findings. Despite marked elevations in IL-6 and IL-8 levels, they could not identify LPS or TNF in the systemic circulation of high-risk trauma patients admitted to their ICU. A criticism of the first described study was that it focused on the portal vein while ignoring that BT may preferentially be spread via the MLNs to the thoracic duct. Several investigators including ourselves, subsequently cultured MLNs in patients requiring emergency trauma laparotomy. Overall, 10 (9%) of the 109 MLNs cultured in these trauma studies were positive. This is not different from the 10% culture positive rate documented in patients undergoing elective general surgery procedures. However, in the trauma studies, positive MLN cultures do not correlate with any adverse outcome. The key issue here is not whether BT to MLNs is occurring early postinjury, but whether it is a pathologic event. It has been proposed that BT to MLNs is a normal response by which the gut-associated lymphoid tissue (GALT) sampled for antigens follows stressful insults.

More recently, laboratory studies implicated that the gut is a cytokine-generating organ after shock-induced gut hypoperfusion, and that gut-associated bacteria may play an important role in this inflammatory response. For instance, Deitch and Chaudry[25] found greater increases in IL-6 and TNF levels in portal versus systemic circulation in rats subjected to hemorrhagic shock and resuscitation. In this study, it is noteworthy that both portal and systemic blood cultures were negative and that BT occurred only to MLNs in a dose-dependent fashion. A subsequent study[26] suggests that the cytokine response generated by gut hypoperfusion can be modulated by alterations in intestinal bacterial flora. In this shock model, plasma IL-6 and TNF levels were lower in rats whose gut flora had been decontaminated by oral antibiotics. Likewise, the induction of intestinal bacterial overgrowth caused a significant rise in plasma IL-6 and TNF after shock when compared to rats with normal gut flora. Recent work by Magnotti[27] and Zallen[28] have renewed interest in the role of mesenteric lymph in the pathogenesis of postinjury MOF. Together they have shown that the mesenteric lymph can be an avenue for gut-derived inflammatory agents, including neutrophil priming, increased neutrophil expression of CD11b, and increased endothelial expression of intracellular adhesion molecule-1 (ICAM-1). Mesenteric lymph diversion before hemorrhagic shock abolishes reperfusion-induced acute lung injury. In addition, posthemorrhagic shock mesenteric lymph but not the portal blood from the same animals increased endothelial cell injury *in vitro*. They propose that mesenteric lymph may contain the key mediators in the development of postinjury SIRS and subsequent MOF.

Based on these and other observations, we conclude that trauma induces gut hypoperfusion in patients at high risk for MOF. With reperfusion, the gut becomes a source of proinflammatory mediators that can amplify the SIRS response, leading to early MOF. Although our early interest was in determining how gut I/R causes remote organ injury, we are now focused on defining the key early events that occur in the gut after an I/R insult. Initial observations led us to propose that with reperfusion, xanthine–oxidase dependent reactive oxygen metabolites, either directly or indirectly, initiated a neutrophil-mediated tissue injury. However, in subsequent studies it was demonstrated that phospholipase A2 activation during ischemia was a necessary proximal step. In fact, very little is known about the early molecular events that initiate and perpetuate gut injury and dysfunction in this setting. We speculate that shock-induced gut I/R activates a cascade of stress-sensitive protein kinases that converge on specific transcriptional factors to regulate expression of proinflammatory genes. These gene products include enzymes such as iNOS, cyclooxygenase, and phospholipase A_2; cytokines, such as TNF-α and IL-1; chemokines (i.e., IL-8); and adhesion molecules. Excessive gene activation can lead to an exuberant proinflammatory response that triggers early MOF.

Because transcription is a central event in this injury cascade, analysis of the events activating key transcription factors and their target genes is critical to the understanding of MOF. Experimental work in the heart and kidney indicate that I/R triggers protein phosphorylation cascades that converge on specific transcription factors to regulate the pattern, timing, and magnitude of expression of pro- or anti-inflammatory genes. Presumably, this occurs via alterations in the cellular redox state that activate families of stress-sensitive protein kinases, such as the Ras–mitogen-activated protein kinases (MAPK) family [comprised of the extracellular-signal-regulated kinases (ERKs), p38/reactivating kinase (p38-MAPK), and the stress-activated protein kinases (SAPK)/c-Jun NH_2-terminal kinases (JNKs)]. These parallel MAPK cascades are activated in response to a number of cellular stresses, including inflammatory cytokines, heat and chemical shock, bacterial endotoxin, ischemia/cellular ATP depletion, and reactive oxygen species. On activation, the MAPKs phosphorylate a variety of nascent transcription factors, such as nuclear factor-$\kappa\beta$ (NF-$\kappa\beta$), CCAAT/enhancer binding protein β (C/EBPβ), and activator protein-1 (AP-1) families that regulate transcription of numerous target genes that encode proteins involved in mediator synthesis. Transcription factors are modular proteins with distinct domains responsible for DNA binding, ligand binding, nuclear localization, and protein–protein interactions. We recently demonstrated that gut I/R activates NF-$\kappa\beta$,[29] which belongs to the Rel family of inducible transcription factors that are activated by a number of stressors relevant to the posttraumatic state. Under basal conditions, NF-$\kappa\beta$ is sequestered in the cytoplasm as a ternary complex tethered with a family of inhibitory proteins known as IκB's whose expression varies in different cell types. Upon stimulation, a large multiprotein signalsome which contains NF-$\kappa\beta$–inducing kinase (NIK) and two homologous IκB kinases (IKK), phosphorylates IκBα and IκBβ, targeting them for ubiquitination and subsequent proteosome-dependent degradation. This rapidly frees the DNA-binding NF-$\kappa\beta$ subunits to translocate to the nucleus where they *trans*-activate target genes.

THE ROLE OF GUT HYPOPERFUSION IN INFECTIONS AND LATE MOF

In the late 1980s, epidemiologic studies by Border et al.[30] and Marshal et al.[31] strongly implicated the gut to be the reservoir for pathogens that cause late MOF-associated infections. There are several lines of evidence that link early gut hypoperfusion to late infections (Figure 37–2). First, in our laboratory model of MOF, gut I/R causes an ileus in both the stomach and small bowel. Clinically, after severe trauma gastric ileus is well documented whereas small bowel ileus is the suspected cause of intolerance to enteral nutrition. In both basic and clinical research, the ileus is known to promote colonization of the upper gastrointestinal tract.[32] Standard ICU therapies (H_2 antagonist, morphine, and broad-spectrum antibiotics) and disuse [i.e., total parenteral nutrition (TPN)] promote further ileus and colonization. Increased intestinal permeability is a marker of gut dysfunction in laboratory models and several investigators[33–35] demonstrated increased permeability early after injury. As this permeability defect worsens, it correlates with the development of infections and MOF.[34] With progressive ileus, increased colonization, increased permeability, and depressed mucosal immunity, bacteria and their toxins escape the bowel lumen. Aspiration of colonized gastric contents is well documented in ICU patients, whereas BT has been implicated to be the source of unexplainable late bacteremias.[31,36] Although the basic and clinical observations that support this

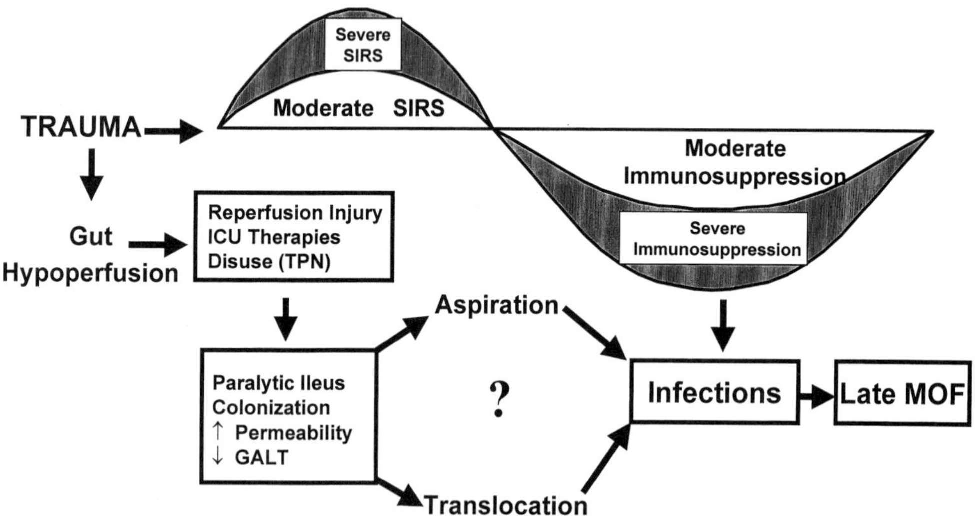

Figure 37–2. Role of gut hypoperfusion in infections and late MOF. ICU: intensive care unit; TPN: total parenteral nutrition; GALT: gut-associated lymphoid tissue.

sequence of events are consistent and logical, it has been difficult to confirm this in the laboratory because there is no chronic animal model. The most convincing evidence that the gut is the reservoir for late infections comes from clinical studies of gut-specific therapies.

It is common ICU practice to use H_2 antagonists for stress gastritis prophylaxis. Although bleeding from stress gastritis was a frequent terminal MOF event in the 1970s, it is distinctly uncommon in trauma ICUs today. Aggressive prophylaxis may be promoting a new role for the stomach in MOF. H_2 antagonists alkalinize the stomach, which facilitates colonization. Aspiration of contaminated gastric contents then sets the stage for pneumonia. Driks et al.[37] suggest that this could be prevented by using sucralfate prophylaxis to maintain gastric acidity. Although the supporting epidemiologic studies and the first two clinical trials are fairly convincing, the subsequent prospective randomized controlled trials (PRCT) by a number of different investigators[38–42] indicate that this strategy does not work in trauma patients. A careful review of these studies reveals an important confounding variable. Patients treated with sucralfate have long periods of time in which intragastric pH is paradoxically high. This may explain why sucralfate prophylaxis does not reduce postinjury nosocomial pneumonias. It also calls into question our basic understanding of gastric acid secretion following trauma.

Selective gut decontamination (SGD) and early total enteral nutrition (TEN) are gut-specific therapies widely practiced in Europe and the United States, respectively. SGD in trauma patients was first reported by Stoutenbeek et al.[43] in 1984, and stimulated numerous studies. A meta-analysis that combined data from 22 PRCTs demonstrates convincingly that this strategy reduces pneumonias.[44] A major criticism of the SGD trials is that although the incidence of pneumonia was decreased, mortality was not. These studies, however, were not designed to look at mortality. The confounding issue in the trauma SGD trials is that they enrolled a high portion of head-injured patients, but head-injured patients die from their brain injury, not as a result of infections. Initial interest in early nutrition was stimulated by Border et al.[30] and Alexander,[45] who emphasized that burns and trauma induce a hypermetabolic state, and that the resulting acute protein malnutrition worsens delayed immunosuppression and is an important cofactor in the development of late infections. Their studies indicated that patients who receive early nutrition (principally via the enteral route) had improved outcomes. Simultaneously, Page and Andrassy[46] demonstrated that patients could receive TEN via a needle catheter jejunostomy immediately after major elective abdominal surgery. This stimulated a series of PRCTs that demonstrated that early TEN following major torso trauma is both feasible and associated with a significant reduction in septic morbidity.[47–50] The important confounding variable in these PRCTs is that the control patients (in all but the first study) received early TPN. Excessive amounts of TPN are immunosuppressive and may account for the increased infections in the control groups. However, the results of more recent PRCTs of early TEN that compare immune-enhancing enteral diets to standard enteral diets indicate that the gut feeding is playing an important role in reducing infections. Although traditional nutritional support emphasized the need to provide early nutrition to prevent acute protein malnutrition, a newer concept is that certain nutrients (glutamine, arginine, Ω-3 fatty acids, and nucleic acids) administered via the gut exert immune-enhancing effects independent of the prevention of acute protein malnutrition. Immunonutrition is well supported by basic laboratory studies. The first PRCT was published by Alexander in 1990. There are now at least 18 published PRCTs, of which 5 involve trauma patients, and 4 of those trauma studies have demonstrated that immune-enhancing diets provide additional clinical benefits by reducing septic morbidity.[52,53]

ACKNOWLEDGMENT

The authors express sincere appreciation to Mary K. Carson for her excellent preparation of the manuscript.

REFERENCES

1. Tilney NL, Bailey GL, Morgan AP. Sequential system failure after rupture of abdominal aortic aneurysms: An unsolved problem in postoperative care. *Ann Surg.* 1973;178:117–124.
2. Eiseman B, Beart R, Norton L: Multiple organ failure. *Surg Gynecol Obstet* 144:323–326, 1977.
3. Fry DE, Pearlstein L, Fulton RL, Polk HC Jr: Multiple system organ failure: The role of uncontrolled infection. *Arch Surg* 1980;115:136–140.
4. Faist E, Baue AE, Dittmer H, Heberer G: Multiple organ failure in polytrauma patients. *J Trauma* 1983;23:775–787.
5. Goris JA, Boekhoerst TP, Nuytinck JK, Gimbrere JS: Multiple organ failure. *Arch Surg* 1985; 120:1109–1115.
6. Moore FA, Sauaia A, Moore EE, Haenel JB, Burch JM, Lezotte DC: Postinjury multiple organ failure: A bimodal phenomenon. *J Trauma* 1996;40:501–510.
7. Sauaia AJ, Moore FA, Moore EE, Norris JM, Lezotte DC, Hamman RF: Multiple organ failure can be predicted as early as 12 hrs postinjury. *J Trauma* 1998;45:291–301.
8. Chang MC, Cheatham ML, Nelson LD, Rutherford EJ, Morris JA Jr: Gastric tonometry supplements information provided by systemic indicators of oxygen transport. *J Trauma* 1994;37: 488–494.
9. Kirton OC, Windsor J, Wedderburn R, Hudson-Civetta J, Shatz DV, Mataragas NR, Civetta JM: Failure of splanchnic resuscitation in the acutely injured trauma patient correlates with multiple organ system failure and length of stay in the ICU. *Chest* 1998;113:1064–1069.
10. Roumen RM, Vreugde JP, Goris JA: Gastric tonometry in multiple trauma patients. *J Trauma* 1994;36:313–316.
11. Ivatury RR, Simon RJ, Islam S, Fueg A, Rohman M, Stahl WM: A prospective randomized study of end points of resuscitation after major trauma: global oxygen transport indices versus organ-specific gastric mucosal pH. *J Am Coll Surg* 1996;183:145–154.
12. Fine J: Current status of the problem of traumatic shock. *Surg Gynecol Obstet* 1965;120:537.
13. Deitch EA, Maejima K, Berg R: Effect of oral antibiotics and bacterial overgrowth on the translocation of the GI tract micro-flora in burned rats. *J Trauma* 1985;25:385.
14. Alexander JW, Boyce ST, Babcock GF, Gionotti L, Peck MD, Dunn DL, Pyles T: The process of microbial translocation. *Ann Surg* 1990;212:496–512.
15. Jiang J, Bahrami S, Leichtfried G, Redl H, Ohlinger W, Schlag G: Kinetics of endotoxin and tumor necrosis factor appearance in portal and systemic circulation after hemorrhagic shock in rats. *Ann Surg* 1995;221:100–106.

16. Rush BF, Sori AJ, Murphy TF, Smith S, Flanagan JJ, Machiedo FW: Endotoxemia and bacteremia during hemorrhagic shock: The link between trauma and sepsis? *Ann Surg* 1988;207:549.
17. Lindberg RB, Wetzler TF, Newton A, Howard JM, Davis JH, Strawitz J: The bacterial flora of the blood stream in the Korean battle casualty. *Ann Surg* 1954;141:366–368.
18. Moore FA, Moore EE, Poggetti RS, Read RA: Postinjury shock and early bacteremia: A lethal combination. *Arch Surg* 1992;127:893–898.
19. Roumen RM, Hendriks T, Wevers RA, Goris JA: Intestinal permeability after severe trauma and hemorrhagic shock is increased without relation to septic complications. *Arch Surg* 1993; 128:453.
20. Endo S, Inada K, Yamada Y, et al: Plasma endotoxin and cytokine concentrations in patients with hemorrhagic shock. *Crit Care Med* 1994;22:949.
21. Moore EE, Moore FA, Franciose RJ, Kim FJ, Biffl WI, Banerjee A: Postischemic gut serves as a priming bed for circulating neutrophils that provoke multiple organ failure. *J Trauma* 1994;37: 881–887.
22. Koike K, Moore EE, Moore FA, Read RA, Carl VS, Banerjee A: Gut ischemia/reperfusion produces lung injury independent of endotoxin. *Crit Care Med* 1994;22:1438–1444.
23. Moore FA, Moore EE, Poggetti RL, McAnena OJ, Peterson VM, Abernathy CM, Parsons PE: Gut bacterial translocation via the portal vein: A clinical perspective with major torso trauma. *J Trauma* 1991;31;629–636.
24. Hoch RC, Rodriguez R, Manning T, Bishop M, Mead P, Shoemaker WC, Abraham E: Effects of accidental trauma on cytokine and endotoxin production. *Crit Care Med* 1993;21:839–845.
25. Deitch EA, Xu D, Franko K, Ayala A, Chaudry IH: Evidence favoring the role of the gut as a cytokine-generating organ in rats subjected to hemorrhagic shock. *Shock* 1994;1:141–146.
26. Mainous MR, Ertel W, Chaudry IH, Deitch EA: The gut: a cytokine-generating organ in systemic inflammation? *Shock* 1995;4:193–199.
27. Magnotti LJ, Upperman JS, Xu DZ, Lu Q, Deitch EA: Gut derived mesenteric lymph but not portal blood increases endothelial cell permeability and promotes lung injury after hemorrhagic shock. *Ann Surg* 1998;228:518–527.
28. Zallen G, Moore EE, Tamura DY, Johnson JL, Biffl WI, Silliman CC: Hypertonic saline resuscitation abrogates neutrophil priming by mesenteric lymph. *J Trauma* 2000;48:45–48.
29. Hassoun HT, Moore F, Kone B, Phan T, Higham S, Weisbrodt N: α Melanocyte stimulating hormone (α-MSH) inhibits NF-κB activation and improves intestinal transit after gut ischemia/reperfusion (I/R). *Neurogastroenterology & Motility* 2000;12:482.
30. Border JR, Hassett J, LaDuca J, et al: The gut origin septic states in blunt multiple trauma (ISS-40) in the ICU. *Ann Surg* 1987;206:427.
31. Marshall JC, Christou NV, Horn R, et al: The microbiology of multiple organ failure. *Arch Surg* 1988;123:309.
32. Nieuwenheijs VB, Verheem A, van Duihvenbode-Beumer H, Visser MR, Verhoef J, Goeszen HG, Akkermans LM: The role of interdigestive small bowel motility in the regulation of gut microflora, bacterial overgrowth, and bacterial translocation in rats. *Ann Surg* 1998;228:188.
33. Pape HC, Dwenger A, Regel G, Auf 'm' Kolck M, Gollub F, Wisner D, Sturm JA, Tscherne H: Increased gut permeability after multiple trauma. *Br J Surg* 1994;81:850–852.
34. Faries PL, Simon RJ, Martella AT, Lee MJ, Machiedo GW: Intestinal permeability correlates with severity of injury in trauma patients. *J Trauma* 1998;44:1031–1036.
35. Epstein MD, Tchervenkov JI, Alexander JW, Johnson JR, Vester JW: Increased gut permeability following burn trauma. *Arch Surg* 1991;126:198–200.
36. Heyland D, Mandell LA: Gastric colonization by gram-negative bacilli and nosocomial pneumonia in the intensive care unit patient: Evidence for causation. *Chest* 1992;101:187–193.
37. Driks MR, Craven DE, Celli BR, Manning M, Burke RA, Gervin GM, Kunches LM, Farber HW, Wedel SA, McCabe WR: Nosocomial pneumonia in intubated patients given sucralfate

as compared with antacids or histamine type 2 blockers: The role of gastric colonization. *NEJM* 1987;317:1376.

38. Simms HH, DeMaria E, McDonald L, Peterson D, Robinson A, Burchard KW: Role of gastric colonization in the development of pneumonia in critically ill trauma patients: Results of a prospective randomized trial. *J Trauma* 1991;31:531–537.
39. Fabien TC, Boucher BA, Croce MA, Kuhl DA, Janning SW, Coffey BC, Kudsk KA: Pneumonia and stress ulceration in severely injured patients. *Arch Surg* 1993;128:185–192.
40. Pickworth KK, Falcone RE, Hoogeboom JE, Santanello SA: Occurrence of nosocomial pneumonia in mechanically ventilated trauma patients: A comparison of sucralfate and ranitidine. *Crit Care Med* 1993;21:1856–1862.
41. Ryan P, Dawson J, Teres D, Celoria G, Navab F: Nosocomial pneumonia during stress ulcer prophylaxis with cimetidine and sucralfate. *Arch Surg* 1993;128:1353–1357.
42. Thomason MH, Payseur ES, Hakenwerth AM, Norton HJ, Mehta B, Reeves TR, Moore-Swartz MW, Robbins PI: Nosocomial pneumonia in ventilated trauma patients during stress ulcer prophylaxis with sucralfate, antacid, and ranitidine. *J Trauma* 1996;41:503–508.
43. Stoutenbeek CP, Van Saene HK, Miranda DR, Zandstra DF: The effect of selective decontamination of the digestive tract on colonisation and infection rate in multiple trauma patients. *Intensive Care Med* 1984;10:185–192.
44. Selective decontamination of the digestive tract trialists' collaborative group: Meta-analysis of randomized controlled trials of selective decontamination of the digestive tract. *Br Med J* 1993;307:525.
45. Alexander JW, MacMillan BG, Stinnett JC, Ogle CK, Bozian RC, Fischer JE, Oates HB, Morris MJ, Krummel R: Beneficial effects of aggressive protein feeding in severely burned children. *Ann Surg* 1980;192:505–517.
46. Page CP, Carlton PK, Andrassy RJ, Feldtman RW, Shield CF: Safe, cost-effective postoperative nutrition: Refined formula diet via needle catheter jejunostomy (NCJ). *Am J Surg* 1979; 133:939.
47. Moore EE, Jones TN: Benefits of immediate jejunal feeding after major abdominal trauma: A prospective randomized study. *J Trauma* 1986;26:874–881.
48. Moore FA, Moore EE, Jones TN, McCroskey BL, Peterson VM: TEN versus TPN following major abdominal trauma: Reduced septic morbidity. *J Trauma* 1989;29:916–923.
49. Moore FA, Feliciano DV, Andrassy R, McArdle AH, Booth FV, Morgenstain-Wagner TB: Enteral feeding reduces postoperative septic complications: The result of a meta-analysis. *Ann Surg* 1992;216:172–183.
50. Kudsk KA, Croce MA, Fabian TC, Minard G, Tolley GA, Poret HA, Kuhl MR, Braun RD: Enteral versus parenteral feeding: Effects on septic morbidity following blunt and penetrating abdominal trauma. *Ann Surg* 1992;215:503–513.
51. Alexander W, Gottschlich MM: Nutritional immunomodulation in burn patients. *Crit Care Med* 1990;18:S149–S153.
52. Moore FA, Moore EE, Kudsk KA, et al: Clinical benefits of an immune-enhancing diet for early postinjury enteral feeding. *J Trauma* 1994;37:607.
53. Kudsk KA, Minard G, Croce MA, et al: A randomized trial of isonitrogenous enteral diets after severe trauma: An immune-enhancing diet reduces septic complications. *Ann Surg* 1996; 224:531.

38

Logical Approach to the Hypercoagulable Patient

David Green, MD, PhD

The hypercoagulable patient may be defined as one who is at risk for thrombosis in circumstances that would not cause thrombosis in a normal subject.[1] For example, a person having a pulmonary embolus after an airplane ride would be suspected of being hypercoagulable because thousands of people fly regularly and do not experience blood clots. However, developing a deep vein thrombosis in the leg after having total hip arthroplasty is not at all unusual in otherwise healthy persons who have not received thromboprophylaxis.

Most hypercoagulable patients are recognized when they suffer one or more episodes of thrombosis. Occasionally, however, individuals may be suspected to be at risk because they have a strong family history of thrombosis or have certain laboratory abnormalities detected by screening tests. In this chapter, the clinical and laboratory features of hypercoagulability are described and a logical approach to the diagnosis and management of the hypercoagulable patient is presented.

THE HEMOSTATIC MECHANISM

Patients develop thrombosis because the factors promoting coagulation overwhelm the anticoagulant mechanisms that maintain blood fluidity (Tables 38–1 and 38–2). When there is an injury, the vessels at the site undergo reflex spasm resulting in an acute decline in blood flow to the affected area. Stimulated endothelial cells release procoagulants, vasoconstrictors, and chemoattractants that promote the arrival of macrophages and polymorphonuclear leukocytes. High shear stress at the site of injury activates platelets and von Willebrand factor, which binds platelets to exposed subendothelial collagen. Platelets become activated and their membranes provide a surface for binding of procoagulant proteins. Tissue factor conveyed to the site by macrophages activates

TABLE 38–1. SOME PROTHROMBOTIC MECHANISMS

Vessel	Platelets	Circulating Factors
Endothelium	**Granules**	Fibrinogen
Endothelin	ADP, serotonin	Factors II–XIII
Thromboxane A_2	Thromboxane A_2	Oxidized LDL–cholesterol
von Willebrand factor	von Willebrand factor	Lp(a)
Subendothelium	Factors V, XI	Hyperhomocysteinemia
Collagens	PAI-1, TAFI	
Tissue factor	**Membrane**	
Rheology	Anionic phospholipids	
Hyperviscosity	**Thrombocythemia**	
Stasis		
High shear		
Red cell rigidity		

Abbreviations: ADP = adenosine diphosphate; PAI-1 = plasminogen activator inhibitor-1; TAFI = thrombin activatable fibrinolysis inhibitor.

clotting factor VII to VIIa, and the tissue factor–VIIa complex activates factors IX and X. Factor Xa and platelet-associated factor V convert prothrombin to thrombin. Thrombin activates platelets and factors V, VIII, and XI, thereby amplifying its own generation. Thrombin, in addition to converting fibrinogen to fibrin, activates factor XIII, which cross-links the polymerizing fibrin strands.

Thrombin activates an inhibitor of fibrinolysis (thrombin-activatable inhibitor of fibrinolysis (TAFI).[2] Platelets release another inhibitor of fibrinolysis, plasminogen activator inhibitor (PAI-1), and these two inhibitors (TAFI and PAI-1) delay fibrinolysis, resulting in the formation of a stable thrombus at the site of injury. Were there no circulating anticoagulants or promotors of fibrinolysis, the uncontrolled generation of fibrin would lead to vascular occlusion, organ necrosis, and death.

TABLE 38–2. SOME ANTITHROMBOTIC MECHANISMS

Vessel	Circulating Factors
Endothelium	**Phospholipid-binding proteins**
Nitric oxide	Annexin-V
Prostacyclin	β_2-glycoprotein-1
Thrombomodulin	**Anticoagulants**
TFPI	Antithrombin
Subendothelium	Protein C
Proteoglycans	Protein S
Dermatan sulfate	Heparin
Heparan sulfate	Heparin cofactor II
Rheology	
Pulsatile, rapid flow	

Abbreviations: TFPI = tissue factor pathway inhibitor.

At virtually every step of the coagulation cascade there are inhibitors to modulate coagulation activation. Activated factor X forms a complex with tissue factor pathway inhibitor (TFPI); this complex inactivates the tissue factor–factor VIIa complex. Heparin-like proteoglycans in the subendothelium activate antithrombin, which then inactivates factors XIa, IXa, Xa, thrombin, and the VIIa–tissue factor complex. The activity of these proteoglycans is neutralized by platelet factor IV, released from activated platelets. Heparin cofactor II is activated by dermatan sulfate and heparin, and may then act as a thrombin inhibitor.

Thrombin forms a complex with endothelial-derived thrombomodulin; this complex activates protein C (aPC). aPC, with free protein S as a cofactor, inactivates factor Va, and the complex of aPC and factor V inactivates factor VIIIa.[3] Phospholipid-binding proteins such as annexin V interfere with the attachment of procoagulants to activated platelets,[4] and β_2-glycoprotein-1 increases the availability of free protein S.[5]

Tissue plasminogen activator released from the endothelium activates fibrin-bound plasminogen to plasmin, initiating clot dissolution. In addition, endothelial cell membrane–associated urokinase plasminogen activator contributes to clot lysis. The fibrinolytic enzymes located within the clot are protected from inhibition by circulating PAI-1 and α_2-antiplasmin. Thus, a variety of mechanisms powerfully limit the extent of thrombus formation. Whether a particular patient ever develops a thrombus depends on a myriad of factors that may tilt the hemostatic balance in favor of thrombosis.

DETECTING HYPERCOAGULABILITY

The first step in the evaluation is to establish that the patient indeed has a thrombosis; in addition to a careful history and physical examination, an imaging study is usually required. Ultrasound is advantageous for detecting occlusion of the carotid arteries and also has high sensitivity and specificity in diagnosing deep vein thrombosis (DVT) of the lower extremities. Magnetic resonance angiography (MRA) is valuable in examining the cerebral circulation, including the venous dural sinuses, and also is used in assessing the vena cavae, portal, mesenteric, and renal veins. Contrast angiography is used for evaluating the coronary and peripheral arterial beds as well as the venous system of the upper and lower extremities. Other studies that indirectly suggest the presence of thrombosis are ventilation/perfusion lung scans and measurements of D-dimer and other products of coagulation, such as prothrombin fragment 1.2, thrombin–antithrombin complexes, and fibrinopeptides.

CLINICAL CHARACTERISTICS OF HYPERCOAGULABILITY

Once it has been established that the patient has a thrombosis, an evaluation for hypercoagulability should be performed. Hypercoagulability is suspected if the patient has one or more of the characteristics described by the **FURY** acronym:

- Family history of thrombosis
- Unusual site for thrombosis, such as venous dural sinuses or axillary or mesenteric veins

- Recurrent episodes of thrombosis, especially when different vessels are affected
- Young: thrombosis prior to the age of 40 with no other obvious risk factors

ETIOLOGY OF HYPERCOAGULABILITY

Once hypercoagulability is suggested by the previously mentioned features, the cause of the thrombosis should be ascertained. Because arterial thrombi often have a very different etiology than venous thrombi, the diagnostic possibilities are considered separately.

Disorders Associated with Arterial Thrombosis

Disorders associated with arterial thrombi are shown in Table 38–3. Hyperlipidemia, hypertension, diabetes, and chronic renal failure are often complicated by atherosclerosis. When the fibrous cap overlying an atheromatous lesion is destabilized through the action of metalloproteinases, the exposed subendothelium acts as a nidus for thrombus formation. Subsequent partial or complete occlusion of the vessel lumen brings the patient to medical attention. Until there is reendothelialization of the ulcerated plaque, thrombosis is recurrent. Thrombi also recur if the vessel becomes stenotic as a result of

TABLE 38–3. DISEASES ASSOCIATED WITH ARTERIAL THROMBOSIS

Atherosclerosis
Hyperlipidemia
Hypertension
Diabetes
Chronic renal failure
Vasculitis
Large vessels: Takayasu arteritis
Medium vessels: Polyarteritis, Kawasaki disease
Small vessels: micropolyarteritis, cryoglobulinemia
Thrombotic microangiopathies
Thrombotic thrombocytopenic purpura
Hemolytic–uremic syndrome
Hemolysis, thrombocytopenia, elevated liver enzymes of pregnancy
Hematologic disorders
Sickle cell disorders
Polycythemia
Essential thrombocythemia
Genetic disorders
Polymorphisms of certain platelet proteins
Inherited thrombophilias in association with other risk factors[a]

[a] Smoking, diabetes, hypercholesterolemia.

previous episodes of thrombosis. These repeated thromboses lead to the diagnosis of hypercoagulability.

Vasculitis of whatever etiology may be associated with thrombosis. In Takayasu disease, the thrombi may be in the aorta or its branches; whereas in polyarteritis, smaller arteries are involved. Thrombotic microangiopathies are a group of disorders characterized by the formation of hyaline thrombi in the arterioles of the brain, kidney, myocardium, and other organs. Platelets are deposited in these thrombi, leading to thrombocytopenia, and red cells are fragmented when traversing thrombosed vessels, causing anemia. Thrombosis of cerebral vessels occurs in sickle cell anemia, resulting in stroke at a young age. Occlusion of small vessels is usually due to aggregates of rigid, sickled red cells. Polycythemia vera and essential thrombocythemia may be associated with thrombotic occlusion of cerebral and retinal vessels, and less commonly affect other arteries such as those in the mesentery.

Because of the involvement of platelets in arterial thrombosis, considerable effort has been expended to determine if there are polymorphisms of platelet proteins that may result in platelet hyperactivity. The best documented polymorphism is in the gene-encoding glycoprotein IIIa (Pl^{A2}), a receptor for fibrinogen and von Willebrand factor (vWf) on the platelet membrane.[6] The original report suggested that this polymorphism was a risk factor for coronary thrombosis, and many, but not all, subsequent studies confirm this. There is also evidence that polymorphisms of the platelet glycoprotein Ib-IX-V complex are associated with arterial disease.[7,8]

Finally, in young patients with stroke or myocardial infarction, associations have been described with inherited thrombophilia traits such as prothrombin 20210 mutation and factor V Leiden.[9–11] In general, these associations have been noted in patients with other risk factors, such as smoking, diabetes, and hypertension.[12] These inherited thrombophilia factors are present in anywhere from 1% to 7% of the population, and the observation that they are only associated with disease in conjunction with other risk factors suggest that their role is ancillary, and not pivotal in arterial thrombus development.

Disorders Associated with Venous Thrombosis (Table 38–4)

Genetic Disorders

Venous thrombosis is associated with a number of gene polymorphisms; these may be classified as producing a gain or loss of function of the protein product (Table 38–5).[13] *Gain of function* applies to those mutations leading to greater activity of specific procoagulants, such as prothrombin and factors V, VIII, and XI; *loss of function* refers to mutations coding for defective or deficient anticoagulants. Loss of function mutations are less prominent but more severe than gain of function mutations. The lifetime risk of developing a thrombosis in patients with either protein C, protein S, or antithrombin deficiencies is around 8%, as compared to 2% for those with gain of function mutations.[14] Furthermore, persons who are homozygous for deficiency mutations either die *in utero* (antithrombin), or develop purpura fulminans shortly after birth (proteins C and S) and die if not transfused with these proteins. Heterozygous individuals usually develop thrombi in the second or third decade of life. Thromboses may occur in the deep veins

TABLE 38–4. DISEASES ASSOCIATED WITH VENOUS THROMBOSIS

- Genetic disorders
  - Deficiencies of antithrombin, protein C, protein S, heparin cofactor II
  - Polymorphisms of genes for factor V (factor V Leiden), prothrombin (G20210A), factors VIII, IX, XI
- Malignancies
  - Adenocarcinomas of breast, lung, prostate, pancreas, etc.
  - Glioblastoma multiforme, neuroblastoma
- Nephrotic syndrome
- Obesity
- Paralysis
  - Spinal cord injury: paraplegia, tetraplegia
  - Stroke: hemiplegia
- Pregnancy and puerpuerium
- Trauma and surgery
  - Long bone fractures
  - Orthopedic procedures: arthroscopy, arthroplasty
  - Neurosurgery
  - Various other types of operations
- Hematologic disorders
  - Myeloproliferative diseases
  - Paroxysmal nocturnal hemoglobinuria
- Inflammatory bowel disease
  - Regional enteritis
  - Ulcerative colitis

TABLE 38–5. MUTATIONS ASSOCIATED WITH VENOUS THROMBOSIS

	Prevalence (%)	Attributable Risk[a] (%)
Loss of function		
Protein C deficiency	0.2	2
Protein S deficiency	<1	<1
Antithrombin deficiency	0.02	<1
Heparin cofactor II deficiency	<0.01	<1
Gain of function		
Prothrombin 20210	4	25
Factor V Leiden	2	4
Factor VIII > 150%	11	16
Factor XI > 110%	10	11

[a] Attributable risk is calculated from the relative risk and the prevalence of the risk factor in the population.
Adapted from Refs. 13, 15.

of the limbs, the mesenteric veins, or the venous dural sinuses. Heparin cofactor II deficiency is only symptomatic when homozygous.

Homozygosity for gain of function mutations is associated with more frequent thrombosis than is heterozygosity, which may be completely asymptomatic, even to age 100![15] The mutation that gives rise to factor V Leiden produces a molecule that is relatively resistant to inactivation by activated protein C, and also does not function well as a cofactor for the protein C–mediated inactivation of factor VIII. The persistence of activated factors V and VIII increases the risk for thrombosis, mostly in the limbs.

Prothrombin G20210A represents a mutation in the promotor sequence of the gene for prothrombin, resulting in prothrombin concentrations that average 130% to 150%. These high levels of prothrombin are associated with an increased risk for DVT, pulmonary emboli (PE), and cerebral vein thrombosis (CVT). Both prothrombin 20210 and factor V Leiden are also associated with an increased risk of superficial thrombophlebitis, as well as obstetric complications, such as early-term miscarriages, preeclampsia, and toxemia. Elevated levels of factor VIII were previously considered to represent nothing more than a stress reaction to thrombosis, but careful studies now show that such elevated concentrations occur prior to these events and appear to be familial.[16,17] This suggests that there are mutations in the genes for factor VIII, and probably for factors IX and XI as well,[18] that modulate increased synthesis of these proteins.

Malignancies

An association between cancer and venous thrombosis is well established.[19] Malignancies promote thromboembolism by a variety of mechanisms, including the elaboration of cancer procoagulants, mucin, induction of tissue factor on activated monocytes and macrophages, generation of phospholipid-rich membrane microparticles, and compression and/or invasion of blood vessel walls.[20] Tumors that may directly induce thrombosis include small cell carcinoma of the lung, renal cell carcinoma, and melanoma; and tumors that indirectly promote thrombosis are non–small cell lung cancer, breast cancer, colon cancer, prostate cancer, and lymphomas.[21] Syndromes associated with malignancy include migratory thrombophlebitis, disseminated intravascular coagulation (DIC), marantic endocarditis, and thrombotic microangiopathy associated with tumor micrometastasis.

An important question is whether patients presenting with venous thrombosis should undergo evaluation for an occult malignancy. The data of Prandoni et al.[22] show that 17% of patients with recurrent thromboses are found to have cancer, so clearly this is a group at high risk. In patients with a first episode of thromboembolism without obvious etiology, cancer should be sought if there are abnormal findings in the history, physical examination, basic laboratory testing, or chest radiograph.[23] These abnormalities can be pursued with appropriate evaluations such as imaging, endoscopy, and serologic studies. In patients whose baseline tests are normal, routine cancer screening with mammography, testing for fecal occult blood, and measurement of prostate specific antigen are all that is currently recommended.

Nephrotic Syndrome

Hypercoagulability associated with the nephrotic syndrome is multifactorial. Evaluation of patients with nephrosis reveals elevated levels of fibrinogen and factor VIII and decreased concentrations of antithrombin. The last has been attributed to urinary loss of this protein. Loss of free water and hyperfibrinogenemia promote hyperviscosity, which further enhances the thrombotic tendency. One-third of patients have renal vein thrombosis; DVT and PE are also common.

Obesity

Obesity is defined as a body mass index (weight in kilograms divided by height in meters squared) >30. Obese patients are at increased risk for thrombosis, and clotting in such patients is often extensive and recurrent. The mechanisms of hypercoagulability in the obese are not well defined; compression of thin-walled veins, increased venous pressure, and poor venous emptying may be important. In addition, there is impaired fibrinolysis due to elevated levels of PAI-1, especially in patients with the metabolic syndrome.

Paralysis

Acutely, after stroke or spinal cord injury, there is dehydration and hyperfibrinogenemia increasing blood viscosity. Subsequently, high levels of factor VIII and PAI-1, reduced venous return due to muscle paralysis, and external compression on the vessels of flaccid limbs lead to venous thromboembolism.

Pregnancy and Puerperium

The risk of thrombosis in pregnancy and the puerperium is small—about 1 in 1000 to 1 in 2000 deliveries.[24] Factors promoting thrombosis are decreased venous return due to compression of the vena cava by the gravid uterus; increases in the levels of factor VIII, vWf, and fibrinogen as pregnancy progresses; and decreased fibrinolytic activity. In addition, levels of protein S and antithrombin decline during pregnancy. The risk of thrombosis is highest in the immediate postpartum period, especially if cesarean section has been performed. Pregnant patients with factor V Leiden or prothrombin 20210 mutations have higher rates of thrombosis (0.2% and 0.5%, respectively), and those with both mutations have a rate as high as 4.6%.[25]

Trauma and Surgery

Trauma and surgery result in raised levels of procoagulants, decreased circulating antithrombin, and impaired fibrinolytic activity. The trauma most associated with thromboembolism is spinal cord injury, followed by long bone fractures,[26] but any injury that leads to prolonged immobilization may be complicated by venous thrombosis. With regard to surgery, postoperative thrombosis occurs most often after joint replacement, especially if there is direct injury to underlying femoral or popliteal veins. Extensive resections for cancer and neurosurgical operations are also high-risk procedures, perhaps because of exposure to large amounts of tissue factor. However, any surgery may be complicated by intra- or postoperative thromboembolism.

Hematologic Disorders

The initial manifestation of myeloproliferative diseases such as polycythemia vera and essential thrombocythemia may be thrombosis of splanchnic or hepatic veins. Recurrent DVT and PE may also occur. Paroxysmal nocturnal hemoglobinuria is often complicated by thrombosis of portal veins or venous dural sinuses. An increased prevalence of venous thrombosis is also observed in hemolytic anemias and thalassemia.

Inflammatory Bowel Disease

Both regional enteritis and ulcerative colitis may be complicated by recurrent superficial or deep venous thrombosis. Acquired deficiency of antithrombin has been identified as a probable risk factor. The low levels of antithrombin are due to loss of this protein in the stool as part of the protein-losing enteropathy that complicates inflammatory bowel disease.[27]

Disorders Associated with Both Arterial and Venous Disease (Table 38–6)

Hyperhomocysteinemia

Homocysteine is a product of amino acid metabolism that, when present in elevated concentrations in the plasma, alters the ability of the endothelium to generate nitric oxide and activate fibrinolysis. Hyperhomocysteinemia is associated with arterial disease (cerebral, coronary, and peripheral arteries) as well as venous thrombosis. The levels may be elevated because of inherited defects in enzymes needed for homocysteine metabolism, nutritional deficiencies of folic acid, vitamin B_{12}, and/or vitamin B_6, and a variety of other disorders, including cancer, kidney disease, and hypothyroidism. If elevated levels of homocysteine are discovered, patients should be examined for the presence of one of these disorders and treatment with folic acid should commence. If homocysteine levels fail to decline with the administration of folic acid, vitamins B_6 and B_{12} are added.

Antiphospholipid Antibody Syndrome

Antiphospholipid antibodies are autoantibodies directed against phospholipid–protein complexes. Their targets include complexes of phospholipid with β_2-glycoprotein-1,

TABLE 38–6. DISORDERS ASSOCIATED WITH BOTH ARTERIAL AND VENOUS DISEASE

Hyperhomocysteinemia
Antiphospholipid antibodies
Cardiac diseases
Mural thrombi
Cardiomyopathy
Atrial fibrillation and other arrhythmias
Medications
Oral contraceptives, estrogens
Chemotherapeutic agents: 5-fluorouracil, tamoxifen, raloxifen, platinum
Heparin-induced thrombocytopenia with thrombosis, warfarin necrosis
Ticlopidine-associated thrombotic thrombocytopenic purpura

annexin V, prothrombin, and protein C. They are detected by anticardiolipin antibody tests (β_2-glycoprotein-1) and coagulation tests (the lupus anticoagulant). Antiphospholipid antibodies are associated with either arterial thrombosis (stroke, placental infarction, peripheral arterial occlusion) or venous thromboembolism. They interfere with the activation of protein C, hinder β_2-glycoprotein-1 from protecting free protein S from C4B binding, and displace annexin V from binding to placental and other coagulant phospholipids.[28]

Cardiac Disorders

Myocardial infarction (MI) may result in mural thrombus adherent to the myocardial scar, with subsequent embolization of disintegrating clot. Stasis of blood within the heart, whether due to cardiomyopathy or arrhythmia, leads to intracardiac thrombus formation. Patients may experience pulmonary, cerebral, splenic, and/or renal infarcts as well as embolization to fingers or toes. Transesophageal echocardiography (TEE) usually identifies valvular or intracardiac thrombi, which must be removed surgically or by interventional radiologic techniques.

Medications

A variety of medications are associated with thrombosis. The use of oral contraceptives may be complicated by DVT, PE, or the development of cerebral infarction. Venous thromboembolism is also reported with the administration of estrogens, tamoxifen, and raloxifene. Chemotherapeutic agents such as 5-fluorouracil have induced coronary spasm, thrombosis, and MI. Of great concern is the paradoxical thrombosis that occurs with warfarin, heparin, and ticlopidine. Each has a different pathogenesis; in the case of warfarin, it is rapid decline in protein C/S prior to reduction in prothrombin, which disturbs the hemostatic balance in favor of thrombosis. Heparin binds to platelet factor IV, and the complex elicits autoantibodies that bind to and activate platelets resulting in vascular occlusion by platelet thrombi and an accompanying thrombocytopenia. Ticlopidine induces a clinical picture characteristic of thrombotic thrombocytopenic purpura, most likely due to the formation of autoantibodies directed against the vWf protease.[29]

LOGICAL APPROACH TO HYPERCOAGULABILITY

A stepwise approach to the patient with thrombosis is recommended.

1. Confirm presence and location of thrombus—arterial vs venous.
2. Are there features consistent with hypercoagulability? Use the FURY acronym (**f**amily history of thrombosis; **u**nusual site of thrombosis; **r**epeated episodes of thrombosis; **y**oung-thrombosis prior to the age of 40).
3. Evaluate for any underlying disorders; for example, inherited or acquired thrombophilia.
4. Management based on etiology and location of thrombosis.

Although the management of thrombosis is beyond the scope of this chapter, specific treatment given for associated conditions, such as hyperlipidemia, hypertension, diabetes, myeloproliferative diseases, and hyperhomocysteinemia, may prevent future episodes of thrombosis. Furthermore, detection of an inherited thrombophilia (factor V Leiden, prothrombin 20210 mutation) may lead to behavioral modifications, such as discontinuation of oral contraceptives and cigarette smoking. Arterial thrombosis is usually treated with inhibitors of platelet function such as cyclooxygenase inhibitors (aspirin, nonsteroidal anti-inflammatory agents), thienopyridine derivatives (clopidogrel, ticlopidine), and phosphodiesterase inhibitors (dipyridamole, cilostazol). Venous thrombosis is controlled with heparins (unfractionated and low-molecular-weight) and warfarin. Thrombolytic therapy is selected for the management of life- or limb-threatening vascular occlusion. For patients with disorders associated with recurrent arterial and venous thrombosis, such as the antiphospholipid antibody syndrome, a combination of a platelet inhibitor and an anticoagulant may be most effective.

REFERENCES

1. Schafer AI. Hypercoagulable states: molecular genetics to clinical practice. *Lancet.* 1994; 344:1739–1742.
2. Von dem Borne PAK, Bajzar L, Meijers JCM, Nesheim ME, Bouma BN. Thrombin-mediated activation of factor XI results in a thrombin-activatable fibrinolysis inhibitor-dependent inhibition of fibrinolysis. *J Clin Invest.* 1997;99:2323–2327.
3. Dahlback B. Procoagulant and anticoagulant properties of coagulation factor V: factor V Leiden (APC resistance) causes hypercoagulability by dual mechanisms. *J Lab Clin Med.* 1999;133:415–422.
4. Rand JH. "Annexinopathies"—a new class of diseases. *N Engl J Med.* 1999;340:1035–1036.
5. Merrill JT, Zhang HW, Shen C, et al. Enhancement of protein S anticoagulant function by β_2-glycoprotein-1, a major target antigen of antiphospholipid antibodies. *Thromb Haemost.* 1999;81:748–757.
6. Weiss EJ, Bray PF, Tayback M, et al. A polymorphism of a platelet glycoprotein receptor as an inherited risk factor for coronary thrombosis. *N Engl J Med* 1996; 334:1090–1094.
7. Gonzalez-Conejero R, Lozano ML, Rivera J, et al. Polymorphisms of platelet membrane glycoprotein Ibα associated with arterial thrombotic disease. *Blood.* 1998;92:2771–2776.
8. Afshar-Kharghan V, Li CQ, Khoshnevis-Asi M, Lopez JA. Kozak sequence polymorphism of the glycoprotein (GP) 1bα gene is a major determinant of the plasma membrane levels of the platelet GP 1b-IX-V complex. *Blood.* 1999;94:186–191.
9. Rosendaal F, Siscovick DS, Schwartz SM, et al. Factor V Leiden (resistance to activated protein C) increases the risk of myocardial infarction in young women. *Blood.* 1997;89:2817–2821.
10. Rosendaal F, Siscovick DS, Schwartz SM, Psaty BM, Raghunathan TE, Vos HL. A common prothrombin variant (20210 G to A) increases the risk of myocardial infarction in young women. *Blood.* 1997;90:1747–1750.
11. Inbal A, Freimark D, Modan B, et al. Synergistic effects of prothrombotic polymorphisms and atherogenic factors on the risk of myocardial infarction in young males. *Blood.* 1999;93:2186–2190.
12. DeStefano V, Chiusolo P, Paciaroni K, et al. Prothrombin G20210A mutant genotype is a risk factor for cerebrovascular ischemic disease in young patients. *Blood.* 1998;91:3562–3565.

with HAAb, the Fc portion of the antibody binds to the platelet FcγIIa receptor leading to platelet activation and aggregation. Patients with HIT have an increased number of FcγIIa receptors on their platelet membranes. The activated platelets lead to platelet thromboses and the generation of thrombin-induced thrombosis.

The interval between the beginning of heparin administration and the onset of thrombocytopenia or heparin-induced complications is 4 to 15 days (mean: 8 days) for patients receiving heparin for the first time. Thrombocytopenia and/or complications usually occur between the second and ninth day (mean: day 5) in the patient who has previously been sensitized to heparin, and may occur as early as the first day of heparin reexposure.

In addition to the thrombocytopenia, patients with HAAb who receive heparin are at risk for thrombosis and, to a lesser degree, hemorrhage.

CLINICAL SPECTRUM

From 2% to 4% of patients receiving any form of heparin develop HAAb. There is no preference as to sex nor is age a factor. HAAb occurs without regard to type, amount, route of administration, or indication for administration of heparin. HAAb occurs more often in patients with multiple exposures to heparin. Walls and associates[7] found HAAb in 1.3% of patients undergoing cardiopulmonary bypass. Patients identified preoperatively and pretreated with platelet-inhibiting drugs before a brief exposure to heparin had no thromboembolic complications or mortality. The patients who were not identified preoperatively had a 32% thromboembolic rate and a 37% mortality rate. Calaitges and associates[8] demonstrated the presence of HAAb in 21% of vascular patients and found these patients to be at a 2.6-fold increased risk for developing postoperative thromboembolic events. In general, only 30% to 40% of the patients with HAAb develop HIT when exposed to heparin.

Because there are no signs or symptoms that allow one to predict which patient will develop HIT, all patients receiving heparin should be monitored. HIT should be suspected when the patient receiving heparin develops a resistance to anticoagulation with heparin, a thrombocytopenia (platelet count $<100{,}000/mm^3$ or a fall in the platelet count of 30%), and/or a new arterial or venous thromboembolic event. Unfortunately, the diagnosis is often made only after the patient develops recurrent or persistent thromboembolism or, rarely, hemorrhage. A few patients develop heparin-induced skin lesions from microvascular thrombosis. The skin lesions may progress to full thickness necrosis, and may not be associated with thrombocytopenia.

In an early report of 62 patients, we reported a mortality and morbidity of 23% and 61%, respectively.[5] Using early detection and prompt cessation of heparin administration to the patient with HAAb, we were able to reduce the mortality and morbidity to 12% and 22%, respectively, and in a later study, 1.1% and 7.4%, respectively.[6] Arterial thrombosis is the most common thromboembolic complication of HIT. The thromboses in patients with HIT often occur in the aorta, iliac, and lower limbs and less often in the mesenteric, renal, cerebral, or coronary systems. Venous thromboembolism is being recognized with increased frequency as a complication of HIT. The venous thrombosis may manifest 4 to 5 days after the cessation of heparin therapy.

DIAGNOSIS

HIT must be suspected in any patient receiving heparin who develops increased resistance to anticoagulation with heparin, new and/or progressive arterial and/or venous thromboembolic events, unexplained bleeding (rare), a falling platelet count, or persistent platelet count $<100{,}000/mm^3$. The HIT must be distinguished from other thrombocytopenias [e.g., disseminated intravascular coagulation (DIC), posttransfusion thrombocytopenia, infectious thrombocytopenia, other drug-induced thrombocytopenias].

The diagnosis of HIT is usually confirmed by the prompt increase of platelet count when all sources of heparin are eliminated. Further confirmation is obtained by the reduction or elimination of the thromboembolic events as the heparin administration is discontinued. When HIT is suspected, blood samples should be sent for analysis for HAAb. Three tests are currently used for the detection with HAAb: platelet aggregation, enzyme-linked immunosorbent assay (ELISA), and serotonin release assay.

The platelet aggregation study is a reliable and widely used test for HAAb. When properly done, aggregation testing establishes the presence of HAAb.[9] It is not generally appreciated that if the patient has sufficient circulating heparin to bind the antibodies, the aggregation test may be negative. Our routine includes daily repeat aggregation studies on suspected patients with negative tests. If the aggregation test remains negative at 96 hr, the patient does not have HIT and may receive heparin if there is indication to continue heparin therapy. We currently test all patients with HAAb against beef and pork unfractionated heparin, dalteparin, and enoxaparin low molecular weight heparins (LMWH), and danaparoid; we often find that the patients' antibodies do not react to all of these anticoagulants.

Although several ELISA assays have been developed to test for HAAb, they are not widely used. We have not found good correlation between ELISA assays and platelet aggregation assays. The serotonin release assay is a sensitive method to determine the presence of HAAb. The difficulty in performing this procedure and the use of radioactive substrates have impeded the widespread use of this method of testing for HAAb.

MANAGEMENT OF HIT

When it is suspected that a patient has HIT, all sources of heparin, including heparin-coated catheters, should be eliminated. A prompt increase in the platelet count suggests the presence of HIT. A positive aggregation test confirms the presence of HAAb. If the patient is HAAb negative, the clinician should search for other reasons for the thrombocytopenia. When continued anticoagulation is needed, the patient is HAAb positive, and anticoagulation with warfarin is not appropriate, alternate forms of anticoagulation are used. These alternate forms include nonreactive LMWH and heparinoids, direct thrombin inhibitors, defibrinogenating agents, and platelet function inhibitors.

If the patient does not require immediate anticoagulation and the diagnostic or surgical procedure can be deferred until the heparin antibodies are no longer present, the patient then safely tolerates, at least, a brief exposure to heparin. We have usually combined this brief exposure to heparin with a platelet function inhibitor (aspirin).[10] It should be noted that although the heparin antibodies tend to disappear in a few weeks to months (like most drug-induced antibodies), we have had a few patients whose antibodies have persisted for years (one patient up to 13 yr) without reexposure to heparin. We recommend that all patients with a history of HAAb be retested for HAAb prior to receiving heparin.

HEPARIN SUBSTITUTES

The LMWH are effective, rapid anticoagulants, and have been used successfully in patients with HIT. Unfortunately, the LMWHs can also react with the HAAb and must be tested against the patient's HAAb before being administered to the patient. We have found the cross-reactivity with enoxaparin to be 34%[11] and dalteparin to be 25.5%.[12] HIT patients who do not cross-react with LMWH can be effectively and safely treated with them.

Danaparoid is a heparinoid compound that is a mix of low molecular weight glycosaminoglycans derived from porcine intestine mucosa. It contains approximately 84% heparan sulfate, 12% dermatan sulfate, and 4% chondroitin sulfate. Danaparoid, like LMWH, predominately inhibits factor Xa but also inhibits, to a lesser degree, factor IIa. Numerous studies have demonstrated danaparoid's effectiveness as an anticoagulant in HIT. One study of 42 patients with HIT reported effective anticoagulation, with 2 related deaths and 3 major hemorrhagic complications (2 patients were also receiving aspirin). The authors concluded that danaparoid was a safe and effective agent for managing patients with HIT.[13] However, because of its potential cross-reaction with HAAb and its long half-life (24 hr), danaparoid is not the ideal anticoagulant for patients with HIT.

DIRECT THROMBIN INHIBITORS

Two direct thrombin inhibitors, lepirudin and argatroban, have been evaluated as anticoagulants in patients with HIT. Lepirudin, a recombinant form of the medicinal leech salivary protein hirudin, was approved for use by the FDA for use in patients with HIT in March 1998. Lepirudin does not require cofactors and is not inhibited by platelet factor IV. These characteristics allow it to act on clot-bound thrombin as well as free thrombin. Presently, there is no antidote for lepirudin. About 40% of patients receiving lepirudin develop an antibody to it that may prolong the activated partial thromboplastin time (aPTT) by reducing the rate of metabolism of lepirudin.[14]

Lepirudin is a 65 amino-acid polypeptide with a molecular weight of 6979 daltons. The circulating half-life of lepirudin is 1.3 hr. Lepirudin is excreted by the kidneys, and dosage must be reduced accordingly in patients with poor renal function. The functional level of anticoagulation is measured with the aPTT, with the goal being prolongation of the aPTT to 1.5 to 2.5 times the control. Lepirudin has been shown to be effective as an anticoagulant in numerous clinical situations, including dialysis, cardiopulmonary bypass, management of venous thromboembolism, and so on.

Fourteen of our patients, 12 of whom were HAAb positive, have received lepirudin. One of the other two patients had a platelet thrombus but did not have HAAb, whereas the other patient had a history of HIT but was currently HAAb negative. Thrombocytopenia promptly resolved in all of these patients; there were no hemorrhagic or thromboembolic complications. Two of the 14 patients received lepirudin during subsequent hospitalizations without complications. We have found lepirudin to be an effective anticoagulant in patients with HIT.

Argatroban, a synthetic analog of hirudin, has recently (June 30, 2000) received FDA approval for managing HIT. It is a small polypeptide with low antigenicity. It has normal excretion in patients with renal dysfunction and may have a greater role in these patients than does lepirudin. Patients with hepatic insufficiency may require reduced dosing.

PLATELET FUNCTION INHIBITORS

Prior to the development of alternate anticoagulants, patients with HIT were treated successfully with platelet function inhibiting agents and limited exposure to heparin. These patients had fewer complications than patients not treated with antiplatelet agents and normal heparin dosage.[10]

Various antiplatelet medications have been evaluated in the treatment of HIT. Aspirin, dipyridamole, and clopidogrel have marginal effect when used alone in patients with HIT because they do not effectively block platelet activation by HAAb. Aspirin, when used in conjunction with danaparoid, has been shown to increase hemorrhagic complications.[13] At high doses, the ADP receptor inhibitor ticlodipine has been shown to reduce platelet aggregation in serum from patients with HIT.[15]

The glycoprotein IIb/IIIa (GP IIb/IIIa) inhibitors may be useful in the treatment of HIT. These drugs block the binding of fibrinogen to platelets and decrease thrombin generation by inhibiting the exposure of procoagulant phospholipid surfaces by platelets.[16] Platelet activation in patients with strong reactivity to heparin is incompletely blocked by GP IIb/IIIa inhibitors as the platelet response in HIT is mediated via the FcγIIa receptor, not the GPIIb/IIIa receptor. GP IIb/IIIa inhibitors have been used in patients with HIT undergoing cardiopulmonary bypass as well as patients with HIT undergoing heart catherization with good results.

Several GPIIb/IIIa inhibitors are available in the United States. Abciximab is a monoclonal antibody to the GPIIb/IIIa receptor with a cleaved Fc portion. Both eptifibatide and tirofiban are peptides that bind to the GPIIb/IIIa receptor. All GPIIb/IIIa inhibitors have complications of bleeding and thrombocytopenia.

OTHER THERAPEUTIC AGENTS

Ancrod, a defibrinogenating agent derived from the Malayan pit viper, has been used to manage HIT.[16] It cleaves fibrinopeptide A from fibrinogen leaving an unstable fibrin compound that is rapidly cleared from the circulation. This drug does not stop, and may even increase, thrombin generation.[17] Studies have shown that ancrod is less effective than danaparoid in preventing thromboembolic complications in patients with HIT.[17] Anticoagulation with ancrod cannot be achieved rapidly, and neutralizing antibodies may develop during this period.[18] Ancrod is not presently approved by the FDA for use in HIT.

Immunoglobulin G has been administered to patients with HIT. High doses of IgG theoretically bind competitively to the platelet FcγIIa receptor, thereby preventing platelet aggregation and activation. No large study has been performed to show its safety and efficacy for routine use in HIT.

Warfarin, an oral vitamin K analog, should not be used as the sole anticoagulant in patients recently diagnosed with HIT. Treatment with warfarin alone may lead to an acute protein C deficiency that contributes to a hypercoaguable state. Warfarin anticoagulation should be started only in conjunction with another agent that provides short-term anticoagulation while the therapeutic effects of warfarin commence to prevent development of a hypercoaguable state.

SUMMARY

From 2% to 4% of patients receiving heparin develop HAAb and are at risk for developing HIT, which may be the most common hypercoagulable disorder encountered in vascular surgery patients. If a patient with HAAb receives a heparin to which he/she is sensitive, the patient is at risk for developing HIT. Therefore, all patients receiving heparin should be monitored for the development of HIT (usually with platelet counts). When HIT is suspected, heparin therapy should be discontinued and the patient tested for HAAb. If the patient is HAAb negative, heparin can be safely given. If the patient has HAAb, management options include: (1) withholding heparin until the antibodies are no longer present; (2) blocking platelet function and offering a brief exposure to heparin; (3) offering the patient a heparin (usually a LMWH) or heparinoid to which he/she is not sensitive; or (4) offering the patient a thrombin inhibitor, such as lepirudin. Our current choice is to offer lepirudin to the patient with HAAb who requires rapid anticoagulation.

REFERENCES

1. Copley AL, Robb TP. The effect of heparin on the platelet count in dogs and mice. *Am J Phys.* 1941;133:248.
2. Gollub S, Ulin AW. Heparin-induced thrombocytopenia in man. *J Lab Clin Med.* 1962; 59:430–435.
3. Johnson RA, Lazarus KH, Henry DH. Heparin-induced thrombocytopenia: a prospective study. *Am J Hematol.* 1984;17(4):349–353.
4. Rhodes GR, Dixon RH, Silver D. Heparin-induced thrombocytopenia with thrombotic and hemorrhagic manifestations. *Surg Gynecol Obstet.* 1973;136(3):409–416.
5. Silver D, Kapsch DN, Tsoi EK. Heparin-induced thrombocytopenia, thrombosis, and hemorrhage. *Ann Surg.* 1983;198(3):301–306.
6. Almeida JI, Coats R, Liem TK, Silver D. Reduced morbidity and mortality rates of the heparin-induced thrombocytopenia. *J Vasc Surg.* 1998;27(2);309–314.

7. Walls JT, Curtis JJ, Silver D, Boley TM. Heparin-induced thrombocytopenia in patients who undergo open heart surgery. *Surgery.* 1990;108(4):686–693.
8. Calaitges JG, Liem TK, Spadone D, Nichols WK, Silver D. The role of heparin-associated antiplatelet antibodies in the outcome of arterial reconstruction. *J Vasc Surg.* 1999;29(5):779–786.
9. Kapsch DN, Adelstein EH, Rhodes GR, Silver D. Heparin-induced thrombocytopenia, thrombosis, and hemorrhage. *Surgery.* 1979;86(1):148–155.
10. Laster J, Elfrink R, Silver D. Reexposure to heparin of patients with heparin-associated antibodies. *J Vasc Surg.* 1989;9(5):677–682.
11. Slocum MM, Adams JG Jr, Teel R, Spadone DP, Silver D. Use of enoxaparin in patients with heparin-induced thrombocytopenia syndrome. *J Vasc Surg.* 1996;23(5):839–843.
12. Kikta MJ, Keller MP, Humphrey PW, Silver D. Can low molecular weight heparins and heparinoids be safely given to patients with heparin-induced thrombocytopenia syndrome? *Surgery.* 1993;114(4):705–710.
13. Tardy-Poncet B, Tardy B, Reynaud J, et al. Efficacy and safety of danaparoid sodium (ORG 10172) in critically ill patients with heparin-associated thrombocytopenia. *Chest.* 1999;115(6): 1616–1620.
14. Huhle G, Hoffmann U, Song X, Wang LC, Heene DL, Harenberg J. Immunologic response to recombinant hirudin in HIT type II patients during long-term treatment. *Br J Haem.* 1999; 106(1):195–201.
15. Polgar J, Eichler P, Greinacher A, Clemetson KJ. Adenosine diphosphate (ADP) and ADP receptor play a major role in platelet activation/aggregation induced by serum from heparin-induced thrombocytopenia patients. *Blood.* 1998;91(2):549–554.
16. Demers C, Ginsberg JS, Brill-Edwards P, et al. Rapid anticoagulation using ancrod for heparin-induced thrombocytopenia. *Blood.* 1992;79(9):2194–2197.
17. Warkentin TE. Limitations of conventional treatment options for heparin-induced thrombocytopenia. *Semin Hematol.* 1998;35(4 suppl 5):17–25.
18. Greinacher A. Treatment of heparin-induced thrombocytopenia. *Thromb Hemost.* 1999;82(2): 457–467.

40

New Anticoagulants

Michael Sobel, MD

WHY ANTICOAGULANTS?

Since the first published use of heparin in arterial surgery in the late 1940s, heparin has been used routinely to prevent thrombosis during the temporary interruption of blood flow in vascular surgery. This is the primary use of heparin by vascular surgeons. Even though efficacy has never been proved in clinical trials, this use of heparin has withstood the test of time. A second major use for anticoagulants like heparin is the treatment of arterial and venous thromboembolism. A third important use for anticoagulants is the prevention of postoperative thrombosis. The optimal methods to prevent postoperative venous thromboembolism have been studied thoroughly. Unfortunately, however, less is known about the ideal antithrombotic regimen to prevent thrombosis of vascular reconstructions in the perioperative period. The new anticoagulants coming into use share the dilemma of heparin—where is the optimal balance between efficacy and bleeding complications? Can new anticoagulants offer a safer balance?

NEW ANTICOAGULANTS OF THE PLASMA COAGULATION CASCADE

Table 40–1 and the following discussion outline the general characteristics of new anticoagulants, beginning with the most familiar types. All but argatroban are currently approved by the FDA. Because of the clinical diversity of indications and applications, only general dosing guidelines are provided here. Clinicians should consult the most recent manufacturer's guidelines before prescribing.

Low Molecular Weight Heparin

Low molecular weight heparins (LMWH) bear the closest resemblance to conventional heparin. They all belong to the family of glycosaminoglycans—long-chain carbohydrate

TABLE 40–1. GENERAL CHARACTERISTICS OF NEW ANTICOAGULANTS

Anticoagulant	Mechanism of Action	Monitoring	Pharmacokinetics`	Antidote
Low molecular weight heparins	Catalyzes antithrombin III neutralization of factor Xa	Empiric dosing; may monitor anti-factor Xa levels	$T_{1/2}$ ~2–4 hr intravenous ~3–6 hr subcutaneously	Protamine may be partially effective
Danaparoid	Glycosaminoglycan mixture that catalyzes antithrombin III and heparin cofactor II	Plasma anti-factor Xa levels	$T_{1/2}$ >12 hr; renal metabolism requires adjustment of dosage	Protamine may be partially effective
Lepirudin	Recombinant hirudin that directly neutralizes thrombin	aPTT, ACT	$T_{1/2}$ ~1.5 hr intravenous; renal metabolism requires adjustment of dosage	None
Argatroban	Small molecular weight synthetic thrombin inhibitor	aPTT, ACT	$T_{1/2}$ <1 hr intravenous; no adjustments needed for renal failure	None

aPTT = activated partial thromboplastin time; ACT = activated clotting time.

polymers with heterogeneous patterns of sulfation. LMWHs are manufactured by depolymerization of the conventional, "unfractionated," pharmaceutical heparins we customarily use and are still heterogeneous in size and structure, but their molecular mass is typically one-half that of standard heparin. Different brands of LMWHs are physicochemically distinct because methods of digestion and refinement differ. Like all true heparins, LMWHs exert their main anticoagulant effects through plasma cofactors. Heparins bind to antithrombin III (and, to a lesser extent, heparin cofactor II), thus accelerating the neutralization of activated factors X (Xa) and thrombin (IIa), as well as other factors. The original hope for LMWHs was that by making smaller, biologically active heparin units, it would be possible to disassociate their antithrombotic properties from their hemorrhagic properties. Targeting the inhibition of factor Xa (positioned earlier in the cascade) might strategically prevent thrombosis with less risk of bleeding. Targeting thrombin activity certainly yields an effective anticoagulant, but theoretically at a higher risk of hemorrhage. The key difference between LMWHs and conventional heparin is that LMWHs have a proportionately greater inhibitory potency against factor Xa than against factor IIa (thrombin). In contrast, longer polymer length heparins have a superiority in neutralizing thrombin. Figure 40–1 illustrates why this is so. In brief, the longer polymer length heparins have more efficient and cooperative interactions between antithrombin III and thrombin, an advantage that is lacking for short-chain heparins. In practice, the ratios of anti-Xa : anti-IIa activity for LMWHs are 2 to 3 times higher than for standard heparins.

This higher anti-Xa : IIa ratio of LMWHs may confer a greater efficacy in preventing thrombosis, but a lower risk of hemorrhage has not been borne out in clinical trials. Still, LMWHs have other benefits. Their smaller size improves absorption and bioavailability

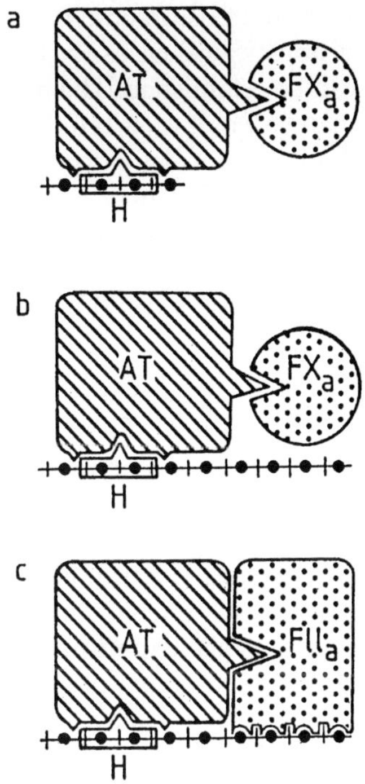

Figure 40–1. The interactions of antithrombin III (AT), standard or low-molecular-weight (LMW) heparins (H), with factor Xa (FX_a) and thrombin (FII_a).

and produces a more predictable anticoagulant response. LMWHs have fewer interactions with other vascular cells and cause less immune sensitization. Because of their more predictable, longer half-life, dosing can be less frequent, with less monitoring.

LMWHs only mildly prolong the activated partial thromboplastin time (aPTT) at high doses. For most venous indications, dosing is weight-based and monitoring is not required, but if desired, therapy can be monitored by laboratory measurement of plasma anti-factor Xa levels. The recommended therapeutic levels for venous thromboembolism are 0.3–0.6 anti-Xa units/mL plasma. LMWHs cannot be used safely to replace standard heparin in the syndrome of heparin-induced thrombocytopenia (HIT). Once the immune sensitization is established, LMWHs usually cross-react with a patient's antibodies and can perpetuate the thrombotic syndrome.

Danaparoid

Orgaran (danaparoid sodium, Org10172, Organon, Inc.) is a heparinoid, a mixture of heparin-like polysaccharides (heparans, dermatans, and chondroitins). It is also a glycosaminoglycan but structurally distinct enough from regular heparins that immune cross-reactivity is low *in vitro* and negligible in clinical use. Although it has been used widely in Europe for a range of indications, its niche in North America is primarily as a substitute for heparin in cases of HIT. Given intravenously or subcutaneously, danaparoid is used like heparin and feels familiar to clinicians. For an acute arterial intervention like embolectomy, a typical intravenous dose would be a bolus of 2500 U followed by a tapering continuous infusion of 150–400 U/hr in the postoperative period. It can also be used intravenously or subcutaneously in nonsurgical cases for the intermediate term until oral anticoagulation with warfarin can be established. The duration of action of danaparoid is longer than heparin. More than half of it is excreted by the kidneys, so dosages must be adjusted in renal failure. Monitoring of drug dosages must be done by measuring plasma anti-factor Xa levels—a service that may not be readily available in all clinical laboratories. There is no official antidote for danaparoid, but protamine injection may partially neutralize its anticoagulant effects. In several large retrospective studies, treatment with danaparoid reduced the mortality and morbidity of HIT.

Thrombin Inhibitors

Instead of working through plasma cofactors, thrombin inhibitors bind and neutralize thrombin's coagulant activity directly. The model thrombin inhibitor is hirudin, a small protein discovered in the salivary gland of the leech. Hirudin is like a molecular mousetrap—it tenaciously binds thrombin at two different molecular sites (Figure 40–2). Hirudin derivatives produced by recombinant protein technology first attracted clinical attention in the treatment of unstable angina and coronary thrombosis. Experimental data suggested that the platelet-rich thrombi forming at unstable coronary plaques were resistant to conventional heparin anticoagulation. Thrombin activity may be an important factor in these arterial thrombi, and clot-bound thrombin may be relatively resistant to antithrombin-III/heparin. Indeed, hirudin derivatives were very effective at blocking this platelet and thrombin-dependent form of arterial thrombosis in experi-

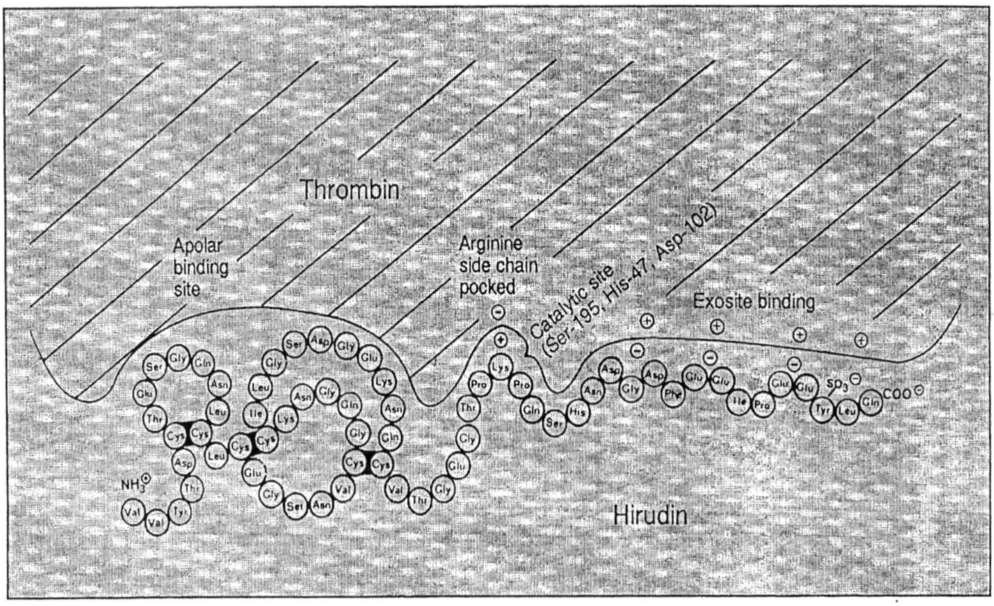

Figure 40–2. How hirudin interacts with two different sites on the thrombin molecule.

mental models. However, in clinical trials, the cost for a more potent anticoagulant was paid in bleeding complications. With fine-tuning of dosages, hirudin derivatives may be just as effective and as safe as heparin. However, hirudins and thrombin inhibitors are not yet widely accepted as primary therapy in acute coronary syndromes. Rather, these drugs have currently found a niche as replacements for heparin in HIT.

The anticoagulant effects of hirudins can be monitored by the aPTT or the activated clotting time (ACT), and they have a predictable dose–response relationship. Hirudins have little effect on the prothrombin time. A more obscure clotting test, the ecarin clotting time, can be adapted to measure drug levels more precisely. There is no antidote for hirudins, so when treatment is associated with surgery or invasive thrombolytic therapy, bleeding can be serious.

The one recombinant hirudin approved for vascular surgery is Refludan (lepirudin rDNA, Hoechst Marion Roussel, Kansas City, MO). For HIT, treatment with lepirudin was found to be an excellent alternative anticoagulant. A large prospective trial showed a 72% reduction in combined adverse events and a significant reduction in HIT-related morbidity and mortality compared to historical controls (25.4% vs. 52.1%). Lepirudin is given as an intravenous bolus (0.4 mg/kg) followed by a continuous infusion (0.15 mg/kg/hr). It has a short half-life like heparin, and dose adjustments must be made in renal failure. The hirudin family of drugs are extremely potent anticoagulants, and bleeding complications can occur, especially in patients with renal failure. Lepirudin has primarily been used in the treatment of nonsurgical patients with HIT. There has been limited experience in cardiopulmonary bypass and still less in peripheral vascular surgery. Thus, dosage guidelines are not as well established for episodic, acute, short-term anticoagulation.

In our own experience with the drug during vascular surgery, we found that bedside (point-of-care) coagulation testing systems are invaluable for providing rapid feedback and tight control of the intensity of anticoagulation perioperatively. Figure 40–3 illustrates the case of a patient with confirmed HIT undergoing aortic aneurysm repair Because of renal insufficiency and concern for perioperative bleeding, a reduced dose of lepirudin (0.1 mg/kg) was given as an intravenous bolus, and the responses of the aPTT and ACT were measured in OR with point-of-care testing apparatus. Those results revealed that the initial dose had not achieved the desired intensity of anticoagulation, so a second dose was given, and the response monitored. Then, the aorta was cross-clamped and the aneurysm repair proceeded. Of note, even 4 hr after lepirudin administration the clotting times had not returned to baseline, although there was no pathologic bleeding.

Argatroban (Novastan, Texas Biotechnology, Houston, TX) is the leading synthetic thrombin inhibitor undergoing trials and is still awaiting FDA approval. This small synthetic molecule binds directly to the active enzymatic site of thrombin (hirudin binds there, plus at an extra site). Thus, argatroban's affinity and specificity for thrombin are slightly less than hirudin. Because it is a small synthetic molecule, it has a short plasma half-life. Dosages do not need to be adjusted for renal failure, and it is likely to be less immunogenic than the hirudin protein. It is a highly effective anticoagulant that, like hirudin, prolongs conventional clotting assays in a predictable, dose-dependent manner.

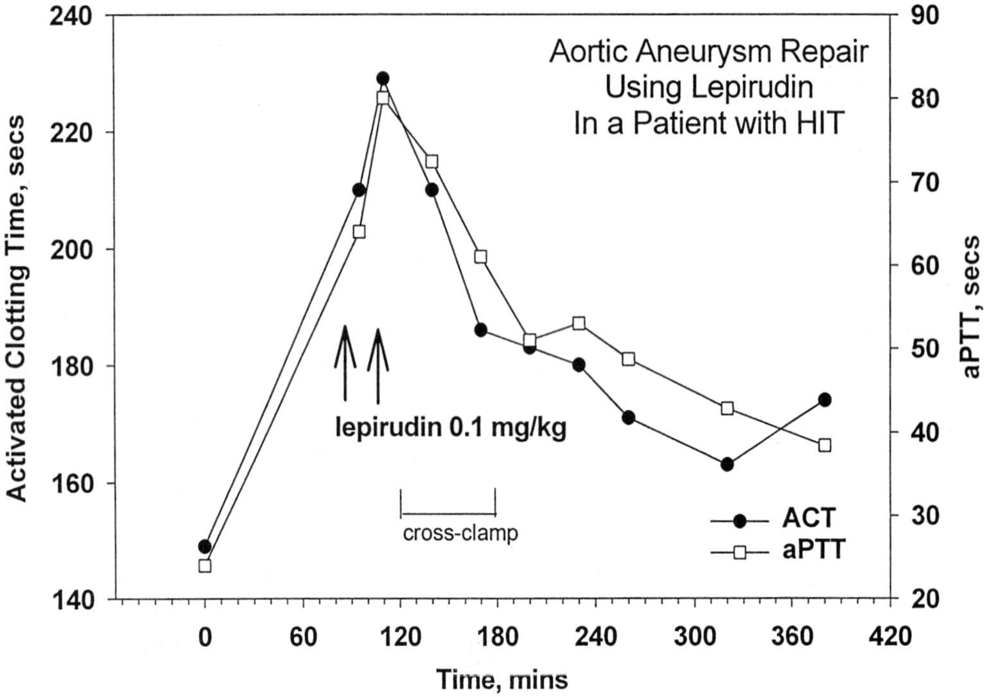

Figure 40–3. Anticoagulant responses to lepirudin during aortic aneurysm repair.

Platelet Receptor Antagonists

Platelet receptor antagonist drugs are no longer new, nor can they be properly considered anticoagulants. However, they are worthy of mention because they represent a unique and extremely potent class of antithrombotic drugs whose applications have not yet entered the realm of vascular surgery practice. This group of drugs shares a basic mechanism of action: They prevent glycoprotein IIb/IIIa, the principal platelet receptor, from binding fibrinogen, the main ligand for platelet aggregation. Platelets have a diversity of interrelated activation pathways; this is why platelet inhibitors such as aspirin or ticlopidine, which target only a single pathway, are only partially effective. The receptor antagonists have the advantage of blocking the final common pathway to which almost all routes of activation lead: the aggregation and consolidation of a platelet thrombus requires fibrinogen binding to this integrin receptor. Rheopro (abciximab, Centocor) is a chimeric, humanized mouse monoclonal antibody that blocks GpIIb/IIIa. At doses of 0.25 mg/kg IV bolus followed by 10 μg/min for 12 hr, more than 80% of GpIIb/IIIa receptors are blocked and platelet aggregation is reduced to <20% of normal. In acute coronary syndromes and interventions, the addition of abciximab treatment offers a 35% to 50% risk reduction for most thrombotic clinical endpoints. The antibody-induced platelet inhibition lasts for several days. Eptifibatide (Integrilin, COR Therapeutics) and tirofiban (Aggrastat, Merck) are both potent intravenous agents that block fibrinogen binding by occupying the receptor with a synthetic peptide or nonpeptide mimetic of fibrinogen. These drugs vary in their half-lives, their selectivity for the platelet integrin receptor, and the incidence of immune sensitization and thrombocytopenia. Such profound platelet inhibition carries an increased risk for hemorrhage, particularly when combined with liberal heparin anticoagulation after arterial procedures. Finally, orally active versions of these receptor antagonists are in clinical trials.

INDICATIONS AND OPPORTUNITIES FOR NEW ANTITHROMBOTIC DRUGS

Prevention or Treatment of Venous Thromboembolism

The LMWHs have excelled in the prophylaxis of postoperative venous thromboembolism, especially in the high-risk patient. A few trials have also suggested that hirudin may be an effective prophylatic drug, but it is not widely accepted. In the treatment of deep venous thrombosis (DVT), LMWH has been shown to be equivalent but not superior to conventional intravenous heparin. Both danaparoid and thrombin inhibitors can also be used with success to acutely treat venous thromboembolism while warfarin therapy is being instituted.

Direct Substitutes for Heparin

If a patient cannot receive heparin because of bleeding risks, then thrombin inhibitors or heparinoids should not be given either. The need for heparin substitutes arises most often when patients develop HIT. To make a firm diagnosis of HIT, Warkentin suggests a patient should have at least one key clinical characteristic and one confirmatory laboratory test. Key clinical signs include unexpected thrombocytopenia, pathologic thrombosis, heparin-induced skin lesions, or an anaphylactoid response to intravenous heparin. Acceptable laboratory tests include the detection of antibodies that activate/aggregate platelets in the presence of heparin or antibodies that recognize the prime antigen, a complex of heparin and platelet factor 4 (PF4, a secreted platelet protein). Once acquired, these antibodies can activate the platelet through its Fc receptor and may also activate endothelial cells.

Most HIT patients should be treated with an alternative anticoagulant, if it can be safely done. Depending on clinical circumstances, this acute anticoagulation with a heparin alternative may be followed by chronic oral anticoagulation with warfarin. There are two major justifications for using an alternative to heparin. First, many HIT patients already have a thrombotic condition; second, HIT is a hypercoagulable state. Even uncomplicated cases with thrombocytopenia alone may later evolve serious thrombotic complications. Treatment with an alternative anticoagulant appears to reduce mortality and morbidity from HIT, regardless of whether their initial presentation was accompanied by thrombosis. In the postoperative state, vascular patients with HIT are up to three times more liable to experience thrombosis of their vascular reconstruction. It is admittedly hard to prescribe a detailed program of management for this heterogeneous group of patients, especially considering that the prevention of thrombosis must be balanced in each case with the risks of postoperative hemorrhage. In all cases, avoidance of heparin exposure is essential; this includes all forms of heparin via all routes.

For the elective preoperative patient with a distant past history of HIT who is now quiescent with a normal platelet count, one can use intravenous boluses and infusions of danaparoid or a thrombin inhibitor as one would use heparin to prevent thrombosis during the vascular surgery. Postoperatively, one might continue lower doses of the alternative anticoagulant for 5 to 7 days. The patient with acute HIT (with or without thrombosis) should be immediately anticoagulated with danaparoid or a thrombin inhibitor. This anticoagulation should be continued for 5 to 7 days until platelet counts have recovered. If vascular surgery is necessary, adjust the intensity of the alternative anticoagulation as appropriate during the perioperative period using bedside monitoring. Continue anticoagulation postoperatively, and consider converting to warfarin, according to the risks of thrombosis.

Prevention of Arterial Thrombosis and Early Graft Failure

Besides aspirin and warfarin, few drugs have proved to be very effective in preventing arterial thrombosis over the long term or in reducing the early closure rate of thrombosis-prone vascular grafts. Less is known about the optimal roles for LMWHs on the arterial side. LMWHs have shown hints of efficacy in preventing thrombotic events in the coronary circulation; therefore, might they be effective in preventing vascular graft closure in the postoperative period? The data so far are inconclusive. The family of platelet receptor antagonist drugs are the most potent inhibitors of platelet function and may have some role in preventing platelet-dominated thrombosis in vascular surgery. *In vitro*, abciximab can totally block the antibody-induced platelet aggregation seen in HIT, although its clinical effectiveness has not been proved. Platelet receptor antagonists may offer some value as pharmacologic adjuncts to high-risk peripheral angioplasty or adjuncts for thrombosis-prone vascular surgical reconstructions. Also, chronic oral therapy with receptor antagonists may improve graft patency. However, these indications are still speculative. The bleeding risks are unknown and may be high. We have now entered a new era in which novel compounds target specific proteins and receptors. The true value of these new anticoagulants will be discovered through carefully conducted clinical trials. We look forward to them.

BIBLIOGRAPHY

Chong PH. Glycoprotein IIb/IIIa receptor antagonists in the management of cardiovascular diseases. *Am J Health Syst Pharm*. 1998;55:2363–2386.

Hirsh J, Warkentin TE, Raschke RA, et al. Heparin and low-molecular-weight heparin. Mechanisms of action, pharmacokinetics, dosing considerations, monitoring, efficacy, and safety. *Chest*. 1998;114:489S–510S.

Hirsh J, Weitz JI. New antithrombotic agents. *Lancet*. 1999;353:(9162)1431–1436.

Greinacher A, Volpel H, Janssens U, et al. Recombinant hirudin (lepirudin) provides safe and effective anticoagulation in patients with heparin-induced thromboyctopenia: a prospective study. *Circulation*. 1999;99:73–80.

Koster A, Kuppe H, Crystal GJ, Mertzlufft F. Cardiovascular surgery without cardiopulmonary bypass in patients with heparin-induced thrombocytopenia type II using anticoagulation with recombinant hirudin. *Anesth Analg.* 2000;90:292–303.

Magnani HN. Heparin-induced thrombocytopenia (HIT): an overview of 230 patients treated with Orgaran (Org 10172.). *Thromb Haemo.* 1993;70:554–561.

Neuhaus KL. New antithrombotic and antiplatelet treatment. *Heart.* 1999;82(1S): 8I–11I.

Warkentin TE. Heparin-induced thrombocytopenia: A ten year retrospective. *Ann Rev Med.* 1999;50:129–147.

Watson HR, Belcher G, Horrocks M. Adjuvant medical therapy in peripheral bypass surgery. *Br J Surg.* 1999;86:981–991.

Wilde MI, Markham A. Danaparoid. A review of its pharmacology and clinical use in the management of heparin-induced thrombocytopenia. *Drugs.* 1997;54:903–924.

Yeghiazarians Y, Braunstein JB, Askari A, Stone PH. Medical progress: unstable angina pectoris. *N Engl J Med.* 2000;342:101–114.

41

Thrombolytic Therapy in the Post-Urokinase Era

Anthony J. Comerota, MD, FACS, and Lori I. Cindrick, MD

INTRODUCTION

Plasminogen activators have played an important role in the treatment of patients with thrombotic/thromboembolic vascular disease. Vascular surgeons and vascular interventionalists have assumed the responsibility to care for these acute and subacute arterial and venous thrombotic complications.

Streptokinase (SK) and subsequently urokinase (UK) were the first two plasminogen activators to be used clinically and were initially approved for the treatment of pulmonary embolism.

Vascular surgeons and interventional radiologists began using streptokinase for arterial thrombotic/embolic occlusions in the late 1970s. They found that direct catheter delivery was more effective than systemic infusion. The allergic and bleeding complications of streptokinase caused physicians to evaluate urokinase as a potential alternative. The collective experience demonstrated that urokinase was a safer and more effective alternative for the treatment of acute arterial and graft occlusion, and was rapidly adopted as the preferred lytic agent for catheter-directed thrombolysis.

Recombinant tissue plasminogen activator (rtPA) was developed and studied in patients suffering acute myocardial infarction (MI). The benefits of the use of plasminogen activators in patients with acute MI became readily apparent. Prior to the thrombolytic era, the 30-day mortality of patients with acute MI was approximately 13%. Since thrombolytic agents have demonstrated that early coronary reperfusion can be achieved, the 30-day mortality of acute MI has decreased by 50%. The benefits of thrombolytic therapy result from rapid reperfusion of the infarct-related artery, which limits infarct size, reduces left ventricular dysfunction, and thereby improves survival.

The numbers of patients entered into trials of thrombolytic therapy for acute myocardial infarction number in the hundreds of thousands. Unfortunately, we who take care of patients with acute peripheral vascular thromboembolic complications do not have the same patient database to draw on. Our collective experience, however, has demonstrated that appropriate use of thrombolytic therapy is an important part of the strategy of management of these patients.

During the late 1980s and throughout the 1990s, urokinase has been the preferred agent for vascular surgeons and vascular interventionalists for the majority of these problems. Contemporary urokinase was manufactured from isolates of human fetal kidney cells. The manufacturing process came under scrutiny by the US Food and Drug Administration (FDA), which recognized deficiencies that might increase the risk of virally transmitted diseases. As a result of concerns about the manufacturing process, urokinase was removed from the market by the FDA.[1]

This chapter addresses the most common peripheral vascular thromboembolic disorders faced by vascular surgeons and vascular interventionalists and how they are being managed in the post-urokinase era. Background information with UK is provided as a basis for comparison. These include:

- Acute arterial and graft occlusion
- Intraoperative intra-arterial lytic therapy
- Thrombosed dialysis access
- Pulmonary embolism
- Deep venous thrombosis (DVT)/iliofemoral DVT
- Axillosubclavian DVT
- Catheter clearance

Before addressing these indications, a short review of the available thrombolytic agents and those likely to be approved by the FDA in the near future seems appropriate.

THROMBOLYTIC AGENTS

Streptokinase

Streptokinase (SK) is a single-chain nonenzymatic protein produced by β-hemolytic streptococci. SK is an indirect activator of plasminogen. It complexes with circulating plasminogen to form the SK–plasminogen complex, which then activates plasminogen.[2]

The half-life of streptokinase is biphasic, one at 16 and one at approximately 80 min. The dose–response relationship of SK appears to vary between patients. The disadvantages of streptokinase have been the observed bleeding complications as well as the pyretic and allergic reactions to the streptococcal antigen.

Urokinase

Urokinase is a serine protease that activates plasminogen directly. It was initially considered to be nonantigenic; however, recent pyretic responses have been observed and are thought to be related to interleukins present that may result from the manufacturing process. Urokinase cleaves plasminogen to plasmin by first-order reaction kinetics. A single bolus of urokinase given intravenously in humans is cleared with a half-life of approximately 14 min, most of which is degraded to inert metabolites by the liver.[3]

Recombinant Tissue Plasminogen Activator

Tissue plasminogen activator (like urokinase) is a naturally occurring activator of plasminogen that has an important physiologic role in the regulation of hemostasis and fibrinolysis. It is normally produced and released by vascular endothelial cells. With the use of recombinant DNA technology, tissue plasminogen activator (tPA) is now genetically produced. Because rtPA is identical to the naturally occurring human tissue plasminogen activator, it is essentially nonantigenic.

Recombinant tissue plasminogen activator has high-affinity binding for fibrin. The activity of rtPA is enhanced by fibrin, and this fibrin specificity should lead to plasminogen activation primarily at the thrombus level.[4]

Tissue plasminogen activator appears to be cleared through the liver, and has a half-life of 3.5 to 4 min.

Reteplase

Reteplase is a new plasminogen activator that was approved for the treatment of acute MI.[5] It is produced by recombinant DNA technology and has a half-life of approximately 19 min. It was specifically designed to be used as bolus therapy (instead of continuous infusion) for acute MI. Reteplase has been used in patients with arterial and venous thromboembolic complications; however, less experience is available with reteplase than with other lytic agents.

Prourokinase

Prourokinase is a zymogen that is inert in circulating plasma. In the presence of fibrin clot, pro-UK becomes active and induces plasminogen activation. Therefore, recombinant prourokinase is a highly fibrin-specific plasminogen activator. In the presence of fibrin, pro-UK is converted to an active, two-chain UK. The freshly generated UK converts plasminogen to plasmin.[6]

It was initially thought that the development of fibrin-specific plasminogen activators would reduce the incidence of distant bleeding complications. It is likely that this was an unrealistic expectation because these agents bind to the hemostatic fibrin plugs that seal vascular defects anywhere in the body. Available data do not support the premise that high-fibrin specificity/avidity reduces bleeding complications.

Tenecteplase

Tenecteplase (TNK-tPA) is a new thrombolytic agent that is a genetically engineered variant of tPA. TNK-tPA is similar to the wild type tPA with amino acid substitutions at 3 different sites on the molecule. This modification leads to a prolonged half-life of the molecule, increased fibrin specificity and increased resistance to inhibition by the circulating plasminogen activator inhibitor−1 (PAI-1).[7]

The plasma half-life of TNK-tPA is approximately the same as reteplase, 14 to 19 min. TNK-tPA is more fibrin specific than rtPA. System fibrinogen and plasminogen levels are much less affected with TNK-tPA compared to the changes observed with rtPA.

It is anticipated that TNK-tPA will be approved by the FDA for the treatment of acute MI using a bolus dose of 30 or 40 mg. The potential advantages of an agent with this high degree of fibrin specificity for patients with peripheral arterial and venous thrombotic occlusion remains to be delineated.

CLINICAL USE OF THROMBOLYTIC THERAPY

Acute Arterial and Graft Occlusion

Vascular surgeons and vascular interventionalists have appreciated the benefits of catheter-directed thrombolysis for the management of acute arterial and graft occlusion. Unfortunately, prospective randomized trials have not demonstrated superiority of thrombolytic agents compared to surgical intervention.[8–10]

Single center studies have demonstrated improved amputation-free survival with catheter-directed thrombolysis for acute arterial occlusion, but no difference in limb salvage.[11]

A subset analysis from the STILE trial demonstrated that patients randomized with acute limb ischemia ($\leq$14 days) had significantly improved limb salvage.[8] There was a significant reduction in the need for surgical intervention, and the duration of hospitalization for patients with acute limb ischemia was shorter for patients randomized to lytic therapy than patients randomized to surgical therapy. The benefits observed in patients with acute limb ischemia were essentially those resulting from patients who had acute graft thrombosis.[12] Because thrombolytic patients entered into the STILE trial were randomized to urokinase or rtPA, this database offered an opportunity to evaluate objectively the efficacy and safety of rtPA compared to UK in similar patients; therefore, the data were recently reanalyzed in greater detail.

The composite clinical outcome was the major end-point evaluated, which included death, major limb amputation, ongoing or recurrent ischemia, and major morbidity (which included bleeding). There was no difference in the composite clinical outcome or any of individual the variables in the patients treated with rtPA compared to those treated with UK.

During the course of the STILE trial, the dose of rtPA was changed from 0.1 mg/kg/hr $\times$ 12 hr to 0.05 mg/kg/hr $\times$ 12 hr. When the higher and the lower doses were compared, there was no difference in efficacy or bleeding complications.

Interestingly, the use of heparin was found to significantly improve efficacy of both UK and rtPA compared to patients who did not receive heparin.

Recent experience has demonstrated that once reconstituted, rtPA can be diluted and delivered in much lower doses than previously anticipated. This observation has led to revised dosage schemes in most centers. We currently treat patients with a 2 to 4 mg bolus followed by 2 mg/hr via intrathrombus catheter delivery of rtPA. Lower doses are also being used with successful outcomes. Heparin is infused through the sheath at a dose of at least 500 U/hr. Observed efficacy and bleeding complications appear to be equivalent to that observed with UK.

A number of clinicians have used reteplase with good clinical results.[13,14] Davidian and colleagues[13] treated 15 patients with catheter-directed reteplase and reported a 73% clinical success rate treating patients with either 0.5 mg/hr or 1.0 mg/hr. The average duration of thrombolysis was 21 hr. Bleeding complications occurred in 12%, which included hemoptysis in 1 patient and a major retroperitoneal bleed in another. Mortality was 6%, and resulted from cardiac arrest and death in the patient suffering the retroperitoneal hemorrhage.

A randomized, double-blind, parallel multicenter trial of pro-UK versus UK in patients with acute arterial and graft occlusion was reported by Ouriel et al.[15] This trial compared three doses of intra-arterial, catheter-directed r-pro-UK (2, 4, or 8 mg/hr for 8 hr, then 0.5 mg/hr) versus one dose of UK (4000 IU/min for 4 hr, then 2000 IU/min) for the treatment of acute lower extremity arterial occlusion (≤14 days). Two hundred forty-one (241) patients were treated, with the primary end-point being complete (>95%) lysis of the occluding thrombus after 8 hr of infusion.

This well-designed and conducted trial demonstrated that the higher the dose of r-pro-UK used the better the lytic response. The frequency of achieving the primary endpoint at 8 hr increased from 39% with 2 mg r-pro-UK to 44% with 4 mg r-pro-UK to 56% with 8 mg r-pro-UK. Forty-nine percent (49%) of the UK group had complete clot lysis at 8 hr. Major bleeding complications were relatively low and were similar between all treatment groups, and as might be expected, the frequency of bleeding complications appeared to follow a dose–response relationship in the r-pro-UK groups.

Intraoperative Intra-Arterial Thrombolytic Therapy

Intraoperative intra-arterial thrombolytic therapy has been used to assist in clearing residual thrombus from the distal vasculature.[16,17] A randomized and blinded evaluation has shown that a bolus dose of 125,000, 250,000, or 500,000 units of UK into the distal arterial bed did not significantly reduce plasminogen or fibrinogen levels and was not associated with bleeding complications.[17] We have routinely used 250,000 units of UK intraoperatively when residual, distal thrombus was suspected following balloon-catheter thrombectomy.

Recombinant tissue plasminogen activator has been substituted during 1999. We used up to 5 mg of rtPA intraoperatively. Once reconstituted, the rtPA is diluted in normal saline to the desired volume. If infused into small arteries with a limited outflow bed (hand or foot), 2 to 5 mg in 3 to 5 cc is used. If a larger outflow bed requires perfusion, such as infusion into the popliteal, superficial femoral, or profunda femoris arteries, volumes of 25 to 50 cc have been used. Although efficacy is difficult to evaluate, we have not experienced additional bleeding complications with this regimen.

Thrombosed Hemodialysis Access

The construction of arteriovenous fistulae, either autogenous or prosthetic, for hemodialysis access is the most common vascular operation performed in the United States. Unfortunately, thrombosis is a major problem, and complications associated with arteriovenous access are the most frequent cause of hospitalization for patients on chronic hemodialysis. Put into perspective, approximately 1 mo of hospitalization each year is required for patients on hemodialysis, half of the time for placement or revision of their arteriovenous fistula. Preservation of each access site is critical to the patient's well-being and long-term care. Infusion of plasminogen activators into the thrombosed access graft has become the preferred method of treating an acutely thrombosed dialysis access. The crossed catheter technique with lacing of the thrombus of 250,000–500,000 IU of UK was widely accepted. The pulsed spray technique using concentrated UK represented an additional refinement over the crossed-catheter technique. Cynamon et al.[18] reported a multicenter randomized study comparing pulse–spray pharmacomechanical thrombolysis versus the "lyse and wait" technique. Eighty-eight patients (88) were randomized. They found that the "lyse and wait" approach was 20 min quicker than the pulsed spray approach with similar success and patency. The lyse and wait technique uses 6 mL of a plasminogen activator (250,000 U/UK, or 6 mg of rtPA) injected into the thrombosed graft via a 22-gauge angiocath. The mixture is allowed to remain in the graft for 30 to 60 min. Contrast evaluation at this point typically shows an underlying venous lesion and an arterial plug, with minimal or no residual clot in the graft. A Fogerty catheter is then used to manipulate the arterial plug and angioplasty of any existing venous stenosis is performed.

Two reports using reteplase showed excellent results. Gibbens et al[19] treated 64 patients with a crossed catheter infusion technique with 1.5 to 2.5 units per catheter. The majority of the patients underwent venous angioplasty subsequent to thrombolysis and 9 patients had stents placed at the venous anastomosis or in the outflow vein. The primary success rate was 98%, with patency at 1, 3, and 6 mo being 86%, 55%, and 27%, respectively.

Flick et al.[20] reported results from treating 18 patients with either 2 or 3 U or reteplase diluted in 7 cc of normal saline. All patients received 3000 U of heparin. Seventeen (17) of 18 grafts (94%) had perfusion restored with lysis and venous angioplasty. No patients experienced bleeding or embolic complications.

Pulmonary Embolism

The early trials of thrombolytic therapy for pulmonary embolism (PE) demonstrated early improvement in the lung scan, arteriographic findings, and pulmonary hemodynamics in patients treated with thrombolytic agents compared to standard anticoagulation alone. Because there was no reduction in overall mortality and the associated bleeding complications with lytic agents were greater than standard anticoagulation, lytic therapy for PE was not widely accepted.

The clinical trials performed in the 1980s and 1990s studied the hemodynamic effects of lytic therapy in patients with PE. These trials evaluated escalating doses of bolus infusions of plasminogen activators and compared those results to standard dose and prolonged infusion of plasminogen activators.

The development of newer lytic agents—specifically rtPA, which was not antigenic—generated an increased interest in the use of lytic agents for PE. Accelerated dosage regimens were explored in an effort to maximize lytic response and minimize bleeding complications.

Intravenous infusion of plasminogen activators remains the standard form of lytic therapy for acute PE. rtPA has been compared to standard-dose and high-dose UK in three prospective randomized trials. Goldhaber and colleagues[21] demonstrated improved early reperfusion with 100 mg of rtPA given over 2 hr compared to standard-dose UK (4400 U/kg bolus followed by 4400 U/kg over the next 12 hr). Interestingly, 9 of the 23 patients randomized to UK had their infusions prematurely terminated because of a significant allergy in 1 and bleeding complications in 8.

Meyer et al.[22] reported the results of a study comparing the rtPA regimen of a 10 mg bolus followed by 90 mg over the next 2 hr to urokinase given at 4400 U/kg bolus followed by 4400 U/kg over the next 12 hr. In the 63 patients randomized, the investigators found more rapid resolution at 2 hr in patients receiving rtPA; however, at the 12-hr time point, angiographic resolution and pulmonary vascular resistance was equivalent between the two groups. Bleeding complications were also equivalent. Goldhaber and colleagues[23] evaluated 100 mg of rtPA given over 2 hr compared to 3 million units of UK (1 million unit bolus followed by 2 million units over the next 2 hr). Repeat pulmonary angiograms demonstrated that 79% of rtPA patients and 67% of UK patients showed significant arteriographic improvement (P = NS). The mean change in lung scans was similar between the two groups at 24 hr. Goldhaber and colleagues[24] addressed the important question of whether thrombolytic therapy for PE improved right ventricular function and pulmonary perfusion compared to anticoagulation alone. One hundred one (101) patients were randomized to receive either rtPA at 100 mg over 2 hr compared to 55 patients treated with heparin. Thirty-nine percent (39%) of rtPA patients versus 17% of heparin-treatment patients had improvement in right ventricular wall motion ($P = 0.005$). There was significantly improved pulmonary perfusion in the rt-PA group. Interestingly, in the heparin-treated group, 2 patients suffered subsequent fatal pulmonary emboli and 3 had nonfatal pulmonary emboli.

Recently, Konstantinides et al.[25] evaluated the results of thrombolytic therapy for PE in patients who were hemodynamically stable. The overall 30-day mortality was significantly lower in the 169 patients receiving thrombolytic agents than the 550 patients receiving anticoagulation alone (4.7 versus 11.1%, $P = 0.016$). Tebbe et al.[26] studied the hemodynamic effects of double-bolus reteplase versus rtPA infusion in patients with massive PE. Patients were randomized to receive reteplase 10 units + 10 units administered 30 min apart, or rtPA, 100 mg over 2 hr. Total pulmonary vascular resistance and mean pulmonary artery blood pressure decreased in both groups and was not significantly different between groups. Bleeding occurred in 57% in the reteplase group and 31% in the rtPA group ($P = 0.14$).

Iliofemoral Deep Venous Thrombosis

Extensive DVT presenting with a painfully swollen extremity often accompanied by cyanosis frequently results in debilitating post-thrombotic symptoms. It is commonly said that the post-thrombotic syndrome requires years for its full manifestation; however, we have observed debilitating symptoms in active individuals from the time of the initial thrombotic event. Although skin changes may take many months to years to manifest, painful swelling resulting from significant venous hypertension is immediate and often persistent.

Because the underlying pathophysiology of the post-thrombotic syndrome is ambulatory venous hypertension, and its components are venous obstruction and valvular incompetence, it is physiologically sound that restoring patency (thereby eliminating obstruction) and/or preservation of valvular function will reduce venous hypertension and therefore reduce post-thrombotic sequelae. The combination of venous obstruction and valvular insufficiency is known to be particularly virulent.

We have adopted a strategy of catheter-directed thrombolysis or venous thrombectomy for the treatment of patients with iliofemoral venous thrombosis.[27] This is based on the principles that elimination of thrombus from the iliofemoral venous system will restore patency in all patients treated successfully and preserve valvular function at least in some patients. Successful therapy has been associated with significantly reduced post-thrombotic symptoms and significantly improved quality-of-life compared to standard anticoagulation.[28] The currently available literature using catheter-directed UK for the treatment of iliofemoral venous thrombosis indicates that 80% to 90% of patients will be successfully treated.[29,30] This is consistent with our observations in 54 patients treated with catheter-directed thrombolysis. Identification and correction of an underlying iliac venous stenosis is important for long-term success. Bleeding complications occur in 7% to 12% of patients. The UK dose commonly used was 250,000 to 350,000 U/hr. With the restriction of urokinase, we have a growing experience with catheter-directed rtPA. Following appropriate catheter positioning (usually ultrasound-guided popliteal vein puncture with antegrade positioning of the catheter into the thrombus), a bolus of 2 to 4 mg of rtPA is given, followed by a continuous infusion of 2 to 4 mg/hr. Heparin is infused through the sheath at a dose of at least 500 U/hr. The concentration of the bolus dose is approximately 1 mg in 1 to 2 cc of saline. The concentration of rtPA in the continuous infusion is 1 mg in 10 to 20 cc of saline. Our initial observations of rtPA appear equivalent to catheter-directed UK, both for efficacy and safety.

Axillosubclavian Vein Thrombosis

Although some physicians believe that axillosubclavian DVT is a benign condition, others believe that more aggressive management techniques of clot removal and full anticoagulation are justified. Untreated, from 25% to 75% of affected patients will have some limitation of activity.[31,32]

Primary axillosubclavian DVT is usually caused by a chronic extrinsic compression of the vein as it crosses the first rib, between the first rib and the clavicle. This extrinsic compression causes stricture of the subclavian vein at the thoracic inlet. Treatment of these patients is designed to remove the acute thrombus, decompress the extrinsic compression, and relieve the intrinsic stricture.

Catheter-directed UK was the standard technique used to achieve thrombolysis at a dose of 250,000 U/hr delivered into the thrombus. We have now substituted a bolus dose of rtPA of 2 to 4 mg followed by an infusion of 1 to 2 mg/hr. Heparin is infused through the sheath at a dose of at least 500 U/hr. Preliminary observations with this technique have been gratifying. Following thrombolysis, repeat phlebography is performed with hyperabduction maneuvers. If the vein is normal, the patient is continued on anticoagulation. If the vein is chronically occluded at the thoracic inlet and a balloon angioplasty catheter cannot be passed across the segmental occlusion, the first rib collaterals may provide adequate drainage if rethrombosis is avoided.

If a stricture of the vein is observed, we perform a temporizing balloon angioplasty followed by 4 to 6 weeks of anticoagulation. At that point, a first rib resection is performed followed by definitive angioplasty and stenting (if needed) of the stenotic subclavian vein. One report indicates that first rib resection can be performed safely and effectively immediately following thrombolysis without the 4 to 6 week delay.[33]

Catheter Clearance

Functioning central venous catheters are important for chemotherapy, hyperalimentation, and hemodialysis. At least 25% of these catheters fail to function as a result of thrombosis. Clinical trials showed that bolus doses of 5000 U of UK restored catheter functioning in the majority of these patients. As a result of these observations, small-dose (5000 U) UK was approved by the FDA to restore patency to occluded catheters.

Haire et al.[34] performed a double-blinded randomized trial evaluating UK versus rtPA in thrombosed central venous catheters. They injected either 2 mg rtPA in 2 cc saline or 10,000 U/UK and allowed both to incubate for 2 hr. A second dose was allowed if catheter function was not restored after the first injection. Thirteen of 22 catheters randomized to UK had full function restored, compared to 25 of 28 randomized to rtPA ($P = 0.13$).

Alternatives to urokinase according to indication are listed in Table 41–1.

TABLE 41–1. SUGGESTED LYTIC AGENTS, DOSES, AND DELIVERY BY INDICATION, ACCORDING TO RECENT REPORTED AND CLINICAL EXPERIENCE

Indication	Agent/Dose	Site/Infusion Duration	Comment
Acute arterial and graft occlusion	rtPA 2–4 mg bolus then 2 mg/hr (diluted to 1 mg/10 cc); Retavase 0.5–1.0/hr	Intrathrombus 12–36 hr intrathrombus up to 20 hr has been reported	Diluted rtPA (in saline) and Retavase appear to be as safe as UK; initial observations suggest similar efficacy
Intraoperative intra-arterial lytic therapy	rtPA 2–5 mg in 3–50 cc saline depending on volume of distal vascular bed	Intra-arterial bolus	2–5 mg bolus rtPA can be repeated if clinically warranted
Pulmonary embolism	rtPA 100 mg over 2 hr; Retavase 20 U; given as two 10-U bolus doses 30 min apart	Intravenous 2 hr Intravenous 30 min.	Early bolus of 10–20 mg rtPA may speed lysis
Iliofemoral DVT	rtPA 2–4 mg bolus, then 2–4 mg/hr	Intrathrombus 12–36 hr	Actual duration depends on thrombus resolution on follow-up phlebograms
Axillosubclavian DVT	rtPA 2–4 mg bolus, then 1–2 mg/hr	Intrathrombus 12–24 hr	Actual duration depends on thrombus resolution on follow-up phlebograms
Catheter clearance	rtPA 2 mg in 2-3 cc saline	Into catheter, incubate 2 hr	Dose can be repeated if catheter function not restored in 2 hr

REFERENCES

1. Zoon KC. Public Health Service, Food and Drug Administration, Center for Biologics Evaluation and Research. Important drug warning. Issued January 25, 1999. Downloaded from ww.fda.gov/cber on September 10, 1999.
2. Rubin RN. Streptokinase. In Comerota AJ, ed. *Thrombolytic Therapy for Peripheral Vascular Disease* 1995;6:87.
3. Verstraete M. Urokinase. In Comerota AJ, ed. *Thrombolytic Therapy for Peripheral Vascular Disease* 1995;7:99–101.
4. Froehlich J, Stump DL. Recombinant Tissue Plasminogen Activator. In Comerota AJ, ed. *Thrombolytic Therapy for Peripheral Vascular Disease* 1995;8:103–114.
5. Fischer S, Kohnert U. Major mechanistic differences explain the higher clot lysis potency of reteplase over alteplase: lack of fibrin biding is an advantage for bolus application of fibrin-specific thrombolytics. *Fibrin Proteo.* 1997;11(3):129–135.
6. Sobolski JC, Sasahara AA, Marcotte PA, Henkin J, Gurewich V. Prourokinase: a new clot-selective thrombolytic agent. In Comerota AJ, ed. *Thrombolytic Therapy for Peripheral Vascular Disease* 1995:10:133–141.
7. Assessment of the safety and efficacy of a new thrombolytic (ASSENT-2) investigators. Single-bolus tenecteplase compared with front-loaded alteplase in acute myocardial infarction: the ASSENT-2 double-blind randomized trial. *Lancet.* 1999;353:716–722.
8. The STILE investigators. Results of a prospective randomized trial, evaluating surgery versus thrombolysis for ischemia of the lower extremity. *Ann Surg.* 1994;220:251–268.
9. Ouriel K, Veith FJ, Sasahara AA, for the TOPAS investigators. Thrombolysis or peripheral arterial surgery: phase I results. *J Vasc Surg.* 1996;23:64–75.
10. Ouriel K, Veith FJ, Sasahara AA. A comparison of recombinant urokinase with vascular surgery as initial treatment for acute arterial occlusion of the legs. *N Engl J Med.* 1998; 338:1105–1111.
11. Ouriel K, Shortell CK, De Weese JA, et al. A comparison of thrombolytic therapy with operative revascularization in the treatment of acute peripheral arterial ischemia. *J Vasc Surg.* 1994;9:1021–1030.
12. Comerota AJ, Weaver FA, Hosking JD, et al. Results of a prospective, randomized trial of surgery versus thrombolysis for occluded lower extremity bypass grafts. *Am J Surg.* 1996;172:105–112.
13. Davidian MM, Powell A, Benenati JF, et al. Initial results of reteplase in the treatment of acute lower extremity arterial occlusions. *J Vasc Interv Radiol.* 2000;11(3):289–295.
14. Laird JR, Dangas G, Jaff M, et al. Intra-arterial reteplase for the treatment of acute limb ischemia. *J Invas Cardiol.* 1999;11:757–762.
15. Ouriel K, Kandarpa K, Schuerr DM, Hultquist M, Hodkinson G, Wallin B. Prourokinase versus urokinase for recanalization of peripheral occlusions, safety and efficacy: the PURPOSE trial. *JVIR.* 1999;10:1083–1091.
16. Comerota AJ, White JV, Grosh JD. Intraoperative, intra-arterial thrombolytic therapy for salvage of limbs in patients with distal arterial thrombosis. *Surg Gynecol Obstet.* 1989;169:283.
17. Comerota AJ, Rao AK, Throm RC, et al. A prospective randomized, blinded and placebo-controlled trial of intraoperative, intra-arterial urokinase infusion during lower extremity revascularization: regional and systemic effects. *Ann Surg.* 1993;218:534.
18. Cynamon J, Lakritz PS, Wahl S, Bakal CW, Sprayregen S. Hemodialysis graft declotting: description of the "lyse and wait" technique. *J Vasc Intervent Radiol.* 1997;8:825–829.
19. Gibbens D, Depalma J, Albanese J, et al. Percutaneous thrombolysis of hemodialysis grafts using reteplase. *J Vasc Interv Radiol.* 2000;11(2 part 2):250 (abstract no. 202).

20. Flick PA, Das M, Horton K, et al. Initial experience with reteplase using the "lyse and wait" technique in thrombosed dialysis grafts. *J Vasc Interv Radiol.* 2000;11(2 part 2):252 (abstract no. 207).
21. Goldhaber SZ, Kessler CM, Heit J, et al. A randomized, controlled trial of recombinant tissue plasminogen activator versus urokinase in the treatment of acute pulmonary embolism. *Lancet.* 1988;2:293.
22. Meyer G, Sors H, Charbonnier B, et al., on behalf of the European Cooperative Study Group for Pulmonary Embolism. Effects of intravenous urokinase versus alteplase on total pulmonary resistance in acute massive pulmonary embolism: a European multicenter double-blind trial. *J Am Coll Cardiol.* 1992;19:239.
23. Goldhaber SZ, Kessler CM, Heit J. et al. Recombinant tissue-type plasminogen activator versus a novel dosing regimen of urokinase in acute pulmonary embolism: a randomized, controlled multicenter trial. *J Am Coll Cardiol.* 1992;20:24.
24. Goldhaber SZ, Haire WD, Feldstein ML, et al. Alteplase versus heparin in acute pulmonary embolism: randomized trial assessing right ventricular function and pulmonary perfusion. *Lancet.* 1993;341:507.
25. Konstantinides S, Geibel A. Association between thrombolytic treatment and the prognosis of hemodynamically stable patients with major pulmonary embolism: results of a multicenter registry. *Circulation.* 1997;96:882.
26. Tebbe U, Graf A, Kamke W, et al. Hemodynamic effects of double bolus reteplase versus alteplase infusion in massive pulmonary embolism. *Am Heart J.* 1999;138(1):39–44.
27. Comerota AJ, Aldridge SA, Cohen G, et al. A strategy of aggressive regional therapy for acute iliofemoral venous thrombosis with contemporary venous thrombectomy or catheter-directed thrombolysis. *J Vasc Surg.* 1994;20:244–254.
28. Comerota AJ, Throm RC, Mathias S, Haughton SH, Mewissen MW. Catheter-directed thrombolysis for iliofemoral DVT improves health related quality-of-life. *J Vasc Surg.* 2000; (In press).
29. Mewissen MW, Seabrook GR, Meissner MH, Cynamon J, Labropoulos N, Houghton SH. Catheter-directed thrombolysis for lower extremity deep venous thrombosis: report of a national multi-center registry. *Radiology.* 1999;211:39–49.
30. Bjarnason H, Kruse JR, Asinger DA, et al. Iliofemoral deep venous thrombosis: safety and efficacy outcome during 5 years of catheter-directed thrombolytic therapy. *J Vasc Intervent Radiol.* 1997;8:405–418.
31. Gloviczki P, Kazmier FJ, Hollier LH. Axillary–subclavian venous occlusion: the morbidity of a nonlethal disease. *J Vasc Surg.* 1986;4:333.
32. Tilney NL, Griffiths HJG, Edwards EA. Natural history of major venous thrombosis of the upper extremity. *Arch Surg.* 1970;101:792.
33. Molina JE. Need for emergency treatment in subclavian vein effort thrombosis. *J Am Coll Surg.* 1995;181:114–120.
34. Haire WD, Atkinson JB, Stephens LC. Urokinase versus recombinant tissue plasminogen activator in thrombosed central venous catheters: a double-blinded, randomized trial. *Thromb Haemost.* 1994;72:543–547.

42

The Role of Venous Valve Surgery in Chronic Venous Insufficiency

Michael C. Dalsing, MD, Ryan D. Nachreiner, MD, and Amardip Bhuller, MD

INTRODUCTION

Chronic venous insufficiency, with its attendant problems, has plagued humankind since antiquity. Prominent Greek and Roman physicians, including Hippocrates and Galen, addressed the treatment of varicose veins. Unfortunately, little was known about the underlying pathology until relatively recently. Investigators began to differentiate the various etiologies of venous insufficiency with the advent of diagnostic testing in the first half of the 20th century. Distinguishing venous obstruction from venous reflux was a critical first step. Venous reflux was further delineated into superficial, perforator, and/or deep venous reflux. The reconstruction of venous valves provides a method of preventing reflux within the axial lower extremity deep venous system.

Although the impact of chronic deep venous insufficiency (CDVI) on modern society is difficult to calculate, estimates place the prevalence around 2% to 4% of the adult population.[1] Certainly, there are millions of affected individuals and consequently billions of dollars in lost work revenue and human resources. The large number of people affected mandates that the physician understand the dynamics of the pathology as well as the potential treatments. Fortunately, an improved understanding of the pathophysiology of CDVI coupled with tremendous advances in diagnostic and surgical technology has led to a logical approach in its management.

The first technological breakthrough that revolutionized the diagnosis of CDVI was the development of venography in the 1940s. Initially, ascending and then descending venography allowed precise identification of the venous anatomy and localization of the pathologic process responsible for CDVI. More recently, duplex ultrasonography and other noninvasive tests have enabled us to evaluate and follow patients serially in a convenient, accurate, and economical fashion. Advances in surgical technology and anticoagulation allow surgeons to now perform delicate, once technically doomed procedures.

When dealing with CDVI, it is essential to distinguish between two primary etiologies: the postthrombotic syndrome (PTS) and primary reflux. PTS is a consequence of venous thrombosis. During recanalization, inflammation extends into the vein wall and valve cusps as the clot undergoes lysis and resorption. The delicate cusps are rendered incompetent by scarring and subsequent retraction. The ultimate result is reflux of venous blood, when the leg is in a dependent position, past these dysfunctional, unreconstructable valves. The postthrombotic syndrome accounts for roughly 60% to 80% of CDVI cases.[1,2] The remaining cases are due to primary reflux or, rarely, valvular agenesis. Primary reflux results from progressive dilatation of the vein wall and elongation of the valve cusps. Eventually, the redundant, malopposed cusps permit reflux. The etiology is presumed to be secondary to structural defects in the vein, either in the extracellular matrix or muscle cells themselves.[1]

ANATOMY AND PHYSIOLOGY

There are three interrelated yet distinct venous systems in the lower extremity. The deep system is composed of veins that parallel the named arteries of the leg and lie deep within the muscle compartments. These veins carry the bulk of venous return from the leg. The superficial system lies within the subcutaneous fat and superficial to the deep investing fascia of the muscles. It consists of the greater and lesser saphenous veins and branches. Finally, perforating veins bridge the deep and superficial systems. Perforating veins are most concentrated in the calf and lower leg, partially explaining the typical "gaiter" distribution of skin changes associated with CDVI. Venous hypertension generated in the deep system is allowed to have an impact on the superficial system in the face of incompetent perforator veins.[3]

Veins, like arteries, have a well-defined intima, media, and adventitia. Compared to arteries, the smooth muscle content is far less prominent, rendering the vein wall much thinner and also less stiff. Veins can collapse completely under normal physiologic conditions when the limb is not in a dependent position. As the lumen refills, with dependency, the vein transforms from an elliptical to a circular shape.[3] This gradual change in shape allows venous volume to increase with minimal elevations in venous pressure until the vein is maximally distended to a circular shape. This feature enables veins to serve as capacitance vessels. Venous hypertension occurs at rest only when the vein has maximally dilated, at which time a change in volume is reflected as a significant change in pressure.

Valves are bicuspid, thin structures that can withstand significant retrograde pressures without leakage. In most instances, these valves direct blood flow from superficial to deep and distal to proximal. They decrease in frequency from distal to proximal.[4] Infrapopliteal veins generally have between 5 and 15 valves, whereas the superficial femoral vein has only 2 to 3 valves. Approximately two-thirds of the time, the common femoral vein has a valve, but valves proximal to this location are the exception rather than the rule.

The energy to propel blood from the distal leg to the right atrium is derived from two sources. Hydrostatic pressure governs flow while at rest, whereas the calf muscle pump generates flow, against gravity, during muscle contraction. The calf muscle pump is composed of the gastrocnemius and soleus muscles, which contain venous sinuses that pool venous blood between muscle contractions. This blood is forced into the venous system proper during contraction and is prevented from reentering the sinuses, or distal veins, by valves. Pressures as high as 300 mmHg can be achieved during maximal muscular contraction. These high pressures are not transmitted to the superficial system if competent valves exist.[4] Following muscle contraction, proximal valves prevent reflux so that the muscle pump fills from distal veins and capillaries while venous conduit blood is directed toward the heart. Failure of the calf muscle pump to function properly can cause venous pooling and stasis, contributing to the development of CDVI.[5]

The codependent interaction between the veins, valves, and muscle pump mandates a comprehensive, systematic approach to the evaluation of a patient with CDVI. A breakdown in any of these components can lead to venous reflux and stasis, and ultimately end-organ damage (edema, skin changes, and ulcers).

PATIENT EVALUATION

Patients with CDVI present with symptoms of venous hypertension and stasis. Less severe manifestations consist of dependent edema after prolonged standing and a feeling of fullness or fatigue in the legs. Progressively more severe symptoms are intractable edema, eczema, cellulitis, hyperpigmentation, and skin ulceration. A careful history and physical examination should be performed with special attention paid to a previous history of deep venous thrombosis (DVT) or other venous disorders, as well as the physical and occupational limitations the disease inflicts on the patient. Stratification of patients with CDVI should follow the guidelines laid out in the CEAP classification system (Table 42–1).[6] Operative candidates are generally those patients with class 5 or 6 disease. However, if lifestyle requirements of the lower extremities are more demanding, exceptions can be made for patients with less severe disease.

Diagnostic evaluation of the venous system should begin with a venous Duplex ultrasound study. This noninvasive test can distinguish refluxive from obstructive venous disease, identify the extent of involvement (including evaluation of the superficial, perforating, and deep systems), and eliminate patients with isolated superficial or perforator reflux from additional, unnecessary invasive testing. Duplex ultrasonography can be used to visualize the entire venous system distal to the inguinal ligament and is suf-

TABLE 42–1. CEAP CLASSIFICATION SYSTEM

C	**Clinical presentation:** Class 0–6, A = asymptomatic, S = symptomatic
E	**Etiology:** C = congenital, P = primary, S = secondary
A	**Anatomic distribution:** S = superficial, D = deep, P = perforator
P	**Pathophysiology:** R = reflux, O = obstruction

ficiently sensitive to detect valve cusps (Figure 42–1). It is performed while the patient is standing upright, with their weight supported on the contralateral leg. Continuous-wave doppler is used to determine blood flow velocity and direction, while B-mode imaging provides a picture of the vein structure. A pneumatic cuff, placed on either the thigh or the calf, is inflated to 80 mmHg or 100 mmHg, respectively, for 3 sec then deflated in <0.3 sec. Reflux that lasts longer than 0.5 sec (a determination of valve closure time) is considered abnormal. Others have used manual compression as the stimulus and consider 1.0 sec to be the critical level for significant reflux.

Patients who are found to have significant deep venous reflux as the source of their disabling symptoms should be referred for venography. Ascending venography delineates the precise anatomy of the venous system. The patient is positioned semi-erect at an approximately 45° to 50° tilt. Intravenous contrast is injected through a cannula placed in a pedal vein. A tourniquet placed at the ankle prevents flow to the superficial system. Contrast outlines the deep system as well as any incompetent perforators. Ambulatory venous pressure measurements can be performed at the same time, with the

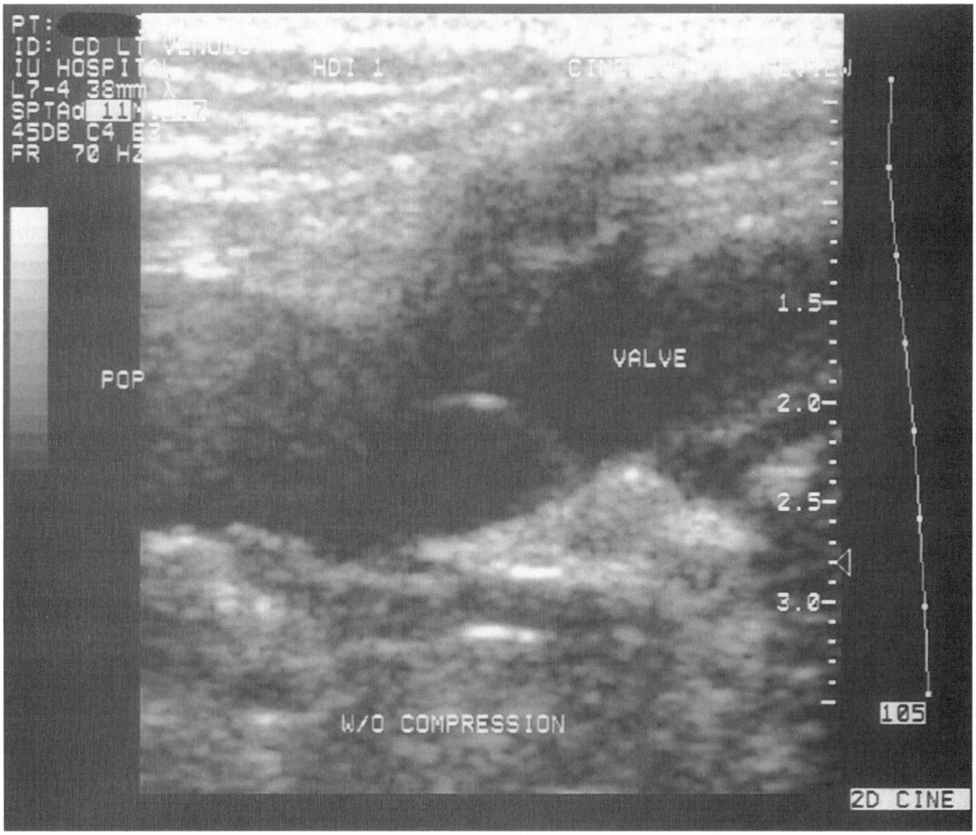

Figure 42–1. The valve cusps of a popliteal vein are clearly seen in the center of this B-mode image taken during duplex ultrasonography.

addition of hyperemic testing to evaluate the role of venous obstruction (comparison to upper extremity pressures) when required.

Descending venography is subsequently performed to define the degree and location of venous valvular reflux. Contrast injected into the common femoral vein (CFV), via a catheter that is inserted at a distant location (contralateral groin or upper extremity), is allowed to cascade down the limb; first with the patient resting quietly in a semi-erect position, and then while the patient performs a Valsalva maneuver. The initial study helps to outline the location of the valve cusps; the latter demonstrates competent valves as contrast pools in the valve sinuses without retrograde flow past the valves. Compromised yet reconstructable (Figure 42–2) or damaged/absent valves (Figure 42–3) allow contrast to reflux down the leg until a competent valve is encountered, if one exists. The test is sufficiently sensitive to distinguish between the scarred, retracted valves involved in PTS and the redundant, floppy valves responsible for primary reflux. Generally, only those patients with reflux noted past the knee during the Valsalva maneuver (grades 3 or 4) should be considered for deep venous valve repair

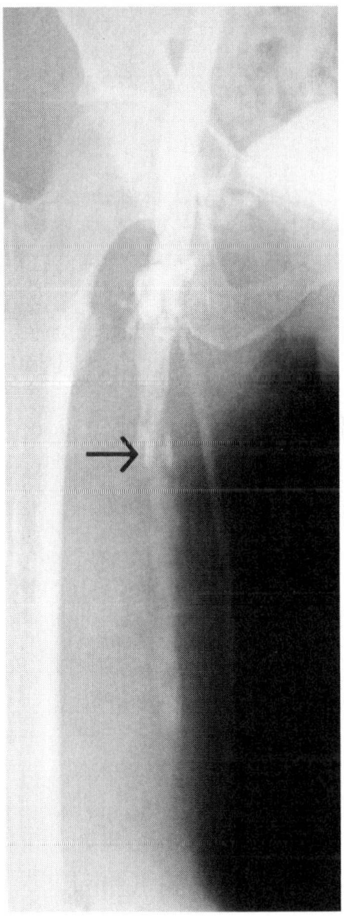

Figure 42–2. Intravenous contrast pools in the valve sinuses during descending venography. This venogram demonstrates the appearance of intact valves (*arrow*), which are incompetent and are amenable to valvuloplasty.

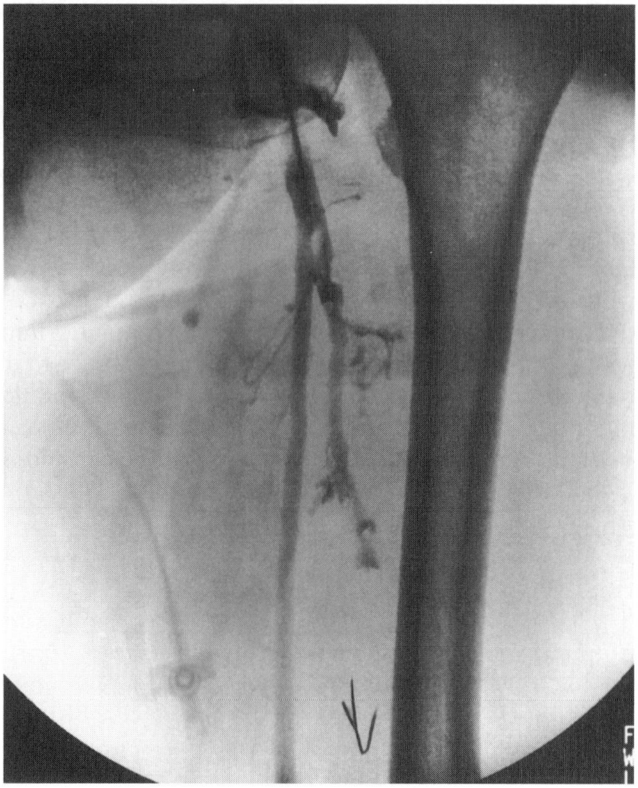

Figure 42–3. Intravenous contrast cascades down the deep venous system of this leg during a Valsalva maneuver demonstrating the lack of identifiable valves following a prior episode of deep venous thrombosis.

or replacement. It is important to document the competency of the profunda femoris vein (PFV) valves during descending venography.[7] The outcome of valve surgery is dependent on the integrity of these valves. If the PFV valves are competent, then repair of a valve in the proximal superficial femoral vein (SFV) is adequate to control SFV deep venous reflux. Reflux throughout the PFV mandates a more distal reconstruction to control all axial reflux or the need to address both the SFV and PFV systems.

Calf muscle pump function and other hemodynamic components of the venous system are evaluated by air plethysmography.[5] A plastic cylinder fitted over the calf is used to measure pressure and volume changes in the calf during standing and after various calf exercises. Venous volume (VV) is the difference in calf volume measured as the patient moves from a supine position with the legs elevated at 45° to a standing position with the weight supported on the opposite leg. Venous filling time 90 (VFT_{90}) is the time it takes to achieve 90% of the VV following standing. The venous filling index (VFI) is calculated by dividing the 90% VV by VFT_{90}. A VFI <2 mL/sec is normal, whereas values greater than that are indicative of valvular reflux. The volume eliminated during a single tiptoe maneuver is the ejection volume (EV). An ejection fraction (EF) can be derived from EV/VV. The residual volume (RV) is the calf volume remaining after 10 rapid tiptoe maneuvers. The residual venous volume (RVF) is determined by RV/VV. Normal calf muscle pump function is denoted by an EF $>60\%$ and a RVF $<35\%$.

MEDICAL THERAPY

Medical therapy directed to alleviate the symptoms of CDVI should be maximized prior to any contemplated surgical repair. This point is emphasized by the fact that multiple factors contribute to the development of CDVI, some of which may not be amenable to surgical intervention, and the clinical presentation may significantly differ from what might be predicted based on diagnostic studies alone.[8] Measures that minimize venous hypertension, which ultimately leads to the changes associated with CDVI, include eliminating prolonged periods of standing, elevating the feet above the heart when resting, and wearing graded compressive stockings at all times while upright. Meticulous care of the skin, especially when preulcerative changes or ulcers are present, is required. Surgical therapy should be pursued when disabling symptoms are intractable to maximal medical therapy.

SURGICAL REPAIR

Patients with superficial axial reflux and varicose veins are treated adequately with vein stripping and varicosectomy alone. If venous hypertension is the result of perforator incompetence, ligation and/or division of the involved perforating veins by either an open technique or subfascial endoscopic perforator surgery (SEPS) addresses the problem. These patients do not require further consideration for valve repair. When these problems coexist with deep venous reflux, they are generally corrected prior to aggressive repair of incompetent deep venous valves.

Internal Valvuloplasty

Primary deep venous reflux can be approached in several different ways. In 1968, Kistner[9] was the first to report successful surgical repair of primary venous valve reflux. He used a longitudinal venotomy through the valve commissure (Figure 42–4). The redundant valve cusps were plicated to the vein wall with 7-O nonabsorbable suture. After closing the venotomy, proper coaptation of the valve cusps prevented reflux. Others have modified the surgical approach. Raju[10] uses a transverse venotomy just proximal to the valve. Sottiurai[11] offers a hybrid approach, with a supravalvular transverse venotomy with distal extension into, but not past, the valve sinus.

Regardless of the approach, several principles should be followed during valve repair. Dissection should be sufficiently extensive to allow for adequate proximal and distal control. The patient should be fully anticoagulated prior to clamping and creating the venotomy. A strip test should be performed to evaluate valve competence prior to and following valve repair. This is performed by milking blood antegrade past the valve while simultaneously occluding inflow, and then by applying retrograde pressure against the valve, either manually or by Valsalva maneuver. Maintenance of the collapsed distal vein during application of the retrograde flow and pressure confirms valve competence, while refilling denotes reflux and an incompetent valve. Valve and venotomy repair are performed with a small-diameter nonabsorbable suture (6-O or 7-O prolene). Plication of approximately 20% of the leaflet length usually restores valve competence (Figure 42–5).[12] Wound drainage should be considered to reduce the risk of

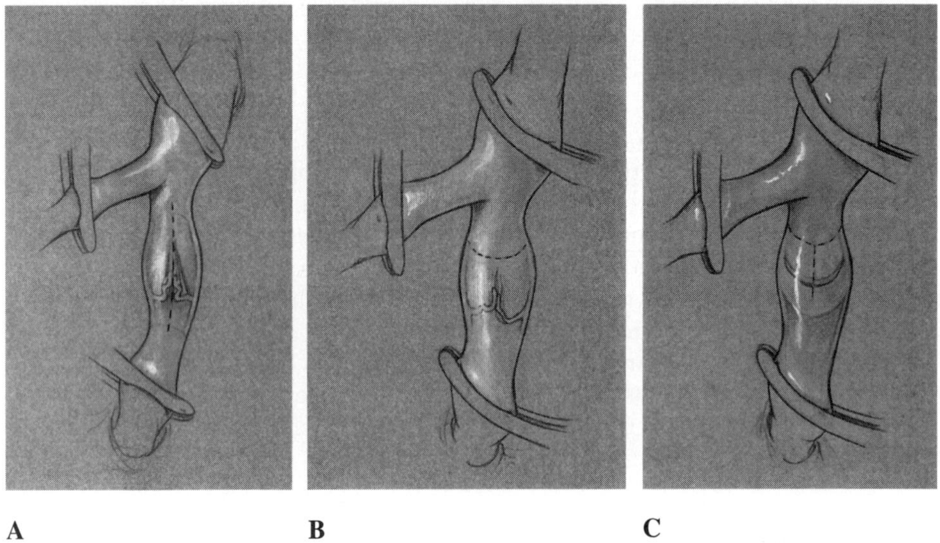

Figure 42–4. The three options for creating a venotomy in preparation for internal valvuloplasty are shown: (A) the transcommissural approach; (B) the supravalvular transverse approach; and (C) the supravalvular "T"-shaped approach.

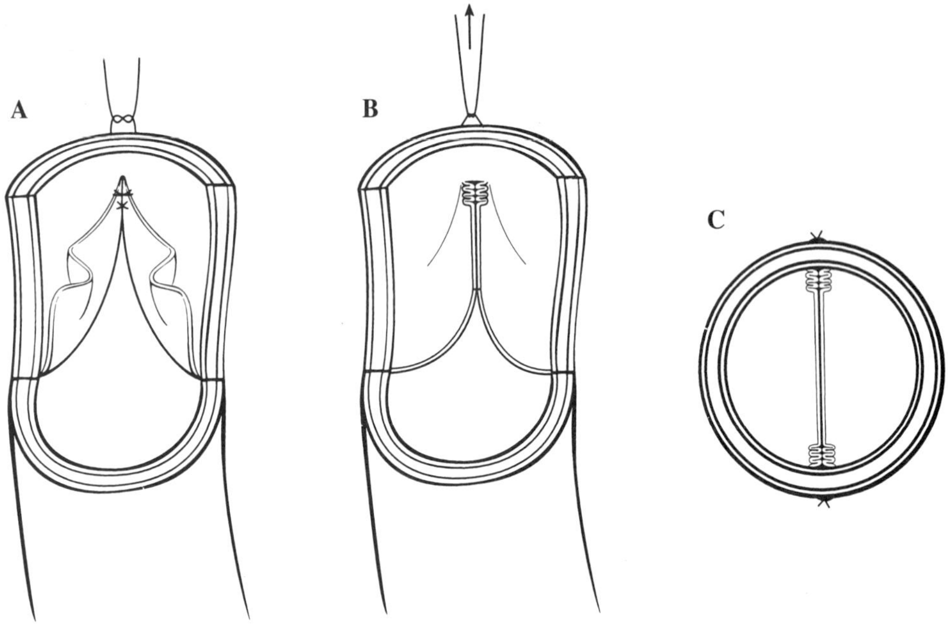

Figure 42–5. Cutaway images through the vein wall and valve demonstrate redundant valve cusps (A) prior to and (B) during plication. The valve (C) is seen following application with the valve cusps in apposition while the redundant valve cusp leading edge has been tacked to the vein wall.

hematoma formation, especially because postoperative anticoagulation is used routinely. Intermittent pneumatic compression should be used in the perioperative period to discourage venous stasis and augment venous blood flow across the valve.

Short-term follow-up from multiple series demonstrates that internal valvuloplasty performed for primary reflux is a durable, effective repair, providing 60% to 75% of the patients prolonged valve competence with a reduction in symptoms and freedom from ulcer recurrence. Masuda and Kistner[13] report similarly good clinical results in 70% of patients with a follow-up as long as 21 yr.

Minimally Invasive Valvuloplasty

As with other surgical procedures, there is always an effort to perform less invasive venous surgery. Kistner[14] introduced the concept of external valvuloplasty in 1990. This approach avoided a venotomy and its attendant complications. Plicating sutures are placed through the vein wall without direct visualization of the valve leaflets. These sutures narrow the commissural angle, drawing the leaflets into proper coaptation. This approach is less time-intensive, requires less dissection, and can be performed without anticoagulation because blood flow is not interrupted. However, because the valve is not visualized, the repair is not as precise as internal valvuloplasty. Limited anterior plication has been championed by Belcaro et al.[15] for patients with mild to moderately severe reflux. This approach limits dissection even further by requiring exposure of only the anterior vein wall rather than circumferential control.

External banding is another approach that avoids the creation of a venotomy. Its use is restricted to a specific operative situation: If valve competence is restored by the venospasm caused during dissection, then banding may be appropriate.[16] In addition, banding is occasionally added to valve transplants to avoid delayed venous dilatation. Banding uses synthetic or autogenous material (Dacron, PTFE, or fascia) to wrap the circumference of the vein for 1 to 2 cm above and below the valve (Figure 42–6). This band is tightened until valve competence is maintained, then it is sutured to itself. The band is also sutured to the venous adventitia to prevent migration.

In 1991, Gloviczki et al.[17] reported angioscopic-assisted valvuloplasty. An angioscope is introduced through a side branch and advanced into the vein directly above the incompetent valve. Proximal and distal control and clamping is mandatory, and therefore the patient is anticoagulated. Heparinized saline solution is used to irrigate the blood from the lumen, allowing visualization of the leaflets. Sutures are placed from outside the vein lumen with intraluminal positioning of the suture through the cusp leading edge being guided by video-enhanced angioscopic visualization. Like external valvuloplasty, venous trauma is minimized because a large venotomy is avoided. The distinct advantage over external valvuloplasty is the more precise repair that results from leaflet visualization. The disadvantage over an external repair is the heparin requirement, with the attendant risk of bleeding.

Internal valvuloplasty seems to be more precise and durable than the other valve repairs discussed previously. Raju et al.[18] ranked the durability of various methods of valve repair, as assessed by venous duplex scanning, following reconstruction of 316 valves. Internal valvuloplasty was the most durable, with external banding a close second. Patients receiving an external valvuloplasty experienced earlier and more frequent

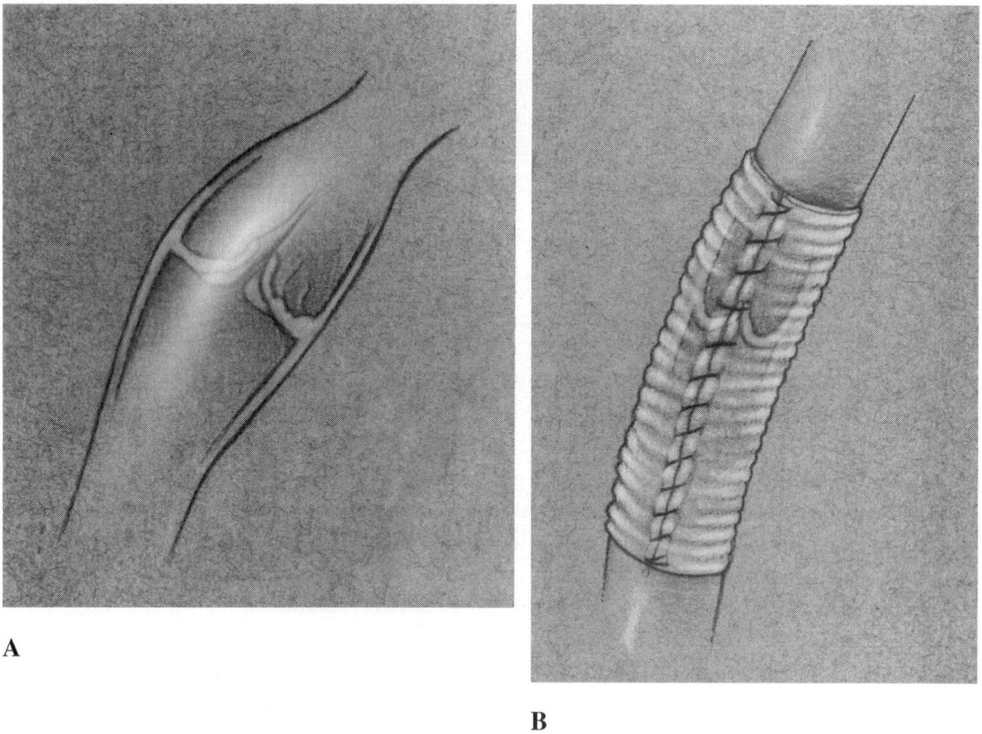

Figure 42–6. Placement of a synthetic band around the circumference of an incompetent vein valve segment (**A**) restores valve competence (**B**) by reducing the diameter and bringing the valve edges into alignment.

recurrence of venous reflux. Angioscopic valvuloplasty, still in its infancy, was not included in the analysis, although preliminary reports are promising.

Primary valve repair is generally well tolerated with acceptably low complication rates. Most importantly, the majority of series report no operative mortality. Hematoma and/or seroma formation occurs in up to 15% of the patients. Wound infection was noted in only 2% to 4% of patients. Once feared to be a common occurrence after venous surgery, DVT is observed in <10% of the patients.

Vein Transposition

As mentioned previously, the inflammatory process that accompanies thrombus lysis and recanalization damages surrounding valve cusps. Valvuloplasty is, therefore, not an option in these cases. In the event that the reflux is isolated to a single axial venous conduit, with competent veins in a parallel system, a vein transposition operation is possible. It reroutes blood flow from the incompetent system through a competent vein valve (Figure 42–7). This is possible in approximately 3% of the patients with CDVI. The most common circumstance involves SFV reflux in the face of a competent PFV valve.

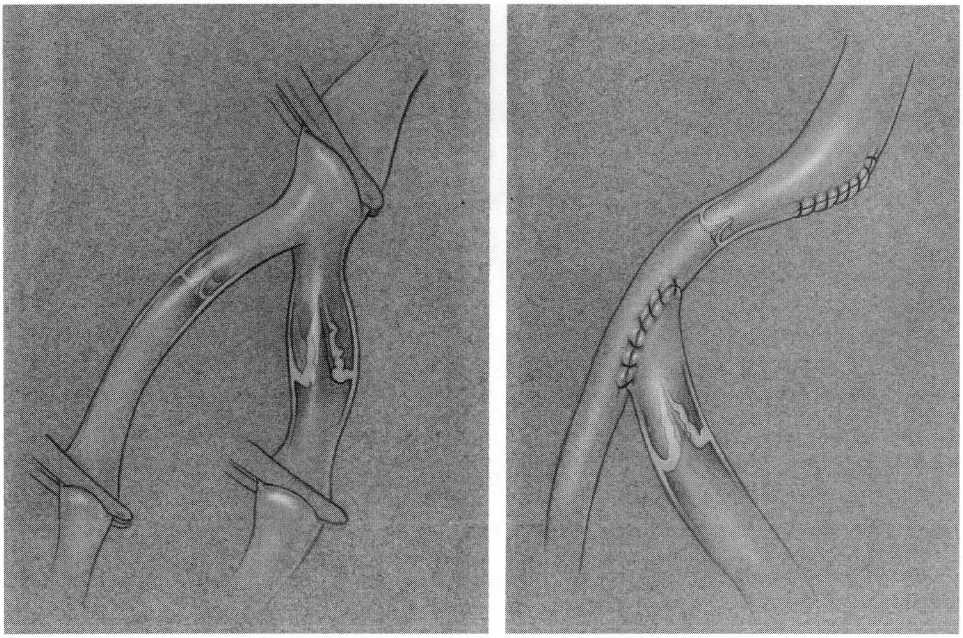

A B

Figure 42–7. (**A**) A competent PFV valve and a scarred, retracted SFV valve. The SFV is ligated at its junction with the CFV and subsequently anastomosed distal to the competent PFV valve (**B**), completing the vein transposition.

The SFV is ligated distal to its junction with the CFV and then anastomosed to the PFV distal to the competent valve. Other less common scenarios include anastomosis of the SFV to the greater saphenous vein (GSV) or an incompetent PFV to a competent SFV or GSV. From 40% to 50% of patients achieve long-term relief from their severe CDVI symptoms following this approach.[19]

Valve Transplantation

When transposition is not practical, valve transplantation is a surgical option. Taheri et al.[20] reported the first successful human venous valve transplants in 1982, although others had previously reported venous valve transplants in canine models. Taheri harvested a 2- to 3-cm segment of axillary vein that included a competent valve. This segment was then transplanted into the lower extremity (Figure 42–8). In the original description, the segment was placed in the SFV just distal to its junction with the PFV. To be ultimately effective, it is currently held that the transplanted valve must be distal to all parallel axial refluxive vein segments. Alternate locations have been described, including the popliteal vein, which may be a preferred location because this vein acts as a "gatekeeper" to the distal lower extremity.[21] As enticing as the universally applicable valve transplant seems, there are several potential problems. From 30% to 40% of

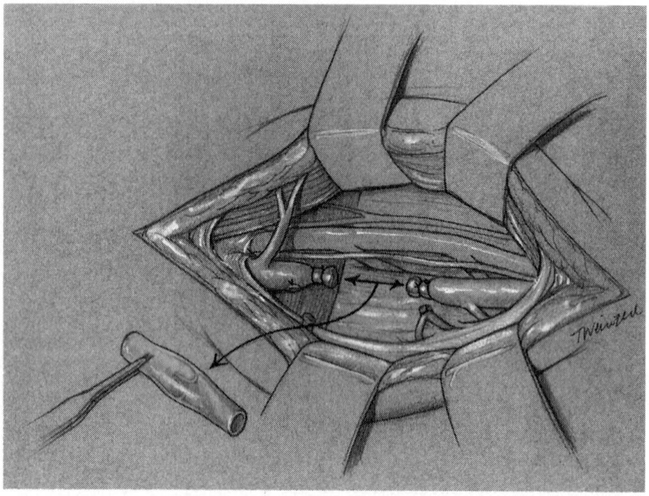

A

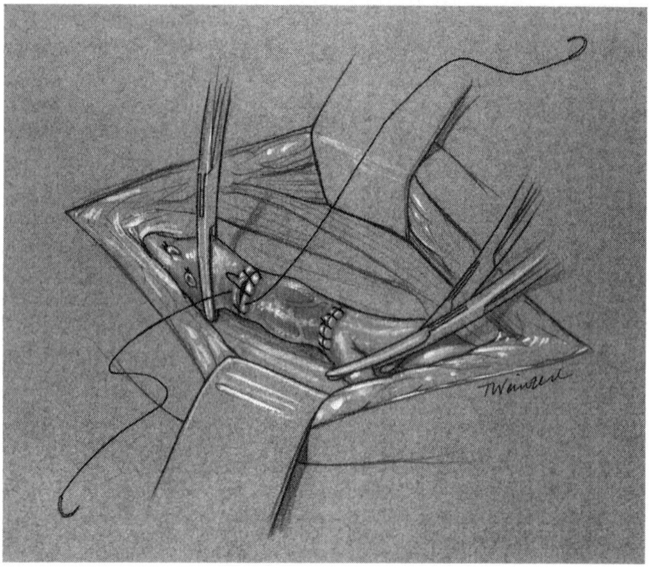

B

Figure 42–8. (**A**) During valve transplantation, a competent valve-bearing segment of axillary vein is harvested, then (**B**) transplanted into the lower extremity distal to all axial reflux.

patients with CDVI have no competent upper extremity valves. When acceptable valves exist, the procedure exposes the patient to a second incision and its attendant complications. Finally, delayed dilatation of the vein segment with resulting cusp malapposition does occur over time. This problem can be anticipated and potentially prevented by wrapping the transplant segment with an external band as described previously.[1] Initial reports were glowing; authors reported between 80% and 90% competency rates with nearly all patients reporting good to excellent clinical outcomes.[21,22] More recent reports, although still acceptable, have outcomes that are slightly less favorable than those of primary valve repairs, with long-term competency rates of between 40% and 50%.[19] Deep venous thrombosis seems to be slightly more common after valve transplantation, with an approximately 15% incidence reported. Site-specific complications, such as hematoma and seroma formation as well as wound infection, are comparable to those of primary valve repairs. The one difference is related to the additional site for potential complications due to the upper-extremity vein harvest.

Extensive research has been conducted into developing a valve substitute for the subpopulation of patients that have CDVI not amenable to any of the previously described methods of valve repair. This primarily describes those patients with PTS lacking an acceptable upper-extremity valve for transplant. Substitutes that have failed in canine trials include fresh and glutaraldehyde-preserved allografts as well as synthetic polymer or titanium valve devices. However, promising outcomes were found when using a cryopreserved allograft in canines.[23]

A recent phase I clinical trial of cryopreserved human allograft venous valves was reported by Dalsing et al.[24] Nine patients had a single valve transplant placed so that it was distal to all lower extremity venous reflux. During this 6-mo feasibility study, a 78% secondary valve patency and 67% secondary valve competence rate was achieved. In a second trial, Raju and Negland[25] reported a 50% competency rate at 1 yr.

SUMMARY

Advances in diagnostic capabilities and surgical technology have paved the way for significant advances in the surgical treatment of CDVI. For primary reflux, internal valvuloplasty remains the surgical gold standard, with good to excellent results in 70% of the patients. As more experience is gained with minimally invasive procedures, particularly angioscopic-assisted valvuloplasty, there may be a trend towards using these techniques. Chronic deep venous insufficiency secondary to PTS is treated with valve replacement, either by transposition or transplantation. Results from these procedures, although not as impressive as those for valvuloplasty, still result in significant improvement of the disabling symptoms these patients have experienced. Finally, the search for valve substitutes to treat patients with no other options continues, with some early success being reported using a cryopreserved allograft.

REFERENCES

1. Raju S. Operative management of chronic venous insufficiency. In: Rutherford RB, ed. *Vascular Surgery*. Philadelphia: WB Saunders; 1995:1851–1862.
2. Cheatle TR, Perrin M. Venous valve repair: early results in fifty-two cases. *J Vasc Surg*. 1994;19:404–413.
3. Nehler MR, Moneta GL. The lower extremity venous disease. Part 1: anatomy and physiology. *Perspect Vasc Surg*. 1991;4:104–116.
4. Browse NL, Burnand KG, Thomas ML. *Disease of the Veins: Pathology, Diagnosis, and Treatment*. London: Edward Arnold; 1988:53–69.

5. Araki CT, Back TL, Padberg FT, et al. The significance of calf muscle pump function in venous ulceration. *J Vasc Surg*. 1994;20:872–877.
6. Porter JM, Moneta GL. An International consensus Committee on Chronic Venous Disease. Reporting standards in venous disease: an update. *J Vasc Surg*. 1995;21:643–645.
7. Eriksson I, Almgren B. Influence of the profunda femoris vein on venous hemodynamics of the limb. *J Vasc Surg*. 1986;4:390–395.
8. Iafrati MD, Welch H, O'Donnell TF, et al. Correlation of venous noninvasive tests with the Society for Vascular Surgery clinical classification of chronic venous insufficiency. *J Vasc Surg*. 1994;19:1001–1007.
9. Kistner R. Surgical repair of a venous valve. *Straub Clin Proc*. 1968;24:41–43.
10. Raju S. Venous insufficiency of the lower limb and stasis ulceration. *Ann Surg*. 1983;197: 688–697.
11. Sottiurai VS. Technique in direct venous valvuloplasty. *J Vasc Surg*. 1988;8:646–648.
12. Raju S, Fredericks R. Valve reconstruction procedures for nonobstructive venous insufficiency: rationale, techniques, and results in 107 procedures with two- to eight-year follow-up. *J Vasc Surg*. 1988;7:301–310.
13. Masuda EM, Kistner RL. Long-term results of venous valve reconstruction: a four- to twenty-one year follow up. *J Vasc Surg*. 1994;19:391–403.
14. Kistner RL. Surgical technique of external venous valve repair. *Straub Found Proc*. 1990;55:15.
15. Belcaro G, Nicolaides AN, Ricci A, et al. External femoral vein valvuloplasty with limited anterior plication (LAP): a 10-year randomized follow-up study. *Angiology*. 1999;50:531–536.
16. Camilli S, Guarnera G. External banding valvuloplasty of the superficial femoral vein in the treatment of primary deep valvular incompetence. *Internat Angiol*. 1994;13:218–222.
17. Gloviczki P, Merrell SW, Bower TC. Femoral vein valve repair under direct vision without venotomy: a modified technique with use of angioscopy. *J Vasc Surg*. 1991;14:645–648.
18. Raju S, Fredericks RK, Neglen PN, et al. Durability of venous valve reconstruction techniques for "primary" and post-thrombotic reflux. *J Vasc Surg*. 1996;23:357–367.
19. Eklof BG, Kistner RL, Masuda EM. Venous bypass and valve reconstruction: long-term efficacy. *Vasc Med*. 1998;3:157–164.
20. Taheri SA, Lazar L, Elias SM, Marchand P. Vein valve transplant. *Surgery*. 1982;91:28–33.
21. O'Donnell TF, Mackey WC, Shepard AD, et al. Clinical, hemodynamic, and anatomic follow-up of direct venous reconstruction. *Arch Surg*. 1987;122:474–482.
22. Taheri SA, Heffner R, Budd T, et al. Five years experience with vein valve transplant. *World J Surg*. 1986;10:935–937.
23. Burkhart HM, Fath SW, Dalsing MC, et al. Experimental repair of venous valvular insufficiency using a cryopreserved venous valve allograft aided by a distal ateriovenous fistula. *J Vasc Surg*. 1997;26:817–822.
24. Dalsing MC, Raju S, Wakefield TW, Taheri S. A multicenter, phase I evaluation of cryopreserved venous valve allografts for the treatment of chronic deep venous insufficiency. *J Vasc Surg*. 1999;30:854–866.
25. Raju S, Neglan P. The cryo-preserved vein valve: clinical application and early results. Presented at the *American Venous Forum*. Phoenix, AZ. Feb 3, 2000.

43

Surgery for Incompetent Perforating Veins at the Turn of the Millennium

A Gentler and Kinder Approach than at the Start of the 20th Century

Thomas F. O'Donnell, Jr., MD, and Moon Kwoun, MD

The ligation of incompetent perforating veins for advanced chronic venous insufficiency (CVI) has undergone a cyclic pattern of utilization.[1] Linton[2] in the United States and Cockett and Elgan Jones[3] in Europe have popularized the concept that interruption of incompetent perforating veins prevents[4] the abnormal transmission of high pressure generated in the deep venous system to the superficial system during walking. During the late 1950s and through the early 1970s, surgeons enthusiastically adopted this concept as the rationale for the surgical eradication of venous ulcer—ligate the perforator and the ulcer will heal.[5] As surgeons became familiar with this surgical technique, modifications were developed to prevent its most morbid complication: wound slough. Dodd[4] had already moved the medial posterior paratibial incision of Linton [2] and Cockett and Elgan Jones[3] to a more posterior location before Rob[6] in Rochester and Lim et al.[7] on the West Coast popularized the posterior stocking seam incision used by Felder et al.[8] that avoids the damaged tissue of the medial calf. Finally, DePalma[9] advocated multiple oblique incisions along Langer's lines to avoid wound slough. Another alternative—making a limited incision over the site of the perforators—was thwarted by the inadequacy of instrumentation for such limited access and the drawbacks of ligating the arborizing branches of the perforating veins extrafascially.

Wound slough combined with growing doubt that interruption of incompetent perforating veins had any long-term value in the management of venous ulcer, especially with deep venous incompetence led to a dormant period for this surgical procedure.[1] There were conflicting results reported in the mid-1980s from various groups regarding the failure rate for the standard subfascial approach to the ligation of incompetent perforating veins. Some groups reported ulcer recurrence rates of only 10% to 25%,[10,11] whereas other surgeons experienced much higher failure rates (Table 43–1) in which the crude recurrence rate averaged 20%. Bowen[12] observed a 34% failure rate in his patients, and while working on the St. Thomas' Hospital professional unit, Burnand et al.[13] reported a 55% recurrence rate of venous ulcers. In this series, the relevance of the deep venous system's status was emphasized. Ulcer recurrence was unusual with incompetent perforating veins and a **competent** deep venous system. By contrast, eventual ulcer recurrence was the usual fate when the deep system evidenced postthrombotic deep venous changes on ascending phlebography. Johnson et al.[14] from the Boston Veterans Administration (VA) noted a similar high ulcer recurrence rate. A subsequent physiologic study by Burnand et al.[15] examined pre- and postoperative venous pressures following superficial venous surgery and correlated these hemodynamics with the anatomic pattern of venous incompetence as judged by ascending phlebography. This study is discussed in detail subsequently, but strikingly it showed only minimal improvement in the percentage decrease in foot venous pressure with ligation of incompetent perforating veins alone, even with a competent deep venous system (Table 43–2). In addition, after interruption of incompetent perforating veins by an open subfascial approach, no statistical improvement in the percentage decrease in foot venous pressure was observed in limbs with phlebographically demonstrated postthrombotic disease. Due to the appreciable incidence of wound morbidity and the questionable value of this approach in venous ulcer, open subfascial ligation of incompetent perforating veins was largely abandoned in the late 1970s.

TABLE 43–1. WOUND COMPLICATIONS AND ULCER RECURRENCE FOLLOWING OPEN SUBFASCIAL VEIN LIGATION

Series	Year	Number of Limbs	Average Follow-Up (Years)	Wound Complications (%)	Recurrence (%)
Field and VanBoxel[52]	1971	57	6	Not given	2
Silver et al.[53]	1971	31	5	13	10
Thurston and Williams[54]	1973	102	3	12	13
Bowen[12]	1974	71	3	44	34
Burnand et al.[13]	1976	53	2	—	55
Blumenberg and Gelfand[55]	1978	25	0.5–6	4	4
DePalma[9]	1979	68		1	6
Hyde et al.[10]	1981	125	10	13	24
Negus and Friedgood[11]	1983	107	4	19	13
Johnson et al.[14]	1985	47	8.5	11	43
Wilkinson and Maclaren[56]	1986	134	5	24	2

TABLE 43–2. THE EFFECTS OF SUPERFICIAL VENOUS SURGERY ON PERCENTAGE REDUCTION IN FOOT VEIN PRESSURE DURING EXERCISE

Group	Number of Limbs	Preoperative (% Reduction)	Postoperative (% Reduction)
Normal	38	68 ± 12	—
SVI	21	45 ± 23	52 ± 13
ICPV alone	11	26 ± 23	39 ± 11
SVI and ICPV	37	31 ± 27	54 ± 18
DVI and SVI and/or ICPV	40	17 ± 18	30 ± 21

ICPV = Incompetent perforating veins; SVI = saphenous vein incompetence; DVI = deep venous incompetence.
From: Burnand KG, O'Donnell TF, Thomas ML, Browse NL. The relative importance of incompetent communicating veins in the production of varicose veins and venous ulcers. *Surgery.* 1977;82:9–14.

The introduction of the minimally invasive approach for the ligation of incompetent perforating veins with its low morbidity rate has lead to a resurgence of the popularity of this surgical strategy.[1] Hauer[16] pioneered endoscopic methods for the ligation of incompetent perforating veins in his landmark paper published in 1985. Hauer made practical the desires of many previous surgeons to "gain optical access to the subfascial region from a healthy area in order to be able to ligate, coagulate or clip the perforating veins" (p. 60). Fisher[17] and other European surgeons[18,19] quickly adopted and modified these minimally invasive techniques. The early instrumentation used existing devices such as a bronchoscope or mediastinoscope as the light source, although the development of the subfascial tunnel was somewhat crude.[17] Other surgeons subsequently developed a single light source with a working port for this procedure.[19] Conventional instrumentation was introduced through the working port. Many surgeons, however, found visualization with this technique limited and the narrowed surgical field a challenge, particularly in gaining access to the lower perforating veins. Moreover, the conventional instrumentation felt clumsy to some of us. In 1991, based on a small series of patients, we suggested an alternative technique that used the laparoscopic approach widely used by general surgeons.[20] This technique used a laparoscopic lightsource for visualization of the perforating veins and a separate incision through which a working port was introduced for dissection and clipping/division of incompetent perforating veins by laparoscopic instruments. A paratibial fasciotomy could also be carried out in a controlled fashion. Due to concerns about potential air/CO_2 embolus, we recommended initially that a fluid medium such as Ringers lactate solution be used to distend the subfascial space.[21] The Australian surgeon Conrad[22] and the Mayo Clinic's Gloviczki et al.[23] both suggested CO_2 insufflation, but it was Gloviczki et al. who popularized both a thigh tourniquet and CO_2 for the laparoscopic approach used by many surgeons in the United States today. It is interesting to note, for the most part, that the techniques follow geographic lines. In the United States the laparoscopic technique appears more popular than the endoscopic approach, whereas the reverse is the rule in Europe.

The minimally invasive subfascial ligation of incompetent perforating veins had two important attributes: (1) it permitted skin incisions to be made distant and above the "underprivileged tissue of the medial calf," and (2) it provided direct visualization of the perforating veins. Perforating vein surgery could now be converted into an ambulatory procedure with the potential for minimal morbidity, while at the same time this approach accomplished the goals of perforator surgery: (1) interruption of abnormal perforating veins with prevention of the transmission of the deleterious high pressure from the deep venous system to the superficial system, and (2) avoidance of tissue damage with minimalization of wound morbidity. The volume of subfascial endoscopic perforator surgery (SEPS) has exploded worldwide and is an excellent example of how new technology drives the use of a surgical procedure.[1] This chapter reviews the anatomy, physiology, and technique of SEPS. The available results in the literature are assessed critically, and finally the future direction of SEPS is discussed.

ANATOMY

Early Work

Most clinicians are familiar with the bas relief or actual statues of the ancient Greeks and Romans that demonstrate varicose veins. Indeed, Leonardo da Vinci graphically demonstrated the anatomy of the superficial venous system in many of his drawings. However, it was left to Von Loder,[24] a Russian anatomist, to draw and describe accurately the calf perforating veins in 1803. In his Lettsomian Lectures more than 50 years later, John Gay[25] described in detail the ankle perforating veins in a clinical case discussion of a 56-year-old man with venous ulcers. In this case, Gay clearly showed the posterior arch vein and three perforating veins, while he also recognized postthrombotic damage to these veins, as evidenced by the scarring and actual thrombi he pictured in these veins. Moreover, Gay intimated that there was a difference between varicose and venous ulcers.

Linton's Contributions

Robert R. Linton[2] of the Massachusetts General Hospital appreciated the anatomic works of Von Loder, which he included in his classic 1938 paper, "The Communicating Veins of the Lower Leg and Their Operative Technique for Ligation." Based on his experience with a series of 50 procedures for the ligation of communicating veins coupled with anatomic dissections of 10 lower legs that had undergone barium sulfate injection, Linton proposed an important role for the perforating veins in the pathogenesis of venous ulcer. He termed the connections between the long and short saphenous systems with the *posterior tibial, anterior tibial, peroneal,* and *popliteal veins*—the communicating veins rather than the perforating veins. Their number was relatively constant and they could occur singly or in pairs. Linton appreciated the difference between pathologic communicating veins, which were thick walled and $\leq$0.5 cm in diameter, and normal veins, which were thin walled and $<$2 mm. Interestingly enough, the latter figure is the cutoff point for the duplex definition of incompetent perforating veins. Linton[26] subsequently recognized that those communicating veins associated with the posterior tibial veins as most important for the genesis of venous ulcer.

The communicating veins are located on the inner medial aspect of the lower leg

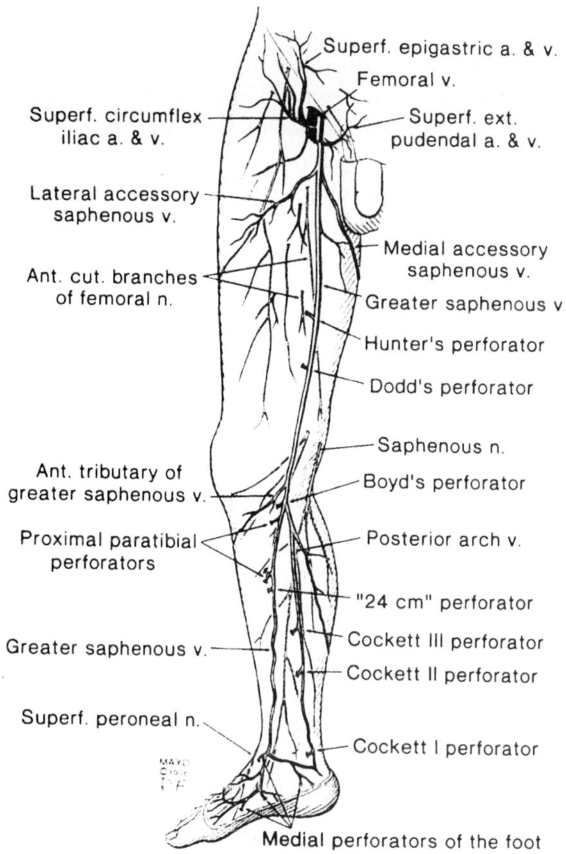

Figure 43–1. Anatomy of medial superficial and perforating veins of the leg.

in three general areas (Figure 43–1). In the upper part of the leg, the communicating veins pass through the intermuscular septum located between the flexor digitorum longus and the soleus muscles. Linton[2] stressed that below the fascia the communicating veins form one trunk, but above the fascia they arborize into a variable number of branches and connect with the long saphenous vein or its tributaries. The communicating veins in the middle third of the leg follow the same course as that of the upper veins, but do not pass through the soleus muscle as they rise below its origin. Finally, in the lower portion of the leg, three or four communicating veins may be found. The upper communicating veins traverse the lamina profunda of the deep fascia of the deep posterior compartment of the leg. This structure separates the posterior tibial vessels and nerves as well as several tendons from the soleus muscle. Linton emphasized the importance of entering the deep posterior compartment to interrupt these lower communicating veins. He described their course as perforating the deep fascia posteriorly at the posteromedial edge of the tibia and proceeding anteriorly to communicate with the long saphenous vein. Linton also called attention to communicating veins associated with the anterior tibial and peroneal veins.

The West Coast Contributions

In 1948, based on both his dissection of 75 cadaver limbs and surgical experience with 465 patients the California surgeon R. Stanton Sherman[27] would build on Linton's contributions. Sherman divided the anatomic location of these perforators into five groups (Figure 43–2). He recognized that two could occur in the lateral aspect of the leg and the foot and another was associated with the short saphenous system. Sherman's work on the perforating veins on the medial aspect of the lower extremity and the muscular perforators in the calf are most germane to this presentation. Sherman described six perforators in the medial calf and located them in centimeters from the sole of the foot. Whereas the upper perforating vein numbers 3, 4, 5, and 6 connect the posterior tibial veins directly with the main long saphenous vein, the lower perforating veins 1 and 2 connect with "secondary veins," which then join with the long saphenous veins. Sherman recognized that the tributaries of the saphenous veins, rather than the main trunks, were the usual drainage point of most of the perforating veins (Figure 43–1). Perforator No. 2 located approximately 18.5 cm above the sole of the foot corresponds to the Cockett 2 perforating vein, and Sherman's 3 and 4 comprise the Cockett 3 perforators, which are at 24 and 30 cm above the sole (Figure 43–2). In addition, Sherman emphasized that the perforating veins branched extensively once they penetrated the fascia and should be ligated subfascially—below where they branch. Sherman also recognized inframalleolar and pedal perforating veins (Figure 43–1).

St. Thomas' Hospital's Early Influences

Frank Cockett carried out anatomic studies of the venous drainage of the leg while a senior lecturer at St. Thomas' Hospital. He stressed that the subcutaneous veins of the leg

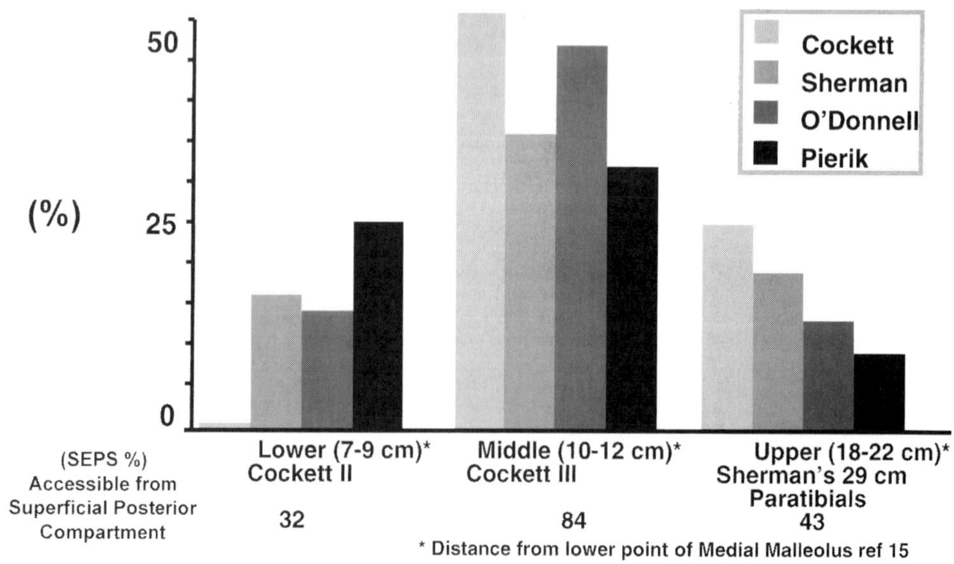

Figure 43–2. Studies of the location of direct medial perforating veins of the leg.

in the ulcer-bearing area do not drain into the saphenous vein, but drain directly into the deep veins through three perforating veins as they perforate the deep fascia. In addition, these veins are anatomically constant, and usually one is larger than the other two. The line through which they perforate the deep fascia usually relates to an area separating the soleus muscle from the deep muscles of the posterior compartment, directly over the course of the posterior tibial veins. Cockett accurately described the joining of the two superficial veins to form a perforating vein. This vessel has a one-way valve that allows flow from the superficial to the deep veins but prevents paradoxical flow of blood in the opposite direction from the deep to the superficial system. He emphasized the importance of valvular competence of the perforating veins in the normal limb and the delicate venous "mesh" in the lower medial calf.[28]

A Modern Day Contribution

A most recent anatomic study of perforating veins by Mozes et al.[29] was carried out in 40 normal limbs from 20 cadavers. These investigators used corrosion cast studies of the leg veins to confirm much described in earlier studies. They distinguished two types of perforating veins: (1) *direct,* which connect the superficial veins to deep axial veins; and (2) *indirect,* which connect superficial veins to muscular veins. Whereas the former are more constant, the latter are more variable in their distribution. The study by Mozes et al.,[29] like that by Sherman,[27] also called attention to the foot-perforating veins, which are valveless and paradoxically direct blood from the deep to the superficial system.

Mozes and coworkers'[29] study showed an average of 13.8 medial calf perforating veins, with a range of 7 to 22 veins. Of these, on average, three veins were dilated to >2 mm in diameter and were considered pathologic, a finding quite consistent with Linton and Cockett's observations. The nomenclature of the medial perforating veins has been based on Cockett's original descriptions.[3,28] Mozes' anatomic study confirmed the four relevant groups of direct perforating veins. The most inferior is found just posterior to the medial malleolus (Figure 43–1). The Cockett II and III perforators—which are of greatest clinical relevance to perforating vein surgery, and particularly SEPS—are located at approximately 7 to 9 cm and 10 to 12 cm above the medial malleolus and approximately 2 to 4 cm posterior to the medial edge of the tibia (Figure 43–1). As observed by Sherman, these veins do not connect directly with the greater saphenous vein superficially, but rather with the posterior arch vein or its tributaries, and they originate deeply from the posterior tibial veins. The highest of the Cockett perforators (No. 4) consists of several groups of perforators, which include the 24-cm perforator of Sherman. Finally, Boyd's perforator, which is just distal to the knee joint, connects the saphenous vein and the posterior tibial, peroneal, or popliteal veins.[28]

The greatest concentration of perforating veins in Mozes' study was located from 25 to 33 cm above the ankle, whereas a second group was from 7 to 13 cm above the ankle. As mentioned previously, Mozes' study was conducted in normal limbs taken from cadavers in contrast with studies by previous surgical investigators who were treating limbs with advanced chronic venous insufficiency. Linton[2] found that the most frequent site of incompetent perforating veins was "the veins at the junction of the middle and lower thirds of the lower leg" (p. 589). He also emphasized the need to divide the lamina profunda of the deep fascia in order to reach the communicating veins in the lower half of the leg. Sherman's study of incompetent veins was based on his surgery on 901 lower limbs demonstrated that perforator No. 2 located at 18.5 cm above the sole of the foot was the most frequent site of incompetence (35%), followed by perforator No. 3 located at 24 cm above the sole of the foot (20%).[27] Perforator No. 2 is approximately in the region of Cockett II and III perforators (Figure 43–2).

St. Thomas' Hospital II

O'Donnell and associates[30] at St. Thomas' Hospital compared in a prospective blinded fashion the value of Doppler ultrasound, ascending phlebography, and clinical examination for the detection of incompetent perforating veins. Surgical findings at an open subfascial ligation procedure were used as the gold standard in the 39 limbs of 26 patients examined for incompetence of perforating veins (ICPV). Of these, 55 PVs (1.8 per limb) were found at surgery, 25 (45%) of the ICPVs were located in an area 10 to 15 cm above the medial malleolus or 15 to 20 cm above the sole of the foot (i.e., in the region of Sherman's perforator Nos. 1 and 2 and Cockett's II and III). An additional 11 (20%) were found in the 20 to 25 cm region, and 14% were in both the 5 to 10 cm and 15 to 20 cm region (Figure 43–2).

Two more recent studies were carried out that used duplex scanning as their primary reference point for detection of incompetent perforating veins. The first, by Pierik et al.,[31] used an open medial subfascial approach and compared the operative findings to duplex examination. Of the 42 ICPVs, 24 were located from 11 to 20 cm above the sole of the foot and an additional 7 ICPVs were located from 21 to 25 cm above the foot (Figure 43–2). Delis and coworkers'[32] duplex ultrasound study failed to use operative findings as a gold standard, so its validity is questioned.

Relevant Anatomy for SEPS Surgery

Although the later anatomic descriptions are of interest when the surgeon has full open access to the subfascial space, the anatomic considerations are different for SEPS. In endoscopic procedures, the operator places the instruments within the superficial posterior compartment underneath the lamina superficialis of the deep fascia (Figure 43–3). In this space, approximately 70% of the Cockett II and 15% of Cockett III perforations are not readily available to the operator (Figure 43–2). This is an extremely important anatomic fact, because the majority of the ICPVs occur at the Cockett II/III level. Thus, only 32% of Cockett II and 74% of Cockett III perforators would be available for interruption at an SEPS procedure through the superficial posterior compartment alone. To access the Cockett II/III perforators, the lamina profunda fascia of the deep posterior compartment must be incised through a paratibial fasciotomy. In addition, the intermuscular septum must be incised and dissected to achieve exposure of the remaining Cockett II/III veins (Figure 43–4). At the distal portion of the subfascial space, the Cockett I perforator cannot be visualized or instrumented because of its position behind the medial malleolus. One must conclude that unless a paratibial fasciotomy is carried out, the operator may miss a significant percentage of incompetent perforating veins through the SEPS approach.

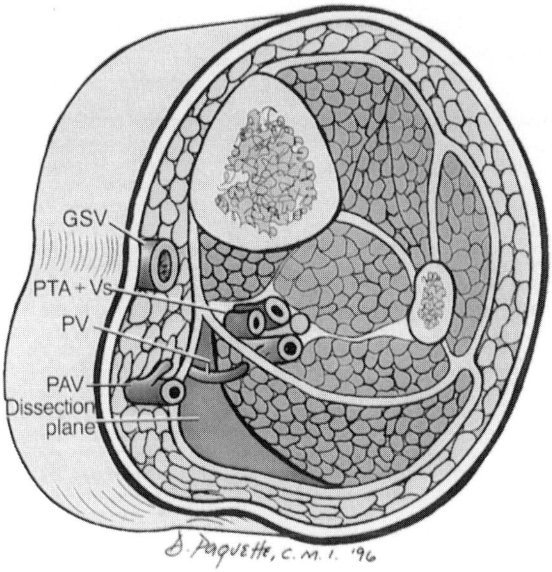

Figure 43–3. Cross-sectional anatomy. The sketch shows a cross-section of the lower leg demonstrating the working space (dissection plane) for SEPS that is created in a subfascial plane within the superficial posterior compartment. The fascia bounds the space (dissection plane), and a perforating vein (PV) is shown crossing the subfacial space connecting the posterior tibial (PTV) and posterior arch veins (PAV). The peroneal and anterior tibial neurovascular bundles are omitted. The greater saphenous vein (GSV) is identified.

PATHOPHYSIOLOGY AND CLINICAL HEMODYNAMIC VALIDATION

In 1916, John Homans[33] described accurately the pathophysiology of perforating veins and their relationship to the production of venous ulcer. Homan's original thesis has dominated the causal relationship for approximately 80 years: "When however they (perforating veins) in turn become dilated, the surface circulation becomes the more embarrassed in that blood may now poor out from the deep veins to the superficial. Under these circumstances ulcers are particularly prone to occur over areas independent of the veins themselves" (p. 301). He further divided causation of venous ulcers into those related to varicose veins in which ulcers usually "ride" on the main varicose trunk and are due to deep venous disease. Only when the perforating veins become involved do the ulcers develop over a wider area. Homans recognized that in the postthrombotic form of venous ulceration, incompetence of the perforating veins is the dominant source of venous hypertension. This classification was entitled "surface varix complicated by varicosity of the perforating veins including especially post phlebitis varix" (Ref. 33, p. 300).

In 1931, the eminent physiologist Beecher and his coworkers[34] were one of the first groups to describe the relationship between ulcerations and ambulatory venous pressure patterns. DeCamp et al.[35] as well as Warren and White[36] measured venous pressures in normal and diseased limbs and demonstrated that ambulatory pressures failed to reduce in diseased limbs. In 1953, Linton[26] clearly shows outward flow from a damaged avalvular deep venous system through incompetent perforating veins to a dilated tortuous superficial system. He argued against the widely held belief that obstruction caused the cutaneous changes associated with the postthrombotic limb. Linton outlined the sequence of events as follows: recanalization of the deep system leads to valvular

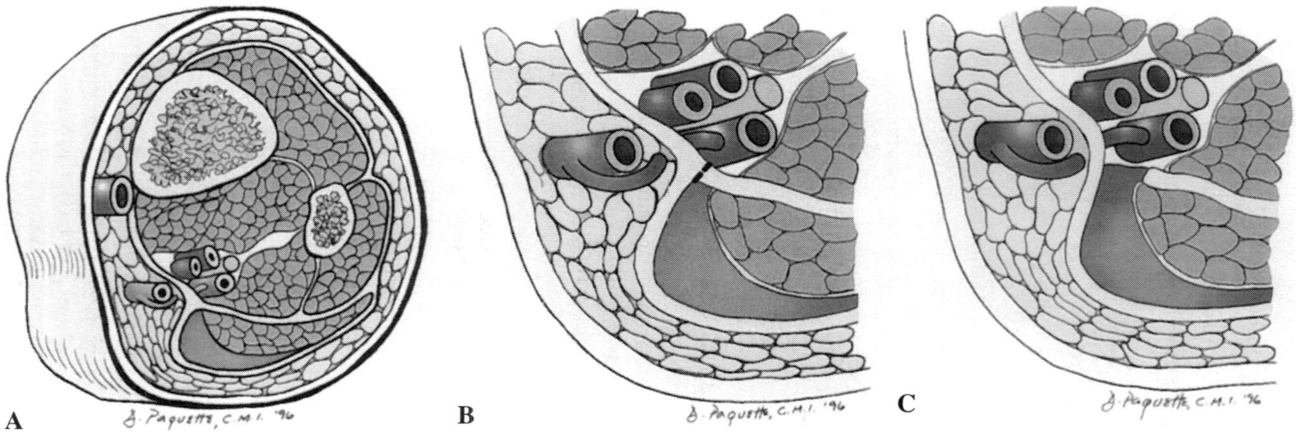

Figure 43–4. Fasciotomy for access to direct perforating veins. (**A**) A perforating vein originating from a subcutaneous axial vein such as the saphenous or posterior arch vein traverses to the posterior tibial vein in the deep posterior compartment without entering the initial dissection plane in superficial posterior compartment. (**B**) A magnified view of a direct perforating vein, outside the initial dissection plane. The dashed line indicated the site of fascial division for access to the deeper posterior compartment. (**C**) An incision in the fascia allows extension of the dissection plane into the deep posterior compartment for control of these direct perforating veins.

destruction and increased deep venous pressures, which in turn are transmitted to the communicating system of veins. These veins, particularly on the "inner side of the lower leg above the ankle become dilated and the valves become incompetent" (Ref. 26, p. 417). The high ambulatory deep venous pressure is transmitted through these incompetent perforating veins to the superficial venous system.

Cockett and Elgan Jones[3] aptly entitled the pathophysiology of the postthrombotic limb the *ankle blowout syndrome*. Their studies emphasized the critical role of the calf muscle pump and its relationship to incompetent perforating veins just above the medial malleolus. These lead to "dilation and tortuosity of the venous mesh" (Ref. 3, p. 20).

Although these studies detail the critical role of superficial venous hypertension and the relative importance of ICPVs, the saphenous vein, and its tributaries, they did not shed light on how each component contributes to the pathophysiology. In a series of clinical studies conducted in 1975, Burnand et al.[15] at St. Thomas' Hospital in London carried out venous pressure measurements in 109 legs of 77 patients and 30 healthy volunteers. The patients were then divided into five anatomic groups based on clinical and phlebographic studies (Table 43–2): they had normal deep systems and saphenofemoral incompetence alone; normal deep systems and saphenopopliteal incompetence; normal deep systems, incompetent lower leg communicating veins, and saphenous incompetence; normal deep systems and incompetent communicating veins alone; and finally, postthrombotic limbs with abnormal deep system and communicating veins.

All patients underwent ligation and stripping alone, subfascial ligation of incompetent perforating veins alone, or a combination of the two procedures. Ambulatory venous pressures were measured before and after surgery (Table 43–2). Preoperatively, there was little difference in the percentage reduction in venous pressure among any of the limbs with incompetent perforating veins alone, with saphenous incompetence, or with deep venous incompetence (Table 43–2). The group with incompetent perforating veins, saphenous incompetence and a normal deep system had an improvement in the percentage reduction of venous pressure following application of a thigh tourniquet, but this change did not reach normal levels. Following subfascial ligation, the group with incompetent perforating veins alone and a normal deep system improved the percentage reduction in venous pressure from a mean of 26 to 39 torr; however, this was still different from that of normal limbs.

Following combined surgery, the limbs with both incompetent perforating veins and saphenous system incompetence reached normal levels. Finally, the pressure patterns in those limbs with ICPVs and deep venous insufficiency failed to change after subfascial ligation. One of the most interesting findings in this study was not in the postthrombotic limbs, but rather in the limbs with phlebographically normal deep systems. These limbs with ICPVs alone failed to show any improvement in their venous pressure pattern after subfascial ligation above that of the limbs with postthrombotic deep systems. This observation implied little hemodynamic benefit, as judged by changes in venous pressure, to ligation of incompetent perforating veins alone even with a normal deep venous system. Treatment of the saphenous system appeared to have a greater hemodynamic benefit.

Similar hemodynamic findings were reported by Bjordal[37] in Scandinavia who carried out direct venous pressure studies and electromagnetic flow probe measurements of both the greater saphenous and the perforating veins in diseased limbs. Bjordal occluded sequentially either the greater saphenous or a large incompetent perforating vein. These maneuvers showed that ambulatory hypertension was only normalized when reflux via the greater saphenous vein was abolished. The abnormal venous pressure pattern did not achieve normal levels with the occlusion of the incompetent perforating vein alone. In limbs with both postthrombotic deep venous systems and incompetent perforating veins, Bjordal observed that occlusion of the saphenous or of the incompetent perforating vein did not normalize ambulatory venous hypertension. These physiologic papers cast doubt that abnormal hemodynamics would improve in limbs with an impaired deep venous system after surgery to the superficial venous system. The lack of a significant improvement in hemodynamics following ligation of incompetent perforating veins alone in limbs with normal deep system was curious and consistent with our findings (Table 43–3).

In an effort to isolate the effect of ligation and stripping of the saphenous vein from that of interruption of ICPVs, Akesson and associates[38] measured hemodynamics following ligation and stripping alone—the first operation; then 3 mo later following perforator interruption—the second operation. Hemodynamics were determined by a battery of tests: foot volumetry, occlusion plethysmography, and ambulatory foot venous pressure measurements. All patients had recurrent venous ulceration. Approximately 85% of the limbs had deep venous involvement, documented by ascending phlebography. Following ligation and stripping alone, the mean ambulatory venous pressure decreased from 82 to 69 torr ($p < .01$). Three months later, after ligation of incompetent perforating veins there was no improvement in the mean ambulatory venous pressure. The authors concluded that ligation of incompetent perforating veins added little hemodynamic benefit (Table 43–3).

A study from the Royal Infirmary at Edinburgh appeared to support the study by

TABLE 43–3. HEMODYNAMIC EFFECTS OF SUBFASCIAL LIGATION (SFL) OF INCOMPETENT PERFORATING VEINS

Series	Year	Number of Limbs	Deep Vein Status	Surgical Method	Technique	Results
Burnand et al.[15]	1977	11	Normal	Open SFL	VP	Still different than normal limbs
		40	Abnormal	Open SFL	VP	
Bjordal[37]	1978	13	Normal	Open SFL	VP and flow with vein occlusion	VP reduced
			Abnormal			VP unchanged
Akesson et al.[38]	1990	30	75% Abnormal	L&S First operation second open SFL	VP Foot volumetry	No improvement in VP or volume with SFL
Rhodes et al.[40]	1998	24	PVI	L&S	Strain guage	Improved
		7	PTS	SEPS	Plethysmography	No change

VP = Ambulatory venous pressure measurement; PVI = primary valvular incompetence; PTS = postthrombotic damage; L&S = ligation and stripping of greater saphenous vein.

Akesson et al.[38] as well as earlier investigators. Stuart et al.[39] used duplex scanning to examine 62 limbs undergoing superficial venous surgery and either ligation and stripping with multiple branch vein avulsions or branch vein avulsions alone. The perforating veins received no direct treatment. Colorflow duplex examinations for the presence of incompetent perforating veins was carried out before and after surgery. Superficial venous surgery without interruption of incompetent perforating veins significantly reduced the number of incompetent perforating veins that were imaged from 65% preoperatively to 37% postoperatively. The proportion of perforators that were incompetent was also reduced from 52% preoperatively to 28% postoperatively. Concomitant reductions in the median perforating vein diameter were also observed. If either superficial or deep reflux was detected postoperatively, incompetent perforating veins persisted. It was the authors' conclusion that interruption of perforating veins might be indicated when superficial reflux persists postoperatively or coexistent deep venous reflux was present, because saphenous surgery alone fails to correct perforator reflux in these clinical situations.

Finally, Rhodes and coworkers[40] assessed the effects of SEPS and concomitant saphenous vein stripping, the latter of which was performed in 22 of 31 limbs, whereas SEPS alone was performed in 7 limbs. Deep venous reflux was present in all limbs, and in 24 of the limbs it was due to primary valvular incompetence and 7 limbs as a result of postthrombotic changes. Two hemodynamic findings were consistent with earlier studies: (1) improvements in calf muscle pump function and venous competence failed to reach significance in the SEPS alone group in contrast to those limbs that underwent both ligation and stripping and SEPS; (2) following superficial venous surgery, no hemodynamic improvement was observed in the seven postthrombotic limbs (Table 43–3).

These series of physiologic studies questions whether interruption of the incompetent perforating veins **alone** is associated with any noticeable hemodynamic benefit. Why should hemodynamics following a minimally invasive approach with its potential limitation to full access to incompetent perforating veins be different than hemodynamics following an open approach. Whether SEPS is important in complimenting ligation and stripping of the greater saphenous is unsettled, and will require a prospective randomized study.

SURGICAL TECHNIQUES

Patient Selection

Our selection process for SEPS relies on several factors. Objective analysis of patients is performed using the 7-point CEAP [clinical, etiologic, anatomic, pathophysiologic (stage 0–6)] scoring of venous disease, according to the updated scale of the Ad Hoc Committee on Reporting Standards in Venous Disease. Patients designated as C3 undergo treatment of their superficial venous system through an extrafascial approach to perforators along with flush ligation and stripping of the saphenous. Patients categorized as C4 through C6 are thought to be potential candidates for SEPS with or without combined ligation and stripping of the saphenous or branch veins because these patients have compromised skin and subcutaneous tissue. We believe that the rational approach to the management of venous ulcer depends on defining the anatomic and hemodynamic reasons for the ulcer, and for this we rely heavily on duplex assessment. Currently, we treat superficial venous incompetence first in C5 and C6 patients and reserve deep venous reconstruction for ulcer recurrence. The presence of an open ulcer should not delay surgery unless actively infected.

Preoperative Assessment

Minimally invasive ablation of incompetent perforating veins requires careful planning and appropriate instrumentation. Duplex ultrasound is useful for not only locating ICPVs, but also for determining the status of the deep veins, which has prognostic significance. ICPVs are usually marked at this examination. Ascending phlebography is not routinely used unless concomitant deep venous reconstruction is done.

Preparation and Positioning

Either general or regional anesthesias are acceptable, although the latter is preferred. Perioperative antibiotics and deep vein thrombosis prophylaxis is indicated. Heparin prophylaxis is strongly recommended when a thigh tourniquet is used. Once the lower leg is prepped out with betadyne, positioning is crucial. Elevating the lower leg parallel to the table provides maximal freedom for instrument mobility (Figure 43–5). Primary considerations for incision/instrument placement are: (1) incisions should be placed in the relatively normal skin of the upper calf, (2) ports placed too close to the knee or tibia limit instrument movement, and (3) ports placed too close to each other result in a "dueling instrument" phenomenon. A thigh tourniquet appropriate to the girth of the leg is placed at the midthigh. Care should be taken to dry the Betadyne underneath the tourniquet to avoid chemical burns. Following esmarch bandage exsanguination of the leg, the tourniquet is inflated to 250 mmHg. We usually sequence concomitant ligation and stripping of the greater saphenous with SEPS as follows: (1) dissection and exposure of the saphenofemoral junction, (2) tourniquet inflation for SEPS, and (3) tourniquet deflation with flush ligation. If the varicosities are large and plump, stripping/branch vein avulsion is carried out under tourniquet control.

Instrumentation Sites

Because the primary impetus for the development of SEPS is the reduction of wound complications, minimizing trauma to the already compromised tissues is imperative. The constraints on instrumentation can be addressed by allowing adequate space between port sites and the bony prominences of the knee and tibia.[51] The relatively small space created by the tunnel is best used by separating the incisions for the scope and instrument ports. This triangulation should diminish the effects of the dueling instrument phenomenon of two parallel instruments in a tight space. The first incision accommodates a 10-mm port and is situated at least 10 cms distal to the tibial tuberosity and 2 cm laterally to the edge of the tibia (Figure 43–6). In making these incisions, care should be taken to avoid necrosis of the skin by the port at the insertion site. The air seal should

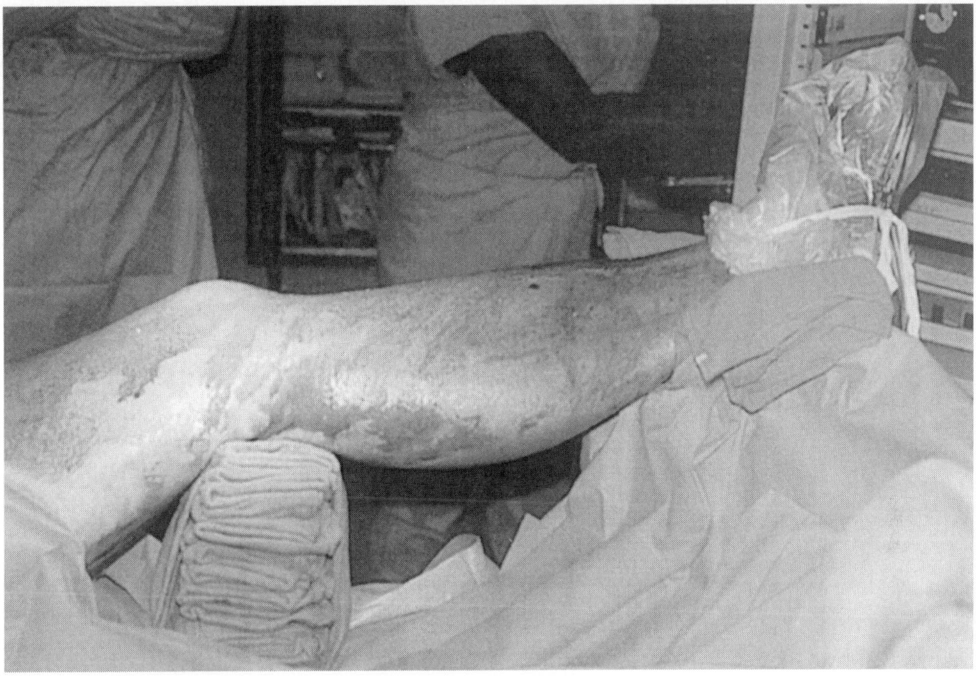

Figure 43–5. SEPS preparation. Photograph of a left leg prepared with betadyne and positioned for the subfascial endoscopic ligation of perforators. The lower leg is elevated and is parallel to the table. A stack of towels at the knee and a padded stand at the ankle maintains this position. Elevation allows for instrument movement unencumbered by either the contralateral leg or ipsilateral thigh and knee.

be at the fascial level, not at the skin level, so that the skin need not be tight around the device. The rubber screw outer sheath guards against an air leak at the skin level. A 5-mm port is then placed under direct visualization after creating and insufflating the subfascial tunnel. This port is positioned 5 cm posterior and at least 5 cm distal to the first incision. Both of these incisions may be placed more distally if healthy skin is available (Figure 43–6) and if the duplex scanning shows more distal perforators. In addition, these incisions may be used for avulsion of branch varicosities or stripping of the greater saphenous vein. In many cases, the stripper may be inserted retrograde to the groin through one of these incisions.

After the primary skin incision is made and following Bovie incision of the subcutaneous tissue, blunt dissection exposes the fascia below. Two opposing finger retractors provide an excellent exposure of the fascia. The fascia is incised and the subfascial space entered. Again, the length of the fascial incision is more critical than that of the skin incision to prevent air leaks. We usually pick up the distal side of the fascial incision with an Allis clamp to facilitate introduction of the port. At this point, numerous options exist. For limited dissections, manual retraction with conventional right angle

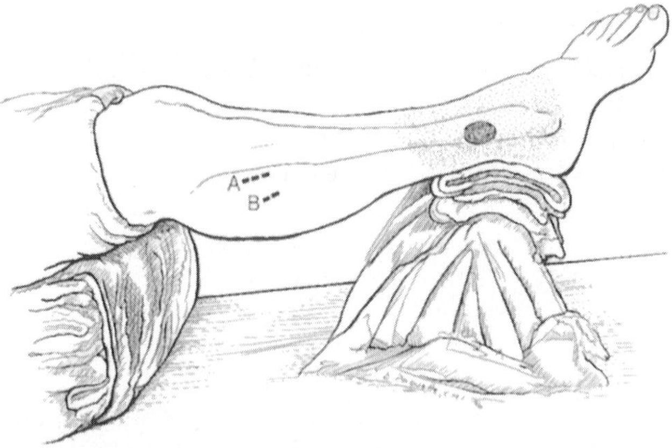

A

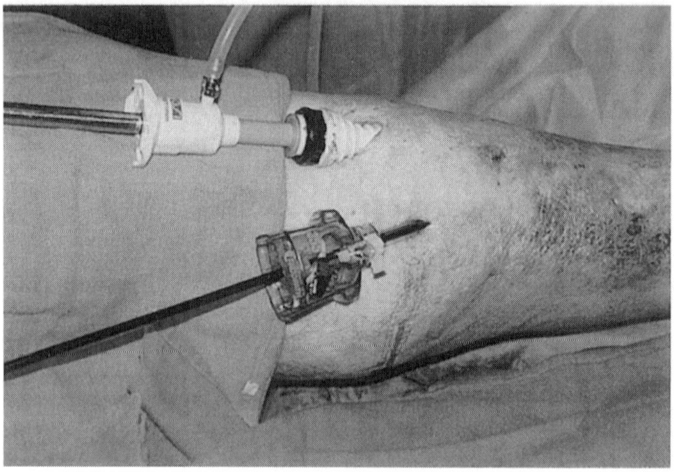

B

Figure 43–6. Incision placement of SEPS. (**A**) Sketch demonstrating the incision sites for port placement in SEPS. Incisions are proximal to the area of lipodermatosclerosis (stipples) and ulceration. Incision (A) accommodates a 10-mm port and is located at least 10 cm distal to the tibial tuberosity and 2 cm lateral to the edge of the tibia. Incision (B) accommodates a 5-mm port and is located 5 cm posterior and distal to the first incision. This incision also may be placed more distally. (**B**) The usual configuration of an anteriorly placed 10-mm port accommodating the scope with a 5-mm port placed posterior and caudal for the operating instruments.

retractors provides exposure for up to 10 cm. Video optics are useful even when this limited approach is used. However, even with improved visualization, complete visual exposure of the subfascial space is not achieved. We strongly advocate different approaches that provide full access to the entire subfascial space. Following insertion of the 10-mm port for videooptics, the 5-mm port can then be introduced under direct visualization through the fascial layer into the superficial posterior compartment, as described previously.

Creation of the Subfascial Tunnel

The subfascial space is a potential space, separating the soleus and gastrocnemius muscles from the overlying fascia and its maintenance is crucial to adequate identification and ligation of perforators. Normally bridged by fatty connective tissue, this potential space may have dense fibrotic changes due to chronic venous disease, especially if overlying ulceration is present. Creation and maintenance of the actual working space in the space is the first unique aspect of the SEPS approach. Figures 43–3 and 43–4 demonstrate the location of the surgically expanded plane.

Although the initial dissection of this subfascial plane may be accomplished without specific dissection aids, we found that the use of a balloon dissector quickly creates a subfascial space that can then be maintained by CO_2 insufflation and occasionally by mechanical retraction. The first type uses an extrusion balloon, packaged in a stiff trocar and covered with a peel-away sheath (U.S. Surgical, Tyco Healthcare Group, L.P., Norwalk, CT). This device also permits insertion of the laparoscope through its obturator. This balloon expander is inserted through the initial incision and is distended with 200 to 300 mL of saline (Figure 43–7). As the balloon deploys along the length of the leg, it can be guided by applying external pressure to the calf. This device provides a consistent working space (Figure 43–8), with most perforators pushed toward the tibia. The balloon usually deflects around dense fibrosis sometimes underneath ulcerations or due to previous surgery. Although the balloon decreases the need for the dissection, it also lessens the potential for injury. An alternative device uses direct visualization and incremental balloon distention to create a working space (Guidant, Menlo Park, CA). We do not have direct experience with this latter device.

We have found that balloon dissection provides a convenient starting point for perforator dissection and expedites the operation. Others, however, have used the laparoscope itself as a blunt dissector. This technique necessitates frequent cleaning of the lens. Scope covers or recessed optics may lessen this problem.

Laparoscopic Alternative—Endoscopic Approach

Although not used at our institution, the endoscopic technique should be described for completeness sake. As detailed by Wolters et al.,[42] the endoscopic approach is performed through a bloodless field, created by a roll-on tourniquet. An open-scope, single-port incision is made 15 to 20 cm proximal to the ulcer, dorsal and posterior to Linton's line. Access is gained to the subfascial space, which is confirmed by digital exam. Surgical halogen light tubes of various lengths are delivered through an overlying sheath with a rigid handle, at which point a video camera is connected to the extreme end of the handle. The cold light tube is then pushed forward to the site of the ulcer and then fixed to the handle. With the help of a 5° optical device, the ICPVs are identified, coagulated, or dissected. Newer instruments allow a working space of 20 mm in diameter with the arc of view up to 80°. The view is also angled 30° to allow for direct view of the paratibial fascia for entrance into the deep posterior compartment, which has become an integral part of the operation. Gas insufflation can be used intermittently for more distal visualization.

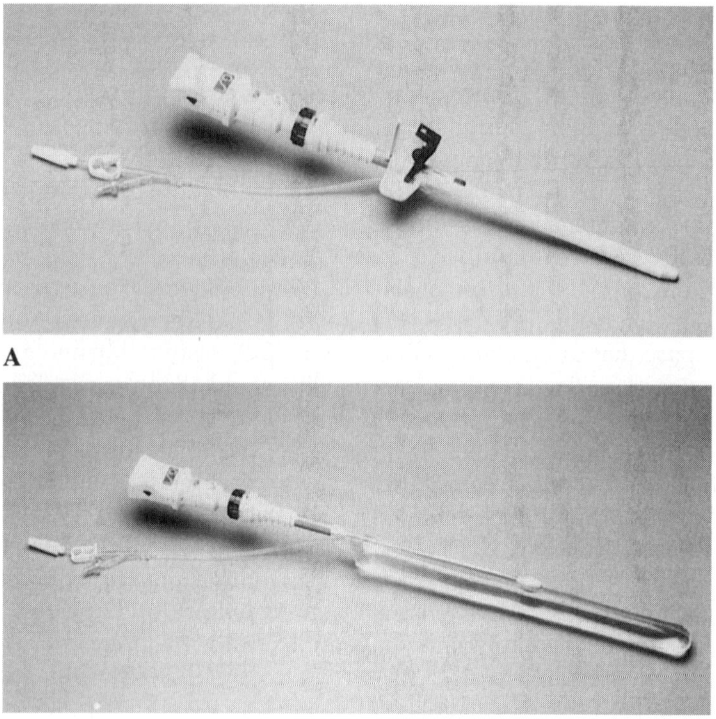

A

B

Figure 43–7. Space maker balloon dissector (USSS, Norwalk, CT). (**A**) This balloon is inserted on a stiff trocar with a covering sheath. (**B**) The sheath is removed and the balloon is distended with saline. The balloon distends longitudinally, creating the subfascial plane. The balloon and trocar are then removed, leaving a 10-mm port in place.

Perforator Dissection

Although the midcalf subfascial working space is often generous (2 × 2 cm in cross-section), the space quickly narrows as the operation is carried down toward the ankle. This small space, combined with noncompliant skin and fibrotic subcutaneous tissue usually associated with CVI, results in an extremely tight working space. Reaching the supramalleolar perforators represents the greatest limitation of our current technology. However, several maneuvers may be used in this situation. Division of the overlying investing fascia may significantly increase the available space. Upward retraction using the scope is a useful maneuver, which may be further enhanced by the use of a 30° lens and a retracting hood. Excessive force should be avoided, as tissue injury at the trocar site is possible, as is injury to the saphenous nerve. These interventions provide some improvement in visualization, but the working space remains confined. Dissection beneath active ulcers on occasion may present some difficulty to balloon expanders because the dense connective tissues can be resistant to most blunt dissection. This situation requires sharp scissor dissection. Fortunately, we have not found reoperative cases,

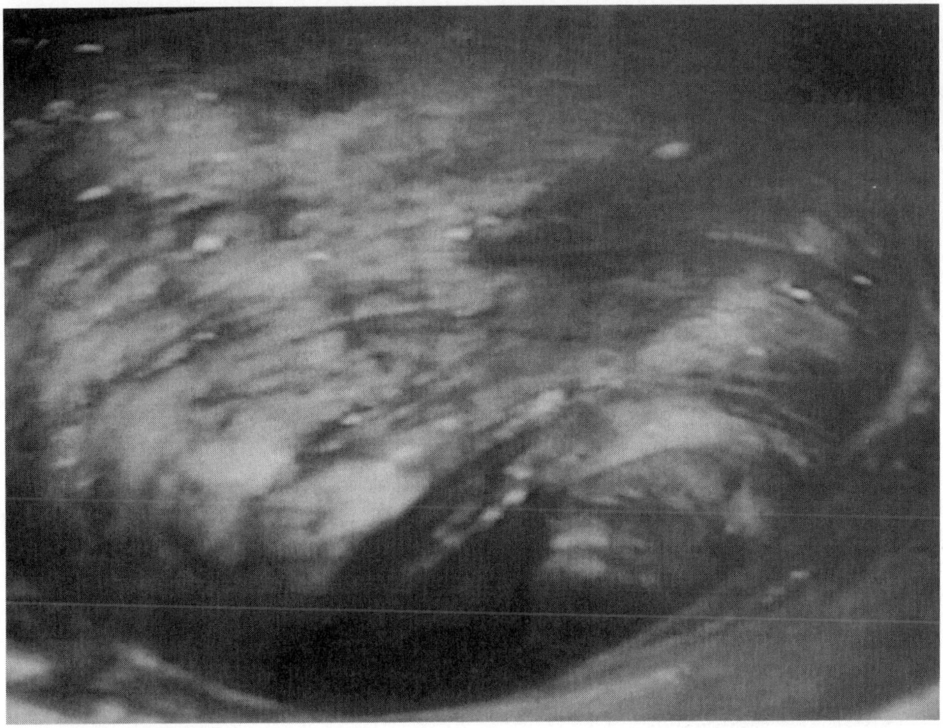

Figure 43–8. Subfascial tunnel. Subfascial working space obtained by the use of balloon dissection and CO_2 insufflation. In this photograph, the tibia and most perforating veins are located along the left.

the majority of which many years after an open approach to be a major problem. Although ICPVs are alleged to occur frequently in the vicinity of ulcers, the duplex study of Hanrahan et al.[50] showed that only 26% of ulcers were situated above perforating veins.

Paratibial Fasciotomy

To this point, we have limited our discussion to exploration of the superficial posterior compartment. Unfortunately, only a minority of direct ICPVs (Cockett and paratibial perforators) can be accessed in the superficial posterior compartment, as discussed in the anatomy section (see Figure 43–2). The majority of Cockett II and III perforators are located either in the deep posterior compartment or they are within a duplication of the deep fascia (intermuscular septum) between the superficial and deep posterior compartments. These perforators are accessed by dividing the fascia (Figure 43–4), which is performed with a laparoscopic scissor, and dissection is carried out bluntly, which exposes the deep posterior compartment and the Cockett perforators. The posterior neurovascular bundle frequently can be encountered during this dissection, and care should be exercised to avoid injury to these structures. The thigh tourniquet may make the vessels and nerves less recognizable than when the limb is perfused. We assiduously avoid electrocautery in this area. In the mid- to upper calf, the fasciotomy exposes paratibial perforators that are immediately adjacent to the tibia or within a duplicated fascial layer (Figure 43–9).

Perforator Disruption

The goal of SEPS is to stop the pathologic flow of blood from the deep venous system through ICPVs to the superficial venous system. Surgical ablative techniques are our

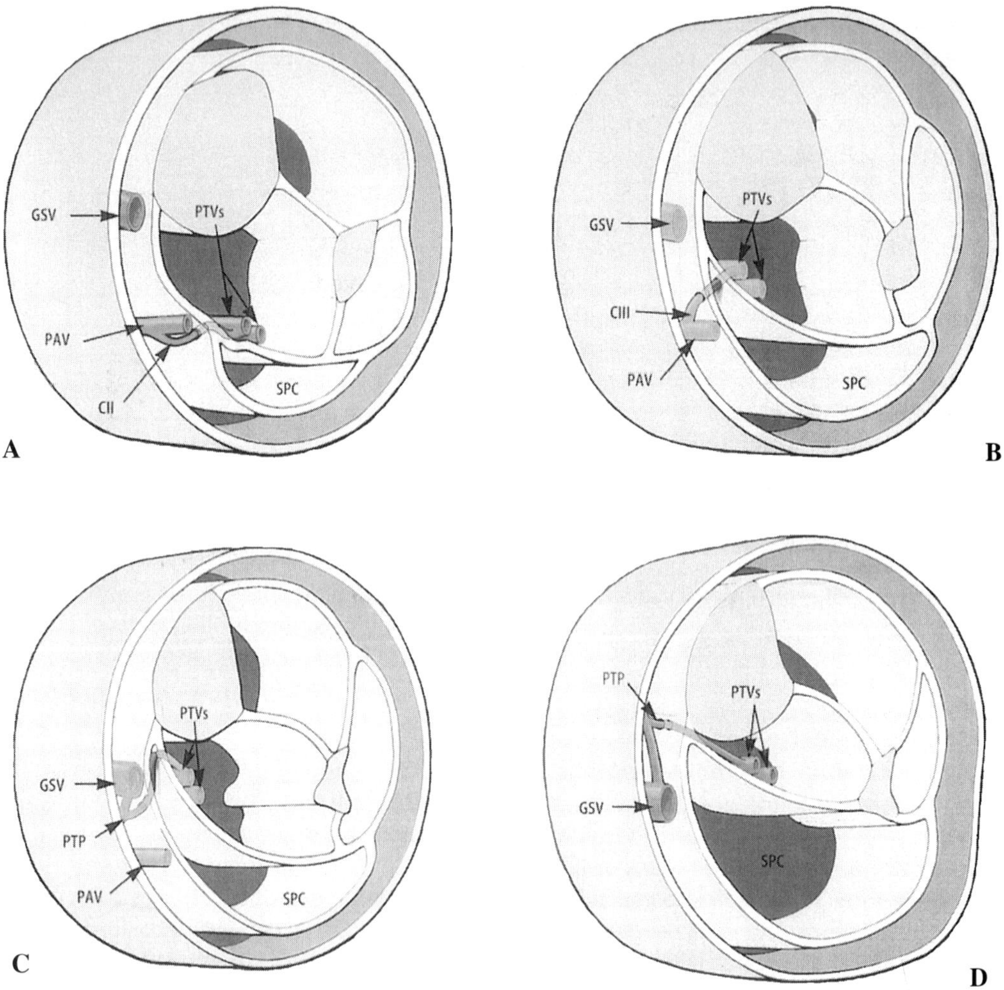

Figure 43–9. Compartments and medial veins of the leg. Cross-sections at the level of Cockett II (A), Cockett III (B), "24-cm" (C), and more proximal paratibial (D) perforating veins. GSV: greater saphenous vein; PAV: posterior arch vein; PTVs: posterior tibial veins; SPC: superficial posterior compartment; CII: Cockett II; CIII: Cockett II; PTP: paratibial perforators. (*Modified from Mozes G, Gloviczki P, Kadar A.* Surgical Anatomy of Perforating Veins. *In Atlas of Endoscopic Perforator Vein Surgery edited by Gloviczki P and Bergan JJ. p. 22. London: Springer, 1998.*)

initial approach to C4 through C6 limbs. Approaches to perforator disruption vary widely and include simple division with subsequent external compression, electrocoagulation, ultrasonic coagulation, and clip application. Because no device is ideal in all circumstance, the merits of each are reviewed.

Uncontrolled disruption of ICPVs provides a rapid and permanent solution. This method is performed in a blind fashion with control of hemorrhage by external compression. This technique is in a sense no different than the shearing method proposed by Edwards,[51] so that injury to the neurovascular bundles is possible. The disruption technique does not allow for direct visualization of perforators and its use is limited to the superficial posterior compartment, which may miss potentially important perforators. We do not favor this approach. When videoscopic techniques are used, simple division of the perforators still may be used, however, the procedure mandates exsanguination and use of a tourniquet to maintain a bloodless operative field—we do not endorse this approach. Although we occasionally use simple perforator division to disrupt the most distal perforator when space limitation precludes other techniques, we advocate the use of hemostatic methods when possible.

Electrocautery devices quickly divide even the largest perforating veins, especially when emptied of blood. Although hemostasis is improved compared to simple uncontrolled division of perforating vessels, electrocautery is less reliable than other techniques for hemostasis and tissue vaporization necessitates frequent lens cleaning. The greatest potential problem with cautery is the dissipation of heat energy to the adjacent nerves and tissues. Injury to nerves are the main concern. Saphenous nerve damage can result in annoying paresthesias whereas posterior tibial nerve trauma can lead to troubling disability that is sometimes permanent. Injury to the posterior tibial veins may predispose to deep venous thrombosis. Collateral damage is minimized by the use of bipolar cautery; however, present-day equipment is cumbersome and energy delivery is not easily regulated. Finally, concern regarding maintenance of hemostasis from the divided vessels is a problem.

Ultrasonic coagulation uses a high-frequency oscillating arm with pincer jaws to coagulate and divide tissue. This device relies on a combination of pressure and harmonic oscillation to hemostatically divide the vessel. The oscillating limb has three surfaces to choose from may be chosen by adjusting the contact surface area, the amount of tissue coagulation may be varied. In general, larger surface contact provides better coagulation but takes more time and causes more vaporization, which results in greater energy transfer. The ability to dissect, divide, and coagulate tissue without exchanging instruments improves the fluidity of the operation. Heat conduction is less than with cautery. Newer ultrasonic coagulators have been developed since 1998 that are able to fit through a 5-mm port. These newer devices remain fairly costly, however, which forces many to use the ultrasonic coagulator with the standard 10-mm shaft. When this device is used for perforator disruption, either the medium or large surfaces should be applied with firm pressure to ensure hemostasis.

Endoscopic clip appliers have been used widely in laparoscopic cholecystectomy and other laparoscopic procedures. They are relatively secure, easy to use, and do not conduct heat. Blunt and sharp dissection along the axis of the vein skelotonizes the perforators and permits more accurate application of the clips for subsequent division of the perforator. Five millimeter devices are currently the device of choice. A variety of clips are available for the SEPS procedure. The Surgiclip (U.S. Surgical, Tyco Healthcare Group, L.P., Norwalk, CT) a 5-mm multifire endo clip applier, allows a successive deployment of clips, therefore streamlining the procedure. The 5-mm Ligaclip Allport (Ethicon Endo-Surgery, Cincinnati, OH), a single use clip applier, has smaller jaws and uses 9-mm clips, which are equivalent in length to most 10-mm devices, therefore allowing easier maneuverability. Perforating veins may be interrupted by placing a single clip across the vessel; however, distal dissection is often facilitated by doubly clipping and then dividing the vein. We have not found clip dislodgment to be a problem. Although the exchange of instruments may be awkward at times, this is our preferred technique for perforator ligation.

Conclusion

The techniques and instrumentation for SEPS have undergone tremendous refinement over the past few years. By using the methods outlined, most incompetent perforating veins can be disrupted. In our experience, paratibial fasciotomy is mandatory; however, dissection and division of the ICPVs near the ankle or under ulcers remains a challenge. With continued improvements in technology and techniques, these difficulties should be mastered.

RESULTS

Preoperative Demographics and Evaluation

We reviewed the available papers in the literature to define patient demographics, preoperative diagnostic studies, surgical techniques, morbidity, and early clinical postoperative results. Sixteen papers published from 1991 through the present were analyzed (Table 43–4). Of the 865 limbs reported, the largest series of 155 limbs was the North American Registry (NA -SEPS Registry) data of Gloviczki et al.[46] and the smallest series is that reported initially by Conrad.[22] Seven of the 16 series contained less than 40 limbs. Fifty-six percent (56%) of the overall series were either at the C5 or C6 clinical stage. The male-to-female ratio was nearly equal (1.1 : 1). Six of the 16 series used ascending phlebography in their preoperative evaluation, whereas 12 of 16 studies used duplex scanning alone or in combination with another modality. Three series used continuous-wave Doppler as the sole preoperative assessment modality. The average number of perforating veins interrupted was 4.96 and ranged from 3 to 11. Disappointingly, only nine papers in the series (585 limbs) commented on the status of the deep system. Of these, 85% had deep venous insufficiency (DVI) with primary valvular insufficiency as the predominant pathology in 72% of these limbs. Postthrombotic changes were found in 28% of those with DVI.

Surgical Technique (Table 43–4)

Of the 15 series that detailed their procedure, only 5 used the laparoscopic approach to some extent. The majority used some form of endoscopic technique. A thigh tourniquet was used in 9 of the 10 series in which this was reported. Three series failed to mention

TABLE 43–4. SUBFASCIAL ENDOSCOPIC PERFORATOR SURGERY[a]

Preoperative Characteristics		
Number of limbs	865	
Ulcer (%)	56	
M : F ratio	1.1:1	
Deep venous involvement (%)		
PVI	62	
PTS	23	
Overall	85	
Operative Techniques		No. of Series Reporting
Endo (%)	70	15
Tourniquet (%)	90	10
CO_2 (%)	88	8
Paratibial *f* (%)	71	5
L&S (%)	52	9
Morbidity		No. of Series Reporting
DVT (%)	0.6	13
PE (%)	0	13
Wound (%)	6.5	13
Cellulitis (%)	3	12
Hematoma (%)	3	12
Follow-Up		No. of Limbs in Series Reporting
Ulcer healing (%)	79	487
Mean follow-up (months)	14.5	N/A
Ulcer recurrence (%)	7	411

[a] Compilation data of 16 series from Refs. 18, 19, 22, 41–49.

whether a thigh tourniquet was applied. CO_2 insufflation was used in 7 series and not used in 1 series. The remaining series failed to mention its use. The most striking lack of technical information was whether a paratibial fasciotomy was performed, which allows access into the deep posterior subfascial compartment. Only 5 series mentioned that this procedure was carried out, whereas 2 series stated that this technique was not performed. The remaining series failed to discuss this essential part of the procedure. Information on concomitant ligation and stripping was included in the reports for 820 limbs, in which 450 (52%) had concomitant ligation and stripping. Clip ligation of incompetent perforating veins was carried out in 4 of the 11 series where reported, and coagulation alone was used in 3 series. Two series used both methods for ablating the perforating veins. Very few series mentioned operative time, but it averaged 36 min, varying from 7.9 to 80 min.

Morbidity

Length of stay was unusually long for what would be considered an ambulatory procedure and averaged 3.2 days in the nine series that reported this factor. The discussion of morbid perioperative complications was unusually incomplete. Thirteen (13) of 16 series (689 limbs) reported whether there was clinical evidence of deep venous thrombosis (DVT). Two limbs (0.6%) developed DVT and no patient sustained a pulmonary embolus (PE). Wound complications occurred in 46 limbs (6.5%), usually at the port insertion site. Twenty-two (22) limbs (3%) developed cellulitis, and an additional 20 limbs sustained hematomas.

Postoperative Follow-up

Ulcers healed postoperatively in 70.8% of limbs. Mean follow-up was available in 14 of 16 papers and averaged a short 14.5 mo. Data on ulcer recurrence was available in 10 series of the 411 limbs that reported on ulcer recurrence. Ulcers recurred in 6.8% of limbs. Postoperatively, 3 of 16 series mentioned the use of elastic stockings, whereas only 5 series had documented postoperative duplex scanning.

Comment

The available literature appears to lack sufficient detail not only on surgical techniques, particularly in the use of a paratibial fasciotomy, but also on the incidence of postoperative ulcer recurrence. Therefore, the NA-SEPS Registry data of Gloviczki et al.[46] and the larger recent paper by Nelzen [49] gain unique significance for judging the efficacy of SEPS. In addition, the retrospective nature of all 16 series severely limits their interpretation. With the exception of the series by Rhodes et al.,[40] there is very little data on the hemodynamic benefits of this procedure. As a model of study design, the prospective randomized study by Pierik et al.[41] stands out and clearly demonstrated the superiority of the endoscopic method over the open technique in avoiding wound complications. The wound complication rate for the open technique was significantly worse, with three superficial and seven deep wound infections versus zero in the endoscopic group ($p = 0.003$). These complications were enough of a concern that no further patients were subsequently enrolled in their "open" study.

Comparison between the NA-SEPS Registry (Gloviczki et al.[46]) Data and New England Medical Center (NEMC) Series (Table 43–5)

Of the 155 patients entered into the NA-SEPS Registry, 85% had preoperative ulcerations (Table 43–5). This proportion is comparable to that observed in the 41 limbs of the

TABLE 43–5. COMPARISON BETWEEN THE NA-SEPS REGISTRY DATA AND THE NEW ENGLAND MEDICAL CENTER (NEMC) SERIES (NUMBER OF LIMBS, PERCENT WHERE INDICATED)

								Methods					Operations	
				Sex		R/o DVI					Post	ICPV		ICPV
Series	Year	Number	Ulcer (%)	M	F	PVI	PTS	Endo/lap	Tourniquet	CO_2	SM	(No.)	L&S	ligation
NA-SEPS Registry Data (Gloviczki et al.[46])	1998	155	126 (85)	67	81	99	45	en66/lap82	112	78	+	3.8	106	clip
NEMC Data (O'Donnell et al.[1])	2000	41	35 (85)	27	15	10	31	lap all	41	41	40	4.3	29	clip

NEMC series. By contrast, the gender ratio differs between the two series, showing that women outnumbered men slightly in the NA-SEPS Registry, whereas in the NEMC series, men outnumbered women in approximately a 2 to 1 ratio. In the NA-SEPS registry, 134 of 155 (86%) limbs had DVI in which PVI was the most common cause of DVI being twice as common as postthrombotic syndrome. In the NEMC series, two-thirds of the patients had postthrombotic syndrome as the cause of their DVI. Although in the NA-SEPS Registry 55% of the patients underwent the laparoscopic technique for ligation of incompetent perforating veins, this technique was used on all patients in the NEMC series. In the NEMC series a thigh tourniquet was used in all cases, and all but one patient had a posterior tibial fasciotomy. More than 60% of the SEPS registry patients had use of a thigh tourniquet, and the actual role of the paratibial fasciotomy is unclear. There was little difference in the number of ICPVs ligated between the two series (Table 43–5). A comparable portion of patients underwent concomitant ligation and stripping in both series (68% NA-SEPS Registry; 70% NEMC). In the NEMC series, 4.8% of patients developed wound complications, which is similar to the 5.1% complication rate in the NA-SEPS Registry data. Although no episodes of cellulitis were observed in our NEMC series, there was a $2^1/_2$% incidence of cellulitis in the SEPS registry. A higher proportion of ulcers healed initially in the SEPS registry series (85%) when compared to the NEMC series.

Long-Term Results

The recently published intermediate follow-up data of the NA-SEPS Registry is quite relevant to the treatment of venous ulcer by superficial venous surgery alone.[58] Of 101 (class VI) patients (open ulcer), 85 healed following SEPS, whereas 16 failed to heal. Of the 85, 10 had a postthrombotic cause of DVI and an additional 4 patients had obstruction. Of the 85 healed ulcers, 26 recurred, for a crude recurrence rate of 31%. The 2-yr life table incidence of recurrence was related to the cause of DVI. Gloviczki et al.[46] observed a significant difference in ulcer recurrence when correlated with the cause of the DVI. Patients with postthrombotic DVI had a twofold greater chance of ulcer recurrence (46%) when compared to patients with primary valvular insufficiency (20%).

The NA-SEPS Registry data outlined factors associated with post-SEPS recurrence of ulcers. Beside the type of DVI (postthrombotic), new or missed perforators were factors leading to recurrence. The latter finding emphasizes the importance of a full ex-

LOS	Morbidity						Ulcers		Follow-up	
(Days)	DVT	PE	Wound	Cellulitis	Hematoma	Cardiac/death	Healing (%)	Recurrence (%)	Elastic Stocking Use	Follow-up Months
2.1	0	0	8	4	0	0	88	6	94/unaboot 15	21
0	0	0	2	0	0	0	71	1	41	11

ploration of both compartments. Non-postthrombotic reflux, level of deep reflux, and patient compliance did not appear to contribute to recurrence.

FUTURE DIRECTION OF SEPS SURGERY

It is apparent from an analysis of the existing series that there are large gaps in our knowledge about the effects of SEPS surgery.[1] This flaw reflects not only the failure of SEPS surgeons to address these questions, but also includes deficiencies in a number of earlier series with the open procedure popularized by Linton. Certain physiologic data in the open series suggests that perforating vein interruption alone has little effect on the hemodynamics of ulcerated limbs, particularly with deep venous involvement. Why should these results then differ when performed by a minimally invasive technique? These findings are important because normalization of hemodynamics may predict long-term clinical results, as it does in other areas of vascular surgery.[1] The improved clinical status of a limb, however, with a permanently healed ulcer is the ultimate criteria for judging therapeutic outcomes following SEPS. Unfortunately, as discussed previously, it is difficult to isolate the various components of the treatment of venous surgery in many series because in the majority of series ligation and stripping of the greater saphenous has been carried out simultaneously with SEPS or, in the past, with the open approach.

Therefore, a randomized prospective study is needed to compare the effects of ligation and stripping of the greater saphenous vein with branch vein avulsion alone versus perforating vein ligation alone. In addition, a nonsurgical treatment arm is required to determine if surgery has any value for patients with C5 through C6 disease. Certainly, these clinical trials will require the enrollment of a large number of patients and therefore should be multicentered in nature. Without this information, one must rely largely on retrospective data so that SEPS will continue to be subject to criticism, as exemplified by the following quotes.

The editorial comment by Porter[58] pointedly focuses this skepticism. "The question remains, however, although one obviously can do a SEPS, why would one want to? . . . There is not one bit of substantial evidence that 'it' [SEPS] accomplished anything." By contrast, Ruckley[59] is less of a surgical nihilist when commenting on SEPS: "it is a *neat* alternative" and then Ruckley[59] hits at the basic unanswered question. "There is a need to confirm the relationship between superficial and especially deep venous incompetence and hemodynamically significant incompetent perforating veins." Ruckley[59] calls into question ultimately the half-century of surgical approach to the venous ulcer: "Perforators—the surgical instinct has been to attack them on the assumption that they are causally related to the skin changes." Without data from a randomized prospective trial, these questions will continue for another century. For now, we are left to follow our own best practices based on implications from the literature and our personal and many times anecdotal experiences.

It has been our approach to treat the superficial venous system first in patients with venous ulcer who fail conservative compression and wound treatment for healing. If these patients develop ulcer recurrence, based on the SEPS registry to date, there is at least a 50% chance in a limb with postthrombotic deep venous changes and an 80% odds in a limb with PVI that the ulcer will remain healed post SEPS. Deep venous reconstruction is reserved for ulcer recurrences following SEPS.

REFERENCES

1. O'Donnell TF. Lessons from the past guide the future: is history truly circular? *J Vasc Surg.* 1999;30:776–786.
2. Linton R. The communicating veins of the lower leg and the operative technic for their ligation. *Ann Surg.* 1938;107:582–593.
3. Cockett FB, Elgan Jones DE. The ankle blow-out syndrome. A new approach to the varicose ulcer problem. *Lancet.* 1953;17–23.
4. Dodd H. The diagnosis and ligation of incompetent ankle perforating veins. *Ann R Coll Engl.* 1964;34:186–196.
5. The hidden perforating vein (editorial). *Br Med J* 1970;1:186.
6. Rob C. Surgery of the vascular system (p. 272). Univ. Minn. Vascular Symposium, 1972.
7. Lim RC, Blaisdell FW, Zubrin J. Subfascial ligation of perforating veins in recurrent stasis ulceration. *Am J Surg.* 1970;119:246–249.
8. Felder DA, Murphy TO, Ring DM. A posterior subfascial approach to the communicating veins in the leg. *Surg Gynecol Obstet.* 1955;100:730–739.
9. DePalma RG. Surgical therapy for venous stasis: results of a modified Linton operation. *Am J Surg.* 1979;137:810–813.
10. Hyde GL, Litton TC, Hull DA. Long term results of subfascial vein ligation for venous stasis disease. *Surg Gynecol Obstet.* 1981;153:683–686.
11. Negus D, Friedgood A. The effective management of venous ulceration. *Br J Surg.* 1983;7:623–627.
12. Bowen FH. Subfascial ligation (Linton operation) of the perforating leg veins to treat post-thrombophlebitic syndrome. *Am Surg.* 1975;41:148–151.
13. Burnand K, O'Donnell T, Thomas ML, Browse NL. The relation between postphlebitic changes in the deep veins and results of surgical treatment of venous ulcers. *Lancet* 1976;I:936–938.
14. Johnson WC, O'Hara ET, Corey C, et al. Venous stasis ulceration effectiveness of subfascial ligation. *Arch Surg.* 1985;120:797–800.
15. Burnand KG, O'Donnell TF, Thomas ML, Browse NL. The relative importance of incompetent communicating veins in the production of varicose veins and venous ulcers. *Surgery.* 1977;82:9–14.
16. Hauer G. The endoscopic subfascial division of the perforating veins—preliminary report (in German). *VASA.* 1985;14:59–61.
17. Fischer R. Surgical treatment of perforating veins: endoscopic treatment of incompetent Cockett veins (in German). *Phlebologie.* 1989;1040–1041.
18. Couto JS, Baptista AL. Endoscopic ligation of perforator leg veins. *Lancet.* 1991;337:1480.
19. Jugenheimer M, Junginger Th. Endoscopic subfascial sectioning of incompetent perforating veins in treatment of primary varicosis. *World J Surg.* 1992;16:971–975.
20. O'Donnell TF. Surgical treatment of incompetent perforating veins. In *Atlas of Venous Surgery,* Bergan JJ, Kistner RL (ed.). Philadelphia:. WB Saunders, 1992.
21. O'Donnell TF. Laparoendoscopic venous surgery. In Veith FJ (ed.), *Current Critical Problems in Vascular Surgery* (Vol. 4). St. Louis: Quality Medical Publishing 1992.
22. Conrad P. Endoscopic exploration of the subfascial space of the lower leg with perforator

vein interruption using laparoscopic equipment: a preliminary report. *Phlebology.* 1994;9: 154–157.

23. Gloviczki P, Cambria RA, Rhee RY, Canton LG, McKusick MA. Surgical technique and preliminary results of endoscopic subfascial division of perforating veins. *J Vasc Surg.* 1996;23:517–523.
24. Von Loder JC. *Anatomische Tafeln* tex (2 vol). Weimar, 1803.
25. On varicose diseases of the lower extremities. Gay, J. Lettsomian Lecture, London, Churchill, 1866.
26. Linton RR. The post-thrombotic ulceration of the lower extremity: its etiology and surgical treatment. *Ann Surg.* 1953;138:415–433.
27. Sherman RS. Varicose veins—further findings based on anatomic and surgical dissections. *Ann Surg.* 1948;130:218–227.
28. Dodd H, Cockett FB. *The Pathology and Surgery of the Veins of the Lower Limb.* Edinbugh, ENS Livingston Ltd., 1956.
29. Mozes G, Gloviczki P, Menawat S, Fisher D, Carmichael S, Kadar A. Surgical anatomy for endoscopic subfascial division of perorating veins. *J Vasc Surg.* 1996;24:800–808.
30. O'Donnell TF, Burnand KG, Clemenson G, et al. A perspective study to compare Doppler examination with clinical and phlebographic detection of the location of incompetent perforating veins. *Arch Surg* 1997;112:31–39.
31. Pierik EGJM, van Urk H, Hop WCJ, Wittens CHA. Endoscopic versus open subfascial division of incompetent perforating veins in the treatment of venous leg ulceration: a randomized trial. *J Vasc Surg.* 1997;26:1049–1054.
32. Delis KT, Ibegbuna V, Nocolaides AN, et al. Prevalence and distribution of incompetent perforating veins in chronic venous insufficiency. *J Vasc Surg.* 1998;28:815–825.
33. Homans J. The operative treatment of varicose veins and ulcers, based upon a classification of these lesions. *Surg Gynecol Obstet.* 1916;22:143–159.
34. Beecher, HK, Field, ME, Krogh A. The effect of walking on the venous pressure at the ankle. *Skand Arch F Physiol.* 1936;73:133–140.
35. DeCamp PT, Ward JA, Ochner A. Ambulatory venous pressure studies in post-phlebitic and other disease states. *Surgery.* 1951;29:365–377.
36. Warren R, White D. Venous pressures in the saphenous system in normal, varicose and post-phlebitic extremities. *Surgery.* 1948;26:435–441.
37. Bjordal R. Circulation patterns in incompetent perforating veins on the calf and in the saphenous system in primary varicose veins. *Acta Chir Scand.* 1972;138:251–200.
38. Akesson H, Brudin L, Cwikiel W, Ohlin P, Plate G. Does the correction of insufficeint superficial and perforating veins improve venous function in patients with deep venous insufficiency? *Phlebology.* 1990;5:113–123.
39. Stuart WP, Adam DJ, Bradbury AW, Ruckley CV. Subfascial endoscopic perforator surgery is associated with significantly less morbidity and shorter hospital stay than open operation (Linton's procedure). *Br J Surg.* 1997;84:1364–1365.
40. Rhodes JM, Gloviczki P, Canton L, Heaser TV, Rooke TW. Endoscopic perforator vein division with ablation of superficial reflux improves venous hemodynamics. *J Vasc Surg.* 1998;28:839–847.
41. Pierik EGJM, Wittens CHA, van Urk H. Subfascial endoscopic ligation in the treatment of incompetent perforating veins. *Eur J Vasc Endovasc Surg.* 1995;9:38–41.
42. Wolters U, Schmitz-Rixen T, Erasmi H, Lynch J. Endoscopic dissection of incompetent perforating veins in the treatment of chronic venous leg ulcers. Vasc Surg 1996;30:481–486.
43. Bergan JJ, Murray J, Greason K. Subfascial endoscopic perforator vein surgery: a preliminary report. *Ann Vasc Surg.* 1996;10:211–219.

44. Chernyshev VN, Krygin SG. The use of endoscopic technology for interruption of the communicating veins of the leg in chronic venous insufficiency. *Angiol Vasc Surg*. 1997;2:94–104.
45. Proebstle TM, Weisel G, Paepcke L, et al. Light reflection rheography and clinical course of patients with advanced venous disease before and after endoscopic subfascial division of perforating veins. *Dermatol Surg*. 1998;24:771–776.
46. Gloviczki P, Bergan JJ, Menawatt SS, et al. Safety, feasibility and early efficacy of subfascial endoscopic perforator surger (SEPS): a preliminary report from the North American Registry. *J Vasc Surg*. 1997;25:94–106.
47. Sato DT, Goff CD, Gregory RT, et al. Subfascial perforator vein ablation: comparison of open versus endoscopic technique. Eastern Virginia Medical School Division of Vascular Surgery. Norfolk, Virginia. (abstract). *J Vasc Surg*. 1998.
48. Illig KA, Shortell CK, Ouriel K, Greenberg RK, Waldman D, Green RM. Photoplethysmography and calf muscle pump function after subfascial endoscopic perforator ligation. *JVS*. 1999;30:1067–1076.
49. Nelzen O. Prospective study of safety, patient satisfaction and leg ulcer healing following saphenous and subfascial endoscopic perforator surgery. *Br J Surg*. 2000;87:86–91.
50. Hanrahan LM, Araki CT, Rodriguez AA, Kechejian GJ, LaMorte WW, Menzoian JO. Distribution of valvular incompetence in patients with venous stasis ulceration. *J Vasc Surg*. 1991;13:805–812.
51. Edwards JM. Shearing operation for incompetent perforating veins. *Br J Surg*. 1976;63: 885–889.
52. Field P, VanBoxel P. The role of the Linton flap procedure in the management of stasis dermatisis and ulceration in the lower limb. *Surgery*. 1971;70:920.
53. Silver D, Gleysteen JJ, Rhodes GR, et al. Surgical treatment of the refractory postphlebitic ulcer. *Arch Surg*. 1971;103:554.
54. Thurston OG, Williams HT: Chronic venous insufficiency of the lower extremity. *Arch Surg* 1973;106:537.
55. Blumenberg RM, Gelfand ML: The posterior stocking seam approach to radial subfascial clipping of perforating veins. *J Surg*. 1978;136:202.
56. Wilkinson GE, Maclaren IF: Long-term review of procedures for venous perforator insufficiency. *Surg Gynecol Obstet*. 1986;163:117.
57. Gloviczki P, Bergan JJ, Rhodes JM, et al. Mid-term results of endoscopic perforator vein interruption for chronic venous insufficiency: lessons learned from the North American Subfascial Endoscopic Perforator Surgery Registry. *J Vasc Surg*. 1999;29:489–502.
58. Porter J. Comment to ref. 23, *Year Book of Vascular Surgery*. 1997, p 439. Mosby, Chicago, 1997.
59. Ruckley CV. Editorial. *Br J Surg*. 1996;83:1492.

44

The Management of Large Vein Occlusions

Peter Gloviczki, MD, Corey Jost, MD, Thomas C. Bower, MD, Michael A. McKusick, MD, and Kenneth J. Cherry, MD

In recent years the more liberal use of endovascular techniques[1–3] has decreased the need for open surgical reconstructions in patients with large vein occlusions. Although early reported results of iliac vein stenting has been promising, long-term results of venous stenting for iliocaval occlusions are still not known. Some stents fail, and long, chronic occlusions are not suitable for stenting. Patient selection for surgical treatment is challenging because valvular incompetence is the most frequent cause of chronic venous insufficiency of the lower limbs, and in <10% of the patients is an associated deep venous obstruction responsible for signs and symptoms of venous congestion. Even if long-term patency of a venous graft is achieved, the patient may have significant residual symptoms due to additional infrainguinal obstruction or valvular incompetence. In this chapter, we discuss graft materials and techniques of large vein reconstructions for pelvic and lower limb occlusive disease and present results of suprapubic femorofemoral crossover bypasses (Palma procedure) and of the in-line prosthetic venous reconstructions.

VENOUS GRAFT MATERIALS

Autologous grafts in the infrainguinal location have a best chance of long-term success. The greater saphenous vein (GSV) has low thrombogenicity, and for crossover femorofemoral bypass it is suitable in size and length in many patients.[4] As a spiral or panel graft, it can be used for direct large vein reconstruction as well, although in our experience these grafts for iliocaval reconstructions do not perform as well as for superior vena cava replacement.[4–6] The contralateral superficial femoral vein (a deep vein!) and arm veins, especially the basilic/brachial/axillary veins, are potential sources for autologous grafts. Harvesting contralateral deep vein in postthrombotic patients, however, may be the source of significant added morbidity. Of the currently available prosthetic materials, the expanded polytetrafluoroethylene (ePTFE) graft has been used most frequently for large vein replacement.[4–10] Because of a large diameter, sufficient length, immediate availability, and the external ring or spiral support associated with relatively low thrombogenicity, ePTFE grafts are currently the best choice for prosthetic replacement of large veins.

FACTORS AFFECTING GRAFT PATENCY

Failure of venous grafts may be due to low flow, low venous pressure, and the increased thrombotic potential of the host. Many patients with previous deep vein thrombosis (DVT) have abnormal coagulation and absent circulating natural anticoagulants. The thrombogenic surface of the prosthetic graft also increases the risk of graft failure. Finally, grafts can collapse under increased abdominal pressure or in tightly confined spaces, such as the area under the inguinal ligament, the retrohepatic space, or when tunneled through the diaphragm.

ADJUNCTS TO IMPROVE PATENCY

The use of adjuncts such as a distal arteriovenous fistula, rigid external support of the prosthetic grafts, perioperative and postoperative anticoagulation, the use of perioperative intermittent compression pumps, and postoperative duplex surveillance have contributed to better patency and improved clinical outcome. Multiple experiments confirmed that a distal arteriovenous fistula, first suggested by Kunlin in 1953, improves patency of grafts placed in the venous system.[4,9] Prosthetic grafts have much higher thrombotic threshold velocity than autologous grafts and require higher flow to maintain patency. Disadvantages of an arteriovenous fistula include an increased operating time needed to perform the fistula and the inconvenience of an additional procedure to close the fistula at a later date, using either endovascular techniques (embolization) or an open surgical cut-down. A potential side effect is an elevated cardiac output, caused by high fistula flow that, when the diameter of the fistula is too large, can also cause venous outflow obstruction. We place a small silastic sheet around the fistula to facilitate localization during a second procedure to occlude it. All prosthetic grafts anastomosed to the femoral vein and all longer (>10 cm) iliocaval grafts have had a femoral arteriovenous fistula added to maintain patency. The fistula is left open for at least 6 mo after the operation, but patients without any side effects benefit from long-term fistula flow to prolong patency. Palma procedures in patients with high pressure gradient (10–20 mmHg) can be performed with good chance of success without a temporary arteriovenous fistula, but patients with a lower pressure gradient and patients with low initial flow (<100 mL/min) benefit from a femoral arteriovenous fistula.[4] Patients with saphenous vein grafts undergo closure of the fistula at 3 months.

PREOPERATIVE EVALUATION

Good-risk symptomatic patients with venous claudication or lower-extremity swelling who have chronic femoral, iliac, or iliocaval occlusive disease are surgical candidates. Short segmental narrowing or short occlusions have been treated in recent years with stents. The patients are evaluated with strain gauge plethysmography, and detailed Duplex scanning is performed to confirm the extent of occlusion and diagnose saphenous or deep venous incompetence. In our practice, contrast venography remained the most important test before reconstruction for iliac or iliocaval occlusions. Magnetic resonance imaging (MRI) with MR venography is performed in patients with malignant disease and vena cava involvement. Ascending and descending venography, iliac venography, and inferior vena cavography is performed. Finally, bilateral femoral vein pressure measurements or femoral central pressure measurements are done to document pressure significant occlusion. A pressure difference of at least 5 mmHg between the two femoral veins in unilateral iliac disease or between the femoral and the central pressures or a two-fold increase in femoral vein pressure after exercise indicates significance of a lesion hemodynamically.

PALMA–DALE PROCEDURE (SUPRAPUBIC SAPHENOUS VEIN TRANSPOSITION)

Described by Palma in Uruguay and popularized by Dale in the United States, the Palma–Dale procedure has remained a useful technique for venous reconstruction in patients with unilateral iliac vein obstruction.[4,7,11–13] Varicose saphenous veins or those <4 mm in size have poor chance of long-term success, although dilation of the vein occurs with time. Results have been better with intact inflow and when the affected limb has no infrainguinal obstruction or deep venous incompetence. Analysis of results of 412 operations published in nine series revealed clinical improvement in 63% to 89% and patency rates between 70% and 85%.[4,9,11–13] However, follow up was variable, and objective graft assessment with imaging was rarely done. Husni[12] reported patency of 47 of 67 grafts followed from 6 mo to 15 yr.

We reported the results of 44 large vein reconstructions performed in 42 patients with benign venous thrombosis or trauma.[14] Thirty-six (36) patients had limb swelling or venous claudication and 38 had pain. Fourteen (14) patients had healed or active ulcers (classes 5 and 6). The etiology of venous obstruction was congenital in 2 and secondary to other causes in 40: of these, DVT was the etiology in 25, trauma in 5, retroperitoneal fibrosis in 4, caval occlusion devices in 4, and others in 2. Eighteen (18) reconstructions were femorofemoral Palma procedures using the greater saphenous vein (Figure 44–1). Patency of the 18 Palma grafts at 4 yr was 83%. Edema decreased, usually after takedown of the arteriovenous fistula. Improvement in clinical signs and symptoms correlated with graft patency.

PROSTHETIC FEMOROFEMORAL BYPASS GRAFTS

In our limited experience, PTFE grafts in this location did not perform well. All three grafts that we implanted occluded early, at 1, 2, and 12 mo after the operation.[14] The ex-

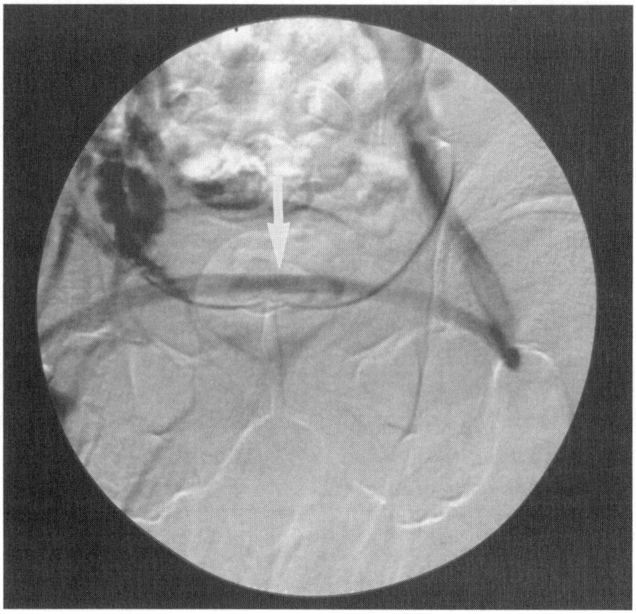

Figure 44–1. Venogram of a right to left femorofemoral crossover vein graft (*arrow*) (Palma procedure). *(With permission from Gloviczki P, Cho J. Surgical treatment of chronic deep venous obstruction. In Vascular Surgery, Rutherford RB, ed. WB Saunders, Co., Philadelphia, 2000: 2049–2065.)*

perience of Eklof[9] and of Eklof and colleagues[15] with PTFE Palma grafts used in 7 patients with acute DVT was only slightly better. Although all 6 surviving patients reported only minimal leg swelling, 5 grafts had thrombosed within 31 mo and only 1 graft remained patent at 36 mo. Comerota et al.[16] used PTFE grafts for similar indication in 3 patients; 2 of the 3 grafts were patent at 40 and 63 mo. We have not favored this technique, and because of our 3 failures we offer in-line femorocaval bypass for those patients who do not have suitable saphenous vein for Palma procedure.

The best results with PTFE were reported by Sottiurai and associates,[17] who observed 100% patency (26/26) at a follow-up ranging from 11 to 139 mo. Gruss and Heimer[7] and Gruss[18] have the largest experience with ePTFE graft in this position, reporting an 85% (27/32) patency rate in a long-term follow-up study. Based on his results and those of others, Gruss now recommends using externally supported ePTFE grafts with AVF for all cross-pubic venous bypasses.

INFERIOR VENA CAVA, ILIOCAVAL, OR FEMOROCAVAL RECONSTRUCTIONS

For in-line reconstruction of iliocaval or caval occlusions, ePTFE graft with external support is the preferred conduit. As mentioned before, all grafts originating from the femoral vein and most long iliocaval grafts are placed with the addition of an arteriovenous fistula. If inflow to the vena cava is satisfactory, an arteriovenous fistula is not added to direct caval replacements because flow is usually high enough to maintain patency.

In our review of 44 large vein reconstructions, performed for benign iliocaval, iliac, or femoral occlusions, 17 patients had ePTFE grafts [femorocaval: 8, iliocaval: 5 (Figures 44–2 and 44–3), cross-femoral: 3, cavoatrial: 1], 6 had spiral vein grafts (5 iliofemoral and 1 cavoatrial), and 1 femoral vein patch angioplasty was performed.[14] Clinical follow-up averaged 3.5 yr (median 2.5 yr), and graft follow-up with imaging studies averaged 2.6 yr (median 1.6 yr). Three patients died of unrelated causes, two with patent grafts. Most patients with prosthetic iliocaval replacement remained on long-term oral anticoagulation. Secondary 3-yr patency rate for all reconstructions was 62% (Figure 44–4). Secondary patency rate of ilio/femorocaval ePTFE bypasses at 2 yr, however, was only 54%. Still, because of the small number in each subgroup, a statistically significant difference between Palma saphenous vein grafts and in-line prosthetic grafts could not be demonstrated (54% vs. 83%. P: NS) Secondary patency was lower in patients with an arteriovenous fistula ($P = 0.023$), although these data probably reflected the more extensive disease in those requiring a fistula to maintain patency.

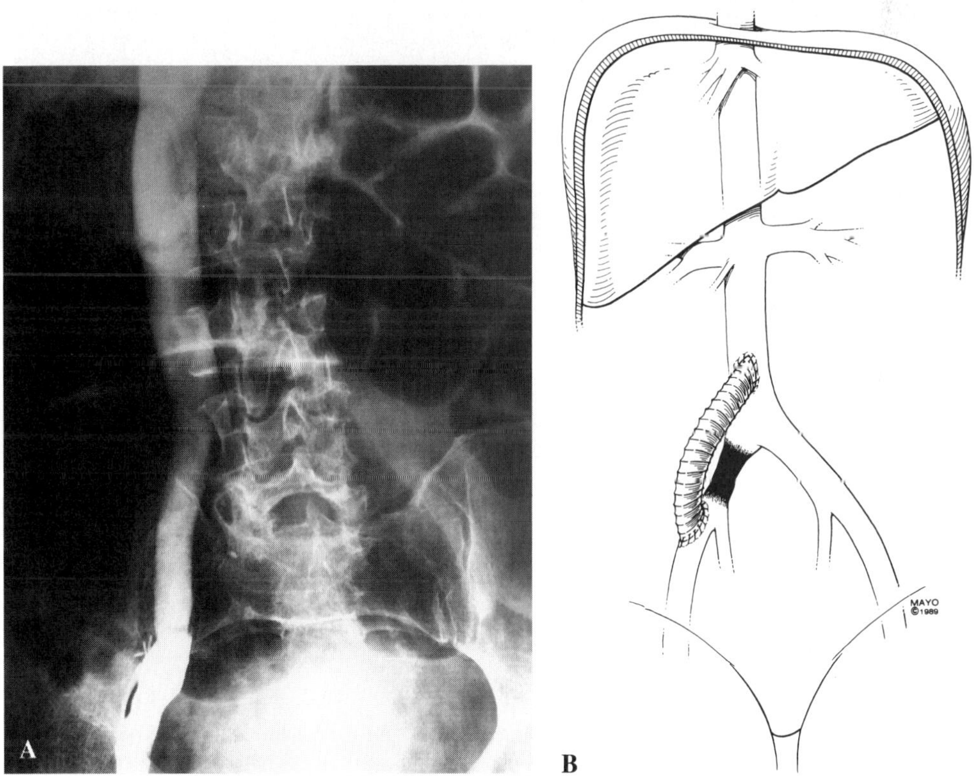

Figure 44–2. (**A**) Illustration of a right external iliac inferior vena cava ringed ePTFE graft. (**B**). Patent graft on venogram 3 mo later. *(With permission from Gloviczki P, Cho J. Surgical treatment of chronic deep venous obstruction. In Vascular Surgery, Rutherford RB, ed. WB Saunders Co., Philadelphia, 2000:2049–2065.)*

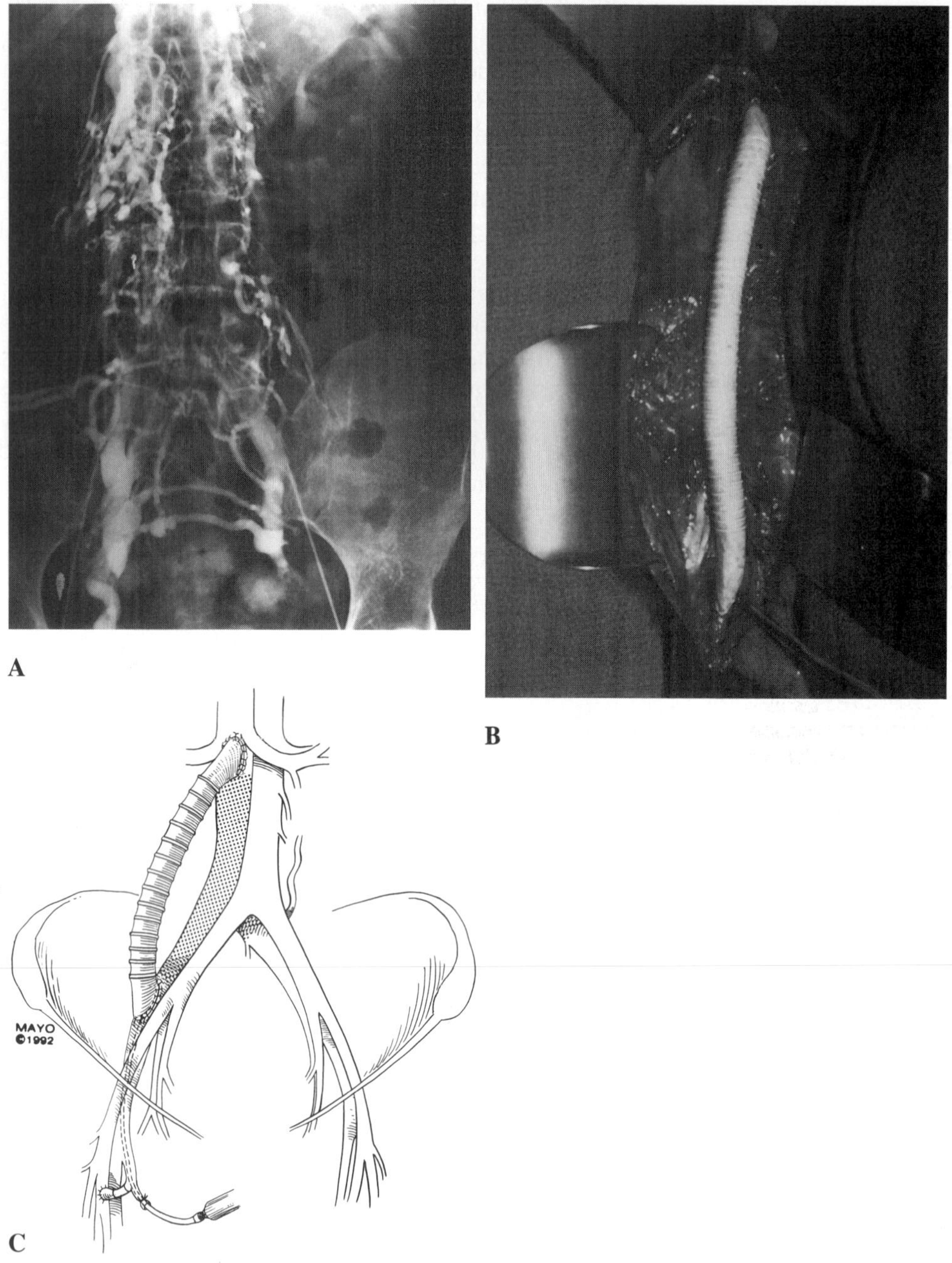

Figure 44–3. (**A, B**) Extensive iliocaval obstruction in a 47-yr-old patient treated with right iliocaval bypass with a right saphenous vein common femoral artery fistula. (**C**) Illustration of a right iliac vein–inferior vena cava externally supported ePTFE graft. Note the arteriovenous fistula at the right groin and a 20-gauge catheter introduced through a tributary of the saphenous vein for perioperative heparin infusion. *(With permission from Gloviczki P, Pairolero PC, Toomey BJ, et al. Reconstruction of large veins for nonmalignant venous occlusive disease. J Vasc Surg 1992;16:750–761.)*

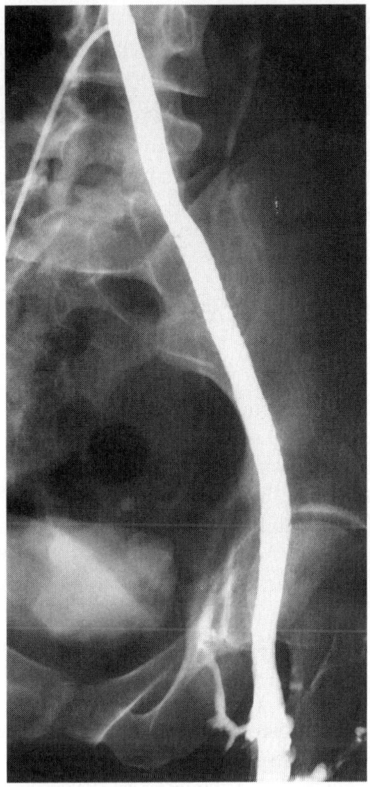

Figure 44–4. Venogram 1.6 yr after implantation confirms widely patent 10 mm femorocaval polytetrafluoroethylene graft. The graft was patent 10 years after the operation. *(With permission from Gloviczki P, Cho J. Surgical treatment of chronic deep venous obstruction. In Vascular Surgery, Rutherford RB, ed. WB Saunders Co., Philadelphia, 2000:2049–2065.)*

If caval reconstruction is performed together with resection of a primary or metastatic tumor, ePTFE graft is used. Early patency of caval reconstruction for malignant disease is excellent, but survival in many patients is limited due to recurrent local tumor or distant metastases. In a recent publication, Bower et al.[10] from our group reported on inferior vena cava replacement with large diameter (>14 mm externally supported PTFE grafts in 28 patients) and with a panel graft of superficial femoral vein in one.[10] Only 3 patients had a femoral arteriovenous fistula. IVC replacement was at the suprarenal segment in 15 patients, at the infrarenal segment in 10, and in both in 4. Thirteen (13) of these patients underwent major hepatic resection as well. Thirty-day mortality was 6.9%. Twenty-five (25) of the 27 patients had a patent graft at a mean follow-up of 2.8 yr (range: 2.7 mo to 6.3 yr).

CONCLUSIONS

Alternatives for venous reconstruction for iliocaval venous occlusive disease includes endovascular stenting and open surgical procedures. Open venous reconstructions for iliofemoral or inferior vena caval obstruction offer 3-yr patency rates of 62%. For unilateral iliac occlusions, the Palma procedure remains the best technique for autologous reconstructions, with a 4-yr patency rate of 83%. Expanded PTFE continues to be the best prosthetic material for reconstruction of the vena cava and short, large-diameter grafts have the best long-term patency. However, patients with significant infrainguinal venous disease have poor chances for long-term success. Although endovascular techniques may limit the need for surgical treatment in the future, carefully selected patients with symptomatic large vein obstruction will continue to enjoy durable benefits of venous reconstructions.

REFERENCES

1. Binkert CA, Schoch E, Stuckmann G, et al. Treatment of pelvic venous spur (May-Thurner syndrome) with self-expanding metallic endoprostheses. *Cardiovasc Intervent Radiol.* 1998;21: 22–26.
2. Akesson H. Venous stents in chronic iliac vein occlusions. *Eur J Vasc Endovasc Surg.* 1997;13:334–336.
3. Liddell RP, Dake MD. Endovascular treatment of chronic occlusion of large veins. In *Vascular Surgery,* Rutherford RB, (ed). WB Saunders Co., Philadelphia, 2000:2066–2077.
4. Gloviczki P, Cho J. Surgical treatment of chronic deep venous obstruction. In *Vascular Surgery,* Rutherford RB, (ed). WB Saunders Co., Philadelphia, 2000:2049–2065.
5. Gloviczki P, Pairolero PC, Toomey BJ, et al. Reconstruction of large veins for nonmalignant venous occlusive disease. *J Vasc Surg.* 1992;16:750.
6. Alimi YS, Gloviczki P, Vrtiska TJ, et al. Reconstruction of the superior vena cava: the benefits of postoperative surveillance and secondary endovascular interventions. *J Vasc Surg.* 1998; 27:298–299.
7. Gruss JD, Heimer W. Bypass procedures for venous obstruction: Palma and May–Husmi bypasses, Raju perforator bypass, prosthetic bypasses, and primary and adjunctive arteriovenous fistulae. In: Raju S, Villavicencio JL (eds). *Surgical Management of Venous Disease.* Baltimore: Williams & Wilkins; 1997:289–305.
8. Lalka SG. Venous bypass graft for chronic venous occlusive disease. In: *Handbook of Venous Disorders,* Gloviczki P, Yao JST (eds). London: Chapman & Hall, 1996:446–470.
9. Eklof B. Temporary arteriovenous fistula in reconstruction of iliac vein obstruction using PTFE grafts. In Eklof B, Gjores JE, Thulesius O, Berqvist D (eds). *Controversies in the Management of Venous Disorders.* London: Butterworths, 1989:280–290.
10. Bower TC, Nagorney DM, Cherry KJ Jr, et al. Replacement of the inferior vena cava for malignancy: an update. *J Vasc Surg.* 2000;31:270–281.
11. Halliday P, Harris J, May J. Femoro-femoral crossover grafts (Palma operation): a long-term follow-up study. In Bergan JJ, Yao JST (eds). *Surgery of the Veins.* Orlando: Grune & Stratton, Inc. 1985:241–254.
12. Husni EA. Clinical experience with femoropopliteal venous reconstruction. In: Bergan JJ, Yao JST (eds.) *Venous Problems.* Chicago: YearBook Medical Publishers, 1978:485–491.
13. AbuRahma AF, Robinson PA, Boland JP. Clinical hemodynamic and anatomic predictors of long-term outcome of lower extremity venovenous bypasses. *J Vasc Surg.* 1991:14:635.
14. Jost CJ, Gloviczki P, Cherry KJ Jr, et al. Surgical reconstruction of iliofemoral veins and the inferior vena cava for nonmalignant occlusive disease. *J Vasc Surg.* In press.
15. Eklof BG, Kistner RL, Masuda EM. Venous bypass and valve reconstruction: long-term efficacy. *Vasc Med.* 1998;3:157–164.

16. Comerota AJ, Aldridge SC, Cohen G, et al. A strategy of aggressive regional therapy for acute iliofemoral venous thrombosis with contemporary venous thrombectomy of catheter-directed thrombolysis. *J Vasc Surg*. 1994;20:244–254.
17. Sottiurai VS, Gonzales J, Cooper M, Lyon R, Hatter D, Ross C. A new concept of arteriovenous fistula in venous bypass requiring no fistula interruption: surgical technique and long-term results. *J Cardiovasc Surg*. In press.
18. Gruss JD, Venous bypass for chronic venous insufficiency. In Bergan JJ, Yao JST, *Venous Disorders*. Philadelphia: WB Saunders, 1991:316–330.

45

Evaluation and Management of the Swollen Limb

Thom W. Rooke, MD

INTRODUCTION

Swollen limbs are, both figuratively and literally, a "big" problem. Not only is limb swelling one of the most common of all human afflictions—for example, the World Health Organization estimates that there are more than 100 million people with lymphedema worldwide, located primarily in tropical regions—but it is also one of the most common problems seen in many vascular practices in North America. During 1999, the diagnosis of edema, including lymphedema, constituted the single most common reason for referral or presentation to the Gonda Vascular Center of the Mayo Clinic. Indeed, in our practice, limb edema is a more common reason for presentation than atherosclerosis, venous disease, or vascular ulcers.

A simplified discussion of the swollen limb involves three parts:

- Classification
- Evaluation
- Treatment

Classification of the Swollen Limb

There are many schemes available for categorizing or classifying swollen limbs. For discussion purposes one can use a very simple approach that combines the most important clinical feature of limb edema (i.e., whether the swelling involves a local process affecting a single limb as opposed to a systemic process that affects more than one limb) with the basic hemodynamic abnormality (i.e., Is too much fluid entering the tissue, or is too little fluid removed from the limb?).

By incorporating these two components, one can create a 2×2 matrix into which virtually all types of limb swelling can be categorized (Table 45–1).

TABLE 45–1. CLASSIFICATION OF THE SWOLLEN LIMBS

	1 Limb	More Than 1 Limb
Not enough fluid removed from tissue	A	C
Too much fluid entry into tissue	B	D

This scheme is admittedly an oversimplification. For example, many limbs have multifactorial edema due to several contributing factors. Conversely, some patients can have a single limb process (for example, deep venous thrombosis or lymphedema) occurring simultaneously in two or more limbs, thus giving the impression that the patient has a diffuse, systemic problem rather than a problem affecting a single limb.

Evaluation of the Swollen Limb

Although a careful history and physical examination are essential for the evaluation of limb edema, most evaluations also require specific tests for completeness. Appropriate venous and/or lymphatic studies are indicated when abnormalities in these systems are suspected. In other cases, clinical findings may lead to the selected performance of tests for cardiac function (echo, nuclear studies, catheterization), liver and kidney function, thyroid (and other endocrine) function, or tests such as urinalysis, serum protein studies, and many others.

If the cause of limb swelling is not readily apparent, the possible tests that can be undertaken are staggering in number. Because of the inherent potential for "diagnostic annihilation," specific tests must be ordered judiciously and only after careful thought has been given as to the most likely diagnostic possibilities. An in-depth discussion of all the possible tests that might be performed on patients with limb edema is beyond the scope of this chapter.

Treatment of the Swollen Limb

The best therapy for a swollen limb is to treat the underlying cause; unfortunately, this is not always possible, or in some cases therapy is ineffective. When necessary, generalized methods for edema control can be used (these are discussed later).

CLASSIFICATION OF LIMB EDEMA

One Limb—"Not Enough Fluid Out"

This quadrant ("A," Table 45–1) contains some of the most common—and certainly the most classic—vascular causes of limb swelling.

Conditions That Cause Swelling

Venous Insufficiency. The term *venous insufficiency* loosely refers to any situation in which the veins fail to transport blood properly from the limbs back to the central veins and right heart. Common causes of venous insufficiency include venous obstruction (from deep venous thrombosis, extrinsic vein compression, venulitis, and other forms of venous inflammation, etc.), venous valvular incompetence (either primary or secondary; the most common secondary cause is valve damage from thrombosis), and failure of the venous calf (or foot) pump.[1] Clinically important venous insufficiency usually requires involvement of the deep venous system, although severe superficial varicose veins, especially with incompetent perforators, can result in significant venous reflux and limb swelling. Because deep venous thrombosis, postphlebitic syndrome, and significant varicose veins are extremely prevalent, venous insufficiency may be the most common vascular cause of edema in North America, with those afflicted numbering in the millions.

Venous insufficiency can often be diagnosed from the history and clinical examination, especially if a history of deep venous thrombosis is noted or if sequela of advanced venous stasis are present along with the edema (such as pigmentation, ulceration, etc.).

Lymphedema[2]. Venous insufficiency may be the most common vascular etiology for limb edema in North America, but the most common vascular cause on the planet is probably lymphedema (primarily tropical forms caused by filariasis associated with *Wuchereria bancrofti* or various *Brugia* spp.). In the United States, malignancy (and perhaps, more likely, the surgery and radiation therapy used to treat malignancy) is the predominant cause of lymphedema, although recurrent infections and cellulitis are also major secondary causes. Primary lymphedema is well recognized but relatively uncommon.

Chronic lymphedema can be clinically diagnosed by the firm, indurated, nonpitting swelling it produces; the edema typically involves the foot and toes (Figure 45–1). These changes may take years to occur. In contrast, the swelling of acute lymphedema tends to be soft and easily reduced (it may even disappear overnight).

Dependent Edema. Any restriction that renders the limb chronically dependent may result in edema, even when the veins and lymphatic vessels are normal. This occurs because gravity opposes the normal flow of fluid out from the limb. Dependent edema is common and may be triggered in countless ways. For example, patients who use wheelchairs as a result of spinal cord (or other neurologic) impairments frequently experience fluid accumulation in their legs as a consequence of their immobility and prolonged, upright posture. People with desk jobs and travelers (especially those trapped on cramped coach-class airline flights) are also subject to this type of leg swelling.[3]

Factitial Edema. This is a relatively uncommon form of edema, although many cases of limb swelling may have (or be aggravated by) a subtle "factitial" component. Extreme cases may be the result of intentional and direct actions such as tourniquet application (Figure 45–2). In less obvious situations, the culprit may be tight clothing, constrictive jewelry, or some other extrinsic cause that binds the limb and prevents the normal egress of venous blood and limb fluid.

Laboratory Evaluations

In addition to the history and physical examination, specific testing modalities may prove helpful in assessing and diagnosing edema of this type. Venous tests include assessments of anatomy (using venogram and/or ultrasound imaging), hemodynamics

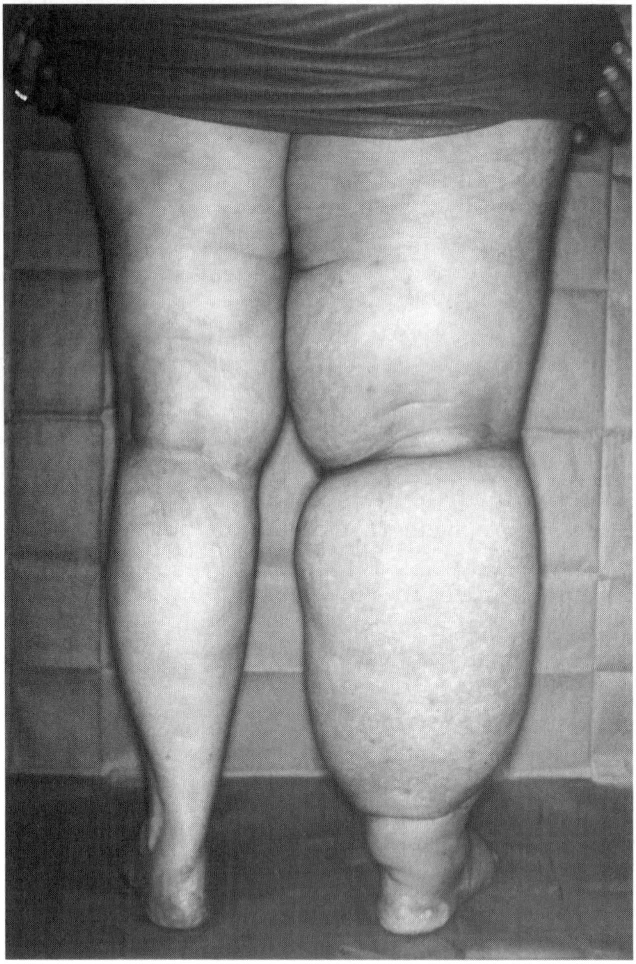

Figure 45–1. Lymphedema. The patient has diffuse right leg swelling caused by lymphatic obstruction. The left leg is normal.

(such as Doppler evaluation of venous blood flow), or functional assessment (including air, photo, or strain-gauge plethysmography, which can be used to measure venous refilling times, calf pump function, etc.). The lymphatic system can be evaluated by lymphangiography (Figure 45–3) or, less invasively, by radionuclear lymphoscintigraphy. The diagnoses of dependency edema and factitial edema are largely diagnoses of exclusion based on history, examination, clinical suspicion, and negative testing.

One Limb—"Too Much Fluid In"

This quadrant ("B," Table 45–1) contains many types of edema that are usually considered nonvascular in etiology, although obvious exceptions (for example, the edema associated with arteriovenous malformation) exist. The potential causes of this type of edema are too numerous to list fully here, but several illustrative examples can be given.

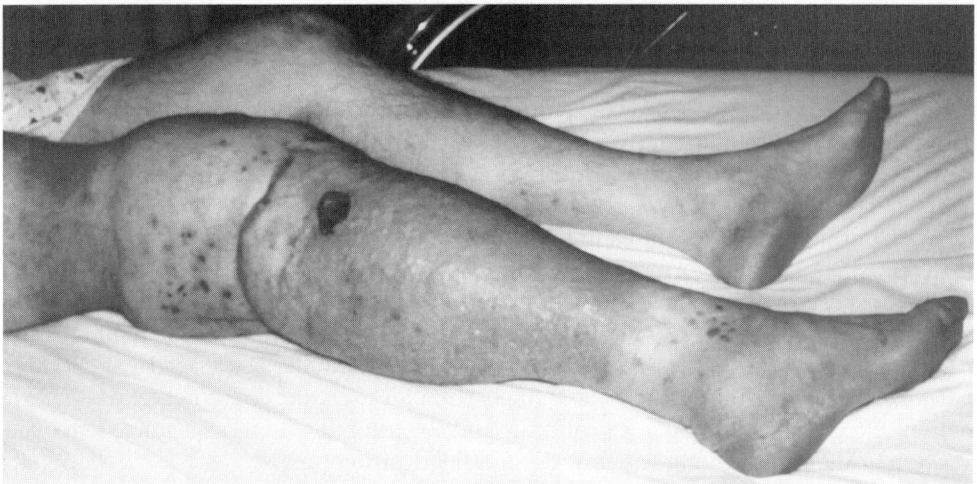

Figure 45–2. Factitial edema. This patient presented with severe, chronic swelling involving the right leg. Notice the mark on the upper thigh where a tourniquet has been self-applied.

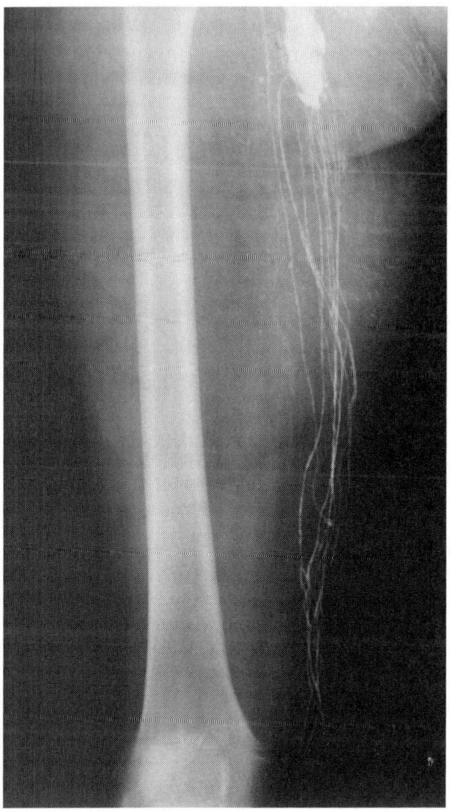

Figure 45–3. Lymphangiogram. Ionic contrast dye can be introduced into the lymphatic system to allow visualization of lymph vessels and nodes. Although this is a good method for imaging the lymphatic system, it has several drawbacks, including the need to perform cutdown on the foot (in order to cannulate and inject lymphatic vessels) and the possibility that the procedure itself may induce lymphangitis.

Conditions That Cause Swelling

Inflammation. When tissues become inflamed, there is typically an associated increase in both blood flow and capillary permeability; these changes may lead to production of edema. Inflammation is commonly seen in association with trauma, autoimmune disorders, or infection. Some cases of trauma-associated edema may have a swelling component caused by hematomas, seromas, or other subcutaneous fluid collections. Infection may take various forms and can cause swelling by different mechanisms. Common types of infection associated with swelling include cellulitis, osteomyelitis, and abscess formation.

In most cases, the cause of the inflammation is apparent by history and physical examination, but this is not always the case. For example, patients with Charcot changes in the feet may experience an episodic aggravation of edema associated with inflammatory changes; at times it can be extremely difficult to determine whether the inflammation reflects infection (such as cellulitis and/or osteomyelitis) or is simply an exacerbation of their underlying (noninfective) bony destruction.

Arthritis. Patients with significant arthritis may experience limb swelling. Some of this may be directly related to inflammation of the joint and surrounding tissues, especially in acute forms of arthritis. However, pain and immobility may lead to limb disuse and dependency, further aggravating the edema through mechanisms discussed previously. In addition, certain types of arthritis (for example, rheumatoid arthritis) may be associated with autoimmune processes that have the potential to affect skin or other tissues directly, producing inflammatory or noninflammatory changes that cause hyperemia and edema.

Thermal Injury. Thermal injury is another quasi-inflammatory cause of edema. Thermal injuries (burns, frostbite, etc.) not only cause direct damage to affected tissue (i.e., they are forms of trauma), but injury may also predispose to infection, which can further inflame the tissues. In addition, thermal injury may directly damage or affect elements in the tissue that control blood flow, capillary permeability, and so on, and in this way aggravate or produce edema.

Tumor. Any malignancy that occurs in the limb may produce localized swelling or edema (indeed, the word *tumor* is derived from a Latin word meaning "swelling"). Local hyperemia, capillary permeability changes, and the direct effects of an expanding mass on the surrounding tissues all contribute to this form of edema.

Sympathetic Dysfunction. Reflex sympathetic dystrophy (RSD) is an uncommon and unusual condition; the pathogenesis is not well understood.[4] During the early phases of reflex sympathetic dystrophy (which often occurs after an injury to the affected limb), there can be a hyperemic phase associated with limb warmth and swelling. Capillary permeability may be increased. Over time, the limb becomes less hyperemic and cooler (in some patients the initial presentation of RSD is a cool limb). However, pain and swelling may persist.

Arteriovenous Malformation (or Fistula). Any acquired or congenital arteriovenous (AV) connection can produce limb hyperemia and edema. In extreme cases, the arterial flow through a peripheral AV connection may be so great as to cause high-output congestive heart failure. If the fistula/malformation cannot be treated adequately, amputation may be necessary to prevent fatal heart failure.

Laboratory Evaluations

Laboratory evaluations for the types of edema found in quadrant "B" are highly variable and depend on the underlying condition. In some cases the work-up is directed at assessing trauma (for example, imaging studies of limbs with fractured bones or crush injuries). The same holds true for patients with suspected arthritis or tumor (i.e., imaging studies are often required). Reflex sympathetic dystrophy can be diagnosed with radionuclear bone scanning[5]; in some cases, specific neuroautonomic and/or sweat test studies are abnormal. Arteriovenous malformations require assessment with some type of vascular imaging and/or functional/hemodynamic study; this may include ultrasound, magnetic resonance imaging (MRI), or angiography.

Two Limbs—"Not Enough Fluid Out"

For all practical purposes, the major causes of edema located in this quadrant ("C," Table 45–1) are right heart failure and renal failure. Other causes, such as inferior vena cava occlusion, are possible, but they remain statistically far less common than heart or renal failure.

Heart Failure

The diagnosis of heart failure is a clinical one, although specific tests may be useful. Two-dimensional echocardiography, radionuclear imaging, and cardiac angiography can provide useful information about the heart (for example, the ejection fraction). In some cases the syndrome of heart failure may be related to restrictive disease or pericardial constriction. Valvular problems, cardiomyopathy, ischemic disease with infarction, and many other disorders can also cause heart failure. Pulmonary hypertension may produce right heart failure and peripheral limb edema; interestingly, episodic pulmonary hypertension associated with sleep apnea is increasingly recognized as an otherwise occult cause of limb swelling.[6]

Renal Disease

Renal failure is an extreme example of inability to remove adequate fluid from the limbs—in this case, the fluid can be transported out of the limbs to the venous and/or lymphatic systems, but it is not adequately removed from the body by the kidneys. The swelling of renal failure resembles that caused by right heart failure, hypoproteinemia, and a variety of other systemic causes. An evaluation of the serum creatinine, blood urea nitrogen, or other tests of kidney function can help to establish this diagnosis.

Two Limbs—"Too Much Fluid In"

This quadrant ("D," Table 45–1) contains a diverse "hodgepodge" of seemingly unrelated disorders that all predispose to edema formation by overloading the limbs with fluid; the fluid enters the tissues through a variety of mechanisms.

Thyroid Dysfunction

Thyroid dysfunction, including both hyper- and hypothyroidism, may produce changes that result in limb swelling. In severe, chronic hypothyroidism, myxedema may occur.[7,8] This condition, which affects many tissues and organs including the heart, periorbital regions, and so on, also causes a classic "indurated" or "woody" swelling of the legs that may closely mimic lymphedema. The pathogenesis of the edema is complex and not entirely understood. Factors may include the interstitial deposition of mucopolysaccharides and proteoglycans (which change oncotic pressure and draw fluid into the interstitial space), changes in cardiac output and peripheral vasodilation, changes in capillary permeability, and so on.[9] Specific tests of thyroid function identify the abnormality.

Hypoproteinemia

When blood proteins, particularly albumin, fall below the level necessary to maintain adequate intravascular oncotic pressure, fluid can no longer be kept from entering the cells and interstitial space, resulting in edema.[10]

Volume Overload

This may be the purest example in which too much fluid causes swelling in more than one limb. The usual example is the postsurgical patient who receives a large amount of intravenous fluid following an operation (such as occurs with aortic surgery) and manifests edema afterwards. Rarely, patients develop edema because of excessive fluid intake PO; the causes for this are numerous, but may include both endocrine and psychological etiologies.

Steroids/Hormones/Drugs

This is a big cause of edema in North America, and the numbers associated with this may be rising. Steroids can trigger edema not only by influencing capillary permeability, but also by exerting mineralocorticoid (or other) effects that triggers volume overload.[11] Certain sex hormones may have similar affects (in particular, estrogen is well known to be associated with the retention of fluid and development of edema). Certain nonsteroid drugs may also cause edema,[12] largely by affecting capillary permeability (calcium channel blockers) and/or the renal exertion of fluid (nonsteroidal anti-inflammatory drugs, ACE inhibitors when bilateral renal artery stenosis is present, etc.).

Cyclic Edema. Some women experience episodic edema in their lower extremities (and, at times, in other areas of the body) that occurs on a cyclic basis.[13,14] This may or may not correspond with the menstrual cycle. This type of swelling is also known as *idiopathic* edema, although it is thought to be associated with an alteration in capillary permeability that allows the interstitial space to become overloaded with fluid from the vascular space. Amphetamines have been shown to be beneficial in this condition.

Capillary Leak. This refers to a wide variety of conditions (including the so-called capillary leak syndrome) in which capillary permeability is increased and interstitial fluid overload occurs, producing edema.[15,16] As noted previously, many conditions are known or suspected to be associated with increased capillary permeability; there appear to be severe, isolated forms of increased capillary permeability that occur in association with infections, drugs, and so on. In many cases, these capillary leak syndromes are idiopathic and poorly understood.

PSEUDOEDEMA

Not all limb "swelling" is caused by edema. Certain conditions may cause limb enlargement that mimics swelling. Classic "look alikes" include entities such as digital clubbing, rheumatoid nodules, and lipedema (Figure 45–4).[17,18] A complete catalog of all the possible causes of pseudoedema is beyond the scope of this work.

TREATMENT OF LIMB EDEMA

It is essential to make an accurate diagnosis as to the etiology of edema because, as mentioned earlier, the most important element of edema control is to treat the underlying cause. In many cases no other therapy is necessary. Unfortunately, in some situations the cause remains unknown despite an extensive evaluation, or once a diagnosis has been made the underlying cause cannot be properly treated. When this occurs, one must still manage the edema. Management can be divided into two steps: reduction and maintenance.

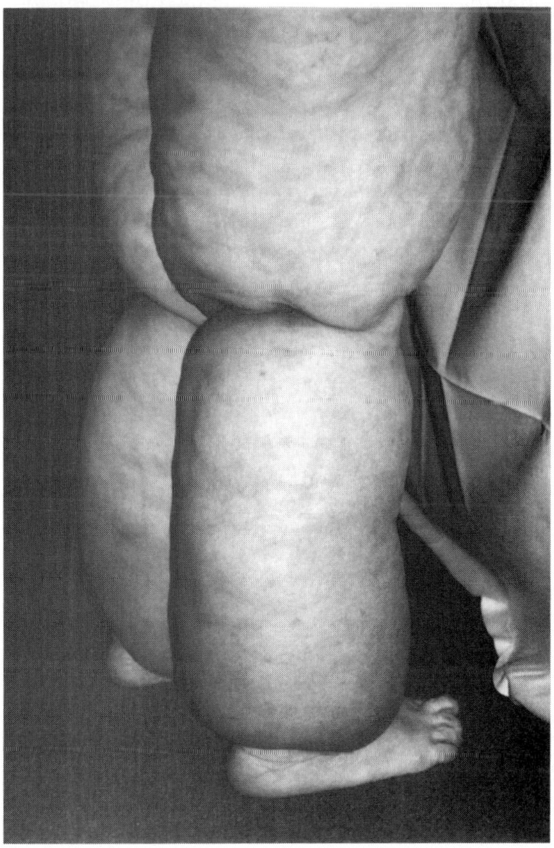

Figure 45–4. Lipedema. These subcutaneous fatty deposits cause limb enlargement. Notice that the feet are relatively spared.

Edema Reduction

Regardless of etiology, edema therapy begins by removing as much fluid as possible from the edematous limb. Traditional modalities for fluid removal include diuretics and restriction of fluids and salt intake; gravity; pumps; and massage.

Diuretics/Fluid Restriction/Salt Restriction

Reducing fluid and salt intake or increasing fluid/salt excretion via the kidneys may help to remove limb fluid in many conditions (for example, congestive heart failure, volume overload, renal failure). In other situations (for example, venous disease and lymphedema) diuretics are notoriously inefficient and play only a minor therapeutic role.

Gravity

Simple limb elevation—the higher, the better—is a surprisingly efficient method for reducing limb edema. This approach enjoyed great popularity in the 1930s to 1970s; patients with severe edema were often admitted to the hospital for aggressive limb elevation (sometimes involving "lymphedema slings"[19]) (Figure 45–5A) and strict bedrest. Most limbs, even those with otherwise intractable severe edema, improve substantially with a few days of in-hospital therapy. Unfortunately, this highly efficient modality became unavailable in the late 1980s and 1990s because third-party payers began to deny payment for this type of hospitalization/treatment. The introduction of special foam wedges (Figure 45–5B) makes aggressive leg elevation at home possible, although in the author's opinion it is not as efficacious as the in-patient form of therapy.

Pumps

Since the late 1960s, pneumatic compression pumps have been the mainstay of edema reduction therapy.[20] Most pumps employ a pneumatic cuff that is placed around the affected limb; this cuff is intermittently inflated by the pump at a pressure that is sufficient to drive edema fluid out of the swollen limb. Patients typically receive therapy as outpatients. Treatment sessions may last from 30 to 90 min and are often performed once or twice daily. An elastic wrap or similar device is applied to the limb between pumping sessions to prevent the reaccumulation of fluid. The limb circumference is measured before and after each session, and pumping is continued until a stable minimal limb circumference (from session-to-session) is achieved. There are several varieties of pumps.

Single-Chamber Pumps. These pumps use large, single-chamber cuffs to compress the swollen limb uniformly. Pressures (which can be varied by the operator) often reach 100 mmHg or more and may be held for 1 min or longer. These pumps can be very effective for certain patients and tend to be lower in price than other types of pumps.

Multichamber, Sequential Pumps. These pumps have multiple chambers (typically 3–12) that inflate sequentially to produce a "milking" affect on the limb.[21,22] They are usually more expensive than single-chamber pumps, but are often more effective.

Cardiac-Gaited Pumps. These pumps typically use a single-chamber cuff that inflates (to 50–100 mmHg) in synchrony with the cardiac cycle. Compression is usually

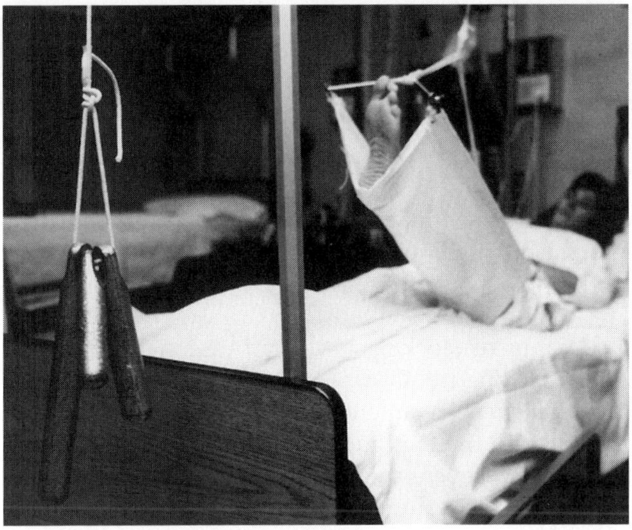

A

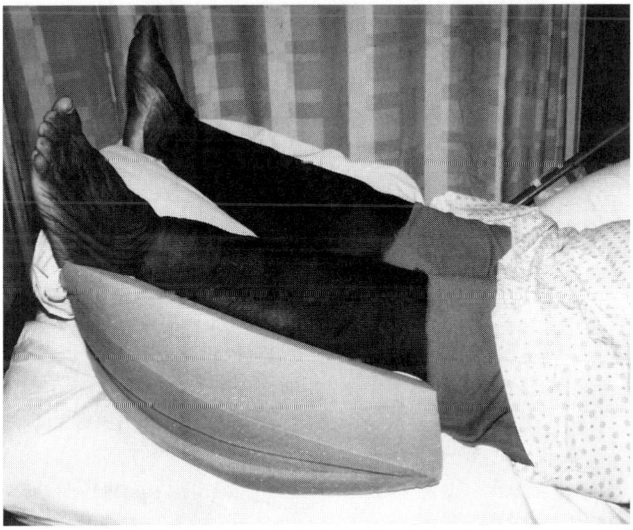

B

Figure 45–5. (**A**) Lymphedema sling. Using this device, the leg can be maintained at a 45° angle while the patient is in bed. (**B**) Foam wedge. The patient can use this device at home to keep the legs elevated while in bed (typically to 30° or more).

timed to occur during cardiac diastole. In some patients these pumps appear to be very effective at mobilizing fluid and reducing limb edema.

Massage

Certain types of edema, especially lymphedema, can be reduced by various types of massage. Manual lymphatic drainage (MLD) is a special technique that uses light massage applied in a central-to-peripheral direction to stimulate lymphatic activity and promote the mobilization of fluid.[23–25] In many practices throughout the world, MLD is considered the optimal approach for reducing lymphedema and certain other types of limb swelling.

Maintenance Therapy

Once a limb has undergone maximum size (fluid) reduction, the benefit must be maintained. This requires less aggressive but still persistent control therapy.

Elastic Compression

Elastic compression in the form of wraps or stockings[26,27] is an essential component of any serious edema control program (Figure 45–6). Compression, often at 30 to 40 mm Hg or more, must be worn whenever the patient is upright. As a rule the compression should be applied beginning with the toes and should cover the limb proximally as far as the swelling extends. With severe swelling (especially lymphedema),

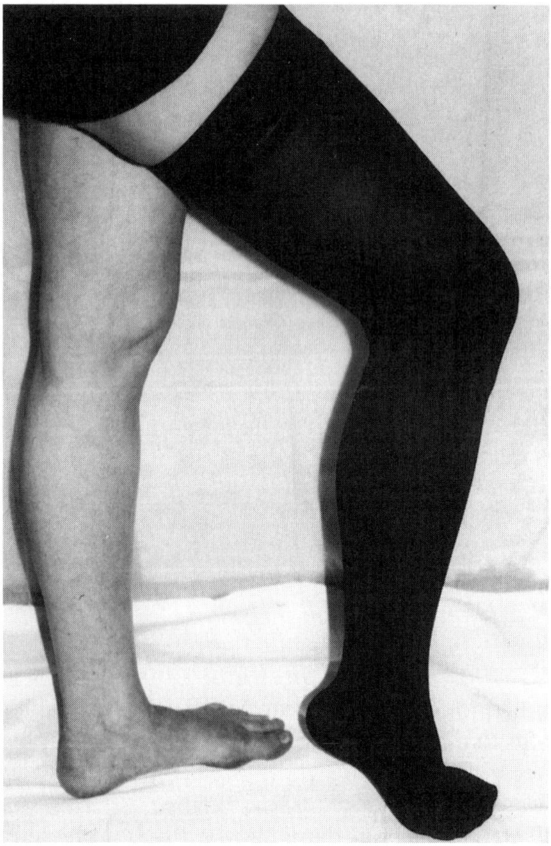

Figure 45–6. Graduated elastic compression stocking. This particular model has a silastic band at the mid-thigh that reduces slipping and rolling.

higher compression pressures (such as 40–50 or even 50–60 mmHg) may be necessary. Foam rubber padding is often placed under wraps to augment and "even out" the compressive forces.

Nonelastic Compression

Some swollen limbs respond best to rigid, nonelastic forms of compression. These include non- or low-stretch wraps and certain nonelastic devices that can be wrapped around the limb and fastened with Velcro straps (i.e., CircAid) (Figure 45–7).

Diuretic/Salt and Fluid Restriction/Pump/Massage

Any of the previously described modalities for achieving the initial fluid reduction can also be used on a chronic—and usually less aggressive—basis as an adjunct measure for keeping fluid out of the limbs. The use of these approaches may be used strictly as needed, or they may be a regular part of various protocols or regimens for maintaining edema control.

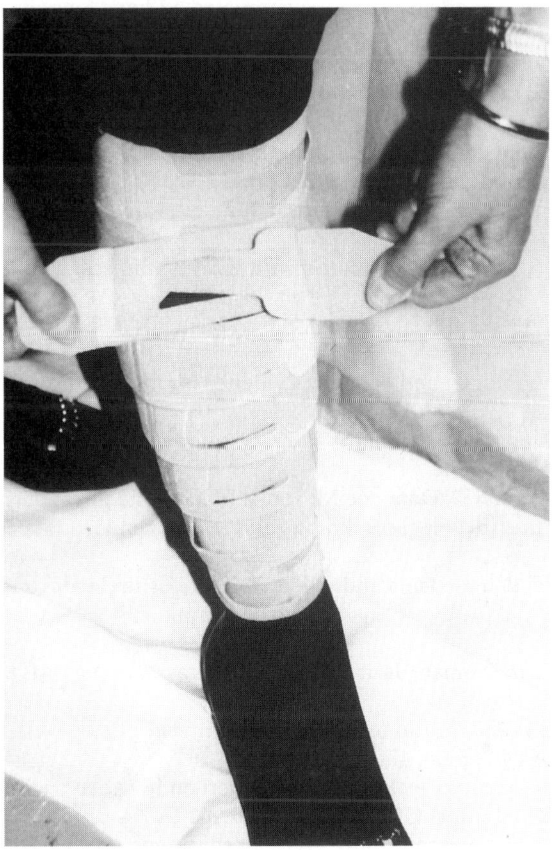

Figure 45–7. CircAid. This device provides nonelastic compression over the lower extremity.

CONCLUSION

The approach used to reduce and control edema must be individualized for each patient, depending on the age, mobility, ability to adhere to complicated programs, associated illnesses and disabilities, and so on. It is a mistake to think that there is a best or optimal method for reducing and controlling edema.[28,29] Programs that insist on employing one (or a few) modalities because they are better than others often fail to satisfy the needs of patients with intractable swelling.

REFERENCES

1. Moneta GL, Nehler MR. The lower extremity venous system: anatomy and physiology of normal venous function and chronic venous insufficiency. In *Handbook of Venous Disorders.* London: Chapman & Hall, 1996:3–26.
2. Cooke JP, Rooke TW. Lymphedema. In *Vascular Medicine: A Textbook of Vascular Biology and Diseases.* Little, Brown & Co. 1996:1133–1146.
3. Landgraf H, Vanselow B, Schulte-Huermann D, Mulmann MV, Bergau L. Economy class syndrome: rheology, fluid balance, and lower leg edema during a simulated 12-hour long distance flight. *Avia Sp Environ Med.* 1994:65:930–935.
4. van der Laan L, Veldman PH, Goris RJ. Severe complications of reflex sympathetic dystrophy: infection, ulcers, chronic edema, dystonia, and myoclonus. *Arch Phys Med Rehab.* 1998: 79(4): 424–429.
5. Schiepers C. Clinical value of dynamic bone and vascular scintigraphy in diagnosing reflex sympathetic dystrophy of the upper extremity. *Hand Clin.* 1997:13(3):423–429.
6. Naughton MT, Bradley TD. Sleep apnea in congestive heart failure. [Review] [97 refs]. *Clin Chest Med.* 1998:19(1):99–113.
7. Ishizawa T, Sugiki H, Anzai S, Kondo S. Pretibial myxedema with Graves' disease: a case report and review of Japanese literature. [Review] [8 refs]. *J Derm.* 1998:25(4):264–268.
8. Hierholzer K, Finke R. Myxedema. [Review] [50 refs]. *Kid Intern.* Supplement. 1997:59:S82–S89.
9. Wheatley T, Edwards OM. Mild hypothyroidism and oedema: evidence for increased capillary permeability to protein. *Clin Endocrin.* 1983:18(6):627–635.
10. Donckerwolcke RA, Vande Walle JG. Pathogenesis of edema formation in the nephrotic syndrome. *Kid Internat.* Supplement. 1997:58:S72–S74.
11. Flynn MD, Shore AC, Sandeman DE, Mawson D, Donohoe M, Tooke JE. Oedema in patients with Addison's disease on replacement therapy: glucocorticoid excess and mineralocorticoid deficiency? *QJM.* 1994:87(7):437–441.
12. Williams SA, Rayman G, Tooke JE. Dependent oedema and attenuation of postural vasoconstriction associated with nifedipine therapy for hypertension in diabetic patients. *Eur J Clin Pharmacol.* 1989:37(4):333–335.
13. Marks AD. Intermittent fluid retention in woman. Is it idiopathic edema? *Postgrad Med.* 1983:73(6):75–83.
14. Streeten DH. Idiopathic edema. Pathogenesis, clinical features, and treatment. [Review] [22 refs]. *Endocrin Metab Clin North Am.* 1995:24(3):531–547.
15. Amoura Z, Papo T, Ninet J, et al. Systemic capillary leak syndrome: report on 13 patients with special focus on course and treatment [see comments]. *Am J Med.* 1997:103(6):514–519.
16. Tahirkheli NK, Greipp PR. Treatment of the systemic capillary leak syndrome with terbutaline and theophylline. A case series. *Ann Intern Med.* 1999:130(11):905–909.

17. Harwood CA, Bull RH, Evans J, Mortimer PS. Lymphatic and venous function in lipoedema. *Br J Derm.* 1996:134(1):1–6.
18. Rudkin GH, Miller TA. Lipedema: a clinical entity distinct from lymphedema. *Plas Recons Surg.* 1994:94(6):841–847; discussion 848–849.
19. Schirger A, Peterson LFA. Lymphedema. In: *Peripheral Vascular Diseases.* WB Saunders Co. 1980:823–851.
20. Tinkham RG, Stillwell GK. The role of pneumatic pumping devices in the treatment of post-mastectomy lymphedema. *Arch Phys Med Rehab.* 1965:46:193–197.
21. Klein MJ, Alexander MA, Wright JM, Redmond CK, LeGasse AA. Treatment of adult lower extremity lymphedema with the Wright linear pump: statistical analysis of a clinical trial. *Arch Phys Med Rehab.* 1988:69:202–206.
22. Richmand DM, O'Donnell TF, Zelikovski A. Sequential pneumatic compression for lymphedema. *Arch Surg.* 1985:120:1116–1119.
23. Foldi E, Foldi M, Weissleder H. Conservative treatment of lymphoedema of the limbs. *Angiol J Vasc Dis.* 1985:171–180.
24. Boris M, Weindorf S, Lasinski B, Boris G. Lymphedema reduction by noninvasive complex lymphedema therapy. *Oncology.* 1994:8(9):95–106.
25. Kasseroller RG. The Vodder school: the Vodder method [Review] [8 refs]. *Cancer.* 1998;83(12 Suppl American):2840–2842.
26. Bowering CK. Use of layered compression bandages in diabetic patients. Experience in patients with lower leg ulceration, peripheral edema, and features of venous and arterial disease. *Adv Wound Care.* 1998:11(3):129–135.
27. Neumann HA. Compression therapy with medical elastic stockings for venous diseases. *Derm Surg.* 1998:24(7):765–770.
28. Johansson K, Lie E, Ekdahl C, Lindfeldt J. A randomized study comparing manual lymph drainage with sequential pneumatic compression for treatment of postoperative arm lymphedema. *Lymphology.* 1998:31(2):56–64.
29. Brennan MJ, Miller LT. Overview of treatment options and review of the current role and use of compression garments, intermittent pumps, and exercise in the management of lymphedema [Review] [51 refs]. *Cancer.* 1998:83(12 Suppl American):2821–2827.

Index

Page numbers followed by *t* and *f* refer to tables and figures, respectively.

Page numbers followed by *t* and *f* refer to tables and figures, respectively.

Page numbers followed by *t* and *f* refer to tables and figures, respectively.

Page numbers followed by *t* and *f* refer to tables and figures, respectively.